Advances in Cancer Immunotherapy

Advances in Cancer Immunotherapy

Editor: Jasmine Johnson

MURPHY & MOORE
www.murphy-moorepublishing.com

www.murphy-moorepublishing.com

MURPHY & MOORE

Cataloging-in-Publication Data

Advances in cancer immunotherapy / edited by Jasmine Johnson.
p. cm.
Includes bibliographical references and index.
ISBN 978-1-63987-016-5
1. Cancer--Immunotherapy. 2. Cancer--Immunological aspects. 3. Cancer--Treatment. I. Johnson, Jasmine.
RC271.I45 A38 2022
616.994 061--dc23

Murphy & Moore Publishing,
1 Rockefeller Plaza,
New York City, NY 10020, USA

ISBN 978-1-63987-016-5 (Hardback)

Contents

Preface VII

Chapter 1 **Modulation of Gut Microbiota: A Novel Paradigm of Enhancing the Efficacy of Programmed Death-1 and Programmed Death Ligand-1 Blockade Therapy** 1
Yiming Wang, Rena Ma, Fang Liu, Seul A. Lee and Li Zhang

Chapter 2 **Combining Immune Checkpoint Inhibitors with Conventional Cancer Therapy** 14
Yiyi Yan, Anagha Bangalore Kumar, Heidi Finnes, Svetomir N. Markovic, Sean Park, Roxana S. Dronca and Haidong Dong

Chapter 3 **PD1-CD28 Fusion Protein Enables $CD4_+$ T Cell Help for Adoptive T Cell Therapy in Models of Pancreatic Cancer and Non-Hodgkin Lymphoma** 27
Felicitas Rataj, Fabian B. T. Kraus, Michael Chaloupka, Simon Grassmann, Constanze Heise, Bruno L. Cadilha, Peter Duewell, Stefan Endres and Sebastian Kobold

Chapter 4 **Biomarkers for Clinical Benefit of Immune Checkpoint Inhibitor Treatment – A Review from the Melanoma Perspective and Beyond** 39
Kristina Buder-Bakhaya and Jessica C. Hassel

Chapter 5 **Metabolic Checkpoints: Novel Avenues for Immunotherapy of Cancer** 56
Ivan Shevchenko and Alexandr V. Bazhin

Chapter 6 **Myeloid-Derived Suppressor Cells Hinder the Anti-Cancer Activity of Immune Checkpoint Inhibitors** 62
Rebekka Weber, Viktor Fleming, Xiaoying Hu, Vasyl Nagibin, Christopher Groth, Peter Altevogt, Jochen Utikal and Viktor Umansky

Chapter 7 **Checkpoint Blockade Rescues the Repressive Effect of Histone Deacetylases Inhibitors on γδ T Cell Function** 71
Sajad A. Bhat, Disha Mohan Vedpathak and Shubhada V. Chiplunkar

Chapter 8 **Interferon-α Up-Regulates the Expression of PD-L1 Molecules on Immune Cells through STAT3 and p38 Signaling** 90
Alexandr V. Bazhin, Katharina von Ahn, Jasmin Fritz, Jens Werner and Svetlana Karakhanova

Chapter 9 **Immune Checkpoint-Mediated Interactions Between Cancer and Immune Cells in Prostate Adenocarcinoma and Melanoma** 103
Angela Rita Elia, Sara Caputo and Matteo Bellone

Chapter 10 **Controlling the Immune Suppressor: Transcription Factors and MicroRNAs Regulating CD73/NT5E** 111
Theresa Kordaß, Wolfram Osen and Stefan B. Eichmüller

Chapter 11 **Successful Anti-CLL1 CAR T-Cell Therapy in Secondary Acute Myeloid Leukemia** 119
Hui Zhang, Wen-Ting Gan, Wen-Ge Hao, Peng-Fei Wang, Zhuo-Yan Li and Lung-Ji Chang

Chapter 12 **Indoleamine 2,3-Dioxygenase Expression Pattern in the Tumor Microenvironment Predicts Clinical Outcome in Early Stage Cervical Cancer** 125
A. Marijne Heeren, Ilse van Dijk, Daniella R. A. I. Berry, Maryam Khelil, Debbie Ferns, Jeroen Kole, René J. P. Musters, Victor L. Thijssen, Constantijne H. Mom, Gemma G. Kenter, Maaike C. G. Bleeker, Tanja D. de Gruijl and Ekaterina S. Jordanova

Chapter 13 **Immune Checkpoint Inhibition for Pancreatic Ductal Adenocarcinoma: Current Limitations and Future Options** 141
Derya Kabacaoglu, Katrin J. Ciecielski, Dietrich A. Ruess and Hana Algül

Chapter 14 **Circulating T Cell Subpopulations Correlate with Immune Responses at the Tumor Site and Clinical Response to PD1 Inhibition in Non-Small Cell Lung Cancer** 165
Nataly Manjarrez-Orduño, Laurence C. Menard, Selena Kansal, Paul Fischer, Bijal Kakrecha, Can Jiang, Mark Cunningham, Danielle Greenawalt, Vishal Patel, Minghui Yang, Ryan Golhar, Julie A. Carman, Sergey Lezhnin, Hongyue Dai, Paul S. Kayne, Suzanne J. Suchard, Steven H. Bernstein and Steven G. Nadler

Chapter 15 **Engineered T Cell Therapy for Cancer in the Clinic** 174
Lijun Zhao and Yu J. Cao

Chapter 16 **Expression of the Circadian Clock Gene *BMAL1* Positively Correlates with Antitumor Immunity and Patient Survival in Metastatic Melanoma** 194
Leonardo Vinícius Monteiro de Assis, Gabriela Sarti Kinker, Maria Nathália Moraes, Regina P. Markus, Pedro Augusto Fernandes and Ana Maria de Lauro Castrucci

Chapter 17 **An IL-4/21 Inverted Cytokine Receptor Improving CAR-T Cell Potency in Immunosuppressive Solid-Tumor Microenvironment** 205
Yi Wang, Hua Jiang, Hong Luo, Yansha Sun, Bizhi Shi, Ruixin Sun and Zonghai Li

Chapter 18 **Mitochondria-Targeting Immunogenic Cell Death Inducer Improves the Adoptive T-Cell Therapy Against Solid Tumor** 215
Qingzhi Jiang, Chi Zhang, Huilan Wang, Tao Peng, Li Zhang, Yang Wang, Weidong Han and Chunmeng Shi

Permissions

List of Contributors

Index

Preface

The world is advancing at a fast pace like never before. Therefore, the need is to keep up with the latest developments. This book was an idea that came to fruition when the specialists in the area realized the need to coordinate together and document essential themes in the subject. That's when I was requested to be the editor. Editing this book has been an honour as it brings together diverse authors researching on different streams of the field. The book collates essential materials contributed by veterans in the area which can be utilized by students and researchers alike.

The stimulation of the immune system through artificial means for the treatment of cancer is known as cancer immunotherapy. It boosts the ability of the immune system to fight cancer cells. It is a subspecialty within oncology. The antibody proteins belonging to the immune system are able to detect the tumor antigens and bind with them. Immunotherapy can be broadly divided into two types, namely, passive immunotherapy and active immunotherapy. The tumor cells are specifically targeted through the immune system in active immunotherapy. Within passive immunotherapy, the cancer cells are not directly attacked by the immunotherapy, but the ability of the immune system to attack cancer cells is enhanced. This book includes some of the vital pieces of work being conducted across the world, on various topics related to cancer immunotherapy. Also included herein is a detailed explanation of the various concepts and applications of this branch of therapy. This book includes contributions of experts and scientists which will provide innovative insights into this field.

Each chapter is a sole-standing publication that reflects each author´s interpretation. Thus, the book displays a multi-facetted picture of our current understanding of application, resources and aspects of the field. I would like to thank the contributors of this book and my family for their endless support.

Editor

1

Modulation of Gut Microbiota: A Novel Paradigm of Enhancing the Efficacy of Programmed Death-1 and Programmed Death Ligand-1 Blockade Therapy

*Yiming Wang, Rena Ma, Fang Liu, Seul A. Lee and Li Zhang**

School of Biotechnology and Biomolecular Sciences, University of New South Wales, Sydney, NSW, Australia

Edited by:
Amedeo Amedei,
Università degli Studi di Firenze, Italy

Reviewed by:
Dr Kawaljit Kaur,
University of California, Los Angeles, United States
Haidong Dong,
Mayo Clinic Minnesota, United States
Sungjune Kim,
Moffitt Cancer Center, United States

***Correspondence:**
Li Zhang
l.zhang@unsw.edu.au

Blockade of programmed death 1 (PD-1) protein and its ligand programmed death ligand 1 (PD-L1) has been used as cancer immunotherapy in recent years, with the blockade of PD-1 being more widely used than blockade of PD-L1. PD-1 and PD-L1 blockade therapy showed benefits in patients with various types of cancer; however, such beneficial effects were seen only in a subgroup of patients. Improving the efficacy of PD-1 and PD-L1 blockade therapy is clearly needed. In this review, we summarize the recent studies on the effects of gut microbiota on PD-1 and PD-L1 blockade and discuss the new perspectives on improving efficacy of PD-1 and PD-L1 blockade therapy in cancer treatment through modulating gut microbiota. We also discuss the possibility that chronic infections or inflammation may impact on PD-1 and PD-L1 blockade therapy.

Keywords: gut microbiota, programmed death 1, programmed death ligand 1, cancer immunotherapy, efficacy

INTRODUCTION

The immune system uses various effector cells and molecules to control and eradicate infectious agents and cancer cells. Cytotoxic T cells (CTL) are the major effector cells in anti-tumor immune responses (1, 2). However, the functions of these effector cells are inhibited in the tumor microenvironment, which contributes to cancer cell immune evasion (3). In recent years, the blockade of immune checkpoint proteins and molecules that deliver inhibitory signals to activated T cells, have shown great promise in cancer treatment. However, the beneficial effects of these treatment strategies were seen only in a subgroup of patients (4). In this review, we summarize the emerging evidence of improving immune checkpoint protein blockade therapy efficacy by modulating gut microbiota and discuss the possibility that chronic infections or inflammation may impact on programmed death 1 (PD-1) and programmed death ligand 1 (PD-L1) blockade therapy.

PD-1 AND ITS LIGANDS

Programmed death 1, also known as cluster of differentiation 279 (CD279), is a cell surface receptor that was discovered in 1992 (5). PD-L1 and PD-L2, the two molecules that interact with PD-1, were identified in the following years (6, 7). PD-L1 is also known as CD274 or B7 homolog 1 (B7-H1) and PD-L2 known as CD273 or B7-DC.

Programmed death 1 is expressed on T, B cells, and myeloid cells (8). PD-L1 is expressed by a variety of cells in the immune system and non-immune cells. However, the expression level of PD-L1 in normal human tissues is low; despite the presence of PD-L1 mRNA, PD-L1 protein is rarely detected on the cell surfaces in most of normal human tissues except for a subset of human tissue macrophages

(6, 9). PD-L2 is predominately expressed by antigen-presenting cells, such as dendritic cells (DCs) and macrophages (10–13). The expression of both PD-L1 and PD-L2 is regulated by cytokines, for example interferon (IFN)-γ greatly increases the expression of PD-L1 and several cytokines are able to induce the expression of PD-L2 in other immune cells and non-immune cells in addition to the DCs and macrophages (9–11, 14–16).

Programmed death 1 and its ligands are members of the immune checkpoint proteins delivering inhibitory signals to activated T cells. The interaction of PD-1 with PD-L1 or PD-L2 leads to suppression of T cells, a regulatory mechanism to prevent overstimulation of immune responses and autoimmunity (6, 7, 9, 16–21). However, such a mechanism is hijacked in the tumor microenvironment, providing opportunities for tumor cells to evade the attack from the immune system.

PD-1 AND PD-L1 BLOCKADE IN CANCER IMMUNOTHERAPY

In anti-tumor immune responses, the tumor antigens generated by gene mutations, are recognized by the immune system and specific CD8+ CTLs targeting tumor antigens are generated (22). These specific effector CTLs recognize the target tumor cells and induce tumor cell apoptosis.

However, tumor cells employ various strategies to escape the attack from the immune system, one of which is to resist the killing effects from the anti-tumor CTLs by increasing PD-L1 expression in tumor tissues (9, 23, 24). Most normal human tissues do not express detectable PD-L1 on their cell surface, in contrast PD-L1 is abundantly expressed by tumor cells, the immune and non-immune cells in various tumor tissues (6, 9, 25–30). IFN-γ released by the anti-tumor CTLs infiltrating into tumor tissues plays a major role in inducing the expression of PD-L1 (9–11, 14–16). Other cytokines, such as tumor necrosis factor (TNF) -α, interleukin (IL)-4, and IL-10 can also increase PD-L1 expression (31, 32).

The interaction of PD-L1 with PD-1 in the tumor microenvironment enables the tumor cells to resist the endogenous anti-tumor activities from the immune system. PD-L1 expressed in tumor tissues interacting with PD-1 expressed on the activated T cells leads to the dysfunction of the effector T cells, *via* multiple mechanisms, such as promoting T cell apoptosis, anergy, and exhaustion (6, 7, 9, 16–21). More recently, it was found that interaction of PD-L1 with PD-1 expressed on tumor-associated macrophages inhibits the phagocytic potency of macrophages against tumor cells (33). The importance of PD-L1 and PD-1 interaction in tumor cell evasion has led scientists to explore the use of these molecules as therapeutic targets in cancer immunotherapy (**Figure 1**).

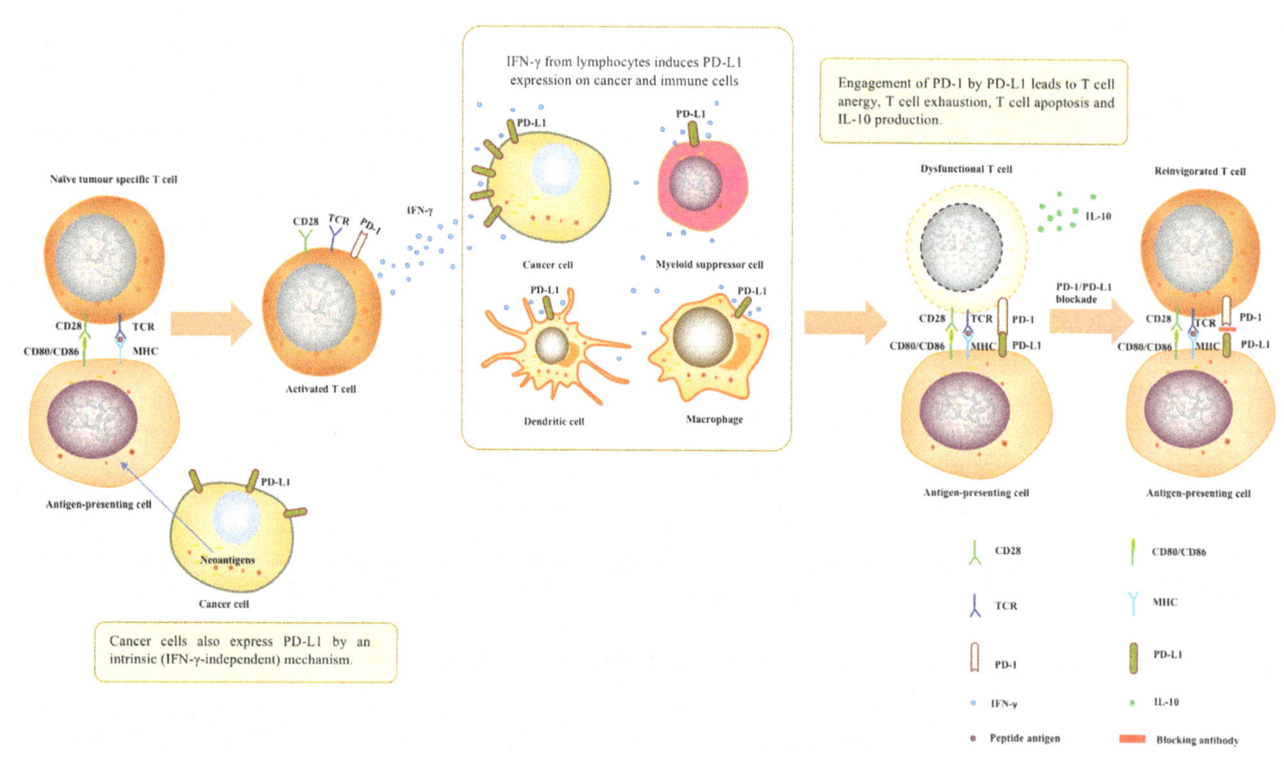

FIGURE 1 | The role of programmed death 1 (PD-1) and programmed death ligand 1 (PD-L1) in tumor evasion and cancer immunotherapy. In the tumor microenvironment, T cells were activated after antigen-presenting cells recognized tumor neoantigens. The IFN-γ produced by activated T cells induced the expression of PD-1 ligands on cancer cells and immune cells. Afterward, the engagement of PD-1 by PD-L1 between T cells and antigen-presenting cells will lead to T cell dysfunction. PD-1/PD-L1 blockade using relevant antibodies can inhibit this process, therefore, offering a chance for T cells to continue being effectors. Abbreviations: TCR, T-cell receptor; MHC, major histocompatibility complex; IFN-γ, interferon gamma; IL-10, interleukin 10.

Dong et al. showed that PD-L1 positive human tumor cells induced apoptosis of co-cultured activated effector T cells and this effect was blocked by an anti-human PD-L1 monoclonal antibody (mAb). They also showed that the growth of PD-L1 positive murine tumors in syngeneic mice was suppressed by an anti-murine PD-L1 mAb (9). Other researchers later reported similar findings in examination of different types of cancer cells using mice models (24, 34–36). These important laboratory observations led to numerous clinical trials of using monoclonal antibodies targeting PD-1 or PD-L1 in cancer immunotherapy for a variety of cancers. In addition to affecting the immunological pathways, PD-L1 and PD-1 blockade may also work in part by disrupting autologous PD-1 and PD-L1 signaling within tumors (37, 38).

To date, the U.S. Food and Drug Administration (FDA) has approved the use of five monoclonal antibodies targeting PD-L1 or PD-1 in cancer treatment. The details of the clinical trials of these five monoclonal antibodies are summarized in **Table 1**. Despite the clear benefits of PD-L1 and PD-1 blockade in treating some cancer patients, not all cases responded to treatment (**Table 1**). Given this, strategies to improve the efficacy of cancer immunotherapy are needed. Emerging evidence suggests that modulation of the gut microbiota is a promising approach.

MODULATION OF GUT MICROBIOTA ENHANCES THE ANTI-TUMOR EFFICACY OF PD-1 AND PD-L1 BLOCKADE THERAPY

A very interesting study by Sivan et al. provided strong evidence that the efficacy of PD-L1 blockage therapy can be improved by the modulation of gut microbiota (70). In this study, Sivan et al. examined the subcutaneous growth of B16.SIY melanoma in genetically similar C57BL/6 mice raised in the Jackson Laboratory (JAX) and Taconic Farms (TAC), and found that the tumor growth was more aggressive in TAC mice as compared to that in JAX mice and that TAC mice had a significantly lower intratumoral CD8+ T cell accumulation. They then conducted various experiments, which demonstrated that gut microbiota contributed to this difference.

They first showed that prophylactic transfer of fecal material from JAX mice to TAC mice was sufficient to delay tumor growth. To examine whether microbial community alone was effective as a therapy, they administered fecal material from JAX mice alone or in combination with anti-PD-L1 mAbs to TAC mice. These experiments showed that fecal material alone was sufficient to significantly inhibit tumor growth and that the combination treatment further improved tumor control. To identify the responsible bacterial species, they used 16S ribosomal RNA (16S rRNA) sequencing and identified *Bifidobacterium* species, particularly *Bifidobacterium breve*, *Bifidobacterium longum*, and *Bifidobacterium adolescentis* as the candidate species. The role of these *Bifidobacterium* species in enhancing protective immunity against tumors were further investigated by administering TAC mice bearing established tumors with a cocktail of *Bifidobacterium* species containing *B. breve* and *B. longum* by oral gavage. This experiment resulted in *Bifidobacterium*-treated mice having significantly improved tumor control as compared to mice that did not receive *Bifidobacterium*. Sivan et al. also showed that the possible mechanisms by which *Bifidobacterium* species inhibited tumor growth were through activating DCs, which in turn, improves the effector function of tumor-specific CD8+ T cells. Given that the enhanced anti-melanoma effect from *Bifidobacterium* species had occurred at the innate immunity level, the authors anticipated that *Bifidobacterium* species also provide anti-tumor beneficial effects to other types of tumors. However, the mechanisms by which *Bifidobacterium* species activated DCs improved the effects of anti-tumor CD8+ cells still need to be clarified.

The findings by Sivan et al. using mice models suggest that it is possible to enhance the anti-tumor efficacy of PD-L1 blockade therapy in treating cancer patients by modulating their gut microbiota and their findings are summarized in **Figure 2**. Interestingly, a very recent study by Matson et al. examining the stool samples collected from patients with metastatic melanoma before anti-PD-1 immunotherapy found that *B. longum*, *Collinsella aerofaciens*, and *Enterococcus faecium* were more abundant in the anti-PD-1 immunotherapy responders, supporting the anti-tumor effects of *Bifidobacterium* species (71).

Several additional studies also compared the gut microbiota in patients with metastatic melanoma receiving anti-PD-1 therapy. A recent study by Frankel et al. using metagenomic shotgun sequencing method showed that melanoma patients who responded to immune checkpoint inhibitors were enriched with *Bacteroides caccae* (72). Furthermore, they showed that the bacteria that are enriched within responders are most likely to be antibody dependent. Patients who responded to nivolumab (PD-1 antibody) were enriched with *Fecalibacterium prausnitzii*, *Bacteroides thetaiotamicron*, and *Holdemania filiformis*, whereas patients who responded to pembrolizumab (another PD-1 antibody), their gut microbiota enriched with *Dorea formicogenerans*. However, the mechanisms responsible for these changes are not clear. Studies comparing the gut microbiota changes prior to and following anti-PD-1 therapy of individual patients are required, which will provide information regarding whether anti-PD-1 antibodies directly affect gut bacterial species.

A study by Wargo et al. examined the human gut microbiota and metabolites of metastatic melanoma patients who received anti-PD-1 therapy using 16S rRNA and whole genome shotgun sequencing (73). They found that bacterial diversity and composition in patients that responded to the therapy were significantly different from that in patients who did not respond to the therapy. The responding patients had a higher diversity of bacteria and a higher abundance of *Clostridiales*, and the non-responders had a higher abundance of *Bacteroidales*. In a very recent study with multiple first authors and J. A. Wargo being the responding author, they further compared the gut microbiota of patients with metastatic melanoma receiving anti-PD-1 therapy (74). They found that patients who responded to anti-PD-1 therapy were associated with a significantly higher bacterial diversity and abundance of bacteria from the *Ruminococcaceae* family, which belongs to the *Clostridiales* order, as compared to patients who did not respond to the therapy. Furthermore, they performed fecal microbiota transplantation experiments in germ-free mice,

TABLE 1 | Five monoclonal antibodies targeting programmed death ligand-1 (PD-L1) or programmed death 1 (PD-1) were approved by the U.S. Food and Drug Association to treat cancer.

Commercial name (active ingredient)	Target	Treatment of disease	Targeting patients	Clinical cases	Clinical phase	Overall response rate (95% CI)	Objective response rate (95% CI)	Clinical study (clinical trial ID)	Reference
Bavencio (Avelumab)	PD-L1	Metastatic MCC	Metastatic MCC patients whose disease had progressed on or after chemotherapy administered	88	Phase 2	33% (23.3%, 43.8%)	Not applicable	JAVELIN Merkel 200 Trial (NCT02155647)	(39, 40)
Tecentriq (Atezolizumab)	PD-L1	Advanced or metastatic urothelial carcinoma	Cisplatin-ineligible patients with locally advanced or metastatic urothelial carcinoma	119	Phase 2	23.5% (16.2%, 32.2%)	Not applicable	IMvigor210 (NCT02951767)	(41)
			Previously treated patients with locally advanced or metastatic urothelial carcinoma	310	Phase 2	14.8% (11.1%, 19.3%)	Not applicable	IMvigor210 (NCT02951767)	(41)
		Metastatic NSCLC	Previously treated patients with metastatic non-small cell lung cancer	22	Phase 2	Not applicable	15% (10%, 22%)	POPLAR (NCT01903993)	(42)
Imfinzi (Durvalumab)	PD-L1	Locally advanced or metastatic urothelial carcinoma	Patients with locally advanced or metastatic urothelial carcinoma in total	182	Phase 1 and 2	Not applicable	17.0% (11.9%, 23.3%)	Study 1108 (NCT01693562)	(43–45)
			Patients with locally advanced or metastatic urothelial carcinoma who showed high PD-L1 expression on tumor cells	95	Phase 1 and 2	Not applicable	26.3% (17.8%, 36.4%)	Study 1108 (NCT01693562)	(43–45)
			Patients with locally advanced or metastatic urothelial carcinoma who showed low or non-PD-L1 expression on tumor cells	73	Phase 1 and 2	Not applicable	4.1% (0.9%, 11.5%)	Study 1108 (NCT01693562)	(43–45)
Keytruda (Pembrolizumab)	PD-1	Melanoma	Patients with Ipilimumab-Naïve melanoma (receive KEYTRUDA at a dose of 10 mg/Kg every 3 weeks)	277	Phase 3	33% (27%, 39%)	Not applicable	KEYNOTE-006 (NCT01866319)	(46, 47)
			Patients with Ipilimumab-Naïve melanoma (receive KEYTRUDA at a dose of 10 mg/Kg every 2 weeks)	279	Phase 3	34% (28%, 40%)	Not applicable	KEYNOTE-006 (NCT01866319)	(46, 47)
			Patients with Ipilimumab-refractory melanoma (receive KEYTRUDA at a dose of 2 mg/Kg every 3 weeks)	180	Phase 2	Not applicable	21% (15%, 28%)	KEYNOTE-002 (NCT01704287)	(48)
			Patients with Ipilimumab-refractory melanoma (receive KEYTRUDA at a dose of 10 mg/Kg every 3 weeks)	181	Phase 2	Not applicable	25% (19%, 32%)	KEYNOTE-002 (NCT01704287)	(48)

(Continued)

TABLE 1 | Continued

Commercial name (active ingredient)	Target	Treatment of disease	Targeting patients	Clinical cases	Clinical phase	Overall response rate (95% CI)	Objective response rate (95% CI)	Clinical study (clinical trial ID)	Reference
		NSCLC	Metastatic NSCLC patients with first-line treatment with a single agent	154	Phase 3	Not applicable	45% (37%, 53%)	KEYNOTE-024 (NCT02142738)	(49)
			Metastatic NSCLC patients with first-line treatment in combination with pemetrexed and carboplatin	60	Phase 1 and 2	55% (42%, 68%)	Not applicable	KEYNOTE-021 (NCT02039674)	(50)
			Previously treated NSCLC patients (all randomized patients who receive KEYTRUDA at a dose of 2 mg/Kg every 3 weeks)	344	Phase 2 and 3	Not applicable	18% (14%, 23%)	KEYNOTE-010 (NCT01905657)	(51)
			Previously treated NSCLC patients (all randomized patients who receive KEYTRUDA at a dose of 10 mg/Kg every 3 weeks)	346	Phase 2 and 3	Not applicable	19% (15%, 23%)	KEYNOTE-010 (NCT01905657)	(51)
		HNSCC	HNSCC patients whose disease had progressed on or after chemotherapy administered	174	Phase 1	16% (11%, 22%)	Not applicable	KEYNOTE-012 (NCT01848834)	(52)
		Urothelial Carcinoma	Cisplatin-ineligible patients with urothelial carcinoma	370	Phase 2	Not applicable	29% (24%, 34%)	KEYNOTE-052 (NCT02335424)	(53)
			Previously treated urothelial carcinoma patients	270	Phase 3	Not applicable	21% (16%, 27%)	KEYNOTE-045 (NCT02256436)	(54)
		cHL	Patients with cHL	210	Phase 2	69% (62%, 75%)	Not applicable	KEYNOTE-087 (NCT02453594)	(55, 56)
		MSI-H	Patients with MSI-H or mismatch repair deficient (dMMR)	149	Phase 1 Phase 2 Phase 1 Phase 2 Phase 2	Not applicable	39.6% (31.7%, 47.9%)	KEYNOTE-012 (NCT01848834) KEYNOTE-016 (NCT01876511) KEYNOTE-028 (NCT02054806) KEYNOTE-158 (NCT02628067) KEYNOTE-164 (NCT02460198)	(52, 57–59)

(*Continued*)

TABLE 1 | Continued

Commercial name (active ingredient)	Target	Treatment of disease	Targeting patients	Clinical cases	Clinical phase	Overall response rate (95% CI)	Objective response rate (95% CI)	Clinical study (clinical trial ID)	Reference
Opdivo (Nivolumab)	PD-1	Unresectable or metastatic melanoma	Previously treated patients with unresectable or metastatic melanoma in the treatment of OPDIVO	316	Phase 3	Not applicable	40% (34%, 46%)	CheckMate-067 (NCT01844505)	(60, 61)
			Previously treated patients with unresectable or metastatic melanoma in the treatment of OPDIVO plus Ipilimumab (anti-CTLA4 antibody)	314	Phase 3	Not applicable	50% (44%, 55%)	CheckMate-067 (NCT01844505)	(60, 61)
		Metastatic NSCLC	NSCLC patients who had experienced disease progressed during or after one prior platinum doublet-based chemotherapy regimen	272	Phase 3	Not applicable	20% (14%, 28%)	CheckMate-017 (NCT01642004)	(62)
			Patients with metastatic non-squamous NSCLC who had experienced disease progressed during or after one prior platinum doublet-based chemotherapy regimen	292	Phase 3	Not applicable	19% (15%, 24%)	CheckMate-057 (NCT01673867)	(63)
		Renal cell carcinoma	Patients with advanced RCC who had experienced disease progressed during or after one or two prior anti-angiogenic therapy regimes	410	Phase 3	Not applicable	21.5% (17.6%, 25.8%)	CheckMate-025 (NCT01668784)	(64, 65)
		cHL	Adult patients with cHL	258	Phase 2 Phase 1	Not applicable	69% (63%, 75%)	CheckMate-205 (NCT02181738) CA209-039 (NCT01592370)	(66, 67)
		Recurrent or metastatic SCCHN	Patients with metastatic or recurrent SCCHN	240	Phase 3	Not applicable	13.3% (9.3%, 18.3%)	CheckMate-141 (NCT02105636)	(68, 69)

Five monoclonal PD-L1 or PD-1 antibodies granted after May 2017 by FDA for cancer treatments were not included in the table.

MCC, metastatic Merkel cell carcinoma; NSCLC, non-small cell lung cancer; HNSCC, head and neck squamous cell cancer; cHL, classical Hodgkin lymphoma; MSI-H, microsatellite instability-high cancer; dMMR, mismatch repair deficient; SCCHN, recurrent or metastatic squamous cell carcinoma of the head and neck.

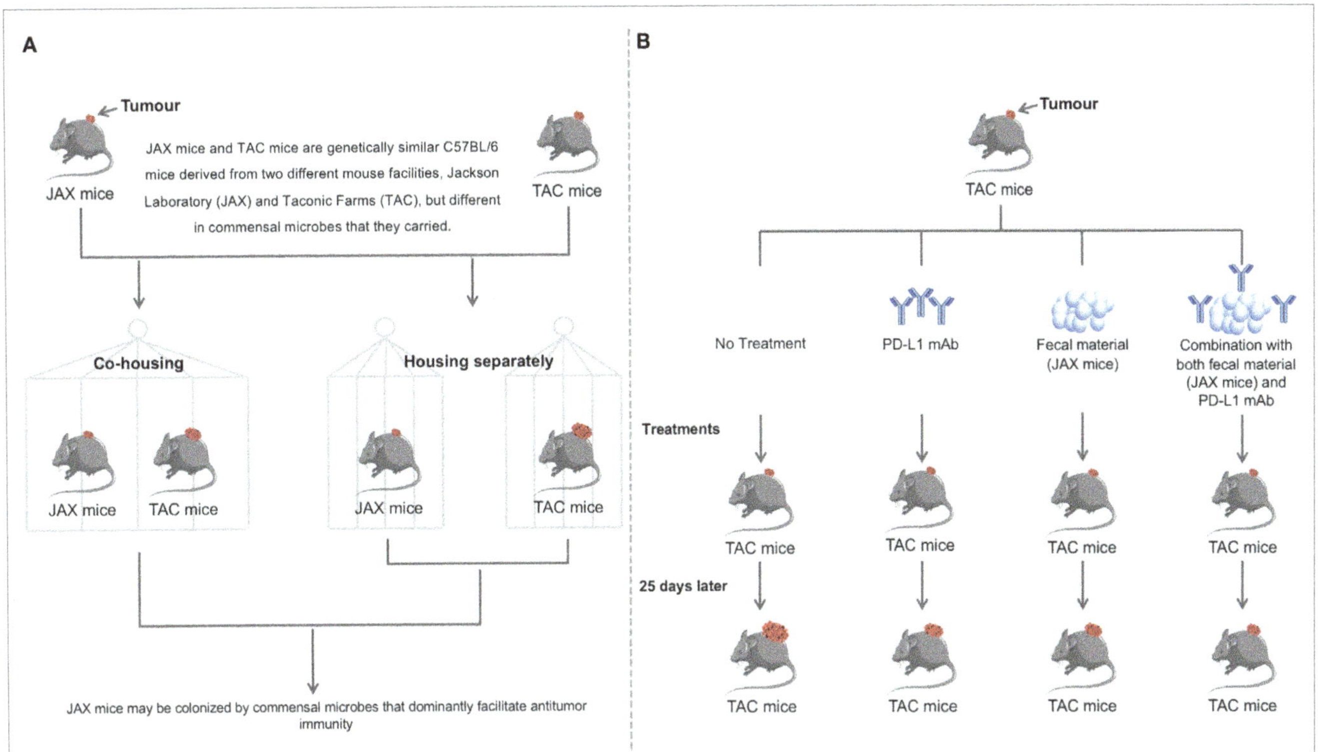

FIGURE 2 | Discovery and validation of the therapeutic significance of commensal microbiota by facilitating anti-programmed death ligand-1 (PD-L1) efficacy. **(A)** Two genetically similar mice, JAX and TAC, differing in commensal microbes carried were cohoused, while another pair was housed separately. Cohousing resulted in the TAC mice obtaining the JAX microbial phenotype, with reduced tumor growth as compared to the TAC mice housed separately. JAX mice had no differences in tumor size when cohoused with TAC mice compared to separate housing. This suggests that JAX mice are colonized by commensal microbes that facilitate anti-tumor immunity. **(B)** TAC mice were treated with PD-L1 mAb, JAX mice fecal material, both the PD-L1 mAb and JAX mice fecal material or not treated. Administration of JAX fecal material alone resulted in slower tumor growth to the same degree as treatment with PD-L1 mAb. Combination treatment with both the PD-L1 mAb and JAX fecal material showed the slowest tumor growth, indicating that commensal microbes play a therapeutic role in anti-tumor immunity. Data were adapted from Sivan et al (38). Further findings in this study have demonstrated that *Bifidobacterium* is the responsible bacterial species that contributes to improving the efficacy of PD-L1 blockade therapy.

in which they showed that germ-free mice transplanted with stool samples from patients who responded to anti-PD-1 and anti-PD-L1 therapy had a significantly reduced tumor growth and improved responses to anti-PD-1 and anti-PD-L1 therapy, coupled with a higher density of CD8+ T cells. However, it is not clear which bacterial species in the *Ruminococcaceae* family has played the role in enhancing the PD-1 blockade therapy.

Another recent study by Routy et al. investigated the effects of gut microbiota in PD-1 blockade therapy (75). In their study, data from 140 patients with advanced non-small-cell-lung cancer, 67 patients with renal cell carcinoma, and 42 patients with urothelial carcinoma were collected, and they found that 69 patients who took antibiotics before or soon after starting the PD-1 blockade therapy had shorter progression-free survival and overall survival. They then explored the composition of the gut microbiota using shotgun sequencing, which showed that *Akkermansia muciniphila* was enriched in patients who responded to anti-PD-1 therapy. This suggests that *A. muciniphila* may enhance patient response to PD-1 blockade therapy. They verified this observation by transplanting the patients stool samples in specific pathogen-free mice or germ-free mice and observed tumor growth in these mice. They also found that *A. muciniphila* alone was able to restore the anti-tumor effects of PD-1 blockade that was inhibited by antibiotics. However, the mechanism by which *A. muciniphila* enhancing PD-1 blockade therapy is not known.

Bacterial species that are positively associated with PD-1 and PD-L1 blockade therapy are summarized in **Table 2**. Some bacterial species have also been demonstrated to affect CTLA-4 blockade immunotherapy, which were not reviewed here (76, 77).

POTENTIAL MECHANISMS OF GUT MICROBES ON IMPROVING THE EFFICACY OF PD-1 AND PD-L1 BLOCKADE THERAPY

Despite the exciting findings in this research field, the underlying molecular mechanisms by which the identified gut bacterial species in the above studies enhance PD-1 and PD-L1 blockade therapy remain largely unknown.

Recently, unmethylated CpG oligodeoxynucleotides, which are abundant in bacterial DNA, were found to enhance CD8+ T cell anti-tumor immunity by downregulating PD-1 expression *via* the IL-12 pathway, suggesting that gut bacterial species that

TABLE 2 | Bacterial species that are positively associated with programmed death 1 (PD-1) and programmed death ligand 1 (PD-L1) blockade therapy.

Bacteria	Model	Methods	Main findings	Reference
Bifidobacterium breve, Bifidobacterium longum, Bifidobacterium adolescentis	Mouse	Fecal transplantation Microbial DNA analysis Bacterial administration Cell sorting Gene expression profiling	• Some *Bifidobacterium* species enhanced the efficacy of anti-PD-L1 therapy *in vivo*	(70)
Fecalibacterium prausnitzii, Bacteroides t hetaiotamicron, Holdemania filiformis, Dorea formicogenerans	Human	Metagenomic shotgun sequencing Gut metabolomic profiling	• Melanoma patients who responded to *nivolumab* (PD-1 antibody) were enriched with *F. prausnitzii*, *B. thetaiotamicron*, and *H. filiformis* • Melanoma patients who responded to pembrolizumab (another PD-1 antibody), their gut microbiota enriched with *D. formicogenerans*	(72)
Clostridiales	Human	16S rRNA gene sequencing Whole genome shotgun sequencing Immunohistochemistry Flow cytometry Cytokines assay Gene expression profiling	• Melanoma patients who responded to anti-PD-1 therapy had a higher diversity of bacteria and a higher abundance of *Clostridiales*	(73)
Ruminococcaceae[a]	Mouse Human	16S rRNA gene sequencing Whole genome shotgun sequencing Immunohistochemistry Flow cytometry Cytokines assay Gene expression profiling Fecal microbiota transplantation	• Melanoma patients who responded to anti-PD-1 therapy had a higher diversity of bacteria and a higher abundance of *Ruminococcaceae* • Germ-free mice transplanted with stool samples from patients responded to anti-PD-1 and anti-PD-L1 therapy had a significantly reduced tumor growth and improved responses to anti-PD-1 and anti-PD-L1 therapy coupled with higher density of CD8+ T cells in tumor	(74)
Akkermansia muciniphila	Mouse Human	Metagenomic shotgun sequencing Fecal microbiota transplantation Immunohistochemistry Flow cytometry Cytokines assay	• 27% cancer patients[b] who took antibiotics before or soon after starting the PD-1 blockade therapy had shorter progression-free survival and overall survival • *A. muciniphila* was found enriched in those patients who respond to anti-PD-1 therapy • *A. muciniphila* alone was able to restore the anti-tumor effects of PD-1 blockade that was inhibited by antibiotics.	(75)
B. longum, Collinsella aerofaciens, Enterococcus faecium	Mouse Human	16S rRNA gene sequencing Metagenomic shotgun sequencing Species-specific quantitative PCR Immunohistochemistry Fecal transplantation	• Melanoma patients who responded to anti-PD-1 therapy had a higher abundance of *B. longum, C. aerofaciens,* and *E. faecium* • Germ-free mice transplanted with fecal material from responding patients could lead to improved tumor control, augmented T cell responses, and greater efficacy of anti-PD-L1 therapy	(71)

[a]*Bacteria of Ruminococcaceae family belongs to the Clostridiales order.*
[b]*Patients here include patients with advanced non-small-cell-lung cancer, renal cell carcinoma, and urothelial carcinoma.*

are positively associated with PD-1 and PD-L1 blockade therapy may release components that directly downregulate PD-1 or PD-L1 expression (78, 79).

It is also possible that the gut bacterial species indirectly affect PD-1 and PD-L1 expression through locally or systematically regulating immune responses, thereby affecting the efficacy of PD-1 and PD-L1 blockade therapy. Gut microbiota has been shown to impact on both innate and adaptive immune cells. Germ-free animals had a reduced number of intestinal DCs and administration of *Escherichia coli* in these animals was able to recruit sufficient DCs to the intestines (80, 81). In Germ-free pigs, systemic circulating macrophages were also reduced and their functions were compromised (82). Germ-free mice had markedly decreased presence of lamina propria CD4+ T cells and absence of lymphocyte zones in spleens and mesenteric lymph nodes (83, 84). Polysaccharide A from *Bacteroides fragilis* was found to induce the Th1 response (83). Reduction of commensal microbiota in mice by using broad-spectrum antibiotics resulted in defective T and B cell responses against influenza infection (85). The findings that gut microbes can affect the immune functions, both locally and systematically suggest that bacterial species positively associated with PD-1 and PD-L1 blockade may enhance PD-1 and PD-L1 immunotherapy through regulation of the immune response. The previous study by Sivan et al. showed that *Bifidobacterium* species that inhibited tumor growth activated DCs, further supporting this view (70).

THE POSSIBLE IMPACT OF CHRONIC INFECTIONS AND INFLAMMATION ON PD-1 AND PD-L1 BLOCKADE THERAPY

Several microbes cause chronic infections in humans, some of which are known to increase host PD-1 and PD-L1 expression (86–94). However, studies have not examined whether existing chronic infections in patients with cancer affect the efficacy of PD-1 and PD-L1 blockade therapy.

An example of a chronic infection is *Helicobacter pylori* infection. *H. pylori* are a Gram-negative bacterium that colonizes the stomach of more than 50% of the world population. While most of the individuals colonized with *H. pylori* are asymptomatic, some may develop chronic gastritis and peptic ulcers, and *H. pylori* colonization is also a risk factor for gastric cancer (95). Previous studies have shown that patients with *H. pylori* infection have a significantly higher level of pro-inflammatory cytokines, such as TNF-α (96–98). Das et al. showed that *H. pylori* increased the gastric epithelial expression of PD-L1 using a gastric epithelial cell line model (86). Furthermore, they showed that gastric epithelial cells exposed to *H. pylori* inhibited the proliferation of CD4+ T cells isolated from blood and the inhibitory effect can be blocked using antibodies PD-L1. Similarly, Wu et al. observed increased PD-L1 expression in gastric biopsies of individuals infected with *H. pylori*, and co-culture of *H. pylori* infected primary gastric epithelial cells with T cells isolated from blood induced T cell apoptosis (87). These results suggest that *H. pylori* infection may cause the non-specific inhibition of circulating T cells, including tumor-specific T cells. In addition to *H. pylori*, several viruses, such as the hepatitis B virus, hepatitis C virus, human papillomavirus, and Epstein–Barr virus are also able to establish chronic infections in humans and increase host PD-1 or PD-L1 expression (88–94). Future studies are needed to examine whether chronic infections or inflammation impact on the efficacy of PD-1 and PD-L1 blockade. A recent study by Kottke et al. using a mouse model showed that pro-inflammatory cytokine TNF-α promoted tumor recurrence, while TNF-α blockade prevented tumor recurrence (99–102). Some bacterial species that are known to reduce chronic inflammation after administration orally may be examined to see whether they can improve cancer treatment (103–108). If chronic infections or inflammation reduce the efficacy of PD-1 and PD-L1 blockade, it would be through mechanisms other than the induction of the PD-1 and PD-L1 expression in the tumor tissues, as previous studies observed better responses to PD-1 blockade in patients with higher expression of PD-L1 in tumor tissues (51).

TABLE 3 | Suggested future directions.

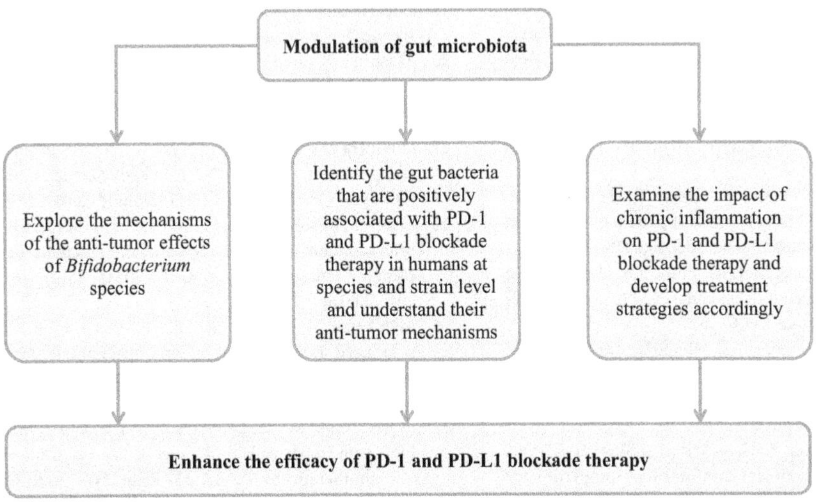

FUTURE DIRECTIONS

As discussed, despite the clear benefits of PD-1 and PD-L1 blockade in treating some cancer patients, the efficacy and the recurrence of tumor are issues that remain to be tackled. Emerging evidence suggests that modulation of the gut microbiota is a promising approach for improving PD-L1 and PD-1 blockade therapy. However, future studies are needed to further develop this research area.

The *Bifidobacterium* species, particularly *B. longum*, increased anti-PD-L1 efficacy in mice models and was positively associated with anti-PD-1 efficacy in metastatic melanoma patients. Future studies are needed to understand the molecular mechanisms of these *Bifidobacterium* species in enhancing PD-1 and PD-L1 blockade therapy. In addition to the *Bifidobacterium* species, various studies reported positive associations of gut microbes with PD-1 and PD-L1 blockade therapy at genus level. These microbes need to be identified at species and strain level and their potential anti-tumor mechanisms require further investigation.

Several bacterial and viral pathogens are known to cause chronic human infections and the pro-inflammatory cytokines are known to induce host PD-1 and PD-L1 expression. In addition, some of these pathogens are known to directly attach immune cells. Whether chronic infections caused by different pathogens impact on PD-1 and PD-L1 blockade therapy should be investigated, and appropriate strategies to enhance PD-1 and PD-L1 blockade therapy in these patients can then be developed accordingly. A suggested course of action is outlined in **Table 3**.

AUTHOR CONTRIBUTIONS

Wrote the paper: YW, LZ. Figures and tables: YW. Revised the paper: YW, LZ, RM, FL, SL. All authors have approved the final version of the manuscript.

ACKNOWLEDGMENTS

The authors would like to thank Dr. Jiezhong Chen (School of Biomedical Sciences, University of Queensland) for reading the manuscript and providing feedback on this article.

REFERENCES

1. Ercolini AM, Ladle BH, Manning EA, Pfannenstiel LW, Armstrong TD, Machiels J-PH, et al. Recruitment of latent pools of high-avidity CD8+ T cells to the antitumor immune response. *J Exp Med* (2005) 201(10):1591–602. doi:10.1084/jem.20042167
2. Melief CJ. Tumor eradication by adoptive transfer of cytototic T lymphocytes. *Adv Cancer Res* (1992) 58:143–75. doi:10.1016/S0065-230X(08)60294-8
3. Zou W. Immunosuppressive networks in the tumour environment and their therapeutic relevance. *Nat Rev Cancer* (2005) 5(4):263–74. doi:10.1038/nrc1586
4. Postow MA, Callahan MK, Wolchok JD. Immune checkpoint blockade in cancer therapy. *J Clin Oncol* (2015) 33(17):1974–82. doi:10.1200/JCO.2014.59.4358
5. Ishida Y, Agata Y, Shibahara K, Honjo T. Induced expression of PD-1, a novel member of the immunoglobulin gene superfamily, upon programmed cell death. *EMBO J* (1992) 11(11):3887.
6. Dong H, Zhu G, Tamada K, Chen L. B7-H1, a third member of the B7 family, co-stimulates T-cell proliferation and interleukin-10 secretion. *Nat Med* (1999) 5(12):1365–9. doi:10.1038/70932
7. Freeman GJ, Long AJ, Iwai Y, Bourque K, Chernova T, Nishimura H, et al. Engagement of the PD-1 immunoinhibitory receptor by a novel B7 family member leads to negative regulation of lymphocyte activation. *J Exp Med* (2000) 192(7):1027–34. doi:10.1084/jem.192.7.1027
8. Keir ME, Butte MJ, Freeman GJ, Sharpe AH. PD-1 and its ligands in tolerance and immunity. *Annu Rev Immunol* (2008) 26:677–704. doi:10.1146/annurev.immunol.26.021607.090331
9. Dong H, Strome SE, Salomao DR, Tamura H, Hirano F, Flies DB, et al. Tumor-associated B7-H1 promotes T-cell apoptosis: a potential mechanism of immune evasion. *Nat Med* (2002) 8(8):793–800. doi:10.1038/nm730
10. Yamazaki T, Akiba H, Iwai H, Matsuda H, Aoki M, Tanno Y, et al. Expression of programmed death 1 ligands by murine T cells and APC. *J Immunol* (2002) 169(10):5538–45. doi:10.4049/jimmunol.169.10.5538
11. Ishida M, Iwai Y, Tanaka Y, Okazaki T, Freeman GJ, Minato N, et al. Differential expression of PD-L1 and PD-L2, ligands for an inhibitory receptor PD-1, in the cells of lymphohematopoietic tissues. *Immunol Lett* (2002) 84(1):57–62. doi:10.1016/S0165-2478(02)00142-6
12. Tseng S-Y, Otsuji M, Gorski K, Huang X, Slansky JE, Pai SI, et al. B7-DC, a new dendritic cell molecule with potent costimulatory properties for T cells. *J Exp Med* (2001) 193(7):839–46. doi:10.1084/jem.193.7.839
13. Shin T, Kennedy G, Gorski K, Tsuchiya H, Koseki H, Azuma M, et al. Cooperative B7-1/2 (CD80/CD86) and B7-DC costimulation of CD4+ T cells independent of the PD-1 receptor. *J Exp Med* (2003) 198(1):31–8. doi:10.1084/jem.20030242
14. Tamura H, Dong H, Zhu G, Sica GL, Flies DB, Tamada K, et al. B7-H1 costimulation preferentially enhances CD28-independent T-helper cell function. *Blood* (2001) 97(6):1809–16. doi:10.1182/blood.V97.6.1809
15. Mazanet MM, Hughes CC. B7-H1 is expressed by human endothelial cells and suppresses T cell cytokine synthesis. *J Immunol* (2002) 169(7):3581–8. doi:10.4049/jimmunol.169.7.3581
16. Selenko-Gebauer N, Majdic O, Szekeres A, Höfler G, Guthann E, Korthäuer U, et al. B7-H1 (programmed death-1 ligand) on dendritic cells is involved in the induction and maintenance of T cell anergy. *J Immunol* (2003) 170(7):3637–44. doi:10.4049/jimmunol.170.7.3637
17. Ghiotto M, Gauthier L, Serriari N, Pastor S, Truneh A, Nunès JA, et al. PD-L1 and PD-L2 differ in their molecular mechanisms of interaction with PD-1. *Int Immunol* (2010) 22(8):651–60. doi:10.1093/intimm/dxq049
18. Chen L. Co-inhibitory molecules of the B7–CD28 family in the control of T-cell immunity. *Nat Rev Immunol* (2004) 4(5):336–47. doi:10.1038/nri1349
19. Zou W, Chen L. Inhibitory B7-family molecules in the tumour microenvironment. *Nat Rev Immunol* (2008) 8(6):467–77. doi:10.1038/nri2326
20. Tsushima F, Yao S, Shin T, Flies A, Flies S, Xu H, et al. Interaction between B7-H1 and PD-1 determines initiation and reversal of T-cell anergy. *Blood* (2007) 110(1):180–5. doi:10.1182/blood-2006-11-060087
21. Goldberg MV, Maris CH, Hipkiss EL, Flies AS, Zhen L, Tuder RM, et al. Role of PD-1 and its ligand, B7-H1, in early fate decisions of CD8 T cells. *Blood* (2007) 110(1):186–92. doi:10.1182/blood-2006-12-062422
22. Engels B, Engelhard VH, Sidney J, Sette A, Binder DC, Liu RB, et al. Relapse or eradication of cancer is predicted by peptide-major histocompatibility complex affinity. *Cancer Cell* (2013) 23(4):516–26. doi:10.1016/j.ccr.2013.03.018
23. Mühlbauer M, Fleck M, Schütz C, Weiss T, Froh M, Blank C, et al. PD-L1 is induced in hepatocytes by viral infection and by interferon-α and-γ and mediates T cell apoptosis. *J Hepatol* (2006) 45(4):520–8. doi:10.1016/j.jhep.2006.05.007
24. Iwai Y, Ishida M, Tanaka Y, Okazaki T, Honjo T, Minato N. Involvement of PD-L1 on tumor cells in the escape from host immune system and tumor immunotherapy by PD-L1 blockade. *Proc Natl Acad Sci U S A* (2002) 99(19):12293–7. doi:10.1073/pnas.192461099

25. Konishi J, Yamazaki K, Azuma M, Kinoshita I, Dosaka-Akita H, Nishimura M. B7-H1 expression on non-small cell lung cancer cells and its relationship with tumor-infiltrating lymphocytes and their PD-1 expression. *Clin Cancer Res* (2004) 10(15):5094–100. doi:10.1158/1078-0432.CCR-04-0428
26. Brown JA, Dorfman DM, Ma F-R, Sullivan EL, Munoz O, Wood CR, et al. Blockade of programmed death-1 ligands on dendritic cells enhances T cell activation and cytokine production. *J Immunol* (2003) 170(3):1257–66. doi:10.4049/jimmunol.170.3.1257
27. Curiel TJ, Wei S, Dong H, Alvarez X, Cheng P, Mottram P, et al. Blockade of B7-H1 improves myeloid dendritic cell–mediated antitumor immunity. *Nat Med* (2003) 9(5):562–7. doi:10.1038/nm863
28. Kuang D-M, Zhao Q, Peng C, Xu J, Zhang J-P, Wu C, et al. Activated monocytes in peritumoral stroma of hepatocellular carcinoma foster immune privilege and disease progression through PD-L1. *J Exp Med* (2009) 206(6):1327–37. doi:10.1084/jem.20082173
29. Liu Y, Zeng B, Zhang Z, Zhang Y, Yang R. B7-H1 on myeloid-derived suppressor cells in immune suppression by a mouse model of ovarian cancer. *Clin Immunol* (2008) 129(3):471–81. doi:10.1016/j.clim.2008.07.030
30. Pardoll DM. The blockade of immune checkpoints in cancer immunotherapy. *Nat Rev Cancer* (2012) 12(4):252–64. doi:10.1038/nrc3239
31. Sznol M, Chen L. Antagonist antibodies to PD-1 and B7-H1 (PD-L1) in the treatment of advanced human cancer. *Clin Cancer Res* (2013) 19(5):1021–34. doi:10.1158/1078-0432.CCR-12-2063
32. Kondo A, Yamashita T, Tamura H, Zhao W, Tsuji T, Shimizu M, et al. Interferon-γ and tumor necrosis factor-α induce an immunoinhibitory molecule, B7-H1, via nuclear factor-κB activation in blasts in myelodysplastic syndromes. *Blood* (2010) 116(7):1124–31. doi:10.1182/blood-2009-12-255125
33. Gordon SR, Maute RL, Dulken BW, Hutter G, George BM, McCracken MN, et al. PD-1 expression by tumour-associated macrophages inhibits phagocytosis and tumour immunity. *Nature* (2017) 545(7655):495–9. doi:10.1038/nature22396
34. Blank C, Brown I, Peterson AC, Spiotto M, Iwai Y, Honjo T, et al. PD-L1/B7H-1 inhibits the effector phase of tumor rejection by T cell receptor (TCR) transgenic CD8+ T cells. *Cancer Res* (2004) 64(3):1140–5. doi:10.1158/0008-5472.CAN-03-3259
35. Petroff M, Chen L, Phillips T, Hunt J. B7 family molecules: novel immunomodulators at the maternal-fetal interface. *Placenta* (2002) 23:S95–101. doi:10.1053/plac.2002.0813
36. Hirano F, Kaneko K, Tamura H, Dong H, Wang S, Ichikawa M, et al. Blockade of B7-H1 and PD-1 by monoclonal antibodies potentiates cancer therapeutic immunity. *Cancer Res* (2005) 65(3):1089–96.
37. Clark CA, Gupta HB, Sareddy G, Pandeswara S, Lao S, Yuan B, et al. Tumor-intrinsic PD-L1 signals regulate cell growth, pathogenesis, and autophagy in ovarian cancer and melanoma. *Cancer Res* (2016) 76(23):6964–74. doi:10.1158/0008-5472.CAN-16-0258
38. Orzechowski A, Dong H. Abstract 5026: B7-H1 confers tumor chemoresistance by regulating MAPK/ERK activation. *Cancer Res* (2014) 74(19 Suppl):5026. doi:10.1158/1538-7445.AM2014-5026
39. Kaufman H, Russell JS, Hamid O, Bhatia S, Terheyden P, D'Angelo SP, et al. Avelumab (MSB0010718C; anti-PD-L1) in patients with metastatic Merkel cell carcinoma previously treated with chemotherapy: results of the phase 2 JAVELIN Merkel 200 trial. *J Clin Oncol* (2016) 34(15):9508. doi:10.1200/JCO.2016.34.15_supll.9508
40. Kaufman HL, Russell J, Hamid O, Bhatia S, Terheyden P, D'Angelo SP, et al. Avelumab in patients with chemotherapy-refractory metastatic Merkel cell carcinoma: a multicentre, single-group, open-label, phase 2 trial. *Lancet Oncol* (2016) 17(10):1374–85. doi:10.1016/S1470-2045(16)30364-3
41. Balar AV, Galsky MD, Rosenberg JE, Powles T, Petrylak DP, Bellmunt J, et al. Atezolizumab as first-line treatment in cisplatin-ineligible patients with locally advanced and metastatic urothelial carcinoma: a single-arm, multicentre, phase 2 trial. *Lancet* (2017) 389(10064):67–76. doi:10.1016/S0140-6736(16)32455-2
42. Spira AI, Park K, Mazières J, Vansteenkiste JF, Rittmeyer A, Ballinger M, et al. Efficacy, safety and predictive biomarker results from a randomized phase II study comparing MPDL3280A vs docetaxel in 2L/3L NSCLC (POPLAR). *J Clin Oncol* (2015) 33(15):8010. doi:10.1200/jco.2015.33.15_suppl.8010
43. Jin C, Zheng Y, Jin X, Mukhopadhyay P, Gupta AK, Dennis PA, et al. Exposure-efficacy and safety analysis of durvalumab in patients with urothelial carcinoma (UC) and other solid tumors. *J Clin Oncol* (2017) 35(15):2568. doi:10.1200/JCO.2017.35.15_suppl.2568
44. Ibrahim R, Stewart R, Shalabi A. PD-L1 blockade for cancer treatment: MEDI4736. *Semin Oncol* (2015) 42:474–83. doi:10.1053/j.seminoncol.2015.02.007
45. Syed YY. Durvalumab: first global approval. *Drugs* (2017) 77(12):1369–76. doi:10.1007/s40265-017-0782-5
46. Ribas A, Hamid O, Daud A, Hodi FS, Wolchok JD, Kefford R, et al. Association of pembrolizumab with tumor response and survival among patients with advanced melanoma. *JAMA* (2016) 315(15):1600–9. doi:10.1001/jama.2016.4059
47. Schachter J, Ribas A, Long GV, Arance A, Grob JJ, Mortier L, et al. Pembrolizumab versus ipilimumab for advanced melanoma: final overall survival analysis of KEYNOTE-006. *J Clin Oncol* (2016) 34(15):9504. doi:10.1200/JCO.2016.34.15_suppl.9504
48. Ribas A, Puzanov I, Dummer R, Schadendorf D, Hamid O, Robert C, et al. Pembrolizumab versus investigator-choice chemotherapy for ipilimumab-refractory melanoma (KEYNOTE-002): a randomised, controlled, phase 2 trial. *Lancet Oncol* (2015) 16(8):908–18. doi:10.1016/S1470-2045(15)00083-2
49. Reck M, Rodríguez-Abreu D, Robinson AG, Hui R, Csőszi T, Fülöp A, et al. Pembrolizumab versus chemotherapy for PD-L1–positive non–small-cell lung cancer. *N Engl J Med* (2016) 2016(375):1823–33. doi:10.1056/NEJMoa1606774
50. Langer CJ, Gadgeel SM, Borghaei H, Papadimitrakopoulou VA, Patnaik A, Powell SF, et al. Carboplatin and pemetrexed with or without pembrolizumab for advanced, non-squamous non-small-cell lung cancer: a random ised, phase 2 cohort of the open-label KEYNOTE-021 study. *Lancet Oncol* (2016) 17(11):1497–508. doi:10.1016/S1470-2045(16)30498-3
51. Herbst RS, Baas P, Kim D-W, Felip E, Pérez-Gracia JL, Han J-Y, et al. Pembrolizumab versus docetaxel for previously treated, PD-L1-positive, advanced non-small-cell lung cancer (KEYNOTE-010): a randomised controlled trial. *Lancet* (2016) 387(10027):1540–50. doi:10.1016/S0140-6736(15)01281-7
52. Seiwert TY, Burtness B, Mehra R, Weiss J, Berger R, Eder JP, et al. Safety and clinical activity of pembrolizumab for treatment of recurrent or metastatic squamous cell carcinoma of the head and neck (KEYNOTE-012): an open-label, multicentre, phase 1b trial. *Lancet Oncol* (2016) 17(7):956–65. doi:10.1016/S1470-2045(16)30066-3
53. Balar AV, Castellano DE, O'Donnell PH, Grivas P, Vuky J, Powles T, et al. Pembrolizumab as first-line therapy in cisplatin-ineligible advanced urothelial cancer: results from the total KEYNOTE-052 study population. *J Clin Oncol* (2017) 35(6):284. doi:10.1200/JCO.2017.35.6_suppl.284
54. Bellmunt J, de Wit R, Vaughn DJ, Fradet Y, Lee J-L, Fong L, et al. Pembrolizumab as second-line therapy for advanced urothelial carcinoma. *N Engl J Med* (2017) 376(11):1015–26. doi:10.1056/NEJMoa1613683
55. Moskowitz CH, Zinzani PL, Fanale MA, Armand P, Johnson NA, Radford JA, et al. Pembrolizumab in relapsed/refractory classical Hodgkin lymphoma: primary end point analysis of the phase 2 Keynote-087 study. *Blood* (2016) 128(22):1107.
56. Chen R, Zinzani PL, Fanale MA, Armand P, Johnson NA, Brice P, et al. Phase II study of the efficacy and safety of pembrolizumab for relapsed/refractory classic Hodgkin lymphoma. *J Clin Oncol* (2017) 35:2125. doi:10.1200/JCO.2016.72.1316
57. Le DT, Yoshino T, Jäger D, Andre T, Bendell JC, Wang R, et al. KEYNOTE-164: phase II study of pembrolizumab (MK-3475) for patients with previously treated, microsatellite instability-high advanced colorectal carcinoma. *J Clin Oncol* (2016) 34(4). doi:10.1200/jco.2016.34.4_suppl.tps787
58. Ott PA, Fernandez MEE, Hiret S, Kim D-W, Moss RA, Winser T, et al. Pembrolizumab (MK-3475) in patients (pts) with extensive-stage small cell lung cancer (SCLC): preliminary safety and efficacy results from KEYNOTE-028. *J Clin Oncol* (2015) 33(15):7502. doi:10.1200/jco.2015.33.15_suppl.7502
59. Ott PA, Bang Y-J, Berton-Rigaud D, Elez E, Pishvaian MJ, Rugo HS, et al. Pembrolizumab in advanced endometrial cancer: preliminary results from the phase Ib KEYNOTE-028 study. *J Clin Oncol* (2016) 34(15):5581. doi:10.1200/JCO.2016.34.15_suppl.5581
60. Wolchok JD, Chiarion-Sileni V, Gonzalez R, Rutkowski P, Grob JJ, Cowey CL, et al. Updated results from a phase III trial of nivolumab (NIVO) combined with ipilimumab (IPI) in treatment-naive patients (pts) with advanced

melanoma (MEL)(CheckMate 067). *J Clin Oncol* (2016) 34(15):9505. doi:10.1200/JCO.2016.34.15_suppl.9505

61. Wolchok JD, Chiarion-Sileni V, Gonzalez R, Rutkowski P, Grob JJ, Cowey CL, et al. Efficacy and safety results from a phase III trial of nivolumab (NIVO) alone or combined with ipilimumab (IPI) versus IPI alone in treatment-naive patients (pts) with advanced melanoma (MEL)(CheckMate 067). *J Clin Oncol* (2015) 33(18). doi:10.1200/jco.2015.33.18_suppl.lba1
62. Spigel DR, Reckamp KL, Rizvi NA, Poddubskaya E, West HJ, Eberhardt WEE, et al. A phase III study (CheckMate 017) of nivolumab (NIVO; anti-programmed death-1 [PD-1]) vs docetaxel (DOC) in previously treated advanced or metastatic squamous (SQ) cell non-small cell lung cancer (NSCLC). *J Clin Oncol* (2015) 33(15):8009. doi:10.1200/jco.2015.33.15_suppl.8009
63. Paz-Ares L, Horn L, Borghaei H, Spigel DR, Steins M, Ready N, et al. Phase III, randomized trial (CheckMate 057) of nivolumab (NIVO) versus docetaxel (DOC) in advanced non-squamous cell (non-SQ) non-small cell lung cancer (NSCLC). *J Clin Oncol* (2015) 33(18). doi:10.1200/jco.2015.33.18_suppl.lba109
64. Motzer RJ, Escudier B, McDermott DF, George S, Hammers HJ, Srinivas S, et al. Nivolumab versus everolimus in advanced renal-cell carcinoma. *N Engl J Med* (2015) 373(19):1803–13. doi:10.1056/NEJMoa1510665
65. Cella D, Grünwald V, Nathan P, Doan J, Dastani H, Taylor F, et al. Quality of life in patients with advanced renal cell carcinoma given nivolumab versus everolimus in CheckMate 025: a randomised, open-label, phase 3 trial. *Lancet Oncol* (2016) 17(7):994–1003. doi:10.1016/S1470-2045(16)30125-5
66. Younes A, Santoro A, Zinzani PL, Timmerman J, Ansell SM, Armand P, et al. Checkmate 205: nivolumab (nivo) in classical Hodgkin lymphoma (cHL) after autologous stem cell transplant (ASCT) and brentuximab vedotin (BV)—A phase 2 study. *J Clin Oncol* (2016) 34(15):7535. doi:10.1200/JCO.2016.34.15_suppl.7535
67. Ansell S, Armand P, Timmerman JM, Shipp MA, Garelik MBB, Zhu L, et al. Nivolumab in patients (pts) with relapsed or refractory classical Hodgkin lymphoma (R/R cHL): clinical outcomes from extended follow-up of a phase 1 study (CA209-039). *Blood* (2015) 126:583.
68. Ferris RL, Blumenschein G Jr, Fayette J, Guigay J, Colevas AD, Licitra L, et al. Nivolumab for recurrent squamous-cell carcinoma of the head and neck. *N Engl J Med* (2016) 2016(375):1856–67. doi:10.1056/NEJMoa1602252
69. Ferris RL, Blumenschein GR, Fayette J, Guigay J, Colevas AD, Licitra LF, et al. Further evaluations of nivolumab (nivo) versus investigator's choice (IC) chemotherapy for recurrent or metastatic (R/M) squamous cell carcinoma of the head and neck (SCCHN): CheckMate 141. *J Clin Oncol* (2016) 34(15):6009. doi:10.1200/JCO.2016.34.15_suppl.6009
70. Sivan A, Corrales L, Hubert N, Williams JB, Aquino-Michaels K, Earley ZM, et al. Commensal Bifidobacterium promotes antitumor immunity and facilitates anti–PD-L1 efficacy. *Science* (2015) 350(6264):1084–9. doi:10.1126/science.aac4255
71. Matson V, Fessler J, Bao R, Chongsuwat T, Zha Y, Alegre M-L, et al. The commensal microbiome is associated with anti–PD-1 efficacy in metastatic melanoma patients. *Science* (2018) 359(6371):104–8. doi:10.1126/science.aao3290
72. Frankel AE, Coughlin LA, Kim J, Froehlich TW, Xie Y, Frenkel EP, et al. Metagenomic shotgun sequencing and unbiased metabolomic profiling identify specific human gut microbiota and metabolites associated with immune checkpoint therapy efficacy in melanoma patients. *Neoplasia* (2017) 19(10):848–55. doi:10.1016/j.neo.2017.08.004
73. Wargo JA, Gopalakrishnan V, Spencer C, Karpinets T, Reuben A, Andrews MC, et al. Association of the diversity and composition of the gut microbiome with responses and survival (PFS) in metastatic melanoma (MM) patients (pts) on anti-PD-1 therapy. *J Clin Oncol* (2017) 35(15):3008. doi:10.1200/JCO.2017.35.15_suppl.3008
74. Gopalakrishnan V, Spencer C, Nezi L, Reuben A, Andrews M, Karpinets T, et al. Gut microbiome modulates response to anti–PD-1 immunotherapy in melanoma patients. *Science* (2018) 359(6371):97–103. doi:10.1126/science.aan4236
75. Routy B, Le Chatelier E, Derosa L, Duong CP, Alou MT, Daillère R, et al. Gut microbiome influences efficacy of PD-1–based immunotherapy against epithelial tumors. *Science* (2018) 359(6371):91–7. doi:10.1126/science.aan3706
76. Vétizou M, Pitt JM, Daillère R, Lepage P, Waldschmitt N, Flament C, et al. Anticancer immunotherapy by CTLA-4 blockade relies on the gut microbiota. *Science* (2015) 350(6264):1079–84. doi:10.1126/science.aad1329
77. Pitt JM, Vétizou M, Gomperts Boneca I, Lepage P, Chamaillard M, Zitvogel L. Enhancing the clinical coverage and anticancer efficacy of immune check point blockade through manipulation of the gut microbiota. *Oncoimmunology* (2017) 6(1):e1132137. doi:10.1080/2162402X.2015.1132137
78. Yin P, Liu X, Mansfield AS, Harrington SM, Li Y, Yan Y, et al. CpG-induced antitumor immunity requires IL-12 in expansion of effector cells and down-regulation of PD-1. *Oncotarget* (2016) 7(43):70223. doi:10.18632/oncotarget.11833
79. Wang S, Campos J, Gallotta M, Gong M, Crain C, Naik E, et al. Intratumoral injection of a CpG oligonucleotide reverts resistance to PD-1 blockade by expanding multifunctional CD8+ T cells. *Proc Natl Acad Sci U S A* (2016) 113(46):E7240–9. doi:10.1073/pnas.1608555113
80. Haverson K, Rehakova Z, Sinkora J, Sver L, Bailey M. Immune development in jejunal mucosa after colonization with selected commensal gut bacteria: a study in germ-free pigs. *Vet Immunol Immunopathol* (2007) 119(3):243–53. doi:10.1016/j.vetimm.2007.05.022
81. Williams AM, Probert CS, Stepankova R, Tlaskalova-Hogenova H, Phillips A, Bland PW. Effects of microflora on the neonatal development of gut mucosal T cells and myeloid cells in the mouse. *Immunology* (2006) 119(4):470–8. doi:10.1111/j.1365-2567.2006.02458.x
82. Zhang W, Wen K, Azevedo MS, Gonzalez A, Saif LJ, Li G, et al. Lactic acid bacterial colonization and human rotavirus infection influence distribution and frequencies of monocytes/macrophages and dendritic cells in neonatal gnotobiotic pigs. *Vet Immunol Immunopathol* (2008) 121(3):222–31. doi:10.1016/j.vetimm.2007.10.001
83. Mazmanian SK, Liu CH, Tzianabos AO, Kasper DL. An immunomodulatory molecule of symbiotic bacteria directs maturation of the host immune system. *Cell* (2005) 122(1):107–18. doi:10.1016/j.cell.2005.05.007
84. Macpherson A, Martinic M, Harris N. The functions of mucosal T cells in containing the indigenous commensal flora of the intestine. *Cell Mol Life Sci* (2002) 59(12):2088–96. doi:10.1007/s000180200009
85. Ichinohe T, Pang IK, Kumamoto Y, Peaper DR, Ho JH, Murray TS, et al. Microbiota regulates immune defense against respiratory tract influenza A virus infection. *Proc Natl Acad Sci U S A* (2011) 108(13):5354–9. doi:10.1073/pnas.1019378108
86. Das S, Suarez G, Beswick EJ, Sierra JC, Graham DY, Reyes VE. Expression of B7-H1 on gastric epithelial cells: its potential role in regulating T cells during *Helicobacter pylori* infection. *J Immunol* (2006) 176(5):3000–9. doi:10.4049/jimmunol.176.5.3000
87. Wu YY, Lin CW, Cheng KS, Lin C, Wang YM, Lin IT, et al. Increased programmed death-ligand-1 expression in human gastric epithelial cells in *Helicobacter pylori* infection. *Clin Exp Immunol* (2010) 161(3):551–9. doi:10.1111/j.1365-2249.2010.04217.x
88. Xie Z, Chen Y, Zhao S, Yang Z, Yao X, Guo S, et al. Intrahepatic PD-1/PD-L1 up-regulation closely correlates with inflammation and virus replication in patients with chronic HBV infection. *Immunol Invest* (2009) 38(7):624–38. doi:10.1080/08820130903062210
89. Peng G, Li S, Wu W, Tan X, Chen Y, Chen Z. PD-1 upregulation is associated with HBV-specific T cell dysfunction in chronic hepatitis B patients. *Mol Immunol* (2008) 45(4):963–70. doi:10.1016/j.molimm.2007.07.038
90. Golden-Mason L, Palmer B, Klarquist J, Mengshol JA, Castelblanco N, Rosen HR. Upregulation of PD-1 expression on circulating and intrahepatic hepatitis C virus-specific CD8+ T cells associated with reversible immune dysfunction. *J Virol* (2007) 81(17):9249–58. doi:10.1128/JVI.00409-07
91. Shen T, Chen X, Chen Y, Xu Q, Lu F, Liu S. Increased PD-L1 expression and PD-L1/CD86 ratio on dendritic cells were associated with impaired dendritic cells function in HCV infection. *J Med Virol* (2010) 82(7):1152–9. doi:10.1002/jmv.21809
92. Yang W, Song Y, Lu YL, Sun JZ, Wang HW. Increased expression of programmed death (PD)-1 and its ligand PD-L1 correlates with impaired cell-mediated immunity in high-risk human papillomavirus-related cervical intraepithelial neoplasia. *Immunology* (2013) 139(4):513–22. doi:10.1111/imm.12101

93. Fang W, Zhang J, Hong S, Zhan J, Chen N, Qin T, et al. EBV-driven LMP1 and IFN-γ up-regulate PD-L1 in nasopharyngeal carcinoma: implications for oncotargeted therapy. *Oncotarget* (2014) 5(23):12189. doi:10.18632/oncotarget.2608
94. Derks S, Liao X, Chiaravalli AM, Xu X, Camargo MC, Solcia E, et al. Abundant PD-L1 expression in Epstein-Barr Virus-infected gastric cancers. *Oncotarget* (2016) 7(22):32925. doi:10.18632/oncotarget.9076
95. Parsonnet J, Friedman GD, Vandersteen DP, Chang Y, Vogelman JH, Orentreich N, et al. *Helicobacter pylori* infection and the risk of gastric carcinoma. *N Engl J Med* (1991) 325(16):1127–31. doi:10.1056/NEJM199110173251603
96. Crabtree J, Shallcross T, Heatley R, Wyatt J. Mucosal tumour necrosis factor alpha and interleukin-6 in patients with *Helicobacter pylori* associated gastritis. *Gut* (1991) 32(12):1473–7. doi:10.1136/gut.32.12.1473
97. Bodger K, Wyatt J, Heatley R. Gastric mucosal secretion of interleukin-10: relations to histopathology, *Helicobacter pylori* status, and tumour necrosis factor-alpha secretion. *Gut* (1997) 40(6):739–44. doi:10.1136/gut.40.6.739
98. Perri F, Clemente R, Festa V, De Ambrosio C, Quitadamo M, Fusillo M, et al. Serum tumour necrosis factor-alpha is increased in patients with *Helicobacter pylori* infection and CagA antibodies. *Ital J Gastroenterol Hepatol* (1999) 31(4):290–4.
99. Kottke T, Evgin L, Shim KG, Rommelfanger D, Boisgerault N, Zaidi S, et al. Subversion of NK-cell and TNFα immune surveillance drives tumor recurrence. *Cancer Immunol Res* (2017) 5(11):1029–45. doi:10.1158/2326-6066.CIR-17-0175
100. Chen J, Jiang C, Jin L, Zhang X. Regulation of PD-L1: a novel role of pro-survival signalling in cancer. *Ann Oncol* (2015) 27(3):409–16. doi:10.1093/annonc/mdv615
101. Gowrishankar K, Gunatilake D, Gallagher SJ, Tiffen J, Rizos H, Hersey P. Inducible but not constitutive expression of PD-L1 in human melanoma cells is dependent on activation of NF-κB. *PLoS One* (2015) 10(4):e0123410. doi:10.1371/journal.pone.0123410
102. Wang X, Yang L, Huang F, Zhang Q, Liu S, Ma L, et al. Inflammatory cytokines IL-17 and TNF-α up-regulate PD-L1 expression in human prostate and colon cancer cells. *Immunol Lett* (2017) 184:7–14. doi:10.1016/j.imlet.2017.02.006
103. Matsumoto S, Hara T, Hori T, Mitsuyama K, Nagaoka M, Tomiyasu N, et al. Probiotic *Lactobacillus*-induced improvement in murine chronic inflammatory bowel disease is associated with the down-regulation of pro-inflammatory cytokines in lamina propria mononuclear cells. *Clin Exp Immunol* (2005) 140(3):417–26. doi:10.1111/j.1365-2249.2005.02790.x
104. Amdekar S, Singh V, Singh R, Sharma P, Keshav P, Kumar A. *Lactobacillus casei* reduces the inflammatory joint damage associated with collagen-induced arthritis (CIA) by reducing the pro-inflammatory cytokines: *Lactobacillus casei*: COX-2 inhibitor. *J Clin Immunol* (2011) 31(2):147–54. doi:10.1007/s10875-010-9457-7
105. Liu Y, Fatheree NY, Mangalat N, Rhoads JM. Human-derived probiotic *Lactobacillus reuteri* strains differentially reduce intestinal inflammation. *Am J Physiol Gastrointest Liver Physiol* (2010) 299(5):G1087–96. doi:10.1152/ajpgi.00124.2010
106. Tien MT, Girardin SE, Regnault B, Le Bourhis L, Dillies MA, Coppee JY, et al. Anti-inflammatory effect of *Lactobacillus casei* on *Shigella*-infected human intestinal epithelial cells. *J Immunol* (2006) 176(2):1228–37. doi:10.4049/jimmunol.176.2.1228
107. Vieira AT, Galvao I, Amaral FA, Teixeira MM, Nicoli JR, Martins FS. Oral treatment with *Bifidobacterium longum* 51A reduced inflammation in a murine experimental model of gout. *Benef Microbes* (2015) 6(6):799–806. doi:10.3920/BM2015.0015
108. Zhang L, Su P, Henriksson A, O'Rourke J, Mitchell H. Investigation of the immunomodulatory effects of *Lactobacillus casei* and *Bifidobacterium lactis* on *Helicobacter pylori* infection. *Helicobacter* (2008) 13(3):183–90. doi:10.1111/j.1523-5378.2008.00595.x

2

Combining Immune Checkpoint Inhibitors with Conventional Cancer Therapy

Yiyi Yan[1], Anagha Bangalore Kumar[2], Heidi Finnes[3], Svetomir N. Markovic[1], Sean Park[4], Roxana S. Dronca[5] and Haidong Dong[2,6]*

[1] Division of Medical Oncology, Mayo Clinic, Rochester, MN, United States, [2] Department of Immunology, Mayo Clinic, Rochester, MN, United States, [3] Department of Pharmacy, Mayo Clinic, Rochester, MN, United States, [4] Department of Radiation Oncology, Mayo Clinic, Rochester, MN, United States, [5] Division of Hematology and Medical Oncology, Mayo Clinic, Jacksonville, FL, United States, [6] Department of Urology, Mayo Clinic, Rochester, MN, United States

Edited by:
Alexandr Bazhin, Klinikum der Universität München, Germany

Reviewed by:
Ivan Shevchenko, Ludwig-Maximilians-Universität München, Germany
Marie-Andree Forget, University of Texas MD Anderson Cancer Center, United States

***Correspondence:**
Yiyi Yan
yan.yiyi@mayo.edu

Immune checkpoint inhibitors (ICIs) have recently revolutionized cancer treatment, providing unprecedented clinical benefits. However, primary or acquired therapy resistance can affect up to two-thirds of patients receiving ICIs, underscoring the urgency to elucidate the mechanisms of treatment resistance and to design more effective therapeutic strategies. Conventional cancer treatments, including cytotoxic chemotherapy, radiation therapy, and targeted therapy, have immunomodulatory effects in addition to direct cancer cell-killing activities. Their clinical utilities in combination with ICIs have been explored, aiming to achieve synergetic effects with improved and durable clinical response. Here, we will review the immunomodulatory effects of chemotherapy, targeted therapy, and radiation therapy, in the setting of ICI, and their clinical implications in reshaping modern cancer immunotherapy.

Keywords: immunotherapy, chemotherapy, targeted therapy, radiotherapy, combination therapy

INTRODUCTION

Deeper understanding in the regulatory mechanisms of antitumor immunity, especially the identification of immune checkpoint pathways, has led to the success of modern immunotherapy. The past decade has witnessed a revolution in cancer therapy since the introduction of immune checkpoint inhibitors (ICIs), including anti-CTLA4 antibody and anti-PD-1/PD-L1 antibody. These antibodies have reshaped the landscape of treatments in various types of cancers, including melanoma, renal cell cancer, colorectal cancer (CRC), and non-small-cell lung cancer (NSCLC). However, it is estimated that up to 60–70% of patients do not respond to single-agent ICI therapy (1–7). To address this clinical challenge, different conventional cancer treatment modalities have been tested in combination with ICIs to achieve synergetic effects and to overcome the resistance to immunotherapy. Although some of these approaches have provided clinical benefits, the lack of knowledge in the functional interactions between conventional cancer therapies and immune checkpoint blockades at the molecular level remains a crucial hurdle in developing rational and optimal combination strategies. In this article, we will review the immune-regulatory effects of conventional cancer treatments and their clinical applications in combination with immune checkpoint blockades and future challenges.

COMBINATION OF IMMUNOTHERAPY AND CHEMOTHERAPY

Immunomodulatory Impact of Cytotoxic Chemotherapy

It has long been speculated that the immunoregulatory properties of conventional cytotoxic chemotherapy contribute to the antitumoral effects of these agents, in addition to direct tumor killing

(8). Although the mechanisms are yet to be fully understood, chemotherapy can regulate antitumor T cell response through increasing tumor antigenicity, inducing immunogenic cell death (ICD), disrupting immune suppressive pathways, and enhancing effector T-cell response (9–12).

Chemotherapy executes direct cancer killing *via* multiple mechanisms, including causing DNA damage, inhibiting DNA replication, and preventing mitosis (13). The induced tumor cell death further elicits systemic and intratumoral immune responses, contributing to the antitumor immunity. Chemotherapy enhances the antigenicity of the tumors through the increase of mutation burden and neoantigen load (such as in NSCLC and other various malignancies), which are correlated with higher responses to ICI therapy (14, 15). Some chemotherapy drugs upregulate MHC class 1 expression to increase antigen presentation (16, 17). In addition, chemotherapy drugs promote dendritic cell maturation and enhance the T cell activation by DCs (18). Chemotherapy also promotes ICD by releasing damage-associated molecular patterns, which can generate effector immune response when bound to pattern-recognition receptor. Experiments in animal models have suggested that some chemotherapy drugs induce the expression of PD-L1 on ovarian cancer cells (19).

Cytotoxic chemotherapy is regarded as immunosuppressive due to its dose-limiting myelosuppression. However, recent studies have demonstrated that it also can disrupt suppressive pathways. These immunosuppressive subsets play critical roles in downregulating the antitumor T-cell response and in promoting resistance to ICI treatments. Lymphodepletion resulted after chemotherapy can potentiate antigen-specific T-cell responses, therefore, augment antitumor immunity, particularly during the recovery phase from lymphopenia. Lymphodepletion can eliminate regulatory T cells (Treg) and other immunosuppressive cell subsets, such as myeloid-derived suppressor cells (MDSCs) (20–22) and tumor-associated macrophages (TAMs) (23). For instances, cyclophosphamide eliminates Treg and improves overall survival when combined with immunotherapy in a colon cancer models (24). Doxorubicin eliminates MDSCs and enhances the efficacy of immunotherapy in breast cancer (25). Reductions of these immunosuppressive populations in the tumor microenvironment of glioblastoma, synergize with anti-PD-1 therapy, and enhance the antitumor immunity (26, 27). The elimination of these immunosuppressive cells will increase the availability of survival and proliferative cytokines for T cells and lower the threshold for T-cell activation. Chemotherapeutic reagents also promote the polarization of Th1/Th2 and enhance the proliferation of T-lymphocytes in patients with advanced solid cancers (such as renal cell carcinoma, colon cancer, and ovarian cancer) (28, 29). Over the past decade, multiple studies have shown that different types of chemotherapy drugs can modulate the antitumor immunity in various mechanisms (9).

Given the extensive roles of chemotherapy in regulating the antitumor immune response, it is safe to hypothesize that the addition of chemotherapy to ICI may further enhance the activities of cytotoxic T cells with improved clinical outcomes. Over the past few years, chemoimmunotherapy (CIT) combination has attracted attention from clinicians and researchers and has been investigated in multiple clinical trials.

Clinical Studies With CIT Combinations

Chemotherapy in combination with immunotherapy (CIT) has been studied in multiple solid tumors, largely in NSCLC, providing broadened treatment options with improved outcomes.

The combination of pembrolizumab with pemetrexed and carboplatin has been evaluated in KEYNOTE-021, a multicenter phase 1/2 study, in patients with NSCLC. In the phase 1 study (30), pembrolizumab in combination with either carboplatin and paclitaxel, or carboplatin and paclitaxel plus bevacizumab, or carboplatin and pemetrexed was investigated, with overall response rate (ORR) of 52, 48, and 71%, respectively, irrespective of PD-L1 expression levels. These results led to the phase 2 study, evaluating the clinical outcome of pembrolizumab in combination with carboplatin and pemetrexed (31). A total of 123 chemotherapy-naïve nonsquamous NSCLC patients were randomized to chemotherapy alone, or chemo-pembrolizumab combination. Indefinite pemetrexed maintenance therapy was allowed for patients in chemotherapy alone group, and maintenance therapy with indefinite pemetrexed and up to 24 months of pembrolizumab was allowed for patients in chemo-pembrolizumab combination group. A significantly higher response rate was observed in the CIT combination group (55%) than in the chemotherapy alone group (29%), with progression-free survival (PFS) of 13 vs. 6 months, respectively. The magnitude of adverse effects (grade 3 or above) in both the groups was comparable (39 vs. 26%, respectively). Based on this study, the FDA granted accelerated approval of pembrolizumab in combination with carboplatin and pemetrexed for the treatment of NSCLC adenocarcinoma in the first-line setting. Updated survival data with median follow-up of 18.7 months showed a PFS of 19.0 months in CIT group vs. 8.9 months in chemotherapy group, with OS in CIT group not reached vs. 20.9 months in the chemotherapy arm (32).

In KEYONOTE-021 study, the tumor cell-associated PD-L1 expression level can impact the response rates in patients who received CIT treatment: response rate of 57% in those with $<1\%$ PD-L1 expression, 54% in those with $\geq 1\%$ PD-L1 expression, 26% in those with 1–49% PD-L1 expression, and 80% in those with $\geq 50\%$ PD-L1 expression (30). Accordingly, higher cutoff of PD-L1 expression was associated with higher response rates. Since pembrolizumab singe-agent is only indicated in NSCLC patients with $\geq 50\%$ PD-L1 expression in the frontline setting (33, 34), this study established CIT as an alternative first-line therapeutic approach for nonsquamous NSCLC patients with $<50\%$ tumor PD-L1 expression, who do not harbor targetable mutations.

The results of the phase 3 trial (KEYNOTE-189) evaluating pembrolizumab in combination with chemotherapy in frontline setting in nonsquamous NSCLC patients without sensitizing EGFR or ALK mutations have been recently reported. A total of 616 patients were randomized in a 2:1 ratio to receive pemetrexed and platinum-based drug plus either pembrolizumab or placebo for 4 cycles, followed by pembrolizumab or placebo (for up to 35 cycles) plus pemetrexed maintenance therapy. With a median follow-up of 10.5 months, the 12-month OS was 69.2% in combination group vs. 49.4% in placebo group, and median PFS was 8.8 vs. 4.9 months, respectively. Interestingly, the survival benefit was seen across all PD-L1 categories (35).

A phase 3 trial evaluating CIT combination in frontline setting is currently ongoing for squamous NSCLC (KEYNOTE-407). The results from a second interim analysis after patients had been followed for a median of 7.8 months were recently presented (36). A total of 559 patients were enrolled and stratified prior to randomization based on tumor PD-L1 expression (<1 vs. ≥1%) as well as the choice of taxane (paclitaxel vs. nab-paclitaxel). Patients were assigned to receive four cycles of carboplatin and paclitaxel/nab-paclitaxel plus either pembrolizumab or placebo, followed by pembrolizumab (for CIT group) or placebo (for placebo group) maintenance therapy. Patients in the placebo group could cross over to receive pembrolizumab monotherapy after disease progression. Significant improvements in OS, PFS, and response rate were observed in CIT group vs. chemo-alone group regardless of PD-L1 expression level: the median OS of 15.9 vs. 11.3 months (HR 0.64, 95% CI [0.49, 0.85]; $p = 0.0008$), PFS of 6.4 vs. 4.8 months (HR 0.56, 95% CI [0.45, 0.70]; $p < 0.0001$), and objective response rate of 58.4 vs. 35.0% at the first interim analysis ($p = 0.0004$), respectively.

Nivolumab has also been tested in multiple clinical trials. In phase 1 CHECKMATE-012 trail, 56 patients with NSCLC received first-line therapy with combination of nivolumab with either gemcitabine and cisplatin, pemetrexed and cisplatin, or paclitaxel and carboplatin, followed by nivolumab maintenance therapy (37). CIT combination demonstrated improved ORR compared with nivolumab monotherapy in the front-line setting, with a manageable, non-overlapping toxicity profile. While nivolumab monotherapy has shown an ORR of 23% in the historical study (38), it demonstrated a higher ORR when combined with gemcitabine and cisplatin (33%), or pemetrexed and cisplatin (47%), or paclitaxel and carboplatin (43%), with acceptable tolerability and toxicity profiles. In addition to that, association between treatment response and PD-L1 expression levels was not observed (ORR 48% in PD-L1 ≥ 1 vs. 43% in PD-L1 < 1%).

A phase 3 study (CHECKMATE-227) is ongoing to evaluate nivolumab in combination with chemotherapy vs. chemotherapy alone in the frontline setting for patients with NSCLC (39). A total of 550 chemo-naive NSCLC patients without known sensitizing EGFR/ALK mutations, with <1% tumor PD-L1 expression were randomized to receive nivolumab 3 mg/kg Q2W + ipilimumab 1 mg/kg Q6W, nivolumab 360 mg Q3W + chemo, or chemotherapy for 2 years. In the recently presented results (40), a total of 177 patients received CIT while 186 received chemotherapy alone. With a minimum follow-up of 11.2 months, an improved PFS was seen in nivolumab-chemo arm vs. chemotherapy alone arm (HR = 0.74, 95% CI [0.58, 0.94]). Part 2 of CheckMate 227 is currently ongoing to evaluate the benefit of nivolumab-chemo combinational irrespective of PD-L1 expression.

The FDA approval of the pembrolizumab-chemotherapy combination in NSCLC has encouraged physicians to investigate various CIT in clinical trials in other types of cancers (**Table 1**). The combination of pembrolizumab with different chemotherapy regimens is being evaluated in PembroPlus study (NCT02331251) for patients with various types of advanced cancers. Pembrolizumab in addition to cisplatin or capecitabine or 5-Fluorouracil is being investigated in KEYNOTE-062 study (NCT02494583) for patients with advanced gastric cancer. Atezolizumab, an anti-PD-L1 antibody, has also been evaluated in combination with chemotherapy in the phase 1 GP28328 study (NCT01633970) in multiple tumor types, demonstrating improved ORR of CIT in patients with NSCLC (41). Phase 3 studies are the currently ongoing to determine the clinical benefit of atezolizumab in combination with chemotherapy (IMpower 130, IMpower132). Durvalumab, another anti-PD-L1 antibody, is also being evaluated in a phase 3 clinical trial (POSEIDON), randomizing untreated NSCLC patients to chemotherapy alone or chemotherapy in combination with durvalumab with or without anti-CTLA4 antibody, tremelimumab (NCT03164616).

Considerations and Challenges

Despite recent clinical success, our limited understanding of the interplay between chemotherapy and immunotherapy hurdles the design of the optimal combination strategy. Different types of chemotherapies execute cytotoxicity against tumors through distinct mechanisms. Similarly, each chemotherapy drug demonstrates unique impact on the systemic and intratumoral immune responses (8). Distinct intrinsic signaling pathways in different types of tumors attribute to the variability in their chemosensitivities. Moreover, the advanced knowledge of immune checkpoint pathways has rapidly expanded the list of ICIs that are acting through different mechanisms (e.g., TIM-3, LAG-3, indoleamine 2,3-dioxygenase, B7-H3). Understanding the impact of chemotherapy in the setting of different types of immunotherapies, as well as the impact of immunotherapy on chemosensitivity (or chemoresistance) of tumors, at both cellular and molecular levels are crucial for the design of rational combination regimens with minimized toxicity.

It is not just the appropriate combination but also the sequence and scheduling of CIT that have to be considered in the clinical scenario. In most of the clinical trials, chemotherapy and immunotherapy are given concurrently, lacking the understanding of the impact of sequencing on the antitumor immunity. Given the fact that antitumor T cell response has different phases that can be targeted by different ICIs (47, 48), and that chemotherapy can modulate immune system while having cytotoxicity against T cells at the same time, it is very likely that the sequence and timing of CIT would significantly impact the treatment outcomes. Both preclinical and clinical studies have shown controversial results regarding the sequence of CIT, and the ideal combination regimens are evolving. Since chemotherapy can cause immunogenic tumor death that promotes T cell priming, some have thought that immunotherapy should be given after chemotherapy to allow maximal T cell proliferation and expansion. In a phase 2 study investigating carboplatin and paclitaxel in combination with concurrent or sequenced ipilimumab in small-cell lung cancer (SCLC), the sequenced treatment is associated with improved PFS compared with chemotherapy alone (49). However, in a mesothelioma mouse model, concurrent treatment with ipilimumab and chemotherapy improved outcomes compared with sequential therapy (50). By contrast, studies in lung cancers and melanoma have shown that chemotherapy administered after immunotherapy can achieve successful clinical responses (51, 52). Our group recently demonstrated that in metastatic melanoma patients who had disease progression after anti-PD1

TABLE 1 | Completed and ongoing clinical trials evaluating chemotherapy in combination with immune checkpoint inhibitors.

Trial	Tumor type	Therapy regimes	Endpoints
Gadgeel et al. (30)	NSCLC (KEYNOTE 021) phase 1	Cohort A: Pembrolizumab (pembro) + carboplatin and paclitaxel (CP) → pembro Cohort B: Pembro + CP + bevacizumab (BEV) → pembro + BEV Cohort C: Pembro + carboplatin + pemetrexed (PEM) → pembro + PEM	Overall response rate (ORR): 52% Progression-free survival (PFS): 10 months ORR: 48% PFS: NR ORR: 48% PFS: 10
Langer et al. (31) Borghaei et al. (32)	NSCLC (KEYNOTE 021) phase 2	Pembro + carboplatin + PEM → pembro + PEM Carboplatin/PEM → PEM	ORR: 55% PFS: 19 months ORR 29% PFS: 8.9 months
Gandhi et al. (35)	NSCLC (nonsquamous) (KEYNOTE-189)	Pembro + platinum + PEM → pembro + PEM Placebo + platinum + PEM → PEM	OS (12 months): 69.2% PFS: 8.8 months OS (12 months): 49.4% PFS: 4.9 months
KEYNOTE-047 (ongoing)	NSCLC (squamous)	Pembro + CP → Pembro Placebo + CP	Primary: OS and PFS Secondary: ORR
Weiss et al. (42)	Advanced, metastatic solid tumors (PEMBRO-PLUS)	Pembrolizumab plus gemcitabine (G), G + docetaxel (D), G + nab-paclitaxel (NP), G + vinorelbine (V), or irinotecan	Standard dose pembrolizumab can be safely combined with G, G + NP, G + V, I, and LD
Rizvi et al. (37)	NSCLC (CHECKMATE 012) phase 1	Nivolumab (Nivo) + gemcitabine (GEM) + cisplatin (CIS) → Nivo Nivo + PEM the + CIS → Nivo Nivo (10 mg/kg) + CP →Nivo Nivo (5 mg/kg) + CP → Nivo	PFS: 5.7 months OS: 11.6 months PFS: 6.8 months OS: 19.2 months PFS: 4.8 months OS: 14.9 months PFS: 7.1 months OS: NR
Paz-Ares et al. (39)	NSCLC (CHECKMATE 227) phase 3 Ongoing	Chemotherapy alone or in combination with Nivo Squamous: CP Nonsquamous: PEM + carboplatin (or cisplatin)	Primary: PFS and OS Secondary: ORR
Liu et al. (41)	NSCLC	Atezolizumab (Atezo) + CP → Atezo Atezo + carboplatin/PEM → Atezo + PEM Atezo + carboplatin + nab-paclitaxel → Atezo	ORR: 36% PFS: 7.1 months OSS: 12.9 months ORR: 68% PFS: 8.4 months OS: 18.9 months ORR: 46% PFS: 5.7 months OS: 17.0 months
NCT02367781 NCT02367794 NCT02657434	IMpower 130 (NSCLC nonsquamous) IMpower 131 (NSCLC Squamous) IMpower 132 (NSCLC nonsquamous) All ongoing	Atezo + carboplatin + nab-paclitaxel → Atezo Atezo + CP → Atezo Atezo + PEM/carboplatin (or cisplatin) → Atezo + PEM	Primary: PFS and OS Secondary: ORR
NCT02537418	NSCLC (PESEIDON) Phase 3 Ongoing	Durvalumab + tremelimumab + chemotherapy (histology-based) Durvalumab + chemotherapy (histology-based) Chemotherapy (histology-based)	Primary: PFS Secondary: OS and ORR
NCT02735239	Metastatic/locally advanced esophageal cancer (neoadjuvant therapy)	Durvalumab in combination with standard of care chemotherapy or chemoradiation	Primary: Adverse events, dose-limiting toxicities Secondary: ORR, PFS, OS
NCT03317496	NSCLC Urothelial Cancer	Avelumab + pemetrexed/carboplatin Avelumab + gemcitabine/cisplatin	Primary: Confirmed OR Secondary: PFS, OS, duration of response, time to tumor response

(Continued)

TABLE 1 | Continued

Trial	Tumor type	Therapy regimes	Endpoints
Govindan et al. (43)	Advanced NSCLC	Ipilimumab + CP Placebo + CP	OS: 13.5 months PFS: 5.6 months (with higher toxicities) OS: 12.4 months PFS: 5.6 months
Patel et al. (44)	Metastatic melanoma	Ipilimumab plus temozolomide	6-month PFS was 45% with median OS of 24.5 months. 10 (15.6%) confirmed partial responses and 10 (15.6%) confirmed complete responses. No deaths/unexpected toxicities
Reck et al. (45)	SCLC	Ipilimumab + etoposide and platinum Placebo + etoposide and platinum	OS: 11.0 months PFS: 4.6 months OS: 10.9 months PFS: 4.4 months
Yamazaki et al. (46)	Melanoma	Ipilimumab + dacarbazine	Was not considered tolerable in the Japanese patient population

monotherapy, the addition of chemotherapy to PD-1 blockade induced a significantly improved clinical response, with an ORR of 65% (CR of 25%) (53–55). Using peripheral blood from patients who benefited from the CIT combination, we identified a novel subset of therapy-responsive $CD8^+$ T cells ($CX3CR1^+$) that can survive chemotherapy toxicity with preserved CTL functions (53). This subset of effector T cells is less actively proliferating during the combination therapy, and hence is spared from chemocytotoxicity. In addition, these $CX3CR1^+CD8^+$ T cells demonstrate the ability to efflux chemotherapy drugs. Our preclinical animal model studies also demonstrate that that CIT combination after previous exposure to immunotherapy provides better tumor control with an increase in $CX3CR1^+CD8^+$ T cells population (53). Our results elucidated mechanisms that are responsible for the success of combination, facilitating the rational design of CIT. This subset of T cells may be used as a biomarker in monitoring and predicting clinical response to CIT, especially when tumor PD-L1 levels fail to show direct correlation with the CIT treatment outcomes in multiple clinical trials. Future studies are warranted to define whether the efficacy of CIT is dependent on certain ICI to recruit immune cells into tumor tissues (like $CX3CR1^+CD8$ effector T cells) or to expand local tumor-infiltrating immune cells to reject tumors.

The scheduling and timing of chemotherapy in CIT are also critical for achieving clinical success. The fluctuation of dynamic systemic immunity in metastatic melanoma patients has been reported. Chemotherapy that was delivered in synchronization with unique phase of dynamic immune response tends to correlate with improved response (56). Some chemotherapy drugs work in cell cycle specific manners (e.g., S phase for drugs inhibiting DNA synthesis), suggesting that their direct tumor-killing activities and immunomodulatory effects can be influenced by the schedule of drug administrations. Platinum-based chemotherapy given in different dosing schedules has shown different antitumor immune responses associated with variable clinical outcomes in an ovarian cancer mouse model (57). Our recent preclinical study further demonstrated that the timing of chemotherapy administration after the immunotherapy initiation can affect the frequencies of $CX3CR1^+$ T cell population and the treatment outcomes (53), suggesting the variable chemo-induced immunomodulation in relationship to the timing of the immunotherapy. With the overwhelming possibility of CIT combinations, further preclinical and clinical research is in need to design rational combinations for different types of cancers, while minimizing the therapeutic toxicities.

COMBINATION OF IMMUNOTHERAPY AND MOLECULAR TARGETED THERAPY

The identification of deregulated cellular signaling pathways that are responsible for tumorigenesis has led to the successful development of molecular targeted therapy in recent decades. Medications inhibiting oncogenic pathways, DNA repair response, and angiogenesis pathways have provided effective treatment options for patients with different types of malignancies, although response durability is often lacking. Recent research has demonstrated that these pathways also have immunomodulatory effects on systemic and intratumoral antitumor immune responses, suggesting that the combination of molecular targeted therapy with ICIs can result in synergistic antitumor effects.

BRAF and MEK Inhibitors

Dysregulations in the RAS/RAF/MAPK pathway are commonly seen in oncogenic transformation and tumorigenesis. Mutations in *BRAF*, a proto-oncogene, are associated with various types of cancers, especially melanoma. In patients with BRAF mutant metastatic melanoma, high response rates are observed after treatment with BRAF/MEK inhibitors, although the duration of response is short lasting due to adaptive therapy resistance. Since ICIs provide durable clinical benefit, combinations of ICIs with BRAF/MEK inhibitors may provide fast and long-lasting disease control.

In melanoma cell models, BRAFV600 mutations can lead to decreased antitumor immunity through upregulation of immunosuppressive factors [e.g., IL-10, vascular endothelial growth factor (VEGF)] (58), elevation of PD-L1 expression levels (59), increased tumor infiltration of immunosuppressive cells (e.g., Treg) (60), and downregulation of melanoma MHC-1 expression (61). In patients with metastatic melanoma, BRAF inhibitors have shown to decrease the immunosuppressive cytokines with resultant increased $CD8^+$ T cell tumor infiltration and antitumor immunity (62). In addition, the treatment response of BRAF inhibitors is $CD8^+$ T-cell dependent (60, 63). Interestingly, in CRC patients, the majority of those who have PD-L1 positive tumor carry BRAF mutations along with microsatellite instability, suggesting that the immunosuppressive tumor microenvironment can be induced by BRAF mutations (64). In a colorectal carcinoma mouse model, MEK inhibitors demonstrated synergistic therapeutic effects with anti-PD-L1 antibody (65). In a melanoma mouse model, dabrafenib treatment alone results in increased TAMs and Treg, while the addition of trametinib further decreases these suppressive cell subsets. When combined with anti-PD-L1 antibody, the triple therapy provides a superior tumor control (66).

The combination of BRAF inhibitors with anti-CTLA-4 antibody has been studied in multiple clinical trials. However, substantial immune-related adverse effects were the main concern in several studies. Liver toxicity and high-grade skin adverse effects were seen in trials with vemurafenib and ipilimumab combination (NCT01400451 and NCT01673854) (67, 68). Severe colitis was seen in patients who received dabrafenib, trametinib, and ipilimumab triple combination (NCT01767454). Anti-PD1/PD-L1 antibodies were also evaluated in combination with BRAF/MEK inhibitors (**Table 2**). In a phase 1 study, the combination of dabrafenib, trametinib, and durvalumab demonstrated tolerable toxicity profiles and encouraging disease response rates (69). Pembrolizumab is also being studied in combination with dabrafenib and trametinib in patients with metastatic melanoma (NCT02130466). Multiple other clinical trials are currently ongoing (NCT01940809; NCT01656642; NCT02027961; NCT02224781) to test similar combinations.

Combining BRAF/MEK inhibitors with ICIs has the potential to overcome resistance to targeted therapy; however, further investigations are needed to understand the underlying molecular interplay and to design the ideal combination regimens. Given the toxicities observed in early trials, the optimum tolerable dose of targeted therapy in combination with ICIs needs to be determined. The rapid development of resistance to BRAF/MEK inhibitors and their dynamic impacts on the tumor microenvironment and systemic antitumor immunity should also be considered to determine the sequencing and scheduling of the combination. One study demonstrated long-term tumor control after short-term targeted therapy with subsequent anti-PD1 antibody in patients with metastatic melanoma, and T cell tumor infiltration was seen in tumor biopsies within 1 week after BRAF/MEK inhibitors administration while less frequent after 2 weeks on therapy (71), suggesting that the timing of combination with PD-1 blockade can impact patient outcomes.

Other oncogenic pathways, such as PI3K–Akt–mTOR pathway and KIT, can also regulate the antitumor immunity in addition to regulating cellular proliferation, providing further options for combination therapy with ICIs. For example, inhibition of PI3kγ can promote T cell infiltration through regulating the balance between stimulatory and suppressive TAMs (72). Inhibition of KIT decreased the INF-γ induced PD-L1 expression (73). Treatments targeting these pathways are also being investigated in combination with ICIs to overcome their limited clinical response. The crosstalk between multiple signaling oncogenic pathways in the setting of immunotherapy should be further investigated to determine the ideal drugs to be combined, with special consideration of the individual's unique intrinsic genetic background.

Poly (ADP-Ribose) Polymerase (PARP) Inhibitors

DNA damage repair machinery plays important roles in cell cycle regulation and tumorigenesis (74). Inhibition of DNA damage repair can potentially increase the tumor mutational burden, especially in tumors with high endogenous DNA damage. PARP plays a critical role in the repair of single-strand DNA break. In tumor cells with BRCA mutations, PARP inhibition can increase the genomic instability and cell death, with resultant increased neoantigen load and antitumor T cell response (75). This synthetic lethality of PARP inhibitors established the foundation for its clinical application in cancer treatment (76). PARP inhibitors also demonstrate immunoregulatory effects in preclinical studies. They can attenuate chronic inflammation and increase T cell infiltration (77).

Olaparib has been recently approved for the treatment of ovarian cancers with BRCA1 and BRCA2 mutations. Olaparib in combination with PD-L1 inhibitor, durvalumab, was recently investigated in a clinical trial for patients with gynecologic

TABLE 2 | Clinical trials of BRAF targeted therapy in combination with immune checkpoint inhibitors.

Trial	Mutation status	Therapy regimens	Outcomes
Puzanov et al. (70)	BRAF V600 mutant melanoma	Dabrafenib ± trametinib + ipilimumab	Triple therapy resulted in severe GI toxicities
Ribas et al. (67)	BRAF V600 mutant melanoma	Vemurafenib + ipilimumab	Combination resulted in severe liver toxicities
Ribas et al. (69)	Both wild-type and BRAF mutant melanoma	Durvalumab + dabrafenib + trametinib Durvalumab + trametinib Trametinib → durvalumab	Tolerable, no unexpected toxicity
Amin et al. (68)	BRAF V600 mutant melanoma	Vemurafenib + ipilimumab	Combination resulted in high-grade GI and skin toxicities
NCT02224781	Metastatic melanoma	Dabrafenib + trametinib followed by ipilimumab + nivolumab at progression vs. ipilimumab + nivolumab followed by dabrafenib + trametinib	Ongoing Primary: OS Secondary: PFS

cancers. Among 26 enrolled women, a disease control rate of 83% was reported, with an acceptable safety profile (78). Several trials evaluating different PARP inhibitors in combination with ICIs are currently ongoing in various solid tumors, including NSCLC and breast cancer (**Table 3**). The combination of niraparib with pembrolizumab was studied in the phase 1/2 TOPACIO/Keynote-162 (NCT02657889) study, and the results from the recurrent ovarian cancer cohort were recently reported (79). Among the 60 evaluable patients, an ORR of 25% was seen in all platinum-resistant ovarian cancer patients with an ORR of 45% in those with BRCA mutations. No new safety concerns were identified.

Given the fact that DNA repair response not only regulates tumorigenesis but also plays role in antitumor immunity, it is imperative to fully understand the interplay between DNA repair inhibitors and ICIs to combine them in a safe and effective manner, since inhibition of DNA repair response can potentially decrease the immune response. Moreover, the intrinsic tumor genetic background and DNA repair response status [e.g., BRCA mutation vs. wild-type (WT)] have positive impact on the PARP inhibitor-induced antitumor immune response during immunotherapy. Furthermore, it is possible that different PARP inhibitors can modulate the antitumor immune response through different mechanisms, which could impact the treatment outcomes when combined with different ICIs.

VEGF Inhibitors

Vascular endothelial growth factor stimulates angiogenesis, tissue remodeling, and fibrosis. Its immunosuppressive effects make VEGF a good target candidate to potentiate the antitumor immune response in combination with ICIs (80, 81). Studies from our group have shown that in patients with stage IV melanoma the baseline Treg concentration positively correlates with baseline VEGF level, which associates with poor clinical outcomes (82). Upregulated VEGF level and chronically Th-2-mediated immune status are observed in patients with metastatic melanoma (83). Animal models have shown that anti-VEGF antibody can increase T cell tumor infiltration with enhanced antitumor response (84). Decreased Treg proliferation and MDSC population are associated with bevacizumab treatment in CRC (85). The hypoxic conditions resulting from anti-VEGF treatment also can upregulate PD-L1 expression.

Tremelimumab in combination with sunitinib has been evaluated in patients with metastatic melanoma. Unfortunately, unexpected dose-limiting renal toxicity was observed (86). High dose of tremelimumab (6 mg/kg) used in this study could contribute to the adverse effects. Bevacizumab was also investigated in combination with ipilimumab in melanoma patients (87). A disease control rate of 67.4% was observed with combination therapy, with increased $CD8^+$ lymphocyte infiltration resulting from more effective lymphocytic trafficking. Multiple clinical trials are currently ongoing investigating the combination of bevacizumab and pembrolizumab in patients with ovarian cancer (NCT02853318) and solid tumor brain metastases (NCT02681549). Other agents targeting VEGF pathway, such as ramucirumab, are also being evaluated in combination regimens (**Table 3**). Lenvatinib, a tyrosine kinase inhibitor, is being studied in combination with pembrolizumab in a phase 1/2 trial (NCT03006926). However, the dynamic immunologic effects of these combinations remain to be elucidated. In a recent report, 10 patients with metastatic renal cell carcinoma were treated with bevacizumab plus atezolizumab after bevacizumab run-in period (88). A partial disease response was observed in four patients, and median time to response was 4.2 months. Following combination therapy, increased intratumoral $CD8^+$ T cells, Th1, and T effector markers are found. Interestingly, increases in intratumoral chemokine, CX3CL1, and peripheral $CX3CR1^+$ (CX3CL1 receptor) $CD8^+$ T cells are observed after combination therapy, similar to the observation in patients received CIT combination (53). Clinical trials are ongoing to evaluate this combination in untreated metastatic renal cell carcinoma (IMmotion151 study)

TABLE 3 | Clinical trials of immune checkpoint inhibitors in combination with poly (ADP-ribose) polymerase inhibitors or vascular endothelial growth factor targeting therapy.

Trial	Tumor type	Treatment regimen	Outcome
Lee et al. (78)	Gynecological cancers	Durvalumab + olaparib Durvalumab + cediranib	83% disease control rate in durvalumab + olaparib group 75% disease control rate in durvalumab plus cediranib group
NCT02734004	Breast, gastric, ovarian and SCLC	Durvalumab + olaparib	Ongoing
NCT02484404	NSCLC, SCLC, breast, ovarian, colorectal, prostate	Durvalumab + olaparib Durvalumab + cediranib Durvalumab + olaparib + cediranib	Ongoing
NCT02657889	Breast and ovarian	Pembrolizumab + niraparib	Ongoing
NCT02944396	NSCLC	Nivolumab + veliparib + platinum-based chemotherapy Veliparib + platinum-based chemotherapy	Ongoing
NCT02849496	Breast	Veliparib Atezolizumab Veliparib + atezolizumab	Ongoing
NCT02443324	Gastric, GEJ adenocarcinoma, NSCLC, transitional cell carcinoma of the urothelium, biliary tract	Pembrolizumab + ramucirumab	Ongoing
NCT02572687	GI or thoracic malignancies	Durvalumab + ramucirumab	Ongoing

(89) and untreated locally advanced or metastatic hepatocellular carcinoma (IMbrave150) (NCT03434379). Further investigation will be critical to design safe and efficacious combinations and to address biomarker selection.

COMBINATION OF IMMUNOTHERAPY WITH RADIOTHERAPY (RT)

Radiotherapy remains to be the backbone modality in the treatment for different types of cancer, either given alone or in combination with chemotherapy. It induces single- and double-strand DNA breaks, triggering multiple signaling pathways including DNA damage responses and activation of cell cycle checkpoints. The RT-induced cell death can further initiate systemic antitumor responses through various immune cell subsets (90). The participation of immune cells is indispensable for the clinical benefit of RT; in turn, RT can also modulate the antitumor immunity. It has been reported that localized tumor radiation can result in distant systemic tumor control in the unirradiated area. This clinical phenomenon, known as the abscopal effect, is a result of RT-induced immune modulations (91). The potential synergistic antitumor activities of RT in combination with ICIs have attracted increased research efforts in this new era of cancer immunotherapy (92).

Increased infiltration of macrophages and monocytes has been observed post-irradiation in multiple humana cancer xenograft models (squamous cell carcinoma, breast, and lung carcinoma), and depletion of the TAMs with antibody to CD11b or inhibitor of SDF-1a receptor CXCR4 (AMD3100) provided further tumor control when combined with irradiation (93, 94). The activation of dendritic cells and their release of type I interferon after irradiation is also critical in CD8^{+} T cell activity and treatment efficacy in mouse colon carcinoma (MC38), lung carcinoma (LLC), and melanoma models (B16F10) (95, 96). In an animal model of Lewis lung carcinoma (LLC), when the local area was exposed to irradiation, distant tumor control was observed only in p53 WT (vs. in p53 null mice), suggesting that the abscopal effect was mediated through pathways downstream of p53 (97). Multiple studies have shown that cytotoxic CD8^{+} T cells are required for RT-induced tumor control in mouse breast cancer (4T1), melanoma (B16), lymphoma (EL4), and lung cancer (98, 99).

Although the myelosuppression after irradiation is thought to be immunosuppressive, RT can regulate T cell-mediated immune responses *via* various mechanisms (100). RT regulates key cell surface molecules for cytotoxic immune cell activation (NKG2D), and antigen presentation machinery (MHC class I expression with antigen peptides), therefore augments T cell tumor recognition and activation (101, 102). RT also enhances T cell priming for activation via activation of antigen-presenting cells (dendritic cells) and releasing of immunogenic antigens (95, 103). RT increases the release of chemokines (CXCL16, a chemokine that binds to CXCR6 on Th1 CD4 and effector CD8 T cells) by mouse breast cancer (4T1) cells, therefore enhances the infiltration of cytotoxic T cells (104). In this situation, blockade of CTLA-4 further promotes tumor regression. Irradiation also alters the immunosuppressive tumor microenvironment to a M1 phenotype, favoring accessibility for T cell infiltration (105). In addition, in melanoma and Kras-mutant lung cancer models, irradiation was found to upregulate PD-L1 expression in tumor microenvironment (106, 107). The synergistic relationship between RT and ICI has been further explored in preclinical models. In mice bearing poorly immunogenic breast carcinoma, treatment with CTLA-4 blockade in combination with RT (vs. CTLA-4 blockade alone) resulted in decreased tumor growth and metastasis with improved survival (108). RT in combination with PD-1 blockade also induced improved and durable tumor control in NSCLC mouse models (107). In melanoma and renal cell carcinoma animal models, PD-1 knockout (KO) mice demonstrated higher survival after stereotactic ablative radiotherapy (SABR) compared with their PD-1 WT little mates. The addition of PD-1 blocking antibody to SABR led to the improved antitumor response and survival in PD-1 WT mice. In addition, treatment with SABR and anti-PD1 antibody combination induced significant reduction of non-irradiate tumor. The increased frequency of CD11a^{high}CD8^{+} tumor-reactive T cells and their enhanced functions were associated with the antitumor response in PD-1 KO mice, suggesting the translation potential of combining RT and PD-1 blockade (109).

Over the recent years, the clinical efficacy of RT in combination with ICIs have been studied in multiple clinical trials were designed to investigate. However, data supporting the routine application of this combination are still limited. The RT and ipilimumab combination demonstrated acceptable toxicity profile in patients with metastatic melanoma, yet failed to provide survival benefit (110). Ipilimumab in combination with radiation was evaluated in a single-arm phase 2 study in melanoma patients with unresectable brain metastases (111). Fifty-eight patients were enrolled in this study; with 1-year OS of 31.8% (95% CI [18.8–44.8%]) that is higher than the historical reported results, without unexpected adverse events.

In a phase 1 KEYNOTE-001 study, 97 patients with advanced NSCLC were enrolled (112). Longer PFS and OS, without higher incidence of grade 3 or above pulmonary toxicity, were seen in patients who underwent RT prior to anti-PD1 therapy compared with those who did not receive RT, supporting the safety and potential synergistic activity of the RT-ICI combination. The phase 3 randomized PACIFIC trial investigated the role of subsequent durvalumab therapy in stage III NSCLC patients after definitive chemoradiation (NCT02125461) (113). A total of 713 patients with locally advanced unresectable NSCLC without disease progression after definitive chemoradiation were randomly assigned in 2:1 to receive durvalumab or placebo irrespective of PD-L1 status. Median progression survival is 16.8 months in durvalumab group vs. 5.6 months in placebo group (16.8 months vs.), with 18-month PFS rate of 44.2 vs. 27.0%, respectively (113). Results from this study led to the FDA approval of durvalumab for the treatment of stage III NSCLC regardless of PD-L1 expression levels. The RT and immunotherapy combination is currently being evaluated in other tumor types, such as metastatic GI malignancies (NCT02830594) and metastatic breast cancer (NCT02730130) (**Table 4**).

Despite the encouraging finding from the PACIFIC trial, future research is urgently needed to define the immunoregulatory mechanisms that cross talk between RT, chemo, and immunotherapy, to design optimized combination strategies. Similar to

TABLE 4 | Clinical trials of immune checkpoint inhibitors in combination with radiotherapy (RT).

Trial	Tumor type	Regimens	Outcomes
Shaverdian et al. (112)	NSCLC (KEYNOTE-001)	Compared patients on pembrolizumab with previous RT to those who did not receive previous RT	Previous treatment with RT results in longer PFS and OS, with an acceptable safety profile
Antonia et al. (113)	NSCLC	Definitive ChemoRT → durvalumab Definitive ChemoRT → placebo	Progression-free survival (PFS): 16.8 months 18 months PFS: 44.2% PFS: 5.6 months 18 months PFS: 27.0%
Levy et al. (114)	Inoperable or metastatic cancers	Concurrent durvalumab + RT	Concurrent palliative RT with the anti-PD-L1 durvalumab was well tolerated
Tang et al. (115)	Metastatic solid tumor	Ipilimumab + stereotactic ablative radiotherapy (SABR)	Combining SABR and ipilimumab was safe with signs of efficacy, peripheral T-cell markers may predict clinical benefit, and systemic immune activation was greater after liver irradiation
Hiniker et al. (116)	Metastatic melanoma	Palliative RT + ipilimumab	Combination therapy was well tolerated without unexpected toxicities. Eleven patients (50.0%) experienced clinical benefit from therapy, including complete and partial responses
NCT03050554	NSCLC	Stereotactic body radiation therapy (SBRT) in combination with Avelumab	Ongoing Tolerability, RFS
NCT02658097	NSCLC	Single fraction nonablative radiation in combination with pembrolizumab	Ongoing RR and best OS
NCT03458455	Brain tumor	Stereotactic radiosurgery plus ipilimumab, nivolumab, or pembrolizumab	Ongoing Treatment response at 18 months
NCT03115801	Metastatic renal cell carcinoma and urothelial carcinoma	Nivolumab/atezolizumab Nivolumab/atezolizumab plus RT	Ongoing Best overall response rate, PFS, toxicities, OS
NCT03176173	NSCLC	Radical-dose image guided radiation therapy daily for up to 10 days (within 2 weeks) while undergoing standard of care immunotherapy Patients who decline to undergo radiation therapy receive standard of care immunotherapy	Ongoing PFS

other combination strategies discussed, the optimum sequencing of the RT and ICI combination has not been elucidated in available studies. In the KEYNOTE-001 study, irradiation prior to pembrolizumab therapy provided improved PFS and OS (112), while in another clinical report palliative RT-induced global disease control in a PD-1 antibody resistant patient (117). In a melanoma mouse model, the addition of adjuvant chemotherapy after ablative RT abrogated the RT-induced $CD8^+$ T cell activation and tumor control, while the addition of immunotherapy can enhance the tumor response (98), suggesting that the treatment modalities and the sequence of their combination need to be carefully investigated to achieve clinical success. In addition, research is needed to identify biomarkers with both predictive and prognostic values in RT-immunotherapy combination.

CONCLUSION

Modern cancer immunotherapies exert their tumor-killing activities through enhancing antitumor immunity while suppressing the tumor-promoting immune process. However, since ICIs do not provide clinical benefits in the majority of cancer patients, it is crucial to design rational and efficacious synergic therapeutic approaches to increase clinical responses to ICI. The combination of chemotherapy, targeted therapy, and RT with ICIs has gained increased attentions from clinicians and researchers over the recent years, given their immunomodulatory effects and potential synergistic antitumor activities. Despite the encouraging clinical results from various clinical studies, further investigations are warranted to elucidate the exact molecular and cellular mechanisms driving these clinical responses. More importantly, the optimal regimens, dose, timing, and schedule of the combination therapy for differently types of tumors are yet to be identified. Molecular interplay between different therapeutic modalities will need to be further investigated given the unlimited possibilities of combining currently available cancer treatments.

AUTHOR CONTRIBUTIONS

YY and HD conceived the outline of the manuscript. YY, HD, AK, HF, and SM wrote and edited the manuscript. SP and RD edited the manuscript.

REFERENCES

1. Topalian SL, Hodi FS, Brahmer JR, Gettinger SN, Smith DC, McDermott DF, et al. Safety, activity, and immune correlates of anti-PD-1 antibody in cancer. *N Engl J Med* (2012) 366(26):2443–54. doi:10.1056/NEJMoa1200690
2. Topalian SL, Sznol M, McDermott DF, Kluger HM, Carvajal RD, Sharfman WH, et al. Survival, durable tumor remission, and long-term safety in patients with advanced melanoma receiving nivolumab. *J Clin Oncol* (2014) 32(10):1020–30. doi:10.1200/JCO.2013.53.0105
3. Rexer H, Bedke J. [First-line therapy in advanced renal cell carcinoma: a randomized, open-label phase III study evaluating the efficacy and safety of pembrolizumab (MK-3475) in combination with axitinib compared to sunitinib monotherapy as first-line treatment for locally advanced or metastatic renal cell carcinoma (mRCC) (Keynote-426) – AN 39/16 of the AUO]. *Urologe A* (2017) 56(3):385–6. doi:10.1007/s00120-017-0335-2
4. Larkins E, Blumenthal GM, Yuan W, He K, Sridhara R, Subramaniam S, et al. FDA approval summary: pembrolizumab for the treatment of recurrent or metastatic head and neck squamous cell carcinoma with disease progression on or after platinum-containing chemotherapy. *Oncologist* (2017) 22(7):873–8. doi:10.1634/theoncologist.2016-0496
5. Pardoll DM. The blockade of immune checkpoints in cancer immunotherapy. *Nat Rev Cancer* (2012) 12(4):252–64. doi:10.1038/nrc3239
6. Robert C, Schachter J, Long GV, Arance A, Grob JJ, Mortier L, et al. Pembrolizumab versus ipilimumab in advanced melanoma. *N Engl J Med* (2015) 372(26):2521–32. doi:10.1056/NEJMoa1503093
7. Larkin J, Hodi FS, Wolchok JD. Combined nivolumab and ipilimumab or monotherapy in untreated melanoma. *N Engl J Med* (2015) 373(13):1270–1. doi:10.1056/NEJMc1509660
8. Coffelt SB, de Visser KE. Immune-mediated mechanisms influencing the efficacy of anticancer therapies. *Trends Immunol* (2015) 36(4):198–216. doi:10.1016/j.it.2015.02.006
9. Galluzzi L, Buque A, Kepp O, Zitvogel L, Kroemer G. Immunological effects of conventional chemotherapy and targeted anticancer agents. *Cancer Cell* (2015) 28(6):690–714. doi:10.1016/j.ccell.2015.10.012
10. Apetoh L, Ladoire S, Coukos G, Ghiringhelli F. Combining immunotherapy and anticancer agents: the right path to achieve cancer cure? *Ann Oncol* (2015) 26(9):1813–23. doi:10.1093/annonc/mdv209
11. Zitvogel L, Galluzzi L, Smyth MJ, Kroemer G. Mechanism of action of conventional and targeted anticancer therapies: reinstating immunosurveillance. *Immunity* (2013) 39(1):74–88. doi:10.1016/j.immuni.2013.06.014
12. Gotwals P, Cameron S, Cipolletta D, Cremasco V, Crystal A, Hewes B, et al. Prospects for combining targeted and conventional cancer therapy with immunotherapy. *Nat Rev Cancer* (2017) 17(5):286–301. doi:10.1038/nrc.2017.17
13. DeVita VT Jr, Chu E. A history of cancer chemotherapy. *Cancer Res* (2008) 68(21):8643–53. doi:10.1158/0008-5472.CAN-07-6611
14. Bezu L, Gomes-de-Silva LC, Dewitte H, Breckpot K, Fucikova J, Spisek R, et al. Combinatorial strategies for the induction of immunogenic cell death. *Front Immunol* (2015) 6:187. doi:10.3389/fimmu.2015.00187
15. Rizvi NA, Hellmann MD, Snyder A, Kvistborg P, Makarov V, Havel JJ, et al. Cancer immunology. Mutational landscape determines sensitivity to PD-1 blockade in non-small cell lung cancer. *Science* (2015) 348(6230):124–8. doi:10.1126/science.aaa1348
16. Sistigu A, Yamazaki T, Vacchelli E, Chaba K, Enot DP, Adam J, et al. Cancer cell-autonomous contribution of type I interferon signaling to the efficacy of chemotherapy. *Nat Med* (2014) 20(11):1301–9. doi:10.1038/nm.3708
17. Liu WM, Fowler DW, Smith P, Dalgleish AG. Pre-treatment with chemotherapy can enhance the antigenicity and immunogenicity of tumours by promoting adaptive immune responses. *Br J Cancer* (2010) 102(1):115–23. doi:10.1038/sj.bjc.6605465
18. Ruffell B, Chang-Strachan D, Chan V, Rosenbusch A, Ho CM, Pryer N, et al. Macrophage IL-10 blocks CD8+ T cell-dependent responses to chemotherapy by suppressing IL-12 expression in intratumoral dendritic cells. *Cancer Cell* (2014) 26(5):623–37. doi:10.1016/j.ccell.2014.09.006
19. Peng J, Hamanishi J, Matsumura N, Abiko K, Murat K, Baba T, et al. Chemotherapy induces programmed cell death-ligand 1 overexpression via the nuclear factor-kappaB to foster an immunosuppressive tumor microenvironment in ovarian cancer. *Cancer Res* (2015) 75(23):5034–45. doi:10.1158/0008-5472.CAN-14-3098
20. Bunt SK, Yang L, Sinha P, Clements VK, Leips J, Ostrand-Rosenberg S. Reduced inflammation in the tumor microenvironment delays the accumulation of myeloid-derived suppressor cells and limits tumor progression. *Cancer Res* (2007) 67(20):10019–26. doi:10.1158/0008-5472.CAN-07-2354
21. Gabrilovich DI, Nagaraj S. Myeloid-derived suppressor cells as regulators of the immune system. *Nat Rev Immunol* (2009) 9(3):162–74. doi:10.1038/nri2506
22. Baba J, Watanabe S, Saida Y, Tanaka T, Miyabayashi T, Koshio J, et al. Depletion of radio-resistant regulatory T cells enhances antitumor immunity during recovery from lymphopenia. *Blood* (2012) 120(12):2417–27. doi:10.1182/blood-2012-02-411124
23. Nakasone ES, Askautrud HA, Kees T, Park JH, Plaks V, Ewald AJ, et al. Imaging tumor-stroma interactions during chemotherapy reveals contributions of the microenvironment to resistance. *Cancer Cell* (2012) 21(4):488–503. doi:10.1016/j.ccr.2012.02.017
24. Ghiringhelli F, Larmonier N, Schmitt E, Parcellier A, Cathelin D, Garrido C, et al. CD4+CD25+ regulatory T cells suppress tumor immunity but are sensitive to cyclophosphamide which allows immunotherapy of established tumors to be curative. *Eur J Immunol* (2004) 34(2):336–44. doi:10.1002/eji.200324181
25. Alizadeh D, Trad M, Hanke NT, Larmonier CB, Janikashvili N, Bonnotte B, et al. Doxorubicin eliminates myeloid-derived suppressor cells and enhances the efficacy of adoptive T-cell transfer in breast cancer. *Cancer Res* (2014) 74(1):104–18. doi:10.1158/0008-5472.CAN-13-1545
26. Sampson JH, Aldape KD, Archer GE, Coan A, Desjardins A, Friedman AH, et al. Greater chemotherapy-induced lymphopenia enhances tumor-specific immune responses that eliminate EGFRvIII-expressing tumor cells in patients with glioblastoma. *Neuro Oncol* (2011) 13(3):324–33. doi:10.1093/neuonc/noq157
27. Ueha S, Yokochi S, Ishiwata Y, Ogiwara H, Chand K, Nakajima T, et al. Robust antitumor effects of combined anti-CD4-depleting antibody and anti PD 1/PD-L1 immune checkpoint antibody treatment in mice. *Cancer Immunol Res* (2015) 3(6):631–40. doi:10.1158/2326-6066.CIR-14-0190
28. Ghiringhelli F, Menard C, Puig PE, Ladoire S, Roux S, Martin F, et al. Metronomic cyclophosphamide regimen selectively depletes CD4+CD25+ regulatory T cells and restores T and NK effector functions in end stage cancer patients. *Cancer Immunol Immunother* (2007) 56(5):641–8. doi:10.1007/s00262-006-0225-8
29. Alizadeh D, Larmonier N. Chemotherapeutic targeting of cancer-induced immunosuppressive cells. *Cancer Res* (2014) 74(10):2663–8. doi:10.1158/0008-5472.CAN-14-0301
30. Gadgeel SM, Stevenson J, Langer CJ, Gandhi L, Borghaei H, Patnaik A, et al. Pembrolizumab (pembro) plus chemotherapy as front-line therapy for advanced NSCLC: KEYNOTE-021 cohorts A-C. *J Clin Oncol* (2016) 34(15_suppl):9016. doi:10.1200/JCO.2016.34.15_suppl.9016
31. Langer CJ, Gadgeel SM, Borghaei H, Papadimitrakopoulou VA, Patnaik A, Powell SF, et al. Carboplatin and pemetrexed with or without pembrolizumab for advanced, non-squamous non-small-cell lung cancer: a randomised, phase 2 cohort of the open-label KEYNOTE-021 study. *Lancet Oncol* (2016) 17(11):1497–508. doi:10.1016/S1470-2045(16)30498-3
32. Borghaei H, Langer CJ, Gadgeel S, Papadimitrakopoulou VA, Patnaik A, Powell SF, et al. Updated results from KEYNOTE-021 cohort G: a randomized, phase 2 study of pemetrexed and carboplatin (PC) with or without pembrolizumab (pembro) as first-line therapy for advanced nonsquamous NSCLC. *Ann Oncol* (2017) 28. doi:10.1093/annonc/mdx440.052
33. Garon EB, Rizvi NA, Hui R, Leighl N, Balmanoukian AS, Eder JP, et al. Pembrolizumab for the treatment of non-small-cell lung cancer. *N Engl J Med* (2015) 372(21):2018–28. doi:10.1056/NEJMoa1501824
34. Reck M, Rodriguez-Abreu D, Robinson AG, Hui R, Csoszi T, Fulop A, et al. Pembrolizumab versus chemotherapy for PD-L1-positive non-small-cell lung cancer. *N Engl J Med* (2016) 375(19):1823–33. doi:10.1056/NEJMoa1606774
35. Gandhi L, Rodriguez-Abreu D, Gadgeel S, Esteban E, Felip E, De Angelis F, et al. Pembrolizumab plus chemotherapy in metastatic non-small-cell lung cancer. *N Engl J Med* (2018) 378(22):2078–92. doi:10.1056/NEJMoa1801005
36. Paz-Ares LG, Luft A, Tafreshi A, Gumus M, Mazieres J, Hermes B, et al. Phase 3 study of carboplatin-paclitaxel/nab-paclitaxel (Chemo) with or without

pembrolizumab (Pembro) for patients (Pts) with metastatic squamous (Sq) non-small cell lung cancer (NSCLC). *J Clin Oncol* (2018) 36(Suppl; abstr 105).
37. Rizvi NA, Hellmann MD, Brahmer JR, Juergens RA, Borghaei H, Gettinger S, et al. Nivolumab in combination with platinum-based doublet chemotherapy for first-line treatment of advanced non-small-cell lung cancer. *J Clin Oncol* (2016) 34(25):2969–79. doi:10.1200/JCO.2016.66.9861
38. Gettinger SN, Hellmann MD, Shepherd FA, Antonia SJ, Brahmer J, Chow LQ, et al. First-line monotherapy with nivolumab (NIVO) in advanced non-small cell lung cancer (NSCLC): safety, efficacy, and biomarker analyses. *Eur J Cancer* (2015) 51:S632.
39. Paz-Ares L, Brahmer J, Hellmann MD, Reck M, O'Byrne K, Borghaei H, et al. CheckMate 227: a randomized, open-label phase 3 trial of nivolumab, nivolumab plus ipilimumab, or nivolumab plus chemotherapy versus chemotherapy in chemotherapy-naive patients with advanced non-small cell lung cancer (NSCLC). *Ann Oncol* (2017) 28. doi:10.1093/annonc/mdx091.064
40. Hossein B, Matthew DH, Luis GPA, Suresh SR, Martin R, Kenneth JB, et al. Nivolumab (Nivo) + platinum-doublet chemotherapy (chemo) vs chemo as first-line (1L) treatment (Tx) for advanced non-small cell lung cancer (NSCLC) with <1% tumor PD-L1 expression: results from CheckMate 227. *J Clin Oncol* (2018) 36(Suppl; abstr 9001).
41. Liu SV, Camidge DR, Gettinger SN, Giaccone G, Heist RS, Hodi FS, et al. Atezolizumab (atezo) plus platinum-based chemotherapy (chemo) in non-small cell lung cancer (NSCLC): update from a phase Ib study. *J Clin Oncol* (2017) 35(15_suppl):9092.
42. Weiss GJ, Waypa J, Blaydorn L, Coats J, McGahey K, Sangal A, et al. A phase Ib study of pembrolizumab plus chemotherapy in patients with advanced cancer (PembroPlus). *Br J Cancer* (2017) 117(1):33–40. doi:10.1038/bjc.2017.145
43. Govindan R, Szczesna A, Ahn MJ, Schneider CP, Gonzalez Mella PF, Barlesi F, et al. Phase III trial of ipilimumab combined with paclitaxel and carboplatin in advanced squamous non-small-cell lung cancer. *J Clin Oncol* (2017) 35(30):3449–57. doi:10.1200/JCO.2016.71.7629
44. Patel SP, Kim DW, Bassett RL, Cain S, Washington E, Hwu WJ, et al. A phase II study of ipilimumab plus temozolomide in patients with metastatic melanoma. *Cancer Immunol Immunother* (2017) 66(10):1359–66. doi:10.1007/s00262-017-2030-y
45. Reck M, Luft A, Szczesna A, Havel L, Kim SW, Akerley W, et al. Phase III randomized trial of ipilimumab plus etoposide and platinum versus placebo plus etoposide and platinum in extensive-stage small-cell lung cancer. *J Clin Oncol* (2016) 34(31):3740–8. doi:10.1200/JCO.2016.67.6601
46. Yamazaki N, Uhara H, Fukushima S, Uchi H, Shibagaki N, Kiyohara Y, et al. Phase II study of the immune-checkpoint inhibitor ipilimumab plus dacarbazine in Japanese patients with previously untreated, unresectable or metastatic melanoma. *Cancer Chemother Pharmacol* (2015) 76(5):969–75. doi:10.1007/s00280-015-2870-0
47. Liu X, Gibbons RM, Harrington SM, Krco CJ, Markovic SN, Kwon ED, et al. Endogenous tumor-reactive CD8(+) T cells are differentiated effector cells expressing high levels of CD11a and PD-1 but are unable to control tumor growth. *Oncoimmunology* (2013) 2(6):e23972. doi:10.4161/onci.23972
48. Pulko V, Harris KJ, Liu X, Gibbons RM, Harrington SM, Krco CJ, et al. B7-h1 expressed by activated CD8 T cells is essential for their survival. *J Immunol* (2011) 187(11):5606–14. doi:10.4049/jimmunol.1003976
49. Reck M, Bondarenko I, Luft A, Serwatowski P, Barlesi F, Chacko R, et al. Ipilimumab in combination with paclitaxel and carboplatin as first-line therapy in extensive-disease-small-cell lung cancer: results from a randomized, double-blind, multicenter phase 2 trial. *Ann Oncol* (2013) 24(1):75–83. doi:10.1093/annonc/mds213
50. Lesterhuis WJ, Salmons J, Nowak AK, Rozali EN, Khong A, Dick IM, et al. Synergistic effect of CTLA-4 blockade and cancer chemotherapy in the induction of anti-tumor immunity. *PLoS One* (2013) 8(4):e61895. doi:10.1371/journal.pone.0061895
51. Ogawara D, Soda H, Iwasaki K, Suyama T, Taniguchi H, Fukuda Y, et al. Remarkable response of nivolumab-refractory lung cancer to salvage chemotherapy. *Thorac Cancer* (2018) 9(1):175–80. doi:10.1111/1759-7714.12543
52. Park SE, Lee SH, Ahn JS, Ahn MJ, Park K, Sun JM. Increased response rates to salvage chemotherapy administered after PD-1/PD-L1 inhibitors in patients with non-small cell lung cancer. *J Thorac Oncol* (2018) 13(1):106–11. doi:10.1016/j.jtho.2017.10.011
53. Yan Y, Cao S, Liu X, Harrington SM, Bindeman WE, Adjei AA, et al. CX3CR1 identifies PD-1 therapy-responsive CD8+ T cells that withstand chemotherapy during cancer chemoimmunotherapy. *JCI Insight* (2018) 3(8): 97828. doi:10.1172/jci.insight.97828
54. Yan Y, Failing J, Leontovich AA, Block MS, McWilliams RR, Kottschade LA, et al. The mayo clinic experience in patients with metastatic melanoma who have failed previous pembrolizumab treatment. *ASCO Meet Abstr* (2016) 34(15_suppl):e21014.
55. Aguilera JV, Paludo J, Bangalore A, Failing J, McWilliams RR, Kottschade LA, et al. Chemoimmunotherapy combination after PD-1 inhibitor failure to improve clinical outcomes in metastatic melanoma patients. *J Clin Oncol* (2018) 36(Suppl; abstr 9558).
56. Leontovich AA, Dronca RS, Suman VJ, Ashdown ML, Nevala WK, Thompson MA, et al. Fluctuation of systemic immunity in melanoma and implications for timing of therapy. *Front Biosci (Elite Ed)* (2012) 4:958–75. doi:10.2741/e433
57. Chang CL, Hsu YT, Wu CC, Lai YZ, Wang C, Yang YC, et al. Dose-dense chemotherapy improves mechanisms of antitumor immune response. *Cancer Res* (2013) 73(1):119–27. doi:10.1158/0008-5472.CAN-12-2225
58. Sumimoto H, Imabayashi F, Iwata T, Kawakami Y. The BRAF-MAPK signaling pathway is essential for cancer-immune evasion in human melanoma cells. *J Exp Med* (2006) 203(7):1651–6. doi:10.1084/jem.20051848
59. Khalili JS, Liu S, Rodriguez-Cruz TG, Whittington M, Wardell S, Liu C, et al. Oncogenic BRAF(V600E) promotes stromal cell-mediated immunosuppression via induction of interleukin-1 in melanoma. *Clin Cancer Res* (2012) 18(19):5329–40. doi:10.1158/1078-0432.CCR-12-1632
60. Knight DA, Ngiow SF, Li M, Parmenter T, Mok S, Cass A, et al. Host immunity contributes to the anti-melanoma activity of BRAF inhibitors. *J Clin Invest* (2013) 123(3):1371–81. doi:10.1172/JCI66236
61. Sapkota B, Hill CE, Pollack BP. Vemurafenib enhances MHC induction in BRAF(V600E) homozygous melanoma cells. *Oncoimmunology* (2013) 2(1):e22890. doi:10.4161/onci.22890
62. Wilmott JS, Long GV, Howle JR, Haydu LE, Sharma RN, Thompson JF, et al. Selective BRAF inhibitors induce marked T-cell infiltration into human metastatic melanoma. *Clin Cancer Res* (2012) 18(5):1386–94. doi:10.1158/1078-0432.CCR-11-2479
63. Cooper ZA, Juneja VR, Sage PT, Frederick DT, Piris A, Mitra D, et al. Response to BRAF inhibition in melanoma is enhanced when combined with immune checkpoint blockade. *Cancer Immunol Res* (2014) 2(7):643–54. doi:10.1158/2326-6066.CIR-13-0215
64. Rosenbaum MW, Bledsoe JR, Morales-Oyarvide V, Huynh TG, Mino-Kenudson M. PD-L1 expression in colorectal cancer is associated with microsatellite instability, BRAF mutation, medullary morphology and cytotoxic tumor-infiltrating lymphocytes. *Mod Pathol* (2016) 29(9):1104–12. doi:10.1038/modpathol.2016.95
65. Ebert PJR, Cheung J, Yang Y, McNamara E, Hong R, Moskalenko M, et al. MAP kinase inhibition promotes T cell and anti-tumor activity in combination with PD-L1 checkpoint blockade. *Immunity* (2016) 44(3):609–21. doi:10.1016/j.immuni.2016.01.024
66. Hu-Lieskovan S, Mok S, Homet Moreno B, Tsoi J, Robert L, Goedert L, et al. Improved antitumor activity of immunotherapy with BRAF and MEK inhibitors in BRAF(V600E) melanoma. *Sci Transl Med* (2015) 7(279):279ra41. doi:10.1126/scitranslmed.aaa4691
67. Ribas A, Hodi FS, Callahan M, Konto C, Wolchok J. Hepatotoxicity with combination of vemurafenib and ipilimumab. *N Engl J Med* (2013) 368(14): 1365–6. doi:10.1056/NEJMc1302338
68. Amin A, Lawson DH, Salama AK, Koon HB, Guthrie T Jr, Thomas SS, et al. Phase II study of vemurafenib followed by ipilimumab in patients with previously untreated BRAF-mutated metastatic melanoma. *J Immunother Cancer* (2016) 4:44. doi:10.1186/s40425-016-0148-7
69. Ribas A, Butler M, Lutzky J, Lawrence DP, Robert C, Miller W, et al. Phase I study combining anti-PD-L1 (MEDI4736) with BRAF (dabrafenib) and/or MEK (trametinib) inhibitors in advanced melanoma. *J Clin Oncol* (2015) 33(15_suppl):3003.
70. Minor DR, Puzanov I, Callahan MK, Hug BA, Hoos A. Severe gastrointestinal toxicity with administration of trametinib in combination with dabrafenib and ipilimumab. *Pigment Cell Melanoma Res* (2015) 28(5):611–2. doi:10.1111/pcmr.12383

71. Deken MA, Gadiot J, Jordanova ES, Lacroix R, van Gool M, Kroon P, et al. Targeting the MAPK and PI3K pathways in combination with PD1 blockade in melanoma. *Oncoimmunology* (2016) 5(12):e1238557. doi:10.1080/2162402X.2016.1238557
72. Kaneda MM, Messer KS, Ralainirina N, Li H, Leem CJ, Gorjestani S, et al. PI3Kgamma is a molecular switch that controls immune suppression. *Nature* (2016) 539(7629):437–42. doi:10.1038/nature19834
73. Seifert AM, Zeng S, Zhang JQ, Kim TS, Cohen NA, Beckman MJ, et al. PD-1/PD-L1 blockade enhances T-cell activity and antitumor efficacy of imatinib in gastrointestinal stromal tumors. *Clin Cancer Res* (2017) 23(2):454–65. doi:10.1158/1078-0432.CCR-16-1163
74. Jackson SP, Bartek J. The DNA-damage response in human biology and disease. *Nature* (2009) 461(7267):1071–8. doi:10.1038/nature08467
75. Farmer H, McCabe N, Lord CJ, Tutt AN, Johnson DA, Richardson TB, et al. Targeting the DNA repair defect in BRCA mutant cells as a therapeutic strategy. *Nature* (2005) 434(7035):917–21. doi:10.1038/nature03445
76. Lord CJ, Ashworth A. PARP inhibitors: synthetic lethality in the clinic. *Science* (2017) 355(6330):1152–8. doi:10.1126/science.aam7344
77. Rosado MM, Bennici E, Novelli F, Pioli C. Beyond DNA repair, the immunological role of PARP-1 and its siblings. *Immunology* (2013) 139(4):428–37. doi:10.1111/imm.12099
78. Lee JM, Cimino-Mathews A, Peer CJ, Zimmer A, Lipkowitz S, Annunziata CM, et al. Safety and clinical activity of the programmed death-ligand 1 inhibitor durvalumab in combination with poly (ADP-ribose) polymerase inhibitor olaparib or vascular endothelial growth factor receptor 1-3 inhibitor cediranib in women's cancers: a dose-escalation, phase I study. *J Clin Oncol* (2017) 35(19):2193. doi:10.1200/JCO.2016.72.1340
79. Konstantinopoulos PA, Waggoner SE, Vidal GA, Mita MM, Fleming GF, Holloway RW, et al. TOPACIO/Keynote-162 (NCT02657889): a phase 1/2 study of niraparib + pembrolizumab in patients (pts) with advanced triple-negative breast cancer or recurrent ovarian cancer (ROC)—results from ROC cohort. *J Clin Oncol* (2018) 36(suppl; abstr 106).
80. Ott PA, Hodi FS, Buchbinder EI. Inhibition of immune checkpoints and vascular endothelial growth factor as combination therapy for metastatic melanoma: an overview of rationale, preclinical evidence, and initial clinical data. *Front Oncol* (2015) 5:202. doi:10.3389/fonc.2015.00202
81. Mansfield AS, Nevala WK, Lieser EA, Leontovich AA, Markovic SN. The immunomodulatory effects of bevacizumab on systemic immunity in patients with metastatic melanoma. *Oncoimmunology* (2013) 2(5):e24436. doi:10.4161/onci.24436
82. Agostino NM, Saraceni C, Kincaid H, Shi W, Nevala WK, Markovic S, et al. A prospective evaluation of the role of vascular endothelial growth factor (VEGF) and the immune system in stage III/IV melanoma. *Springerplus* (2015) 4:186. doi:10.1186/s40064-015-0951-5
83. Nevala WK, Vachon CM, Leontovich AA, Scott CG, Thompson MA, Markovic SN, et al. Evidence of systemic Th2-driven chronic inflammation in patients with metastatic melanoma. *Clin Cancer Res* (2009) 15(6):1931–9. doi:10.1158/1078-0432.CCR-08-1980
84. Manning EA, Ullman JG, Leatherman JM, Asquith JM, Hansen TR, Armstrong TD, et al. A vascular endothelial growth factor receptor-2 inhibitor enhances antitumor immunity through an immune-based mechanism. *Clin Cancer Res* (2007) 13(13):3951–9. doi:10.1158/1078-0432.CCR-07-0374
85. Terme M, Pernot S, Marcheteau E, Sandoval F, Benhamouda N, Colussi O, et al. VEGFA-VEGFR pathway blockade inhibits tumor-induced regulatory T-cell proliferation in colorectal cancer. *Cancer Res* (2013) 73(2):539–49. doi:10.1158/0008-5472.CAN-12-2325
86. Rini BI, Stein M, Shannon P, Eddy S, Tyler A, Stephenson JJ Jr, et al. Phase 1 dose-escalation trial of tremelimumab plus sunitinib in patients with metastatic renal cell carcinoma. *Cancer* (2011) 117(4):758–67. doi:10.1002/cncr.25639
87. Hodi FS, Lawrence D, Lezcano C, Wu X, Zhou J, Sasada T, et al. Bevacizumab plus ipilimumab in patients with metastatic melanoma. *Cancer Immunol Res* (2014) 2(7):632–42. doi:10.1158/2326-6066.CIR-14-0053
88. Wallin JJ, Bendell JC, Funke R, Sznol M, Korski K, Jones S, et al. Atezolizumab in combination with bevacizumab enhances antigen-specific T-cell migration in metastatic renal cell carcinoma. *Nat Commun* (2016) 7:12624. doi:10.1038/ncomms12624
89. Motzer RJ, Powles T, Atkins MB, Escudier B, McDermott DF, Suarez C, et al. IMmotion151: a randomized phase III study of atezolizumab plus bevacizumab vs sunitinib in untreated metastatic renal cell carcinoma (mRCC). *J Clin Oncol* (2018) 36(6_suppl):578. doi:10.1200/JCO.2018.36.6_suppl.578
90. Formenti SC, Demaria S. Systemic effects of local radiotherapy. *Lancet Oncol* (2009) 10(7):718–26. doi:10.1016/S1470-2045(09)70082-8
91. Siva S, Callahan J, MacManus MP, Martin O, Hicks RJ, Ball DL. Abscopal [corrected] effects after conventional and stereotactic lung irradiation of non-small-cell lung cancer. *J Thorac Oncol* (2013) 8(8):e71–2. doi:10.1097/JTO.0b013e318292c55a
92. Sharabi AB, Lim M, DeWeese TL, Drake CG. Radiation and checkpoint blockade immunotherapy: radiosensitisation and potential mechanisms of synergy. *Lancet Oncol* (2015) 16(13):e498–509. doi:10.1016/S1470-2045(15)00007-8
93. Ahn GO, Tseng D, Liao CH, Dorie MJ, Czechowicz A, Brown JM. Inhibition of Mac-1 (CD11b/CD18) enhances tumor response to radiation by reducing myeloid cell recruitment. *Proc Natl Acad Sci U S A* (2010) 107(18):8363–8. doi:10.1073/pnas.0911378107
94. Kozin SV, Kamoun WS, Huang Y, Dawson MR, Jain RK, Duda DG. Recruitment of myeloid but not endothelial precursor cells facilitates tumor regrowth after local irradiation. *Cancer Res* (2010) 70(14):5679–85. doi:10.1158/0008-5472.CAN-09-4446
95. Gupta A, Probst HC, Vuong V, Landshammer A, Muth S, Yagita H, et al. Radiotherapy promotes tumor-specific effector CD8+ T cells via dendritic cell activation. *J Immunol* (2012) 189(2):558–66. doi:10.4049/jimmunol.1200563
96. Burnette BC, Liang H, Lee Y, Chlewicki L, Khodarev NN, Weichselbaum RR, et al. The efficacy of radiotherapy relies upon induction of type I interferon-dependent innate and adaptive immunity. *Cancer Res* (2011) 71(7):2488–96. doi:10.1158/0008-5472.CAN-10-2820
97. Camphausen K, Moses MA, Menard C, Sproull M, Beecken WD, Folkman J, et al. Radiation abscopal antitumor effect is mediated through p53. *Cancer Res* (2003) 63(8):1990–3.
98. Lee Y, Auh SL, Wang Y, Burnette B, Wang Y, Meng Y, et al. Therapeutic effects of ablative radiation on local tumor require CD8+ T cells: changing strategies for cancer treatment. *Blood* (2009) 114(3):589–95. doi:10.1182/blood-2009-02-206870
99. Takeshima T, Chamoto K, Wakita D, Ohkuri T, Togashi Y, Shirato H, et al. Local radiation therapy inhibits tumor growth through the generation of tumor-specific CTL: its potentiation by combination with Th1 cell therapy. *Cancer Res* (2010) 70(7):2697–706. doi:10.1158/0008-5472.CAN-09-2982
100. Barker HE, Paget JT, Khan AA, Harrington KJ. The tumour microenvironment after radiotherapy: mechanisms of resistance and recurrence. *Nat Rev Cancer* (2015) 15(7):409–25. doi:10.1038/nrc3958
101. Kim JY, Son YO, Park SW, Bae JH, Chung JS, Kim HH, et al. Increase of NKG2D ligands and sensitivity to NK cell-mediated cytotoxicity of tumor cells by heat shock and ionizing radiation. *Exp Mol Med* (2006) 38(5):474–84. doi:10.1038/emm.2006.56
102. Reits EA, Hodge JW, Herberts CA, Groothuis TA, Chakraborty M, Wansley EK, et al. Radiation modulates the peptide repertoire, enhances MHC class I expression, and induces successful antitumor immunotherapy. *J Exp Med* (2006) 203(5):1259–71. doi:10.1084/jem.20052494
103. Gameiro SR, Ardiani A, Kwilas A, Hodge JW. Radiation-induced survival responses promote immunogenic modulation to enhance immunotherapy in combinatorial regimens. *Oncoimmunology* (2014) 3:e28643. doi:10.4161/onci.28643
104. Matsumura S, Wang B, Kawashima N, Braunstein S, Badura M, Cameron TO, et al. Radiation-induced CXCL16 release by breast cancer cells attracts effector T cells. *J Immunol* (2008) 181(5):3099–107. doi:10.4049/jimmunol.181.5.3099
105. Klug F, Prakash H, Huber PE, Seibel T, Bender N, Halama N, et al. Low-dose irradiation programs macrophage differentiation to an iNOS(+)/M1 phenotype that orchestrates effective T cell immunotherapy. *Cancer Cell* (2013) 24(5):589–602. doi:10.1016/j.ccr.2013.09.014
106. Deng L, Liang H, Burnette B, Beckett M, Darga T, Weichselbaum RR, et al. Irradiation and anti-PD-L1 treatment synergistically promote antitumor immunity in mice. *J Clin Invest* (2014) 124(2):687–95. doi:10.1172/JCI67313
107. Herter-Sprie GS, Koyama S, Korideck H, Hai J, Deng J, Li YY, et al. Synergy of radiotherapy and PD-1 blockade in Kras-mutant lung cancer. *JCI Insight* (2016) 1:e87415. doi:10.1172/jci.insight.87415

108. Demaria S, Kawashima N, Yang AM, Devitt ML, Babb JS, Allison JP, et al. Immune-mediated inhibition of metastases after treatment with local radiation and CTLA-4 blockade in a mouse model of breast cancer. *Clin Cancer Res* (2005) 11(2 Pt 1):728–34.
109. Park SS, Dong H, Liu X, Harrington SM, Krco CJ, Grams MP, et al. PD-1 restrains radiotherapy-induced abscopal effect. *Cancer Immunol Res* (2015) 3(6):610–9. doi:10.1158/2326-6066.CIR-14-0138
110. Barker CA, Postow MA, Khan SA, Beal K, Parhar PK, Yamada Y, et al. Concurrent radiotherapy and ipilimumab immunotherapy for patients with melanoma. *Cancer Immunol Res* (2013) 1(2):92–8. doi:10.1158/2326-6066.CIR-13-0082
111. Lopez-Martin JA, Arance AM, De La Cruz-Merino L, Illescas A, Valduvieco I, Berrocal A, et al. Ipilimumab and radiation in patients with unresectable melanoma brain metastases: a multicenter, open label, phase-2, Spanish melanoma group (GEM) study (NCT-2013-001132-22). *J Clin Oncol* (2018) 36(Suppl; abstr 9546).
112. Shaverdian N, Lisberg AE, Bornazyan K, Veruttipong D, Goldman JW, Formenti SC, et al. Previous radiotherapy and the clinical activity and toxicity of pembrolizumab in the treatment of non-small-cell lung cancer: a secondary analysis of the KEYNOTE-001 phase 1 trial. *Lancet Oncol* (2017) 18(7):895–903. doi:10.1016/S1470-2045(17)30380-7
113. Antonia SJ, Villegas A, Daniel D, Vicente D, Murakami S, Hui R, et al. Durvalumab after chemoradiotherapy in stage III non-small-cell lung cancer. *N Engl J Med* (2017) 377(20):1919–29. doi:10.1056/NEJMoa1709937
114. Levy A, Massard C, Soria JC, Deutsch E. Concurrent irradiation with the anti-programmed cell death ligand-1 immune checkpoint blocker durvalumab: single centre subset analysis from a phase 1/2 trial. *Eur J Cancer* (2016) 68:156–62. doi:10.1016/j.ejca.2016.09.013
115. Tang C, Welsh JW, de Groot P, Massarelli E, Chang JY, Hess KR, et al. Ipilimumab with stereotactic ablative radiation therapy: phase I results and immunologic correlates from peripheral T cells. *Clin Cancer Res* (2017) 23(6):1388–96. doi:10.1158/1078-0432.CCR-16-1432
116. Hiniker SM, Reddy SA, Maecker HT, Subrahmanyam PB, Rosenberg-Hasson Y, Swetter SM, et al. A prospective clinical trial combining radiation therapy with systemic immunotherapy in metastatic melanoma. *Int J Radiat Oncol Biol Phys* (2016) 96(3):578–88. doi:10.1016/j.ijrobp.2016.07.005
117. Yuan Z, Fromm A, Ahmed KA, Grass GD, Yang GQ, Oliver DE, et al. Radiotherapy rescue of a nivolumab-refractory immune response in a patient with PD-L1-negative metastatic squamous cell carcinoma of the lung. *J Thorac Oncol* (2017) 12(9):e135–6. doi:10.1016/j.jtho.2017.04.029

3

PD1-CD28 Fusion Protein Enables CD4+ T Cell Help for Adoptive T Cell Therapy in Models of Pancreatic Cancer and Non-Hodgkin Lymphoma

Felicitas Rataj [1†], Fabian B. T. Kraus [1†], Michael Chaloupka [1], Simon Grassmann [1], Constanze Heise [1], Bruno L. Cadilha [1], Peter Duewell [1], Stefan Endres [1,2] and Sebastian Kobold [1,2]*

[1] *Center of Integrated Protein Science Munich (CIPS-M) and Division of Clinical Pharmacology, Department of Medicine IV, Klinikum der Universität München, Member of the German Center for Lung Research (DZL), Munich, Germany,* [2] *German Cancer Research Center (DKTK), Partner Site Munich, Heidelberg, Germany*

Edited by:
Svetlana Karakhanova, Universität Heidelberg, Germany

Reviewed by:
Junko Matsuzaki, Roswell Park Cancer Institute, United States
Amorette Barber, Longwood University, United States
Per Thor Straten, Herlev Hospital, Denmark

***Correspondence:**
Sebastian Kobold
sebastian.kobold@med.uni-muenchen.de

† *These authors have contributed equally to this work*

Background: Interaction of the programmed death receptor 1 (PD-1) and its ligand, PD-L1, suppresses T cell activity and permits tumors to evade T cell-mediated immune surveillance. We have recently demonstrated that antigen-specific CD8+ T cells transduced with a PD1-CD28 fusion protein are protected from PD-1-mediated inhibition. We have now investigated the potential of PD1-CD28 fusion protein-transduced CD4+ T cells alone or in combination with CD8+ T cells for immunotherapy of pancreatic cancer and non-Hodgkin lymphoma.

Methods: OVA-specific CD4+ and CD8+ were retrovirally transduced with the PD1-CD28 fusion protein. Cytokine release, proliferation, cytotoxic activity, and phenotype of transduced T cells were assessed in the context of Panc02-OVA (murine pancreatic cancer model) and E.G7-PD-L1 (murine T cell lymphoma model) cells.

Results: Stimulation of PD1-CD28 fusion protein-transduced CD4+ T cells with anti-CD3 and recombinant PD-L1 induced specific T cell activation, as measured by IFN-γ release and T cell proliferation. Coculture with Panc02-OVA or E.G7-PD-L1 tumor cells also led to specific activation of CD4+ T cells. Cytokine release and T cell proliferation was most effective when tumor cells simultaneously encountered genetically engineered CD4+ and CD8+ T cells. Synergy between both cell populations was also observed for specific tumor cell lysis. T cell cytotoxicity was mediated via granzyme B release and mediated enhanced tumor control *in vivo*. Transduced CD4+ and CD8+ T cells in co-culture with tumor cells developed a predominant central memory phenotype over time. Different ratios of CD4+ and CD8+ transduced T cells led to a significant increase of IFN-γ and IL-2 secretion positively correlating with CD4+ T cell numbers used. Mechanistically, IL-2 and MHC-I were central to the synergistic activity of CD4+ and CD8+ T cells, since neutralization of IL-2 prevented the crosstalk between these cell populations.

Conclusion: PD1-CD28 fusion protein-transduced CD4+ T cells significantly improved anti-tumoral effect of fusion protein-transduced CD8+ T cells. Thus, our results indicate that PD1-CD28 fusion protein-transduced CD4+ T cells have the potential to overcome the PD-1-PD-L1 immunosuppressive axis in pancreatic cancer and non-Hodgkin lymphoma.

Keywords: adoptive T cell transfer, cancer immunotherapy, costimulation, PD-1-CD28 fusion protein, CD4+ T cells

INTRODUCTION

Cytotoxic T cells specifically recognize tumor antigens presented on major histocompatibility complex-1 (MHC-I). After binding to the tumor antigen in the context of MHC, T cells are activated, which results in the secretion of cytotoxic factors and target cell lysis (1, 2). This concept is utilized therapeutically for adoptive T cell therapy (ACT). Patient-derived, tumor-specific T cells are expanded *ex vivo* or, to further enhance tumor-specificity, are genetically modified. T cell engineering usually follows two main approaches; either by introducing a T cell receptor specific for a given tumor-associated antigen or by equipping T cells with chimeric antigen receptors (CAR), which are synthetic receptors enabling tumor recognition. Following expansion, T cells are infused back to the patient in therapeutic intention (3). Pioneering work for ACT utilized tumor-infiltrating lymphocytes (TIL) for melanoma treatment yielding consistent durable response rates in subsets of patients. The challenges to generate these cells from tumor tissue of individual patients or even across entities has so far refrained this strategy from large scale clinical testing (4). Based on compelling preclinical and clinical data in hematological malignancies, ACT holds great promise for cancer immunotherapy. In 2017, the Food and Drug Administration (FDA) approved the first cellular therapy for refractory B-cell acute lymphoblastic leukemia (B-ALL) and diffuse large B cell lymphoma. Anti-CD19-CAR T cells are now part of the standard of care in the US, based on unparalleled remission rates and prolonged overall survival for patients with an otherwise very poor prognosis (5). In addition, ACT is under investigation for the treatment of other hematologic as well as more frequent non-hematological malignancies. Typically, ACT is performed with a mixture of CD4+ and CD8+ T cells, which is dictated by the patient's own peripheral blood T cell ratio and the differential expansion status in cell culture. Some protocols also adjust for defined ratios, based on own evidence that this might be more beneficial (6–8). When being transduced for tumor specificity both cell types are being modified and in the case of CAR T cells, both cell populations are thought to be therapeutically relevant (9).

However, CD8+ T cells are generally considered more potent and more central for ACT efficacy. CD4+ T cells have a distinct functional and secretory phenotype from CD8+ T cells which is neither redundant nor overlapping. Importantly, CD4+ T cell-derived cytokines play an important role in anti- but also in pro-tumoral immunity (10, 11). While it is established that CD4+ T cells can be cytotoxic on their own, a major function lays in regulating trafficking, activation, proliferation, differentiation, and persistence of tumor-infiltrating cytotoxic CD8+ T cells (12–15). Several studies have confirmed the helper function of tumor-specific CD4+ T cells and showed that the anti-tumor activity of combined treatment with CD4+ and CD8+ T cells is more pronounced than that seen when using individual cell types. The exact mechanism of this synergy remains to be elucidated (16–18).

Despite the clinical success of ACT in defined indications, ACT is inherently limited by antigen-loss variants of tumor cells, side effects resulting from on- and off-target expression of the chosen antigen and low T cell infiltration into the tumor tissue. ACT failure is often associated with an increased expression of the programmed death-1 receptor (PD-1), a marker protein for T cell anergy, on previously activated T cells (19, 20). PD-1 signaling mediates T cell suppression that prevents autoimmunity under physiological conditions and is therefore a key immune checkpoint on CD4+ and CD8+ T cells (21, 22). PD-L1, one of the two known ligands for PD-1, is broadly expressed on epithelial as well as hematological cells and shields these cells from T cell overactivation (23). Along these lines, tumors usurp this mechanism to evade anti-tumor immune responses (24). It is thereby not surprising, that undulating PD-L1 expression is found in most if not all human cancers at different levels and its expression is associated with dismal prognosis in the pre-immunotherapy era (25). Paradoxically, recognition of tumor cells by T cells transferred for ACT will result in T cell activation, upregulation of PD-1 on the said T cell, but also of PD-L1 on the tumor cell. This will ultimately end in abrogation of T cell activity and thereby ACT failure (26). Clinical evidence that this state of anergy might be reverted when antagonizing the PD-1-PD-L1 axis has been shown in several phase III clinical trials testing anti-PD-1 or anti-PD-L1 antibodies in melanoma or non-small cell lung cancer (27–31). Based on these studies, it seems likely that a similar approach might also be of value for ACT. As both checkpoint blockade and ACT have severe side effects on their own, it might be advisable to develop more targeted strategies to overcome T cell anergy than systemically blocking important immune checkpoints.

To overcome PD-1 suppression selectively and to improve ACT, we have developed a therapeutic concept that converts tumor-associated immunosuppression via the PD-1-PD-L1 axis into stimulation of tumor-specific T cells (32). We created a fusion receptor consisting of the extracellular domain of the PD-1 receptor fused to the intracellular, T cell-activating domain of CD28. In the tumor tissue, PD-1-CD28 fusion protein-expressing CD8+ T cells recognize tumor-derived PD-L1 and get locally activated. This results in tumor cell lysis and therapeutic benefit. It, however, remained unclear if the benefit is specific to CD8+ T cells, and particularly if adding this fusion protein to CD4+ T cells would further accelerate therapeutic activity. We hypothesized that our PD-1-CD28 fusion protein is not only functional in antigen-specific CD4+ T cells but also that simultaneous introduction in CD8+ T cells would further enhance T cell function. Here, we demonstrate that primary murine CD4+ T cells, expressing PD1-CD28 fusion protein, overcome PD-L1-induced T cell anergy in murine models of pancreatic cancer and non-Hodgkin lymphoma. Coculture experiments demonstrate a synergism of gene-modified CD4+ and CD8+ T cells for anti-tumor activity, which was dependent on IL-2 secretion from CD4+ T cells. Our results indicate the potential of PD1-CD28 fusion protein-transduced CD4+ T cells to further improve ACT.

MATERIALS AND METHODS

Cell Lines

Panc02-OVA, a murine pancreatic cancer cell line and E.G7-OVA, a murine T cell lymphoma cell line, were previously described (32, 33). Panc02-OVA-PD-L1 and E.G7-OVA-PD-L1 were generated by transduction of Panc02-OVA or E.G7-OVA cells with pMXs-puro or pMXs (a generous gift from Toshio Kitamura, M.D., PhD, the Institute of Medical Science, University of Tokyo, Japan) encoding the full-length murine PD-L1 (Swiss-Prot accession number Q9EP73). Panc02-OVA-PD-L1 cells were selected based on puromycin resistance. E.G7-OVA-PD-L1 cells were obtained by fluorescence activated cell sorting. Panc02-OVA and Panc02-OVA-PD-L1 were cultured in DMEM3+ (DMEM with 10 % fetal bovine serum [FBS, Life Technologies, USA), 100 U/ml penicillin and streptomycin (PS), and 2 mM L-glutamine (all from PAA, Germany)]. E.G7-OVA-PD-L1 were cultured in RPMI 1,640 supplemented with 10% FBS, 100 U/ml PS and 2 mM L-glutamine, 1 mM sodium pyruvate (PAA, Germany), and 1 mM HEPES (Sigma Aldrich, Germany).The retroviral ecotrophic packaging cell line Platinum-E was purchased from Cell biolabs (USA). DMEM3+ medium for Platinum-E cells additionally contained 10 μg/ml puromycin and 1 μg/ml blasticidin (both from Sigma, Germany). Primary murine T cells were cultured in RPMI 1640 supplemented with 10% FBS, 100 U/ml PS and 2 mM L-glutamine, 1 mM sodium pyruvate (PAA, Germany), 1 mM HEPES (Sigma Aldrich, Germany), and 50 μM β-mercaptoethanol.

Mice

Mice transgenic for a T cell receptor specific for ovalbumine (OT-1 or OT-2) were obtained from the Jackson laboratory (Bar Harbor, ME) (stock number 003831 for OT-1 and 004194 for OT-2) and were bred in our animal facility under SPF conditions. Both mouse strains served as T cell donors for primary murine T cell transduction.

Animal Experiments

For *in vivo* studies wild type C57/Bl6 mice were purchased from Charles River. Tumors were induced by subcutaneous injection of 4×10^5 E-G7-OVA-PD-L1 tumor cells. Mice were randomized with regard to tumor size and treated via serial transfer of PTM-transduced or untransduced T cells: First, CD8+ T cells were injected i.v. 48 h later, CD4+ T cells were injected i.v. Tumor growth was assessed every other day in a blinded fashion and tumor volume was estimated according to the following formula: $4/3 \times \pi \times L_1^2 \times L_2$ (with L_1 defined as maximal diameter and L_2 as the diameter perpendicular to L_1). All experiments were approved by the local regulatory agency (Regierung von Oberbayern).

T Cell Transduction

The PD1-CD28 fusion protein was described previously (32). The retroviral vector pMP71 (kindly provided by Christopher Baum, M.D., Institute of Experimental Hematology, Medizinische Hochschule Hannover, Germany) was utilized for all transduction experiments. Detailed protocols for murine T cell transduction have been published (34–37). In brief, pMP71 PD1-CD28 vector was transfected into Platinum-E cells and retrovirus-containing supernatants were collected for transduction of murine T cells. Primary murine T cells were first stimulated with anti-CD3e and anti-CD28 antibody (eBioscience, clones 145-2C11 and 37.51, respectively) and recombinant IL-2 (Novartis, Switzerland). Priot to transduction, anti-CD3- and anti-CD28 beads (Life technologies, USA) were added. Recombinant IL-15 (Peprotech, Germany) was used for T cell expansion. The CD4+ T cell fraction was purified on the day of spleen extraction by magnetic activated cell sorting using a CD4+ T cell isolation kit (Miltenyi Biotec, Germany).

Flow Cytometry

For multi-color flow cytometry, a BD FACS Canto II (BD bioscience, Germany) together with the following antibody panels was used. For purity testing and analysis of transduction efficiencies, anti-PD-1 (APC, clone RMP-30, BioLegend, USA), anti-CD8 (Pacific Blue^{TM}, clone 53-6.7, BioLegend, USA) and anti-CD4 (Pacific Blue^{TM} e, clone GK1.5, BioLegend, USA) were used. For analysis of MHC I-, MHCII-, and PD-L1-expression, tumor cells were stained with anti-MHCI (PE, clone M1/42.3.9.8, Elabscience, USA), anti-MHCII (APC, clone M5/114.15.2, eBioscience, USA) and anti-CD274 (PE/Cy7, clone 10F.9G2, BioLegend, USA). Rat IgG2a– (PE, clone #54447, R&D Systems, USA), Rat IgG2b kappa—(APC, clone eB149/10H5, eBioscience, USA) and Rat IgG2b kappa—antibodies (PE/Cy7, clone RTK4530, BioLegend, USA) were applied as isotype control. For proliferation analysis in antibody-stimulation assays, T cells were stained with anti-PD-1 (APC, clone RMP-30, BioLegend, USA), anti-CD28 (APC, clone 37.51, BioLegend, USA), anti-CD4 (Pacific Blue^{TM}, clone GK1.5, BioLegend, USA), and Zombie aqua fixable viability dye (BioLegend, USA) prior to fixation and permeabilization with FoxP3/Transcription Factor Staining Buffer Set (eBioscience, USA). For staining of intracellular proteins, anti-Ki67 (PE, clone 16A8, BioLegend, USA) and anti-EOMES (PE/Cy7, clone DAN11mag, eBioscience, USA) were added. Cells were washed and resuspended in PBS (Lonza, Switzerland) containing count bright absolute counting beads (Life technologies, USA). For proliferation analysis in cocultures of T cells and tumor cells, T cells were stained with anti-PD-1 (APC, clone RMP-30, BioLegend, USA), anti-CD4 (Pacific Blue^{TM}, clone GK1.5, BioLegend, USA), anti-CD8 (APC/Cy7, clone 53-6.7, BioLegend, USA), and Zombie aqua fixable viability dye (BioLegend, USA). Equal amounts of counting beads (Life technologies, USA) were added to each sample. The antibody panel for T cell phenotyping consisted of anti-PD-1 (FITC, clone 29F.1a12, BioLegend, USA), anti-CD8 (APC/Cy7, clone 53-6.7, BioLegend, USA), anti-CD4 (PE/Cy7, clone RM4-5, BioLegend, USA), anti-CD62L (Pacific Blue^{TM}, clone MEL-14, BioLegend, USA), anti-CCR7 (PerCP/Cy5.5, clone 4B12, BioLegend, USA), and Zombie aqua fixable viability dye (BioLegend, USA).

MHC I-, MHC II-, and PD-L1-Profiling of Tumor Cells

For the analysis of MHC I-, MHC II-, and PD-L1-expression on Panc02-OVA and E.G7-OVA-PD-L1, 5×10^4 tumor cells were stimulated for 48 h with recombinant murine IFN-γ (Peprotech, USA) at increasing concentrations of 2, 20, or 100 ng/ml respectively and analyzed by flow cytometry as described above.

Antibody-Stimulation Assays

For antibody-stimulation assays, T cells were stimulated with anti-CD3 antibody (100 ng/ml, clone 145-2C11, eBioscience), anti-CD3 antibody and recombinant PD-L1-Fc chimera protein (5 μg/ml, R&D Systems) or anti-CD3 antibody and anti-CD28 antibody (2 μg/ml, clone 37.51, eBioscience) for 48 h. Mitotic activity and CD28 surface expression was analyzed by flow cytometry. Cells were stained as indicated and cell numbers were normalized with counting beads (Life Technologies, Germany). Cytokine release was quantified by ELISA (IL-2 and IFN-γ, both BD).

Cocultures of T Cells and Tumor Cells

For T cell-tumor cell cocultures, CD8+ and CD4+ T cells (in a 3:1, 1:1, or 1:3 cell ratio) were prestimulated with anti-CD3 antibody (100 ng/ml, clone 145-2C11, eBioscience) and recombinant PD-L1-Fc chimera protein (5 μg/ml, R&D Systems) for 24 h, as described above. T cells were then cocultured for 16 h with either E.G7-OVA-PD-L1, Panc02-OVA, or Panc-OVA-PD-L1 tumor cells in a 10:1 effector to target cell ratio. Cytokine release was quantified by ELISA (IL-2 and IFN-γ). For cytotoxicity assays, tumor cell-derived LDH release was quantified after 16 h using CytoTox 96® Non-Radioactive Cytotoxicity Assay (Promega, USA). Granzyme B secretion was determined using Mouse Granzyme B DuoSet® ELISA (R&D systems, USA). For T cell phenotyping and proliferation assays, T cells were cocultured with Panc-OVA-PD-L1 for 36 h, as described above. T cell phenotype and proliferation was analyzed by flow cytometry as described above.

MHC I, MHC II, and IL-2 Neutralization Assays

For MHC I, MHC II, and IL-2 neutralization experiments, CD8+ and CD4+ T cells (in a 1:1 ratio) were prestimulated with anti-CD3 antibody and recombinant PD-L1-Fc chimera for 24 h. Subsequently, T cells and Panc02-OVA cells were cocultured at a 10:1 effector to target cell ratio. Anti-mouse MHC class I antibody (10 μg/ml, clone M1/42.3.9.8, *InVivo*MAb), anti-mouse MHC class II antibody (10 μg/ml, clone M5/114.15.2, eBioscience) and LEAF purified anti-mouse IL-2 antibody (10 μg/ml, clone JES6-1A12, BioLegend) were added during prestimulation and co-culture. Supernatants were analyzed for IFN-γ by ELISA.

Statistical Analysis

For statistical analysis, GraphPad Prism software version 7.04 was used. Reported values are continuous. Differences between experimental conditions were analyzed using the unpaired two-sided Student's *t*-test. *P*-values < 0.05 were considered as significant. Data shown are mean values ± SEM of at least three biological replicates representative for three independent experiments as indicated.

RESULTS

Functional Analysis of PD1-CD28 Fusion Protein (PTM) in CD4+ T Cells

To characterize the functionality of PTM in CD4+ T cells, we transduced PTM into primary murine CD4+ T cells. PTM-transduced and untransduced T cells were then stimulated with anti-CD3 antibody, anti-CD3 antibody and recombinant PD-L1 or anti-CD3 antibody and anti-CD28 antibody for 48 h. CD4+ PTM-transduced T cells showed significantly higher IFN-γ release as compared to untransduced T cells (**Figure 1A**). T cell activation was paralleled by an increase in T cell viability and T cell proliferation (**Figures 1B,C**). Untransduced CD4+ T cells were more strongly stimulated by anti-CD3 than PTM-transduced CD4+ T cells, while combination with anti-CD28 antibodies brought PTM-transduced T cells to a similar level of stimulation as untransduced T cells in this control condition. Similarly, expression of the mitogenic marker Ki67 was higher in PTM-transduced T cells than in untransduced T cells (**Figure 1D**). Expression of Eomesodermin (EOMES), a T cell differentiation marker, was highest for anti-CD3 and PD-L1-stimulated, transduced T cells compared to untransduced cells (**Figure 1E**). Together, these results demonstrate that PTM is functional in CD4+ T cells and enhances their functionality.

Functional Analysis of PTM-Transduced T Cells Cocultured With Tumor Cells

To assess the therapeutic potential of PTM-transduced CD4+ T cells *in vitro*, we prestimulated antigen-specific CD4+ or CD8+ PTM-transduced or untransduced T cells at a ratio of 1:1 with anti-CD3 antibody and recombinant PD-L1 for 24 h. Prestimulation was performed to mimic primary antigen contact and to induce partial anergy of the cells, as expected in the tumor environment. CD4+ or CD8+, untransduced, or transduced T cells were then cocultured alone or in different combinations with either Panc02-OVA cells or E.G7-PD-L1 cells. PTM-transduced CD4+ and CD8+ T cells produced more IFN-γ in contact with either cell line compared to untransduced T cells (**Figure 2A**). Highest IFN-γ secretion was measured for both tumor cell lines when PTM-transduced CD4+ and PTM-transduced CD8+ were combined. The same effect was observed

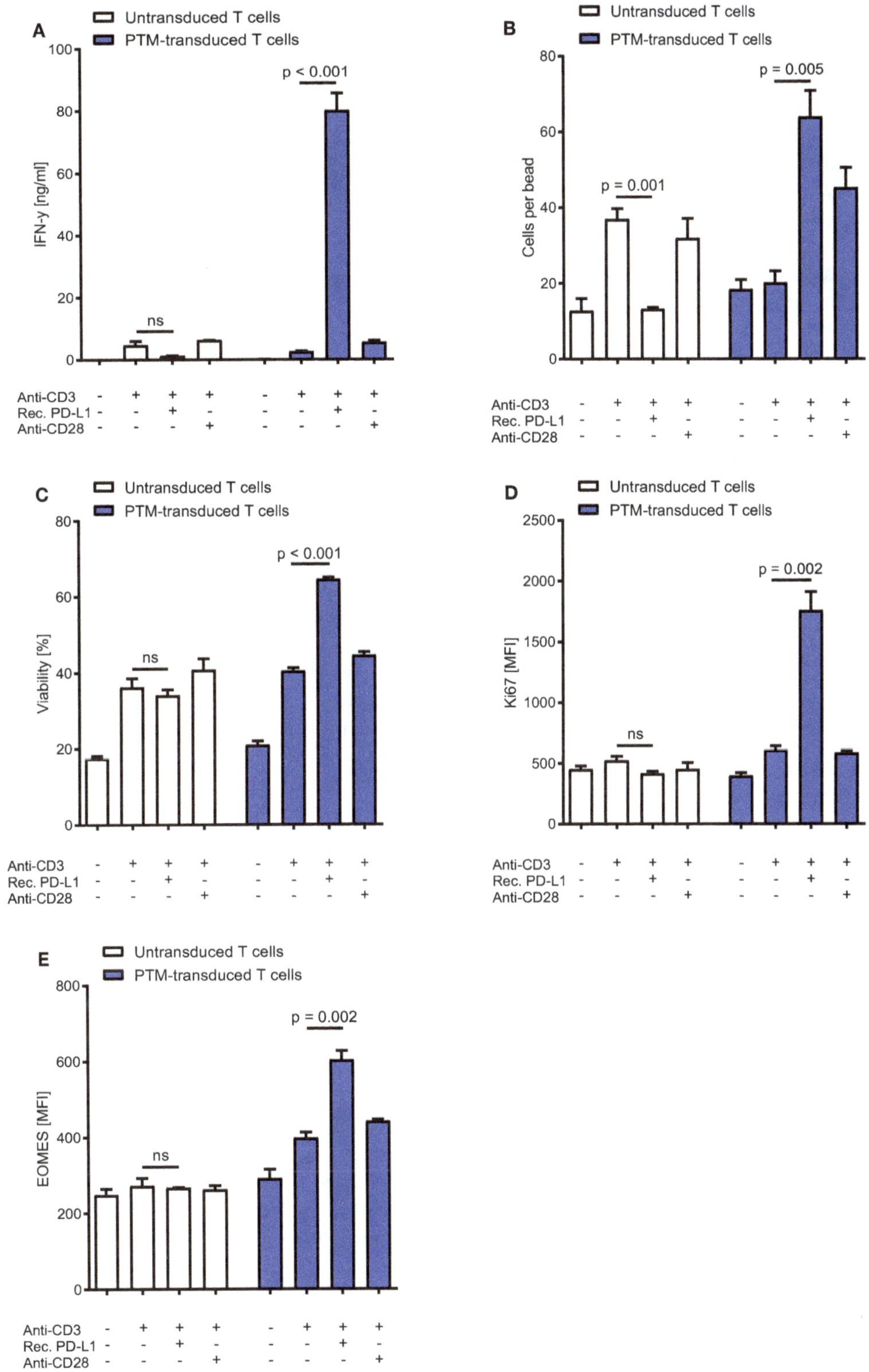

FIGURE 1 | *In vitro* characterization of PD1-CD28 fusion protein (PTM)-transduced CD4+ T cells. PTM-transduced or untransduced primary murine CD4+ T cells were either stimulated with anti-CD3 antibody, anti-CD3 antibody, and recombinant PD-L1 or anti-CD3 antibody and anti-CD28 antibody. **(A)** Interferon-γ (IFN-γ) secretion was measured by enzyme linked immunosorbent assay (ELISA). **(B)** T cell number was analyzed by flow cytometry and normalized to standardized counting beads. **(C)** Viability of T cells was assessed by flow cytometry. **(D)** After 48 h of stimulation T cells were intracellularly stained for Ki67, a mitosis marker or **(E)** for the differentiation marker eomesodermin (EOMES). Experiments **(A–E)** are representative of three independent experiments each performed in triplicates. Bars represent SEM and P values from Student's t-test are shown. All tests are two-sided.

for IL-2 release (**Figure 2B**). T cell activation was followed by a similar effect on T cell-mediated cytotoxicity. CD4+ and CD8+ PTM-transduced T cells, prestimulated individually, induced significant lysis of Panc02-OVA and E.G7-PD-L1 cells as compared to untransduced T cells (**Figure 2C**). Similar to cytokine production, cytotoxic activity was highest, when CD4+ and CD8+ PTM-transduced T cells were cocultured with tumor cells as compared to control conditions. Mechanistically, T cell cytotoxicity correlated with granzyme B release indicating that T cell degranulation is the mode of action, which is boosted by PTM transduction (**Figure 2D**). T cell cytotoxicity was accompanied by an increase in the number of CD8+ T cells in coculture with CD4+ T cells and Panc02-OVA (**Figure 2E**). PTM-transduced CD4+ T cells in coculture with Panc02-OVA-PD-L1 cells developed a predominant central memory phenotype, defined by CCR7+ and CD62L+ expression, over time (**Supplementary Figure 1A**). The effect on CD4+ T cells was strongest in the presence of untransduced or PTM-transduced CD8+ T cells. However, PTM-expression on CD8+ T cells alone, did not have an influence on the CD4+ T cell phenotype. CD8+ T cells, in contrast, differentiated into central memory T cells within the same experimental setting (**Supplementary Figure 1B**). In these cocultures, the amount of effector memory T cells was reduced in both, CD4+ and CD8+ T cells transduced with PTM (**Supplementary Figures 1C,D**). Our results suggest that CD4+ PTM-transduced T cells have therapeutic activity *in vitro* and point toward a synergistic collaboration of CD4+ and CD8+ T cells. Of note, this effect was highest when PTM was expressed by both T cell subsets. *In vivo,* combined treatment of OT1-PTM with OT2-PTM T cells mediated enhanced tumor control over PTM-transduced OT1 T cells, OT1 plus OT2 T cells and OT1 plus PTM-OT2 T cells in the EG7-PD-L1 model (**Figure 2F**). These results indicate the potential value of the strategy *in vivo.*

CD4+ to CD8+ T Cell Ratio Positively Influence the Activity of PTM-Transduced T Cells via IL-2 in Coculture With Tumor Cells

To test the CD4+ to CD8+ T cell ratio with the highest synergistic potential, we prestimulated antigen-specific, untransduced, or PTM-transduced CD8+ T cells and increasing numbers of antigen-specific, untransduced, or PTM-transduced CD4+ T cells with anti-CD3 antibody plus recombinant PD-L1. CD4+- or CD8+-, untransduced or transduced T cells were then cocultured alone or in different combinations with either Panc02-OVA or E.G7-PD-L1. In both tumor models, IFN-γ secretion, as indicator for T cell activation, was highest when PTM+ CD4+ and PTM+ CD8+ T cells were combined (**Figures 3A,B**). IFN-γ level positively correlated with the number of CD4+ T cells present in the coculture, accompanied by comparable IL-2 levels (**Figures 3C,D**). IL-2 levels were highest when PTM+ CD4+ and PTM+ CD8+ were cocultured with target cells. IL-2 production was tightly correlated with the number of CD4+ cells, pointing toward a potential role of IL-2 in their collaborative activity. To test this hypothesis, T cells were prestimulated and incubated with Panc02-OVA cells in the presence of anti-IL-2 neutralizing antibody. T cell activation, measured by IFN-y release, was almost abrogated through neutralization of IL-2 (**Figure 3E**). Similarly, synergy in T cell cytotoxicity was also blocked by anti-IL-2 neutralizing antibody in cocultures of Panc02-OVA cells with PTM+ CD4+ and PTM+ CD8+ T cells (**Supplementary Figure 2**). Taken together, our results demonstrate that the synergistic effect of transduced CD4+ and CD8+ T cells is dose-dependent and is mediated by IL-2.

Synergistic Activity Is Dependent on PD-L1 and MHC I but Not on MHC II Expression

To further delineate the synergistic action of OT1-PTM and OT2-PTM T cells, we addressed the expression of potential components of the system on the tumor cell side. We therefore analyzed MHC I for OT1 T cell recognition, PD-L1 for PTM-T cell activation and MHC II for OT2 T cell activation. In both models—Panc02-OVA and EG7-PD-L1—we found strong expression of MHC I but not of MHC II (**Figures 4A,B**). Not surprisingly, PD-L1 was constitutively overexpressed on EG7-PD-L1 and could be induced on Panc02-OVA upon IFN-γ stimulation (**Figures 4A,B**). Functionally, the observed synergy on EG7-PD-L1 of OT1-PTM and OT2-PTM T cells (**Figure 4C**) was entirely abrogated on OVA negative EL4 T cells (**Figure 4D**). Importantly this was not due to lack of MHC I or PD-L1 expression (not shown). Identical results were found when EG7-PD-L1 were pretreated with MHC I-blocking antibodies. As in the absence of OVA, T cell activity was entirely abrogated (**Figure 4E**). In contrast, MHC II-blockade did not impact on T cell recognition by combined OT1-PTM and OT2-PTM T cells (**Figure 4F**). These results indicate that both PD-L1 and MHC I but not MHC II are essential for the activity of our proposed strategy.

DISCUSSION

ACT, especially for solid tumors, is often limited by the immunosuppressive tumor milieu. Tumor cells evade an efficient tumor immune response especially via the PD-1-PD-L1 axis. Here, we report that CD4+ T cells, expressing a PD1-CD28 fusion receptor, have the potential to overcome PD-L1-mediated T cell suppression. We hypothesized that PTM-transduced CD4+ T cells might further boost the efficacy of CD8+ T cells *in vitro*, pointing toward potential avenues for translation of the approach.

Inhibitory receptors, such as PD-1 and CTLA-4, are important checkpoint molecules that prevent autoimmunity under physiological conditions. However, when expressed by tumor-infiltrating T cells these molecules strongly prevent an effective anti-tumor response. Following a similar strategy, a costimulatory CTLA-4–CD28 fusion receptor was shown to induce large amounts of IL-2 and high proliferation of CD4+ T cells when introduced in the latter, strengthening the idea of such fusion proteins to support CD4+ T cell activity (38). We previously described a PD1-CD28 fusion protein

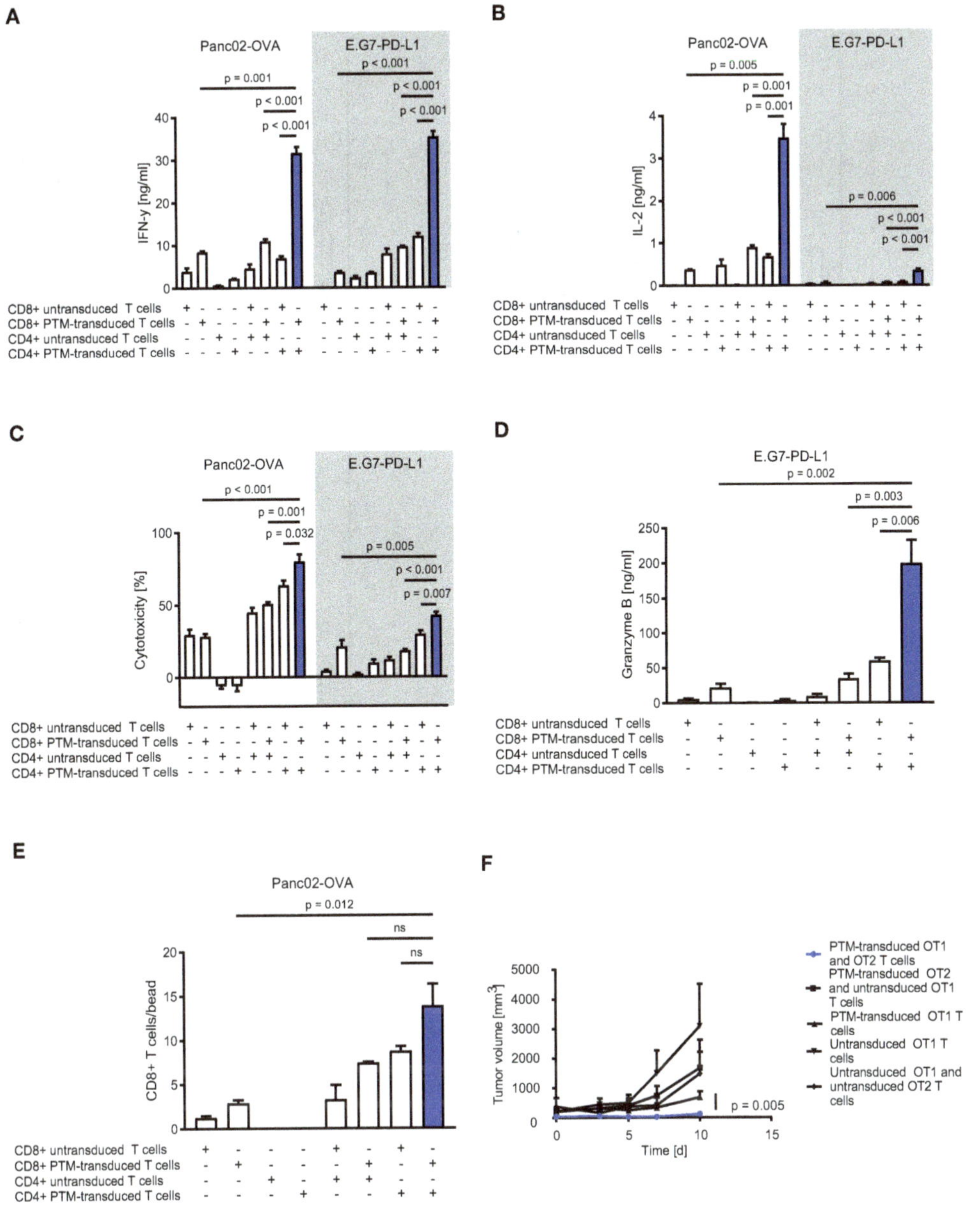

FIGURE 2 | *In vitro* and *in vivo* assessment of anti-tumor efficacy of PD1-CD28 fusion receptor (PTM receptor)-transduced CD4+ and CD8+ T cells. **(A)** PTM-transduced, untransduced primary murine OT-1, PTM-transduced, untransduced primary murine OT-2 T cells, or OT-1 together with OT-2 T cells were prestimulated for 24 h with anti-CD3 antibody plus recombinant PD-L1. T cells were then cocultured with Panc02-OVA or E.G7-PD-L1 cells. Interferon-γ (IFN-γ) secretion was measured by enzyme linked immunosorbent assay (ELISA). **(B)** Interleukin-2 (IL-2) release was measured by ELISA. **(C)** PTM-transduced, untransduced primary murine OT-1, PTM-transduced, untransduced primary murine OT-2 T cells, or OT-1 together with OT-2 T cells were prestimulated for 24 h with anti-CD3 antibody and recombinant PD-L1. In the meantime, Panc02-OVA or E.G7-PD-L1 cells were seeded and grown prior to the addition of T cells. LDH release measurement from lysed tumor cells was performed after 16 h of coculture. **(D)** Granzyme B secretion by T cells cocultured with E.G7-PD-L1 cells for 16 h measured by ELISA. **(E)** PTM-transduced, untransduced primary murine OT-1, PTM-transduced, untransduced primary murine OT-2 T cells or OT-1 together with OT-2 T cells were prestimulated for 24 h with anti-CD3 antibody plus recombinant PD-L1 and then cocultured with Panc02-OVA cells. T cell numbers were analyzed by flow cytometry and normalized to standardized counting beads. **(F)** 30 mice were subcutaneously injected with E.G7-OVA-PD-L1 tumor cells in two independent experiments. As soon as all tumors were established, the mice were randomized, assigned to five different treatment groups and treated with either PTM-transduced ($n = 6$) or untransduced primary murine OT1 T cells ($n = 7$) or with PTM-transduced ($n = 4$) or untransduced ($n = 4$) primary OT2 T cells in combination with OT1 T cells or PTM-transduced OT-1 T cells ($n = 9$). Tumor growth was assessed every other day in a blinded fashion and tumor volume was calculated as indicated. Pooled data from two independent experiments is shown here. Curves are censored by the time the first mice had to be taken out of the experiment either due to tumor size or ulceration (day 10). Experiments **(A–E)** are representative of three independent experiments each performed in triplicates. Experiment **(F)** represents pooled data of two independent experiments. Bars represent SEM and *P* values from Student's *t*-test are shown. All tests are two-sided.

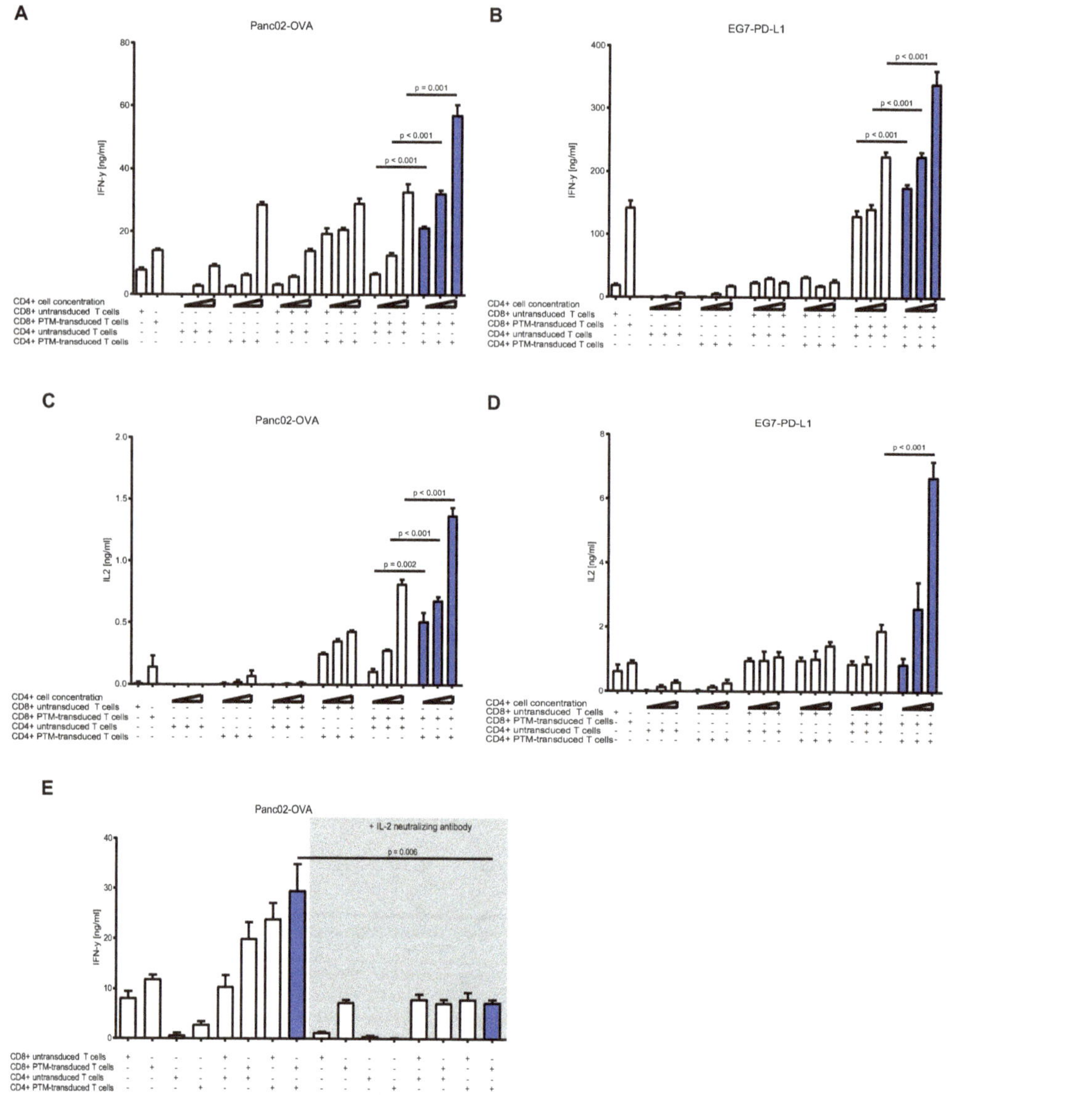

FIGURE 3 | *In vitro* characterization of PD1-CD28 fusion protein (PTM)-transduced CD4+ and CD8+ T cells in T cell-tumor cell cocultures at different CD4+ to CD8+ T cell ratios in the presence or absence of a neutralizing anti-IL-2-antibody. **(A,B)** PTM-transduced or untransduced primary murine OT-1, PTM-transduced or untransduced primary murine OT-2 T cells or combinations of these were prestimulated for 24 h with anti-CD3 antibodies plus recombinant PD-L1. Three different ratios of CD4+ to CD8+ T cells were applied (i.e., 3:1, 1:1, or 1:3 CD4+ to CD8+ T cell ratio). After prestimulation, the T cells were cocultured with Panc02-OVA or E.G7-PD-L1 cells for a further 48 h. The resulting Interferon-γ (IFN-γ) release was measured by enzyme linked immunosorbent assay (ELISA). **(C,D)** The concentration of interleukin-2 (IL-2) in the supernatants was measured by ELISA. **(E)** PTM-transduced or untransduced primary murine OT-1, PTM-transduced or untransduced primary murine OT-2 T cells or combinations of these were prestimulated for 24 h with anti-CD3 antibodies plus recombinant PD-L1. T cells were then cocultured with Panc02-OVA. In the blocking condition, a neutralizing anti-IL-2 antibody was present during the period of prestimulation and coculture. The resulting IFN-γ release was measured by ELISA. Experiments **(A–E)** are representative of three independent experiments each performed at least in triplicates. Bars represent SEM and *P* values from Student's *t*-test are shown. All tests are two-sided.

that rendered antigen-specific CD8+ T cells resistant to PD-1-PD-L1-mediated anergy. Thus, we wondered if this would also apply to CD4+ T cells in a similar fashion (32). In the present manuscript, we could indeed transfer the activity of PTM to CD4+ T cells boosting T cell proliferation and cytokine production in the presence of cancer cells, which further underlines underpinning previous data using a CTLA-4-CD28 fusion receptor.

CD4+ T cells exert potent anti-tumoral effects on their own right (10, 15). This can be mediated either through direct recognition of MHC II+ tumor cells or indirectly through secretion of IFN-γ and activation of bystander myeloid cells (15). In addition, CD4+ T cells can support and contribute to CD8+ T cell function (39–42). If transferred adoptively, CD4+ T cells can even rescue anergic tumor infiltrating CD8+ T cells by T cell help (43). As our fusion protein essentially

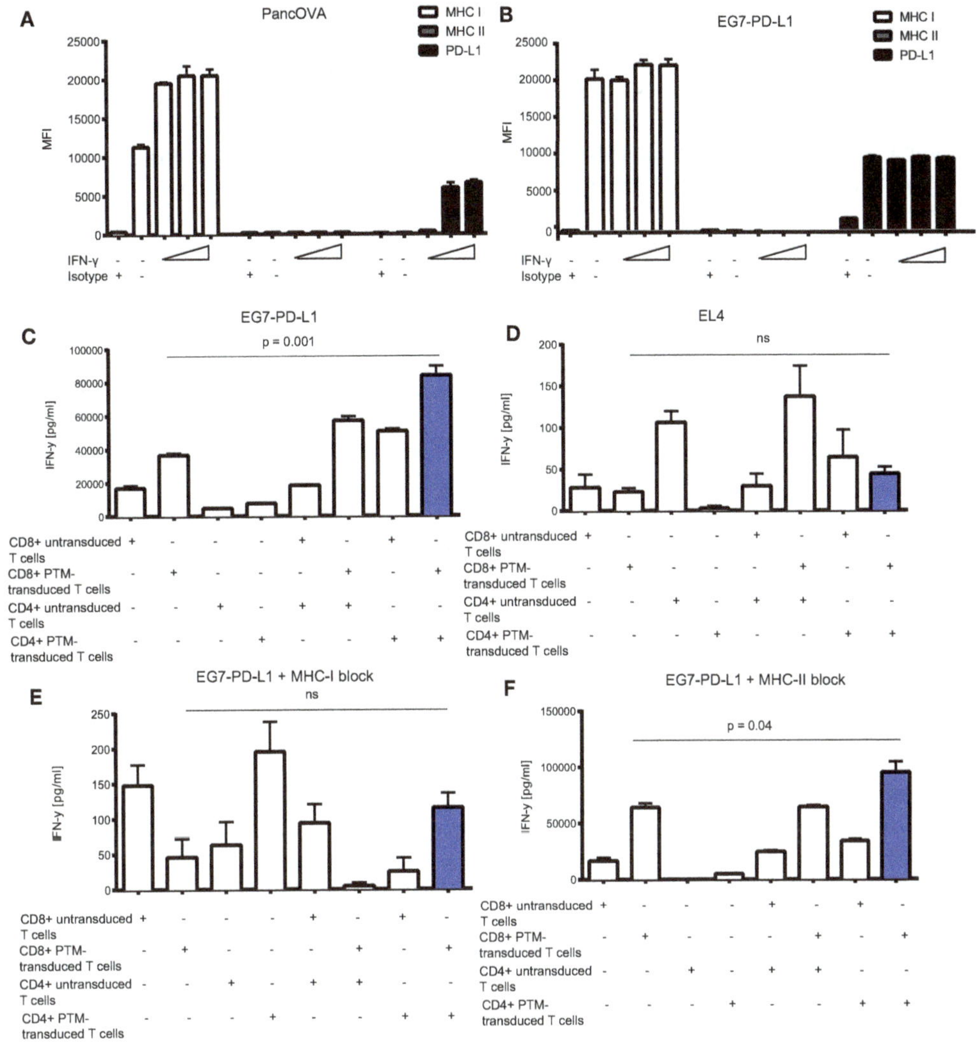

FIGURE 4 | *In vitro* characterization of the MHC I, MHC II, and PD-L1 expression on tumor cells and its effect on interferon-γ (IFN-γ) release by PD1-CD28 fusion protein (PTM)- transduced CD4+ and CD8+ T cells in T cell-tumor cell cocultures. **(A)** Panc02-OVA or **(B)** E.G7-OVA-PD-L1 cells were stimulated with increasing concentrations of recombinant murine IFN-γ (2, 20, 100 ng/ml) during a 48 h period. MHC I, MHC II, and PD-L1 expression was assessed by flow cytometry. **(C–F)** PTM-transduced or untransduced primary murine OT-1, PTM-transduced or untransduced primary murine OT2 T cells or OT1 plus OT-2 T cells were prestimulated for 24 h with anti-CD3 antibody plus recombinant PD-L1. T cells were then cocultured with EL4 **(D)** or with E.G7-OVA-PDL-1 in the absence **(C)** or presence of neutralizing anti-MHC. I antibody **(E)** or of neutralizing anti-MHCII-antibody **(F)**. The resulting interferon-γ (IFN-γ) release was measured by enzyme-linked immunosorbent assay (ELISA). Experiments **(A–F)** were performed in triplicates. Experiments **(C–F)** are representative of two independent experiments. Bars represent SEM and *P* values from Student's *t*-test are shown. All tests are two-sided.

seems to further boost the function of the cell subsets either alone or in combination, we indeed observed that also the collaboration between CD4+ and CD8+ T cells was enhanced through introduction of PTM in both cell types. Interestingly, this effect was dependent on an optimal CD4+ to CD8+ T cell ratio, which is also in line with clinical observations observed with CAR T cells (7, 8). This is further confirmed in multiple studies dealing with mixtures of CD4+ and CD8+ T cells for ACT (16–18). Notwithstanding the role of PD-1-mediated anergy, we argue and show that this brake is released by our PD1-CD28 fusion protein. Similar observations were reported with CTLA-4-CD28-expressing CD4+ and CD8+ T cells (38). Mechanistically, IL-2 derived from CD4+ T cells seems to mediate the synergistic effect of PD1-CD28 fusion receptor-transduced CD4+ and CD8+ T cells. As IL-2 improves CD8+ T cell activation, proliferation, and persistence one could assume that the additional transfer of CD4+ T cells would allow a lower dose of CD8+ T cells per patient. This would come with the additional advantage, that systemic IL-2 administration which often accompanies ACT protocols and causes significant side effects, could be prevented (44, 45). CD4+ T cells are also important for long-term protective anti-tumoral immunity

(46, 47). In our hands, transduced CD4+ and CD8+ T cells predominantly developed a central memory phenotype. At least for CD8+ T cells longer persistence of CD8+ clones isolated from central memory T cells as compared to clones from CD8+ effector cells was observed *in vivo* after T cell transfer. This further indicates the importance of specific T cell subset functions for effective adoptive immunotherapy (48). An open question remains how CD4+-T cells would sense their antigen *in vitro*. We could demonstrate that OVA expression by the tumor cells, MHC I presentation and recognition of MHC I presented peptide by cocultured CD8+ T cells was mandatory for CD4+ T cell action. CD4+ T cells in general and OT-2 T cells in particular can be stimulated MHC II independently in the presence of large amounts of soluble antigen (49). OVA is known to be secreted by cells stably transfected with it and additional antigen release by CD8+-OT-1-T cells might lead to the level of antigen required for CD4+ T cells *in vitro*. The exact role of this known mechanism *in vivo* is currently unclear but has been repeatedly shown in several models (15). In any case, the *in vivo* activity observed strongly suggests translational potential for this strategy. An open question is how much data from the OT-1-OT-2 system will be transferrable to endogeneous antigens and to TCRs with different affinities. This antigen system is one of the most widely tested systems in T cell research. A significant amount of our knowledge has been generated in these models. Several studies suggest that data gathered from such preclinical studies will actually translate to clinical studies, corroborating the value of the OT-1-OT-2 system for translational T cell research (50, 51).

Antibodies, such as nivolumab, targeting the PD-1-PD-L1 axis can revive exhausted CD8+ T cells and have demonstrated impressive clinical activity (52, 53). However, more than 50% of PD-L1-positive tumors do not respond to anti-PD-L1/PD-1 antibody treatment (54). In addition, treatment protocols using those antibodies often require multiple injections and cause significant toxicities to the patient (55). Based on our previous data we assume that a single dose of PD1-CD28 fusion receptor-transduced CD4+ and CD8+ T cells would induce tumor regression *in vivo*, significantly lowering potential side effects due to systemic T cell activation (32). Even PD-L1 negative tumors could be targeted by our combinatorial approach. Transduced CD4+ T cells can also be activated by interaction with PD-L2, another ligand of PD-1, expressed on antigen-presenting cells present in the tumor microenvironment.

In summary, our results indicate that PD1-CD28 fusion protein transduced CD4+ T cells have the potential to overcome the PD-1-PD-L1 immunosuppressive axis in pancreatic cancer and non-Hodgkin-lymphoma. Collectively, inhibiting PD-1 signaling in both CD4+ and CD8+ T cells might be the most effective way to enhance antitumor immunity. This data will need to be further investigated in other models while moving the approach toward translation.

AUTHOR CONTRIBUTIONS

FR designed experiments, supervised experiments, discussed data, and wrote the manuscript. FK designed experiments, conducted experiments, analyzed data, and wrote the manuscript. MC, SG, CH, and BC conducted experiments. PD and SE wrote the manuscript; SK designed and conceptualized the research, supervised the experiments, discussed data, and wrote the manuscript.

SUPPLEMENTARY MATERIAL

Supplementary Figure 1 | Differentiation of PD1-CD28 fusion protein (PTM)-transduced CD4+ and CD8+ T cells in T cell-tumor cell cocultures. **(A–D)** PTM-transduced, untransduced primary murine OT-1, PTM-transduced, untransduced primary murine OT-2 T cells or OT-1 together with OT-2 T cells were prestimulated for 24 h with anti-CD3 antibody and recombinant PD-L1. T cells were then cocultured with Panc02-OVA-PD-L1. CCR7 and CD62L expression on T cells was analyzed prior to and after 36 h of coculture by flow cytometry. Experiments **(A–D)** are representative of three independent experiments each performed at least in duplicates. Bars represent SEM.

Supplementary Figure 2 | Cytotoxic activity of PD1-CD28 fusion protein (PTM)-transduced CD4+ and CD8+ T cells in T cell-tumor cell coculture in the presence of an Interleukin-2 (IL-2) neutralizing antibody. PTM-transduced, untransduced primary murine OT-1, PTM-transduced, untransduced primary murine OT-2 T cells or OT-1 together with OT-2 T cells were prestimulated for 24 h with anti-CD3 antibody and recombinant PD-L1. T cells were then cocultured with Panc02-OVA in the presence or absence of neutralizing anti-IL-2 antibody and LDH release from lysed tumor cells was measured. The experiment was performed in quadruplicates. Bars represent SEM and *P* values from Student's *t*-test are shown. All tests are two-sided.

REFERENCES

1. Ioannides CG, Whiteside TL. T cell recognition of human tumors: implications for molecular immunotherapy of cancer. *Clin Immunol Immunopathol.* (1993) 66:91–106. doi: 10.1006/clin.1993.1012
2. Kobold S, Duewell P, Schnurr M, Subklewe M, Rothenfusser S, Endres S. Immunotherapy in Tumors. *Dtsch Arztebl Int.* (2015) 112:809–15. doi: 10.3238/arztebl.2015.0809
3. Rosenberg SA, Restifo NP. Adoptive cell transfer as personalized immunotherapy for human cancer. *Science* (2015) 348:62–8. doi: 10.1126/science.aaa4967
4. Geukes Foppen MH, Donia M, Svane IM, Haanen JB. Tumor-infiltrating lymphocytes for the treatment of metastatic cancer. *Mol Oncol.* (2015) 9:1918–35. doi: 10.1016/j.molonc.2015.10.018

tumor infiltrating lymphocytes and peripheral blood lymphocytes in patients with metastatic melanoma. *J Natl Cancer Inst.* (1989) 81:1709–17. doi: 10.1093/jnci/81.22.1709

20. Bourquin C, von der Borch P, Zoglmeier C, Anz D, Sandholzer N, Suhartha N, et al. Efficient eradication of subcutaneous but not of autochthonous gastric tumors by adoptive T cell transfer in an SV40 T antigen mouse model. *J Immunol.* (2010) 185:2580–8. doi: 10.4049/jimmunol.0903231
21. Riella LV, Paterson AM, Sharpe AH, Chandraker A. Role of the PD-1 pathway in the immune response. *Am J Transplant* (2012) 12:2575–87. doi: 10.1111/j.1600-6143.2012.04224.x
22. Arasanz H, Gato-Canas M, Zuazo M, Ibanez-Vea M, Breckpot K, Kochan G, et al. PD1 signal transduction pathways in T cells. *Oncotarget* (2017) 8:51936–45. doi: 10.18632/oncotarget.17232

5. Liu Y, Chen X, Han W, Zhang Y. Tisagenlecleucel, an approved anti-CD19 chimeric antigen receptor T-cell therapy for the treatment of leukemia. *Drugs Today* (2017) 53:597–608. doi: 10.1358/dot.2017.53.11.2725754
6. Riddell SR, Sommermeyer D, Berger C, Liu LS, Balakrishnan A, Salter A, et al. Adoptive therapy with chimeric antigen receptor-modified T cells of defined subset composition. *Cancer J.* (2014) 20:141–4. doi: 10.1097/PPO.0000000000000036
7. Turtle CJ, Hanafi LA, Berger C, Gooley TA, Cherian S, Hudecek M, et al. CD19 CAR-T cells of defined CD4+:CD8+ composition in adult B cell ALL patients. *J Clin Invest.* (2016) 126:2123–38. doi: 10.1172/JCI85309
8. Turtle CJ, Hanafi LA, Berger C, Hudecek M, Pender B, Robinson E, et al. Immunotherapy of non-Hodgkin's lymphoma with a defined ratio of CD8+ and CD4+ CD19-specific chimeric antigen receptor-modified T cells. *Sci Transl Med.* (2016) 8:355ra116. doi: 10.1126/scitranslmed.aaf8621
9. Gardner RA, Finney O, Annesley C, Brakke H, Summers C, Leger K, et al. Intent-to-treat leukemia remission by CD19 CAR T cells of defined formulation and dose in children and young adults. *Blood* (2017) 129:3322–31. doi: 10.1182/blood-2017-02-769208
10. Tran E, Turcotte S, Gros A, Robbins PF, Lu YC, Dudley ME, et al. Cancer immunotherapy based on mutation-specific CD4+ T cells in a patient with epithelial cancer. *Science* (2014) 344:641–5. doi: 10.1126/science.1251102
11. Voigt C, May P, Gottschlich A, Markota A, Wenk D, Gerlach I, et al. Cancer cells induce interleukin-22 production from memory CD4(+) T cells via interleukin-1 to promote tumor growth. *Proc Natl Acad Sci USA.* (2017) 114:12994–9. doi: 10.1073/pnas.1705165114
12. Baxevanis CN, Voutsas IF, Tsitsilonis OE, Gritzapis AD, Sotiriadou R, Papamichail M. Tumor-specific CD4+ T lymphocytes from cancer patients are required for optimal induction of cytotoxic T cells against the autologous tumor. *J Immunol.* (2000) 164:3902–12. doi: 10.4049/jimmunol.164.7.3902
13. Marzo AL, Kinnear BF, Lake RA, Frelinger JJ, Collins EJ, Robinson BW, et al. Tumor-specific CD4+ T cells have a major post-licensing role in CTL mediated anti-tumor immunity. *J Immunol.* (2000) 165:6047–55. doi: 10.4049/jimmunol.165.11.6047
14. Hunziker L, Klenerman P, Zinkernagel RM, Ehl S. Exhaustion of cytotoxic T cells during adoptive immunotherapy of virus carrier mice can be prevented by B cells or CD4+ T cells. *Eur J Immunol.* (2002) 32:374–82. doi: 10.1002/1521-4141(200202)32:2<374::AID-IMMU374>3.0.CO;2-9
15. Haabeth OA, Tveita AA, Fauskanger M, Schjesvold F, Lorvik KB, Hofgaard PO, et al. How do CD4(+) T cells detect and eliminate tumor cells that either lack or express MHC class II molecules? *Front Immunol.* (2014) 5:174. doi: 10.3389/fimmu.2014.00174
16. Moeller M, Haynes NM, Kershaw MH, Jackson JT, Teng MW, Street SE, et al. Adoptive transfer of gene-engineered CD4+ helper T cells induces potent primary and secondary tumor rejection. *Blood* (2005) 106:2995–3003. doi: 10.1182/blood-2004-12-4906
17. Kennedy R, Celis E. T helper lymphocytes rescue CTL from activation-induced cell death. *J Immunol.* (2006) 177:2862–72. doi: 10.4049/jimmunol.177.5.2862
18. Wang LX, Shu S, Disis ML, Plautz GE. Adoptive transfer of tumor-primed, in vitro-activated, CD4+ T effector cells, (TEs) combined with CD8+ TEs provides intratumoral TE proliferation and synergistic antitumor response. *Blood* (2007) 109:4865–76. doi: 10.1182/blood-2006-09-045245
19. Griffith KD, Read EJ, Carrasquillo JA, Carter CS, Yang JC, Fisher B, et al. *In vivo* distribution of adoptively transferred indium-111-labeled
23. Gibbons Johnson RM, Dong H. Functional expression of programmed death-ligand 1, (B7-H1) by immune cells and tumor cells. *Front Immunol.* (2017) 8:961. doi: 10.3389/fimmu.2017.00961
24. Dong H, Strome SE, Salomao DR, Tamura H, Hirano F, Flies DB, et al. Tumor-associated B7-H1 promotes T-cell apoptosis: a potential mechanism of immune evasion. *Nat Med.* (2002) 8:793–800. doi: 10.1038/nm730
25. Wang X, Teng F, Kong L, Yu J. PD-L1 expression in human cancers and its association with clinical outcomes. *Onco Targets Ther.* (2016) 9:5023–39. doi: 10.2147/OTT.S105862
26. Abate-Daga D, Hanada K, Davis J, LYang JC, Rosenberg SA, Morgan RA. Expression profiling of TCR-engineered T cells demonstrates overexpression of multiple inhibitory receptors in persisting lymphocytes. *Blood* (2013) 122:1399–410. doi: 10.1182/blood-2013-04-495531
27. Daud AI, Wolchok JD, Robert C, Hwu WJ, Weber JS, Ribas A, et al. Programmed death-ligand 1 expression and response to the anti-programmed death 1 antibody pembrolizumab in melanoma. *J Clin Oncol.* (2016) 34:4102–9. doi: 10.1200/JCO.2016.67.2477
28. Alsaab HO, Sau S, Alzhrani R, Tatiparti K, Bhise K, Kashaw SK, et al. PD-1 and PD-L1 checkpoint signaling inhibition for cancer immunotherapy: mechanism, combinations, and clinical outcome. *Front Pharmacol.* (2017) 8:561. doi: 10.3389/fphar.2017.00561
29. Iafolla MAJ, Juergens RA. Update on programmed death-1 and programmed death-ligand 1 inhibition in the treatment of advanced or metastatic non-small cell lung cancer. *Front Oncol.* (2017) 7:67. doi: 10.3389/fonc.2017.00067
30. Malhotra J, Jabbour SK, Aisner J. Current state of immunotherapy for non-small cell lung cancer. *Transl Lung Cancer Res.* (2017) 6:196–211. doi: 10.21037/tlcr.2017.03.01
31. Abdin SM, Zaher DM, Arafa EA, Omar HA. Tackling cancer resistance by immunotherapy: updated clinical impact and safety of PD-1/PD-L1 inhibitors. *Cancers* (2018) 10:32. doi: 10.3390/cancers10020032
32. Kobold S, Grassmann S, Chaloupka M, Lampert C, Wenk S, Kraus F, et al. Impact of a new fusion receptor on PD-1-mediated immunosuppression in adoptive T cell therapy. *J Natl Cancer Inst.* (2015) 107:146. doi: 10.1093/jnci/djv146
33. Duewell P, Kisser U, Heckelsmiller K, Hoves S, Stoitzner P, Koernig S, et al. ISCOMATRIX adjuvant combines immune activation with antigen delivery to dendritic cells in vivo leading to effective cross-priming of CD8+ T cells. *J Immunol.* (2011) 187:55–63. doi: 10.4049/jimmunol.1004114
34. Leisegang M, Engels B, Meyerhuber P, Kieback E, Sommermeyer D, Xue SA, et al. Enhanced functionality of T cell receptor-redirected T cells is defined by the transgene cassette. *J Mol Med.* (2008) 86:573–83. doi: 10.1007/s00109-008-0317-3
35. Mueller K, von Massenhausen A, Aichele U, Starck L, Leisegang M, Uckert W, et al. Protective capacity of virus-specific T cell receptor-transduced CD8 T cells *in vivo*. *J Virol.* (2012) 86:10866–9. doi: 10.1128/JVI.01472-12
36. Kobold S, Steffen J, Chaloupka M, Grassmann S, Henkel J, Castoldi R, et al. Selective bispecific T cell recruiting antibody and antitumor activity of adoptive T cell transfer. *J Natl Cancer Inst.* (2015) 107:364. doi: 10.1093/jnci/dju364
37. Rapp M, Grassmann S, Chaloupka M, Layritz P, Kruger S, Ormanns S, et al. C-C chemokine receptor type-4 transduction of T cells enhances interaction with dendritic cells, tumor infiltration and therapeutic efficacy of adoptive T cell transfer. *Oncoimmunology* (2016) 5:e1105428. doi: 10.1080/2162402X.2015.1105428
38. Shin JH, Park HB, Oh YM, Lim DP, Lee JE, Seo HH, et al. Positive conversion of negative signaling of CTLA4 potentiates antitumor efficacy of adoptive T-cell therapy in murine tumor models. *Blood* (2012) 119:5678–87. doi: 10.1182/blood-2011-09-380519
39. Keene JA, Forman J. Helper activity is required for the in vivo generation of cytotoxic T lymphocytes. *J Exp Med.* (1982) 155:768–82. doi: 10.1084/jem.155.3.768
40. Matloubian M, Concepcion RJ, Ahmed R. CD4+ T cells are required to sustain CD8+ cytotoxic T-cell responses during chronic viral infection. *J Virol.* (1994) 68:8056–63.
41. Bos R, Sherman LA. CD4+ T-cell help in the tumor milieu is required for recruitment and cytolytic function of CD8+ T lymphocytes. *Cancer Res.* (2010) 70:8368–77. doi: 10.1158/0008-5472.CAN-10-1322
42. Schietinger A, Philip M, Liu RB, Schreiber K, Schreiber H. Bystander killing of cancer requires the cooperation of $CD4^+$ and $CD8^+$ T cells during the effector phase. *J Exp Med.* (2010) 207:2469–77. doi: 10.1084/jem.20092450
43. Arina A, Karrison T, Galka E, Schreiber K, Weichselbaum RR, Schreiber H. Transfer of allogeneic CD4+ T cells rescues CD8+ T cells in anti-PD-L1-resistant tumors leading to tumor eradication. *Cancer Immunol Res.* (2017) 5:127–36. doi: 10.1158/2326-6066.CIR-16-0293
44. Bindon C, Czerniecki M, Ruell P, Edwards A, McCarthy WH, Harris R, et al. Clearance rates and systemic effects of intravenously administered interleukin 2, (IL-2) containing preparations in human subjects. *Br J Cancer* (1983) 47:123–33. doi: 10.1038/bjc.1983.15

interaction with dendritic cells, tumor infiltration and therapeutic efficacy of adoptive T cell transfer. *Oncoimmunology* (2016) 5:e1105428. doi: 10.1080/2162402X.2015.1105428

38. Shin JH, Park HB, Oh YM, Lim DP, Lee JE, Seo HH, et al. Positive conversion of negative signaling of CTLA4 potentiates antitumor efficacy of adoptive T-cell therapy in murine tumor models. *Blood* (2012) 119:5678–87. doi: 10.1182/blood-2011-09-380519
39. Keene JA, Forman J. Helper activity is required for the in vivo generation of cytotoxic T lymphocytes. *J Exp Med.* (1982) 155:768–82. doi: 10.1084/jem.155.3.768
40. Matloubian M, Concepcion RJ, Ahmed R. CD4+ T cells are required to sustain CD8+ cytotoxic T-cell responses during chronic viral infection. *J Virol.* (1994) 68:8056–63.
41. Bos R, Sherman LA. CD4+ T-cell help in the tumor milieu is required for recruitment and cytolytic function of CD8+ T lymphocytes. *Cancer Res.* (2010) 70:8368–77. doi: 10.1158/0008-5472.CAN-10-1322
42. Schietinger A, Philip M, Liu RB, Schreiber K, Schreiber H. Bystander killing of cancer requires the cooperation of $CD4^+$ and $CD8^+$ T cells during the effector phase. *J Exp Med.* (2010) 207:2469–77. doi: 10.1084/jem.20092450
43. Arina A, Karrison T, Galka E, Schreiber K, Weichselbaum RR, Schreiber H. Transfer of allogeneic CD4+ T cells rescues CD8+ T cells in anti-PD-L1-resistant tumors leading to tumor eradication. *Cancer Immunol Res.* (2017) 5:127–36. doi: 10.1158/2326-6066.CIR-16-0293
44. Bindon C, Czerniecki M, Ruell P, Edwards A, McCarthy WH, Harris R, et al. Clearance rates and systemic effects of intravenously administered interleukin 2, (IL-2) containing preparations in human subjects. *Br J Cancer* (1983) 47:123–33. doi: 10.1038/bjc.1983.15
49. Li M, Davey GM, Sutherland RM, Kurts C, Lew AM, Hirst C, et al. Cell-associated ovalbumin is cross-presented much more efficiently than soluble ovalbumin *in vivo*. *J Immunol* (2001) 166:6099–103. doi: 10.4049/jimmunol.166.10.6099
50. Graef P, Buchholz VR, Stemberger C, Flossdorf M, Henkel L, Schiemann M, et al. Serial transfer of single-cell-derived immunocompetence reveals stemness of $CD8^+$ central memory T cells. *Immunity* (2014) 41:116–26. doi: 10.1016/j.immuni.2014.05.018
51. Neuenhahn M, Albrecht J, Odendahl M, Schlott F, Dossinger G, Schiemann M, et al. Transfer of minimally manipulated CMV-specific T cells from stem cell or third-party donors to treat CMV infection after allo-HSCT. *Leukemia* (2017) 31:2161–71. doi: 10.1038/leu.2017.16
52. Robert C, Long GV, Brady B, Dutriaux C, Maio M, Mortier L, et al. Nivolumab in previously untreated melanoma without BRAF mutation. *N Engl J Med.* (2015) 372:320–30. doi: 10.1056/NEJMoa1412082
53. Zheng P, Zhou Z. Human cancer immunotherapy with PD-1/PD-L1 blockade. *Biomark Cancer* (2015) 7(Suppl 2):15–8. doi: 10.4137/BIC.S29325
54. Topalian SL, Hodi FS, Brahmer JR, Gettinger SN, Smith DC, McDermott DF, et al. Safety, activity, and immune correlates of anti-PD-1 antibody in cancer. *N Engl J Med.* (2012) 366:2443–54. doi: 10.1056/NEJMoa1200690
55. Postow MA, Chesney J, Pavlick AC, Robert C, Grossmann K, McDermott D, et al. Nivolumab and ipilimumab versus ipilimumab in untreated melanoma. *N Engl J Med.* (2015) 372:2006–17. doi: 10.1056/NEJMoa1414428

4

Biomarkers for Clinical Benefit of Immune Checkpoint Inhibitor Treatment — A Review from the Melanoma Perspective and Beyond

*Kristina Buder-Bakhaya and Jessica C. Hassel**

Section of Dermatooncology, Department of Dermatology and National Center for Tumor Diseases (NCT), University Hospital Heidelberg, Heidelberg, Germany

Edited by:
Alexandr Bazhin, Klinikum der Universität München, Germany

Reviewed by:
Ekaterina Jordanova, Center for Gynaecologic Oncology Amsterdam, Netherlands
Rodabe N. Amaria, University of Texas MD Anderson Cancer Center, United States

***Correspondence:**
Jessica C. Hassel
jessica.hassel@med.uni-heidelberg.de

Background: Immune checkpoint inhibition (ICI) with anti-CTLA-4 and/or anti-PD-1 antibodies is standard treatment for metastatic melanoma. Anti-PD-1 (pembrolizumab, nivolumab) and anti-PD-L1 antibodies (atezolizumab, durvalumab, and avelumab) have been approved for treatment of several other advanced malignancies, including non-small-cell lung cancer (NSCLC); renal cell, and urothelial carcinoma; head and neck cancer; gastric, hepatocellular, and Merkel-cell carcinoma; and classical Hodgkin lymphoma. In some of these malignancies approval was based on the detection of biomarkers such as PD-L1 expression or high microsatellite instability.

Methods: We review the current status of prognostic and predictive biomarkers used in ICI for melanoma and other malignancies. We include clinical, tissue, blood, and stool biomarkers, as well as imaging biomarkers.

Results: Several biomarkers have been studied in ICI for metastatic melanoma. In clinical practice, pre-treatment tumor burden measured by means of imaging and serum lactate dehydrogenase level is already being used to estimate the likelihood of effective ICI treatment. In peripheral blood, the number of different immune cell types, such as lymphocytes, neutrophils, and eosinophils, as well as different soluble factors, have been correlated with clinical outcome. For intra-tumoral biomarkers, expression of the PD-1 ligand PD-L1 has been found to be of some predictive value for anti-PD-1-directed therapy for NSCLC and melanoma. A high mutational load, particularly when accompanied by neoantigens, seems to facilitate immune response and correlates with patient survival for all entities treated by use of ICI. Tumor microenvironment also seems to be of major importance. Interestingly, even the gut microbiome has been found to correlate with response to ICI, most likely through immuno-stimulatory effects of distinct bacteria. New imaging biomarkers, e.g., for PET, and magnetic resonance imaging are also being investigated, and results suggest they will make early prediction of patient response possible.

Conclusion: Several promising results are available regarding possible biomarkers for response to ICI, which need to be validated in large clinical trials. A better understanding of how ICI works will enable the development of biomarkers that can predict the response of individual patients.

Keywords: biomarker, checkpoint inhibition, PD-1 antibody, PD-L1 antibody, CTLA-4 antibody, cancer, melanoma

INTRODUCTION

In the last decade, treatment of metastatic melanoma and other malignancies has improved significantly. In addition to targeted treatment options, immunotherapy with immune checkpoint inhibitors (ICI) has contributed greatly to this development.

The anti-CTLA-4 antibody (CTLA4ab) ipilimumab was first approved by the U.S. Food and Drug Administration (FDA) for the treatment of metastatic melanoma in 2011 (1), followed by the anti-PD-1 antibodies (PD1ab) pembrolizumab and nivolumab in 2014 (2–4). Combined ICI with CTLA4ab and PD1ab for melanoma was introduced with enormous success, but was also accompanied by significant immune-related adverse events (irAEs) (5, 6). PD1ab treatment is currently approved for treatment of several other advanced malignancies including non-small-cell lung cancer (NSCLC), urothelial cancer, renal cell carcinoma (RCC), squamous cell carcinoma of head and neck (SCCHN), gastric carcinoma, hepatocellular carcinoma, and classical Hodgkin lymphoma (7–12). The anti-PD-L1 antibodies (PD-L1ab) atezolizumab (urothelial carcinoma and NSCLC), durvalumab (urothelial carcinoma), and avelumab [Merkel-cell carcinoma (MCC) and urothelial carcinoma] have also recently been approved by the FDA (13–18). In 2017 the FDA also announced a biomarker-based approval for pembrolizumab for patients with unresectable or metastatic solid tumors, and for colorectal carcinoma (CRC) with high microsatellite instability or mismatch repair deficiency (dMMR) (19).

Despite this enormous success, ICI does not achieve long-lasting responses for all patients. Response varies between different entities, and between different patients. For melanoma, PD1ab monotherapy can achieve a response of 26–32% (2, 4) and the combination of PD1ab and CTLA4ab achieves a response as high as 60% (5). Some subsets of patients achieve durable responses with PD1ab monotherapy and do not require combined ICI, and could therefore be protected from the higher risk of irAEs.

There remains the medical need to find reliable biomarkers that could help to identify both, the patients who would benefit from ICI and the primary resistant patients. Biomarkers are also needed to help decide the type of first-line treatment, e.g., whether BRAF-mutant melanoma should be treated by use of targeted or immunotherapy, therapy sequencing, and/or by a combination of treatments. Here, we review biomarkers in the field of ICI therapy for metastatic melanoma and other malignancies. We have not performed a review of pre-analytic, analytic, and clinical validation techniques for biomarkers because these have been reviewed elsewhere (20, 21).

CLINICAL BIOMARKERS

Tumor Burden

Tumor burden and metastatic site, e.g., liver or brain metastases, significantly affect patient prognosis, particularly in terms of overall survival (OS), as described in the TNM classification (22). Because the prognostic effect of tumor burden and metastatic site is well known, they are used to stratify clinical trials and are the object of sub-group analyses. Several authors have found an association between metastatic site and incidence of response, progression-free survival (PFS), and OS for PD1ab treatment of melanoma (23–26) (**Table 1**). Response to PD1ab therapy is better for lung and skin metastases than for metastases in other organs, particularly those in the liver. Response for melanoma brain metastases is lower compared with response for extracranial sites, particularly for PD-1ab monotherapy (27). This could be because T cell infiltrate in cerebral metastases is less dense compared with other anatomic sites (28). For combined ICI with ipilimumab and nivolumab, response for brain metastases that were asymptomatic was similar to response for extracranial sites (27, 29). Peripheral blood biomarkers which correlate with tumor burden, such as serum lactate dehydrogenase (LDH), circulating tumor cells (CTCs), and circulating tumor DNA (ctDNA), are of significance for biomarker investigations, as described below.

Clinical Condition (Performance Status)

A good clinical condition expressed by the ECOG (Eastern Cooperative Oncology Group) performance status (ECOG PS 0) is associated with prolonged OS for patients receiving PD1ab treatment, as well as for patients receiving other melanoma treatments such as BRAF inhibitors (30, 70). For other entities such as NSCLC (71), association between performance status and OS is also well known. Because of its prognostic character, performance status is frequently used as a biomarker in enrichment designs of clinical trials, i.e., only biomarker-positive patients are included, in this case only patients with good performance status. Because patients with poorer performance are not included and are therefore unavailable for further analysis, enrichment design prevents information from being gathered on the prognostic versus predictive value of performance status (20). Significance of other patient characteristics for ICI response, such as sex and age, has only been found in single studies with PD1ab for melanoma (24).

Immune-Related Adverse Events

Immune-Related Adverse Events are side effects caused by the activated immune system and are, therefore, a possible sign of successful immune checkpoint blockage. Several retrospective analyses have reported an association between CTLA4ab-induced irAE and a more favorable clinical outcome (**Table 1**). From a cohort of 86 patients, occurrence of irAE $\geq$ grade 2 CTC-AE was associated with improved response, PFS, and OS (31). In contrast, other studies focusing on irAE of any grade could not find this association for large ipilimumab-treated cohorts (37, 38). The development of autoimmune hypophysitis was found to be associated with prolonged OS (33). It has been observed in retrospective analyses of several groups receiving PD1ab therapy that incidence of irAEs is associated with a more favorable outcome. In a large cohort of 576 PD1ab-treated patients, response but not PFS was associated with irAE manifestation of any grade (32). For certain adverse events, vitiligo was found to be associated with response (34) and, similar to exanthema, with longer OS (35). Arthralgia of any grade was associated with response and significantly longer PFS (36). Here, median onset of arthralgia was 100 days after start of treatment and was caused by either arthritis or reactivated osteoarthritis in pre-damaged joints. It is worth noting that all these analyses were performed retrospectively and that there is a risk of guarantee-time bias, i.e., patients with early progression are less likely to develop irAEs because of

TABLE 1 | Clinical, blood, and stool biomarkers for clinical outcome under checkpoint blockage for metastatic melanoma patients.

Biomarker	Number of patients	Treatment	Results	Reference
Clinical Biomarkers				
Metastatic sites	$n = 177–593$	Pembrolizumab, nivolumab	Liver metastases associated with lower response rate and shorter PFS	(26) (24) (25)
	$n = 177–257$	Pembrolizumab	Soft-tissue and/or lung metastases associated with longer OS	(23)
ECOG performance status	$n = 50$	Nivolumab	ECOG PS ≥ 1 associated with shorter OS	(30)
Immune-related adverse events (irAEs)	$n = 86$	Ipilimumab, nivolumab	irAEs associated with response	(31) (32)
	$n = 154$	Ipilimumab	Hypophysitis associated with longer OS	(33)
	$n = 65–118$	Pembrolizumab, nivolumab	Vitiligo associated with response and longer OS	(34) (35)
	$n = 196$	Pembrolizumab, nivolumab	Arthralgia associated with response and longer OS	(36)
	$n = 298–833$	Ipilimumab	No association of irAEs with response or survival	(37) (38)
Blood Biomarkers				
LDH	$n = 50–257$	Ipilimumab, nivolumab, pembrolizumab, ipilimumab + nivolumab, or pembrolizumab	Elevated LDH associated with shorter OS	(39) (40) (41) (31) (30) (42) (23) (43) (44)
CRP	$n = 95–196$	Ipilimumab	CRP within normal limits associated with longer OS	(43) (45)
	$n = 50$	Nivolumab	CRP not significant for OS in multivariable analysis	(30)
Neutrophils	$n = 50–720$	Ipilimumab	Elevated neutrophils associated with shorter OS	(40) (30) (46)
Lymphocytes	$n = 50–257$	Ipilimumab, pembrolizumab, nivolumab	Absolute lymphocyte counts (LC) ≥1,000/ml, high relative LC or increasing LC with treatment associated with longer OS	(45) (23) (30) (41, 47)
NLR	$n = 58–720$	Ipilimumab, nivolumab	Baseline NLR ≥ 3–4 associated with shorter OS	(46) (48) (49)
	$n = 90$	Nivolumab	Baseline NLR ≥ 2.2 associated with non-response	(50)
Eosinophils	$n = 59$	Ipilimumab	Increase in eosinophil count (week 3) associated with response	(51)
	$n = 177–209$	Ipilimumab, pembrolizumab	High eosinophils associated with longer OS	(41) (23)
Monocytes, mo-MDSCs	$n = 20–209$	Ipilimumab, nivolumab, pembrolizumab	Elevated mo-MDSCs/monocytes associated with non-response and shorter PFS/OS	(51) (41) (52) (49) (53)
T cell subsets	$n = 95–209$	Ipilimumab	High Treg count associated with longer OS	(45) (41)
	$n = 67–82$	Ipilimumab	Relative numbers of $CD4^+$ and $CD8^+$ T cells correlated with response and longer OS	(47) (54)
	$n = 37–190$	Ipilimumab	Higher PD-L1 expression on peripheral T cells correlated with non-response, shorter PFS and OS	(55)
	$n = 67$	Nivolumab, pembrolizumab	NK cell subsets associated with response to PD1ab	(54)

(Continued)

TABLE 1 | Continued

Biomarker	Number of patients	Treatment	Results	Reference
Human leukocyte antigen class I genotype (HLA-I)	$n = 1535$ (mainly melanoma, NSCLC)	Ipilimumab ± nivolumab, nivolumab, pembrolizumab	Maximum heterozygosity at HLA-I loci correlated with longer OS, melanoma only: HLA-B44 supertype associated with longer OS, HLA-B62, or somatic loss of heterozygosity at HLA-I associated with shorter OS	(56)
T cell receptor (TCR) repertoire	$n = 12$	Ipilimumab	TCR repertoire richness prior to therapy correlated with clinical benefit	(57)
sCTLA4	$n = 14$	Ipilimumab	sCTLA4 higher in responders, associated with longer OS	(58)
sPD-L1	$n = 251$	Ipilimumab (±bevazizumab or sargramostim), pembrolizumab	High pretreatment levels associated with disease progression	(59)
sULBP-1, sULBP-2	$n = 194$ (ICI) $n = 65$ (other treatments)	Ipilimumab ± nivolumab or pembrolizumab, nivolumab	sULBP-1 and 2 associated with disease control and longer OS in ICI, but not in other treatments	(44)
sCD25	$n = 27$	Ipilimumab	High baseline sCD25 associated with shorter OS	(60)
CXCL11	$n = 48–247$	Ipilimumab or gp100 peptide vaccine	Pre-treatment elevated serum CXCL11 level associated with shorter OS	(61)
Cytokine levels	$n = 35$	Nivolumab	Serum IFN-γ, IL-6, and IL-10 levels higher for responders	(62)
Protein signature (multimarker assay)	$n = 119–170$	Ipilimumab ± nivolumab, nivolumab, nivolumab ± vaccine, pembrolizumab	Baseline protein signature of 209 proteins discovered by use of MALDI–TOF and computational algorithms correlated with OS	(63)
CTC count	$n = 7$ (ICI) $n = 42$ (other treatments)	Ipilimumab, chemotherapy, targeted therapy	CTC count correlated with OS	
CTC (droplet digital PCR)	$n = 49$	Ipilimumab, nivolumab, pembrolizumab	Decrease in CTC within the first 7 weeks of ICI was linked to longer PFS and OS	(64)
Plasma ct-DNA: BRAF V600E/K, NRAS Q61K/R	$n = 19$ (ICI) $n = 29$ (targeted therapy)	Ipilimumab, nivolumab, pembrolizumab, targeted therapy	Pre-treatment ctDNA <10 copies/ml associated with response and longer PFS, decrease in ctDNA levels in responders of targeted therapy but not immunotherapy	(65)
Stool Biomarkers				
Gut microbiome	$n = 26$	Ipilimumab	Faecalibacterium and other Firmucutes associated with improved response, higher representation of Bacteroidetes related to poor response	(66)
	$n = 89$	PD1ab, not specified	Enrichment of Ruminococcaceae and Clostridiales found in responders, Bacteriodales in non-responders; Bacteroidales associated with shorter PFS	(67)
	$n = 39$	Ipilimumab + nivolumab, pembrolizumab	Enrichment of *Bacteroides caccae* in responders	(68)
	$n = 39$	PD1ab, not specified	Relative abundance of *Bifidobacterium longum*, *Collinsella aerofaciens*, and *Enterococcus faecium* in responders	(69)

CRP, C-reactive protein; CTLA4ab, anti-CTLA-4 antibody; LDH, lactate dehydrogenase; MALDI–TOF, matrix-assisted laser desorption/ionization–time-of-flight; mo-MDSCs, monocytic myeloid-derived suppressor cells; NLR, neutrophil-to-lymphocyte ratio; PD1ab, anti-PD-1 antibody; PFS, progression-free survival; OS, overall survival; TNF-α, tumor necrosis factor-alpha; CTC, circulating tumor cells; ctDNA, circulating tumor DNA; sCTLA4, soluble CTLA4; sPD-L1, soluble PD-L1; sCD25, soluble CD25.

a shorter treatment period. This bias can be controlled to some degree by use of landmark analysis, which was used in the above-mentioned reports.

BLOOD BIOMARKERS

Blood-based biomarkers have several preferential characteristics and are, therefore, the focus of biomarker research. First, they are easily accessible, which enables analysis at several time-points. Second, they might be independent from intra and inter-tumor heterogeneity. Third, they might reflect multiple sites of interest, e.g., tumor cells, tumor microenvironment, and the patient's immune system.

Serum Biomarkers Correlating With Tumor Load

Lactate dehydrogenase (LDH) is a house-keeping enzyme which is released by rapidly growing tumors. Serum LDH therefore correlates with tumor burden. For melanoma, the prognostic significance of this biomarker is expressed by its inclusion in the American Joint Committee on Cancer classification (72). Serum LDH levels correlate with patients' OS in various treatment regimens (73), including ICI (**Table 1**) (23, 30, 31, 39–45). Nearly all studies have found no correlation between baseline LDH and response. Only a dynamic change in LDH from baseline to week 12 was found to be associated with response (31, 45). Hence, despite the prognostic value of LDH, patients with elevated serum

LDH can respond to ICI; LDH elevation does not, therefore, lead to an exclusion of patients from ICI treatment. Patients with very high levels of more than twice the upper limit of normal, however, did not benefit from either CTLA-4ab or PD1ab monotherapy (23, 31, 39). Importantly, even though targeted treatments by use of BRAF/MEK inhibitors are known to lead to fast tumor responses in highly advanced patients with BRAF-V600-mutated melanoma, patients with normal LDH still achieve the better clinical outcome from treatment (74). Hence, the best treatment sequencing of targeted and immunotherapy for patients with BRAF-mutated melanoma and normal LDH is not clear.

Another serum biomarker which correlates with tumor burden is the acute-phase protein C-reactive protein (CRP). It is a prognostic marker for melanoma, and elevated concentrations are linked to worse PFS and OS (75). CRP also significantly affects prognosis for other malignancies such as renal, gastrointestinal, lung, pancreas, hepatocellular, and bladder cancer (76). For ICI, only retrospective analyses are available. A normal CRP level at the start of treatment was associated with longer OS for ipilimumab-treated melanoma patients (43). Decreasing CRP levels from baseline to week 12 of CTLA4ab therapy were, as for LDH, associated with longer PFS and OS (45). In multivariate analysis of a small study of PD1ab-treated melanoma patients, baseline CRP levels were no independent biomarkers for OS (30). For PD1ab treatment of NSCLC, in contrast, elevated baseline CRP levels were shown to be associated with shorter PFS (77).

Differential Blood Count Biomarkers

Immune checkpoint inhibition works *via* activation of T lymphocytes. Hence, the number of lymphocytes and other immune cells circulating might affect its efficacy. Several retrospective analyses have focused on this question. The role of neutrophils, which can display heterogeneous phenotypes and diverse functionality, is also important (78). Increased levels of neutrophils have been found in the peripheral blood of cancer patients; they might possibly be induced by cytokines such as granulocyte-colony stimulating factor (G-CSF), although no definite cause for neutrophilia in malignancies has been clearly shown (78). Pretreatment elevation of neutrophil count has been found to correlate with worse OS in ICI treatment of melanoma (**Table 1**). Increasing lymphocyte counts, in contrast, correlated with prolonged OS in ICI-treated patients (**Table 1**). The neutrophil-to-lymphocyte ratio (NLR) has been more frequently reported to be of prognostic, and potentially predictive, value by several authors using various cutoffs (NLR $>$ 2–5). For ipilimumab-treated melanoma patients, high baseline NLR was associated with shorter PFS and OS (46, 48). For PD1ab treatment, high baseline NLR was linked to non-response (50) and to worse OS for melanoma (49, 79) and for several other types of cancer being investigated in phase I studies with PD1ab/PD-L1ab treatment (79). For example, NLR was associated with lower incidence of response, poor PFS, and OS for NSCLC (71, 80) and for RCC (81). It is worth noting that an association was also found between NLR and prognosis for melanoma patients treated by use of BRAF inhibitors (82). Overall, NLR certainly has prognostic value but is probably not treatment specific and no predictive ability has been observed so far. It has, however, also been shown that eosinophils correlate with clinical outcome in ICI treatment of melanoma. A high pre-ICI absolute or relative eosinophil count was associated with prolonged OS (23, 41). Dynamically, for melanoma patients treated by use of ipilimumab, eosinophil counts that increased with treatment correlated with response to ipilimumab (51).

Myeloid-derived suppressor cells (MDSCs) are important in melanoma and other malignancies. MDSCs have immunosuppressive potential, particularly by inhibiting activated T cells, and can be divided into two subgroups: granulocytic and monocytic myeloid-derived suppressor cell (mo-MDSC) (78). The number of mo-MDSC in the peripheral blood in particular has been correlated with prognosis for melanoma patients (51). In CTLA4ab treatment, the number of mo-MDSC has been found to negatively affect incidence of response and survival (41, 47, 51). In addition, mo-MDSC was negatively correlated with OS for CTLA4ab-pretreated melanoma patients receiving PD1ab (52) (**Table 1**). The development of cytometry by time-of-flight (CyTOF) has enabled in-depth analysis of peripheral blood immune cells. CyTOF can measure up to 50 proteins per cell. Use of CyTOF for ICI patients has shown that high incidence of classical monocytes ($CD14^{+}CD16^{-}HLA\text{-}DR^{hi}$) are associated with response and improved PFS in PD1ab therapy for melanoma (53).

It is worth mentioning that all these potential markers have been found by retrospective exploratory analyses. They potentially have prognostic features but their predictive potential remains unclear. Furthermore, the above-mentioned publications used several different cutoffs. Prospective studies are needed to investigate a possible predictive value of these biomarkers.

Biomarkers on Peripheral T Cells

T cells are the effector cells of ICI treatment. Therefore, in addition to the pure cell number of several subsets of T cells in the peripheral blood, a more detailed analysis might be beneficial. Retrospective examination of peripheral blood T cell subsets in ipilimumab-treated melanoma patients revealed that higher pre-treatment $CD4^{+}/CD25^{+}/FoxP3^{+}$ Tregs was associated with favorable survival (41, 45) (**Table 1**). Tregs express high levels of CTLA-4 and might, therefore, be one of the main targets of ipilimumab. It was shown that more melanoma-reactive $CD8^{+}$ cytotoxic T cells in the peripheral blood were detected in patients after treatment than before treatment (83). Preexisting immune responses were only infrequently boosted.

Most studies have focused on PD-L1 expression on tumor cells and macrophages in the tumor microenvironment, whereas PD-L1-expression on peripheral T cells has been studied to a lesser extent. High PD-L1 expression on peripheral T cells ($CD4^{+}$ and $CD8^{+}$) has been shown to be associated with worse PFS and OS for CTLA4ab treatment of melanoma (55). For an NSCLC cohort treated mainly by chemotherapy, high PD-1/PD-L1/PD-L2 expression on peripheral blood T cells was associated with shorter OS (84). PD-L1 expression on peripheral T cells might, therefore, be a mechanism for tumor immune escape. Expression of co-stimulatory molecules on peripheral T cells was also studied. Detectable levels of $CD137^{+}CD8^{+}$ cytotoxic T cells in the peripheral blood were found in patients with relapse-free status after adjuvant combined ICI, but this was not investigated in the therapeutic setting (55). CyTOF analysis revealed that high pre-treatment incidence of memory T cells was a potential marker for response to CTLA4ab, whereas higher incidence of distinct NK cell subsets was found to be associated with response to PD1ab treatment for melanoma (54).

Tumor antigen presentation by human leukocyte antigen class I (HLA-I) molecules is a prerequisite for cancer cell attack by cytotoxic T cells. Maximum heterozygosity at HLA-I loci (A, B, C) opposed to homozygosity for at least one HLA locus was shown to be associated with longer OS after ICI for mainly NSCLC and melanoma (56). Furthermore, HLA-B44 supertype was linked to prolonged OS, whereas the HLA-B62 supertype or somatic loss of heterozygosity at HLA-I were associated with worse OS for melanoma (56). Although assessed in test and validation cohorts, these biomarkers have also not been prospectively tested for their potential predictive versus prognostic value. Nevertheless, this investigation indicates that diversity in antigen presentation might improve tumor defense. Tumor cell antigens presented on MHC molecules are recognized by T cells *via* the T cell receptor (TCR). The TCR is, therefore, of great interest in ICI. TCR diversity and clonality can be investigated by use of sequencing methods. Most investigations focus on TCR sequencing in tumor tissue specimens (see "Tissue Biomarkers"). TCR sequencing data in the peripheral blood are limited. In ipilimumab-treated melanoma patients, patients with a positive clinical outcome had a higher degree of TCR repertoire richness prior to therapy (57). In patients with urothelial carcinoma, TCR sequencing in peripheral blood was done before and after atezolizumab administration. Here, a pretreatment TCR clonality below the median was associated with improved PFS and OS (85). Furthermore, a long-lasting clinical benefit was found in patients with a more substantial expansion of tumor-associated TCR clones after three weeks (85). T cells carrying the γδ-TCR-subtype—as opposed to the more common αβ-subtype—play a distinct role in anti-tumor immunology. A study found that higher incidence of $V\delta2^+$ cells (versus $V\delta1^+$ cells) was linked to longer OS in melanoma patients, and suggested that $V\delta2^+$ cells potentially have tumor-killing capability (86). However, this has not yet been investigated for ICI.

In summary, T cells as the effector cells of ICI are the focus of biomarker research for melanoma and other malignancies. Some approaches are promising, but no biomarker has yet been evaluated in a prospective clinical setting. Their predictive ability therefore remains to be determined.

Soluble Serum Biomarkers

Soluble serum biomarkers that might correlate with clinical benefit of ICI treatment include immune regulatory molecules such as cytokines or soluble checkpoint receptors and binding partners. Biomarker potential in ICI treatment of melanoma (**Table 1**) and other malignancies has been found for several soluble serum factors.

Soluble CTLA-4 (sCTLA4), which is mainly secreted by regulatory T cells (Tregs), has inhibitory effects on T cell immune responses (87). An association has been found between higher sCTLA4 levels and both response and prolonged OS for a small cohort of ipilimumab-treated melanoma patients; this was not found for patients who did not receive ipilimumab (58). In view of its inhibitory function on T cells, neutralization by CTLA4ab therapy might be responsible for this finding. Higher levels of soluble PD-L1 (sPD-L1) can be found in tumor patients compared with healthy individuals (88, 89). Its physiological role has not yet been identified (89). It holds some prognostic value because high pre-treatment concentrations are associated with shorter OS for NSCLC (88), and for hepatocellular carcinoma (90), and it is linked to disease progression in ICI for melanoma (59). sPD-L1 is, however, likely to be only prognostic and not predictive for melanoma, because assessments pre- and during early ICI did not reveal significant associations with response or OS (59). In addition to sPD-L1, a soluble form of PD-1 (sPD-1) also exists (89) which is currently being investigated in a clinical trial (NCT03197636).

Soluble ligands of the transmembrane receptor NKG2D (sULBP-1, sULBP-2), which affect induction or reactivation of T cell responses, were associated with OS for ICI-treated but not for BRAF inhibitor-treated melanoma patients (44). They are interesting biomarkers with treatment-specific potential. Further data are, however, needed to confirm the significance of these markers. In addition, soluble CD25 (sCD25), the alpha unit of the IL-2 receptor, was found to be a biomarker in ipilimumab therapy. The interleukin (IL)-2/IL-2 receptor pathway is essential for the antitumor activity of CTLA4ab (91). High pre-treatment serum levels of sCD25 were shown to be associated with shorter OS for CTLA4ab-treated patients (60). A possible explanation for this finding could be direct binding of sCD25 to IL-2, which would amplify Tregs and inhibit tumor immune response.

It has been shown that other serum factors including vascular epithelial growth factor and chemokines such as C-X-C chemokine motif ligand (CXCL)8 are of prognostic significance for PFS and OS of melanoma of different stages, regardless of treatment (92). For CTLA4ab therapy, elevated pre-treatment levels of CXCL11 were associated with poor OS (61). The gene expression of CXCL11 is induced by interferon-(IFN)-γ, and CXCL11 binds to its chemokine receptor CXCR3, which is mainly expressed on activated T cells. CXCR3 is highly important for the migration of cytotoxic T cells, and its tissue expression correlates with poorer prognosis for several malignancies (93). Elevated CXCL11 in blood has been linked to poorer outcome for ipilimumab-treated melanoma (61). For PD1ab treatment, serum IFN-γ, IL-6 and IL-10 levels were significantly higher for responders than for non-responders (62).

In contrast to single-biomarker searches, serum-based multi-marker assays are of current and future interest. One group developed a test based on 119 patients with pre-PD1ab therapy for metastatic melanoma using matrix-assisted laser desorption/ionization-time of flight (MALDI–TOF) mass spectrometry, which was validated in four independent cohorts (63). Computational algorithms were used for data analysis, resulting in a protein signature of 209 proteins that appears to differentiate patients with three-year OS of over 50% from patients with three-year OS of less than 20%. Further analysis revealed that acute phase proteins, complement, and wound healing pathways were associated with poor outcome (63). Because this test has also not been prospectively evaluated yet, distinction of prognostic versus predictive ability is warranted.

Liquid Biopsy

Liquid biopsy, including CTCs, ctDNA, and circulating tumor RNA (ctRNA) has only been studied in small patient cohorts treated by use of ICI (mainly CTLA4ab) for melanoma. An association between treatment response and a decrease in CTCs and ctDNA has been found for targeted therapy, but not for ICI (94). Methodological improvements offer new opportunities for CTC detection, as has been very recently described for microfluidic enrichment of melanoma CTCs combined with RNA-based droplet digital PCR quantitation (64). That study found that a decrease in CTCs within the first seven weeks of ICI was linked to prolonged PFS and OS in CTLA4ab or PD1ab-treated melanoma patients (64). Another approach to CTCs is characterization of subsets of CTCs that express specific markers. The heterogeneity of melanoma CTCs and the significance of CTC subsets (e.g., receptor activator of NF-κβ (RANK) expressing CTCs) as biomarkers has been found to affect targeted treatment; this was not, however, observed for ICI (65). For NSCLC, high expression of carcinoembryonic antigen and telomerase reverse transcriptase was linked to non-response to nivolumab (95). For urothelial carcinoma, CTCs with high PD-L1 expression were associated with worse OS (96), and for chemotherapeutically treated SCCHN, high levels of CTCs with PD-L1 expression were linked to poor PFS and OS (97). CTCs are being studied as part of a recruiting clinical trial on prospective biomarkers for melanoma, and this will hopefully shed light on a potential predictive function of CTCs for ICI.

Not only CTCs but also ctDNA has been investigated in PD1ab therapy. A proof-of-concept study found that detectable levels of ctDNA in week 8 of PD1ab therapy were linked to worse PFS and OS for NSCLC, uveal melanoma, and microsatellite-instable colorectal cancer (98). Furthermore, an association was found between high hypermutated ctDNA levels and response, PFS, and OS for diverse malignancies treated by use of ICI (99).

Other Blood Biomarkers

Several other blood biomarkers have been investigated in ICI patients; for example, blood-based testing of gene-expression profiles of cathepsin D, phopholipase A2 group VII, thioredoxin reductase 1, and interleukin 1 receptor-associated kinase 3 were found to be associated with OS for CTLA4ab-treated patients (100). Ongoing studies on blood biomarkers for ICI treatment of melanoma include assessment of different T cell subsets, cytokines, and CTCs (**Table 1**). The challenge is to select the most promising biomarkers, ideally identified by several different investigators, and to study them in prospective clinical trials.

STOOL BIOMARKERS

The effect of gut microbiota on anti-tumor response has recently been observed in both murine and human studies for several cancers, including melanoma, NSCLC, and RCC. Unsurprisingly, microorganisms are prevalent in primary CRC, but distant metastases are also colonized with Fusobacterium and its associated microbiome, including Bacteroides, Selenomonas, and Prevotella species (101). Gut flora composition can stimulate or inhibit immune response. Immunostimulatory effects of Bacteroidales, particularly *Bacteroides fragilis*, have been observed for CTLA4ab therapy in mice (102). Similarly, Bifidobacterium improved anti-tumor responses for PD-1/PD-L1 blockade in a murine melanoma model (103). In contrast, ICI treatment itself can affect the population of gut microbiota (102). Baseline gut microbiota have been investigated in small CTLA4ab-treated melanoma cohorts (**Table 1**). Enrichment with Faecalibacterium and other Firmucutes was associated with improved response and with development of colitis, whereas a higher representation of Bacteroidetes was related to poorer response to CTLA4ab therapy (66). For melanoma patients receiving PD1ab therapy, enrichment of Ruminococcaceae and Clostridiales was found in responders whereas Bacteriodales were enriched in non-responders (67). Shortened PFS was observed for patients with high abundance of Bacteroidales, which is in agreement with another publication on melanoma patients treated with CTLA4ab (66). Another analysis found enrichment of *Bacteroides caccae* in all ICI responders, and specifically *Faecalibacterium prausnitzii*, *Bacteroides thetaiotaomicron*, and *Holdemania filiformis* if treated with ipilimumab plus nivolumab combination therapy. *Dorea formicogenerans* was enriched in pembrolizumab responders (68). Other authors found relative abundance of *Bifidobacterium longum*, *Collinsella aerofaciens*, and *Enterococcus faecium* in PD1ab responders with melanoma (69). An imbalance in gut microbiota correlating with impaired immune cell activity was observed for non-responders. Treatment by use of antibiotics before or shortly after ICI was associated with poorer response and worse OS for patients with RCC and NSCLC; in this analysis, a higher percentage of non-responders (69%) had a particularly low level of *Akkermansia muciniphila* compared with responders (34%) (104). It is worth nothing that in a mouse model, fecal transplants of responders into germ-free mice restored the anti-tumor effect of PD-1/PD-L1 blockade (67, 69, 104).

In summary, gut microbiota affect anti-tumor immune response. However, there is only partial overlap between the potentially relevant microorganisms (**Table 1**). It is unclear if this is because of methodological reasons, or if it depends on the individual tumor entity, or the geographical region and associated dietary habits of the investigated patients. Further prospective studies are needed to evaluate the prognostic or predictive effect of gut microbiota on ICI outcome (currently ongoing: NCT02960282, NCT03370861). A study on fecal microbiota transplantation for metastatic melanoma patients who failed ICI is also being conducted (NCT03353402).

TISSUE BIOMARKERS

PD-L1 Expression

In the initial phase I study of nivolumab for patients with solid tumors, an association between PD-L1 expression and probability of response was observed for NSCLC, melanoma, and RCC (105, 106) (**Table 2**). Because clinical significance was greatest for NSCLC, this led to further PD1ab studies using enrichment designs with different antibodies and expression cutoffs (107–109). Because patients with PD-L1 negative (or PD-L1 expression below cutoff) value cannot be followed in clinical trials of enriched design, it is not possible to distinguish between

TABLE 2 | Tissue and imaging biomarkers for clinical outcome under checkpoint blockage for metastatic melanoma patients.

Biomarker	Number of patients	Treatment	Results	Reference
Tissue Biomarkers				
PD-L1 expression	*n* = 41–43 (melanoma, NSCLC, renal cell carcinoma, and others)	Nivolumab, atezolizumab	PD-L1 expression on tumor or TILs associated with response	(105) (106) (113)
	n = 945 (stratified for PD-L1 expression)	Ipilimumab, nivolumab, ipilimumab plus nivolumab	Patients with PD-L1 negative tumors had longer PFS and OS under combined ICI compared to nivolumab monotherapy	(5) (114)
Tumor-infiltrating lymphocytes (TILs)	*n* = 82	Ipilimumab	High baseline FoxP3 and IDO expression and increase in TILs from week 0 to week 3 associated with disease control	(115)
	n = 20	Nivolumab, pembrolizumab	Partially exhausted (PD-1^{high}CTLA-4^{high}) tumor-infiltrating $CD8^+$ T cells correlated with response and longer PFS	(116)
	n = 16–46	Pembrolizumab	Cytotoxic T cells at tumor margins associated with response, higher clonal expansion of TCR in responders	(117)
	n = 32–33	Nivolumab, pembrolizumab, atezolizumab	TCR clonality not associated with outcome	(118, 119)
Mutational load, neoantigen load	*n* = 38–110	Ipilimumab, tremelimumab, nivolumab, pembrolizumab	High mutational and neoantigen load associated with clinical benefit (response, DCR > 6 months, PFS, OS)	(85, 120) (121) (122) (123) (124)
	n = 68	Nivolumab	Mutational and neoantigen load decreased with treatment in responders	(125)
Single mutations	*n* = 229	IL-2, CTLA4ab, PD1ab, PD-L1ab, not specified	NRAS mutation correlated with disease control and longer PFS	(126)
	n = 32–33	Nivolumab, pembrolizumab, atezolizumab	NF-1 mutation associated with mutational load and response, NRAS-mutations not associated with clinical outcome	(118, 119)
	n = 38	Nivolumab, pembrolizumab	Tumors from responders were enriched for BRCA2 mutations	(122)
Histological subtype	*n* = 60 (desmoplastic melanoma)	Nivolumab or pembrolizumab ± ipilimumab, PD-L1ab, not specified	Desmoplastic melanoma showed higher response rates as reported in the literature (probably because of high mutational burden)	(127)
MHC-I/II expression	*n* = 23–30	Nivolumab, pembrolizumab, atezolizumab	MHC-II positivity on tumor cells associated with response, PFS, and OS	(118, 119)
Gene expression	*n* = 21–45	Ipilimumab	High IFN-γ expression and of IFN-γ-inducible genes (e.g., CXCL9, CXCL10, and CXCL11) correlated with longer PFS, OS	(128) (129)
	n = 43 (melanoma only)	Atezolizumab	Expression of baseline T helper type 1, CTLA4, and IFN-inducible genes (e.g., IDO1, CXCL9) as well as the absence of CX3CL1 associated with response	(113)
Imaging Biomarkers				
Tumor burden measured by CT (RECIST1.1)	*n* = 593	Pembrolizumab	Lower baseline tumor burden (RECIST 1.1) associated with longer OS	(26)
FDG-PET/CT	*n* = 22	Ipilimumab	FDG-PET/CT (EORTC criteria) at week 5 predicts disease progression while response could not be identified	(130)
	n = 20	Ipilimumab (*n* = 16), nivolumab (*n* = 1), PD-L1ab BMS-936559 (*n* = 3)	FDG-PET/CT at week 3–4 predicted best response at ≥4 months [using RECIST 1.1, immune-related response criteria, EORTC criteria, and PET response criteria in solid tumors (PERCIST)]	(131)
	n = 41	Ipilimumab	Cutoff of four newly emerged FDG-avid lesions on PET/CT after 12 weeks indicates treatment failure, SUV changes did not correlate with clinical outcome	(132)
FDG-PET/MRI (PERCIST)	*n* = 10	PD1ab, not specified	Metabolic response at week 2 might indicate response at 3 months	(133)

CT, computerized tomography; CTLA4ab, anti-CTLA-4 antibody; FDG, ^{18}F-fluoro-deoxy-glucose; MRI, magnetic resonance imaging; PET, positron emission tomography; PD1ab, anti-PD-1 antibody; PFS, progression-free survival; OS, overall survival; SUV, standard uptake value; DCR, disease control rate; TCR, T cell receptor.

prognostic and predictive value (20). It is worth mentioning that in a retrospective analysis of metastatic melanoma patients, PD-L1 expression was linked to improved OS irrespective of treatment type; this raises the possibility of a prognostic rather than a predictive value for ICI (28). Throughout several clinical trials for NSCLC and urothelial cancer, no association was observed between PD-L1 expression and ICI therapy outcome (8, 110, 111). There was one exception: for urothelial carcinoma, a composite biomarker of either ≥25% positive tumor cells or ≥25% positive immune cells indicated tumor response to durvalumab, and is a pre-requisite for treatment according to FDA-approval (15). PD-L1 positivity was also associated with higher probability of response in a subgroup analysis of PD-L1ab therapy for MCC (14). In addition, PD-L1 expression on tumor and immune cells was linked to higher incidence of response for SCCHN (112). There is growing evidence that response is associated more with PD-L1 expression on tumor-infiltrating immune cells than it is with tumor cell PD-L1 expression (113).

PD-L1 expression on tumor cells was used to stratify the design of the Checkmate-067 trial investigating the combination of ipilimumab plus nivolumab compared with nivolumab and ipilimumab monotherapies (5). Although not designed for this purpose, this study revealed that patients with tumors expressing PD-L1 had similar PFS and OS compared with PD1ab monotherapy and the combination of CTLA4ab plus PD1ab (5, 114). Response to combined ICI was still higher, however, compared with response to PD1ab monotherapy. The study was not designed to compare the two nivolumab-containing treatment arms, but it shows possible limitations of PD-L1 as a biomarker for treatment decisions for melanoma.

General problems associated with PD-L1 as a biomarker are: use of different immunohistochemical (IHC) assays, different cut-offs, intra-tumor heterogeneity, and dynamic changes of PD-L1 expression. In summary, there are conflicting data in diverse tumor entities. It is worth noting that treatment responses can be found in PD-L1-negative tumors.

Tumor-Infiltrating Lymphocytes (TIL)

The presence of TILs has prognostic potential for different tumor entities regardless of tumor stage (134, 135). For patients with metastatic melanoma, TILs were associated with a better outcome for primary melanoma and metastatic disease, irrespective of treatment type (28, 136). A prospective biomarker study of ipilimumab-treated patients with melanoma found an association between early increase in TILs and disease control (115) (**Table 2**). A more detailed assessment of the T cell infiltrate at baseline revealed an association between high baseline FoxP3$^+$ Tregs and indoleamine-2,3-dioxygenase (IDO) expression and favorable outcome (115). For PD1ab-treated melanoma patients, no association was found between baseline TILs and response to PD1ab (106). Abundance of partially exhausted (PD-1^{high}CTLA-4^{high}) tumor-infiltrating CD8$^+$ T cells correlated with response and PFS in PD1ab therapy (116). Cytotoxic T cells at tumor margins were also linked to response to PD1abs (117). Preliminary investigations on TCR clonality of TILs in melanoma metastases revealed higher clonal expansion of TCR for PD1ab-responders compared with non-responders (117). This finding was not, however, confirmed by other authors (119).

Interferon-γ is one of the cytokines secreted by activated T cells and is known to upregulate PD-L1 expression. This might be one reason why PD-L1 expression could be co-localized with TIL infiltrates in melanoma metastases (117, 137). In a retrospective analysis, pretreatment tumor samples from NSCLC and melanoma patients treated with PD1ab were evaluated for IFN-γ expression (129). A significantly longer PFS and OS were observed for patients with high IFN-γ expression. High pre-treatment expression of IFN-inducible genes (e.g., IDO1, CXCL9, CXCL10, and CXCL11 among others) was associated with response and prolonged OS for PD-L1ab treatment of melanoma, but this was less pronounced for NSCLC or RCC (113, 128). Primary mutations in IFN-γ signaling pathways (e.g., JAK1 and JAK2 mutations) have been described for several tumor entities. For cutaneous melanomas, JAK1/2 mutations were detected before treatment in 21% of tissue specimens (138). Interestingly, patients with resistance to ICI were found to harbor JAK mutations with consecutive loss of IFN-γ pathways (139, 140).

The following challenges apply for all potential tissue biomarkers described above: possible dependency on biopsy site, the specific time of the biopsy, and intratumor-heterogeneity. It should be noted that, when considering multiple potential biomarkers, large multivariable analyses are required to exclude a significant overlap of markers (138). Moreover, future models might include transcriptome-derived stromal and immune cell scores exceeding a pure TIL assessment (141).

Mutational Analysis

The first notion that mutational changes might affect tumor response came with the observation that melanoma patients with a high mutation rate benefitted more from ipilimumab treatment than patients with a low one, resulting in longer OS (120). In agreement with this, tumors with a naturally high mutation rate because of exogenous cancerogens, such as UV light, smoking, and alcohol (melanoma, lung cancer, SCCHN, and bladder cancer), belong to the entities that respond best to ICI treatment (123, 142–145). A small biomarker-stratified trial was performed for non-colorectal CRC and mismatch-repair deficient cancers. Stratification according to mismatch repair deficiency and mismatch-repair proficiency revealed a 40% response for patients with mismatch-repair deficiency (MSI high, dMMR), whereas mismatch-repair proficient patients did not respond at all (146). Whereas mismatch-repair deficiency can be found in gastro-intestinal and genitourinary tumors (147, 148), it is of minor significance for melanoma. Colli et al. suggested a cutoff of 192 nonsynonymous mutations for a potential clinical benefit of ICI (149). Here, a high mutational load seems to result in prolonged OS in particular, whereas no correlation with response to PD1ab was observed (122). This is in agreement with the observation that melanoma patients treated with PD1ab survive longer even when not responding to the treatment (150). This was found to change, however, for ipilimumab treatment prior to PD1ab therapy; in contrast to ipilimumab-naïve patients, no association between tumor mutational burden and response/OS was observed (125). Most likely, the difference is not because of the number of mutations, but because of the increasing chance of tumor neoepitopes which might be easier recognized by the immune system. Clonal neoantigens in particular might significantly affect ICI outcome (120, 123).

A considerable difficulty of using mutational load as a biomarker is its practical implementation in clinical routine. In addition to the high costs incurred by whole exome sequencing, most neoantigens are probably patient-specific and not recurrent (121). Specific types of mutations might be more frequent, e.g., the frameshift insertion and deletion count was found to be associated with ICI response for melanoma (124). Furthermore, several groups have proposed fitness models to describe neoantigen qualities that could be possibly employed as biomarkers in the future (151, 152). It is not clear, however, that neoantigen burden will add significant value to mutational burden testing, as shown in the examples of urothelial carcinoma and melanoma (85, 153).

Tumor antigen presentation is essential for the immune defense of cancer, and mutations affecting pathways important for antigen presentation, e.g., beta-2-microglobuline (B2M) loss, might result in ICI resistance (139). B2M mutations are more frequent for melanoma, bladder, gastric, and lung cancer in particular, with 27–50% found for these cancers in The Cancer Genome Atlas dataset compared with 1.8% across all tumor types (138). The MHC-II-expression itself (HLA-DR$^+$) was found to be associated with PD1ab/PD-L1ab response in melanoma (118).

It would be easy to use biomarkers for mutations that are routinely assessed in clinical care. BRAF-V600 mutations, which are found in 40–50% of melanomas, are not associated with ICI outcome (154–157). A subgroup survival analysis of combined ipilimumab plus nivolumab versus PD1ab monotherapy showed a trend toward longer OS for combined ICI treatment of BRAF-mutant patients, but this needs to be addressed further (114). In a retrospective analysis from the pre-ICI era, NRAS mutations, which are seen in up to 20% of melanomas, were found to be associated with worse OS (158). After introduction of ICI, a retrospective study investigating patients treated by immunotherapy, including IL-2, CTLA4ab, PD1ab, and PD-L1ab revealed greater disease control and longer PFS for NRAS-mutant melanoma (126). This result was not, however, found for a smaller cohort of patients with PD1ab/PD-L1ab therapy (119). The NF-1 mutation, which is associated with UV damage and high mutational load, was linked to higher incidence of response and prolonged survival for PD1ab-treated patients (119). A more favorable response to PD1ab therapy was observed for desmoplastic melanomas which are characterized by a high mutational load and frequent NF-1 mutations (127); it should be mentioned that this observation was also made from retrospective assessment. For NSCLC, single-gene mutation analysis showed that the presence of an EGFR-mutation seems to be a negative predictor for PD1ab response (159). NGS data, however, revealed a lower mutational burden for EGFR-mutant NSCLC, which could be one reason for this finding (160).

Objectives for the future include exploration and validation of a panel of genetic biomarkers detected by next-generation sequencing. Definition of cutoffs is a current challenge because absolute values depend on the depth of sequencing. Furthermore, gene translocations/fusions and other variants will not be detected by use of targeted sequencing techniques. Development of multi-marker assays is more complex and specific computational algorithms must be used for validation (20).

IMAGING BIOMARKERS

Anatomic Imaging

The use of imaging enables non-invasive assessment of tumor dimensions and can also provide biologic tumor data. The current standard assessment procedure for metastatic melanoma and other advanced malignancies is computerized tomography (CT) with iodine contrast dye, evaluated according to response evaluation criteria in solid tumors (RECIST) 1.1 (161). It has been shown that the size of baseline tumor lesions is associated with OS (26, 162). This is probably of prognostic value because it correlates with tumor load. However, RECIST 1.1 might be insufficient to evaluate response to ICI therapy, in particular cases of initial tumor progression or occurrence of new lesions during ICI. To overcome this problem, immune-related response criteria (irRC and irRECIST) have been introduced as alternative response criteria (163). Pure anatomic imaging is, however, unlikely to be sufficient to predict tumor response to ICI. New imaging biomarkers for metabolic and immune imaging are discussed below.

Metabolic Imaging

In addition to anatomic imaging, metabolic imaging by use of ^{18}F-fluoro-deoxy-glucose-positron emission tomography (FDG-PET) can add clinically meaningful data when imaging malignancies. Two different response criteria for FDG-PET imaging are currently used in clinical routine: European Organisation for Research and Treatment of Cancer (EORTC) criteria and positron emission tomography response criteria in solid tumors (PERCIST) (164, 165). It has been shown that FDG-PET combined with CT is of clinical value for assessment of ICI responses in melanoma (130–132) (**Table 2**). The assumption for metabolic imaging is that metabolic changes in tumors occur prior to anatomic changes, which might enable prediction of response to ICI earlier during the course of treatment. This can be prevented by the failure to discriminate between inflammation and tumor metabolism (166). For ipilimumab, one clinical trial showed that FDG-PET/CT 5 weeks after treatment initiation could predict disease progression to CTLA4ab; patients responding to treatment could not be identified at this time (130). In another trial it was possible to predict best response by use of PERCIST and EORTC criteria (131). To evaluate ICI response, a new PET-CT classification, the PET response evaluation criteria for immunotherapy criteria, was developed to reflect the fact that single new lesions do not define disease progression. The absolute number of new lesions was, however, more important than changes in standardized uptake values (SUV) (132). During PD1ab therapy for melanoma, use of FDG-PET/magnetic resonance imaging (MRI) as early as 2 weeks after the start of treatment might identify patients with complete response at the 3-month time-point (133). For FDG-PET/CT for NSCLC, maximum SUV at 4 weeks after commencement of PD1ab therapy was associated with PFS and OS (167). However, these are case series and small prospective studies. Larger prospective trials are needed to investigate these findings further.

^{18}F-fluorothymidine-PET (FLT-PET) uses a thymidine analog that accumulates in proliferating tissues, including malignant and immune cells (168). Positive findings were published for e.g., differentiation of cerebral radionecrosis from glioma progression (169), and correlation of mean SUV with OS for resectable pancreatic carcinoma (170). In contrast, no association was found between early changes in FLT uptake after the first cycle of chemotherapy for CRC and the response evaluated from subsequent CT scans (171). Its value as a biomarker for ICI in melanoma has only been reported in one case of FLT-PET/MRI; this precludes general conclusions (172). Further clinical evaluation of FLT-PET in ICI is, therefore, warranted. O-(2-[18F]fluoroethyl)-L-tyrosine (FET-)PET can be used to specifically image primary brain tumors and metastases to the brain which can be differentiated from healthy, inflamed, and radionecrotic tissue (173, 174). FET-uptake correlates with ki-67 expression and could be a potential biomarker for early response assessment (175). For melanoma, a case report showed that pseudo-progression of melanoma brain metastases could be detected by use of FET-PET (176) but more data are needed to assess the value of FET-PET in ICI.

Modern MRI techniques, including dynamic contrast-enhanced MRI, are also available for high resolution imaging of tumor perfusion or cell-membrane permeability (177). This technique could be particularly useful for assessment of specific metastatic sites, e.g., hepatic metastasis (178). Another potential application could be MRI-based immune-cell tracking and assessment of drug delivery (179).

With the exception of FDG-PET/CT, all the methods described above have been studied in only a few patients, and rarely in the setting of ICI. Results of ongoing studies will reveal a potential prognostic or predictive value of PET-biomarkers.

Immuno-Imaging

Several immuno-PET tracers, namely monoclonal antibodies, scaffold proteins, or peptides have been evaluated in preclinical tumor models. Potential targets are, for example, CD8$^+$ cytotoxic T cells, PD-1, and PD-L1. Immuno-PET tracers have been studied in preclinical models. A ^{89}Zr-labeled PEGylated single-domain anti-CD8 antibody was used for longitudinal evaluation of CTLA4ab treatment in the B16-melanoma mouse model. A homogeneous distribution of the anti-CD8 PET signal was observed for responding animals, whereas a heterogeneous signal was associated with lower response and faster tumor growth (180). Another group studied a ^{89}Zr-desferrioxamine-labeled anti-CD8 cys-diabody in PD1ab treatment of Balb/c mice with CRC. They found a higher SUV in responding animals compared with non-responding ones. They also found that uptake for responders tended to be intra-tumoral, whereas uptake for non-responders was in the margins of the tumor (181); this is in agreement with the role of intra-tumoral CD8$^+$ cytotoxic T cells in PD1ab response.

Another T cell imaging approach is *via* visualization of PD-1. The feasibility of this method has been proven in murine studies. Natarajan et al. developed the anti-PD-1 tracers ^{89}Zr-keytruda and ^{64}Cu-keytruda; these were evaluated in a humanized NOD-scid mouse model, and uptake in tumors and lymphoid tissue was observed for human melanoma tumors (182). Other groups developed radiotracers which target PD-L1 expressed on tumor cells and on immune cells of the tumor microenvironment (183–185). The feasibility of PD-L1 imaging was shown by use of ^{64}Cu-atezolizumab in mice with tumors constitutively expressing PD-L1, and in two breast cancer mouse models (183). Investigation of irradiated versus non-irradiated tumors in a HPV + SCHNN and a B16F10 melanoma mouse models by use of an ^{89}Zr-labeled anti-PD-L1 monoclonal antibody revealed PD-L1 upregulation in irradiated tumors specifically (184). In a patient-derived xenograft model of NSCLC, the ^{89}Zr-C4-PD-L1 antibody revealed PD-L1 changes after chemotherapy (185).

These immuno-PET tracers have been investigated in animal models, which can certainly improve understanding of response or non-response mechanisms to ICI treatment. Studies in humans are under way. A possible predictive ability of immuno-PET in the setting of ICI, however, needs to be explored in the future (NCT03313323, NCT02760225).

CONCLUSION

Several factors might affect response to ICI treatment, including mutational load, tumor microenvironment, and stool microbiome. Upfront exclusion of metastatic melanoma patients from ICI therapy on the basis of biomarkers is not currently possible. It also remains unclear which patients will need combined ICI and which patients will benefit from use of PD1ab only. Although there are several potential biomarkers, their predictive versus prognostic abilities have not yet been validated by prospective clinical trials. In particular, the best sequence of treatment to follow, e.g., targeted versus immunotherapy for melanoma, cannot be answered on the basis of the biomarker data currently available.

Peripheral blood immune-cell analysis, e.g., by use of CyTOF, enables investigation of multiple markers, and will hopefully reveal predictive biomarkers in future. A multi-marker assay is more likely than a single biomarker. Future challenges include the development and validation of multi-marker assays, which will require detailed pre-analytics, computation algorithms, and, most importantly, well-designed clinical trials with large numbers of patients.

AUTHOR CONTRIBUTIONS

KB-B and JH contributed to the conception and design of the article, acquisition and interpretation of data, drafting of the article, critical revision, and final approval. Both are accountable for the content of this manuscript.

REFERENCES

1. Robert C, Thomas L, Bondarenko I, O'Day S, Weber J, Garbe C, et al. Ipilimumab plus dacarbazine for previously untreated metastatic melanoma. *N Engl J Med* (2011) 364:2517–26. doi:10.1056/NEJMoa1104621
2. Robert C, Ribas A, Wolchok JD, Hodi FS, Hamid O, Kefford R, et al. Anti-programmed-death-receptor-1 treatment with pembrolizumab in ipilimumab-refractory advanced melanoma: a randomised dose-comparison cohort of a phase 1 trial. *Lancet* (2014) 384:1109–17. doi:10.1016/S0140-6736(14)60958-2
3. Robert C, Long GV, Brady B, Dutriaux C, Maio M, Mortier L, et al. Nivolumab in previously untreated melanoma without BRAF mutation. *N Engl J Med* (2015) 372:320–30. doi:10.1056/NEJMoa1412082
4. Weber JS, D'Angelo SP, Minor D, Hodi FS, Gutzmer R, Neyns B, et al. Nivolumab versus chemotherapy in patients with advanced melanoma who progressed after anti-CTLA-4 treatment (CheckMate 037): a randomised, controlled, open-label, phase 3 trial. *Lancet Oncol* (2015) 16:375–84. doi:10.1016/S1470-2045(15)70076-8
5. Larkin J, Chiarion-Sileni V, Gonzalez R, Grob JJ, Cowey CL, Lao CD, et al. Combined nivolumab and ipilimumab or monotherapy in untreated melanoma. *N Engl J Med* (2015) 373:23–34. doi:10.1056/NEJMoa1504030
6. Hassel JC, Heinzerling L, Aberle J, Bahr O, Eigentler TK, Grimm MO, et al. Combined immune checkpoint blockade (anti-PD-1/anti-CTLA-4): evaluation and management of adverse drug reactions. *Cancer Treat Rev* (2017) 57:36–49. doi:10.1016/j.ctrv.2017.05.003
7. Borghaei H, Paz-Ares L, Horn L, Spigel DR, Steins M, Ready NE, et al. Nivolumab versus docetaxel in advanced nonsquamous non-small-cell lung cancer. *N Engl J Med* (2015) 373:1627–39. doi:10.1056/NEJMoa1507643
8. Brahmer J, Reckamp KL, Baas P, Crino L, Eberhardt WE, Poddubskaya E, et al. Nivolumab versus docetaxel in advanced squamous-cell non-small-cell lung cancer. *N Engl J Med* (2015) 373:123–35. doi:10.1056/NEJMoa1504627
9. Garon EB, Rizvi NA, Hui R, Leighl N, Balmanoukian AS, Eder JP, et al. Pembrolizumab for the treatment of non-small-cell lung cancer. *N Engl J Med* (2015) 372:2018–28. doi:10.1056/NEJMoa1501824
10. Armand P, Shipp MA, Ribrag V, Michot JM, Zinzani PL, Kuruvilla J, et al. Programmed death-1 blockade with pembrolizumab in patients with classical Hodgkin lymphoma after brentuximab vedotin failure. *J Clin Oncol* (2016) 34:3733–9. doi:10.1200/JCO.2016.67.3467
11. El-Khoueiry AB, Sangro B, Yau T, Crocenzi TS, Kudo M, Hsu C, et al. Nivolumab in patients with advanced hepatocellular carcinoma (CheckMate 040): an open-label, non-comparative, phase 1/2 dose escalation and expansion trial. *Lancet* (2017) 389:2492–502. doi:10.1016/S0140-6736(17)31046-2
12. Kasamon YL, De Claro RA, Wang Y, Shen YL, Farrell AT, Pazdur R. FDA approval summary: nivolumab for the treatment of relapsed or progressive classical Hodgkin lymphoma. *Oncologist* (2017) 22:585–91. doi:10.1634/theoncologist.2017-0004
13. Fehrenbacher L, Spira A, Ballinger M, Kowanetz M, Vansteenkiste J, Mazieres J, et al. Atezolizumab versus docetaxel for patients with previously treated non-small-cell lung cancer (POPLAR): a multicentre, open-label, phase 2 randomised controlled trial. *Lancet* (2016) 387:1837–46. doi:10.1016/S0140-6736(16)00587-0
14. Kaufman HL, Russell J, Hamid O, Bhatia S, Terheyden P, D'Angelo SP, et al. Avelumab in patients with chemotherapy-refractory metastatic Merkel cell carcinoma: a multicentre, single-group, open-label, phase 2 trial. *Lancet Oncol* (2016) 17:1374–85. doi:10.1016/S1470-2045(16)30364-3
15. Massard C, Gordon MS, Sharma S, Rafii S, Wainberg ZA, Luke J, et al. Safety and efficacy of durvalumab (MEDI4736), an anti-programmed cell death ligand-1 immune checkpoint inhibitor, in patients with advanced urothelial bladder cancer. *J Clin Oncol* (2016) 34:3119–25. doi:10.1200/JCO.2016.67.9761
16. Apolo AB, Infante JR, Balmanoukian A, Patel MR, Wang D, Kelly K, et al. Avelumab, an anti-programmed death-ligand 1 antibody, in patients with refractory metastatic urothelial carcinoma: results from a multicenter, phase Ib study. *J Clin Oncol* (2017) 35:2117–24. doi:10.1200/JCO.2016.71.6795
17. Gulley JL, Rajan A, Spigel DR, Iannotti N, Chandler J, Wong DJL, et al. Avelumab for patients with previously treated metastatic or recurrent non-small-cell lung cancer (JAVELIN solid tumor): dose-expansion cohort of a multicentre, open-label, phase 1b trial. *Lancet Oncol* (2017) 18:599–610. doi:10.1016/S1470-2045(17)30240-1
18. Ning YM, Suzman D, Maher VE, Zhang L, Tang S, Ricks T, et al. FDA approval summary: atezolizumab for the treatment of patients with progressive advanced urothelial carcinoma after platinum-containing chemotherapy. *Oncologist* (2017) 22:743–9. doi:10.1634/theoncologist.2017-0087
19. Overman MJ, Mcdermott R, Leach JL, Lonardi S, Lenz HJ, Morse MA, et al. Nivolumab in patients with metastatic DNA mismatch repair-deficient or microsatellite instability-high colorectal cancer (CheckMate 142): an open-label, multicentre, phase 2 study. *Lancet Oncol* (2017) 18:1182–91. doi:10.1016/S1470-2045(17)30422-9
20. Dobbin KK, Cesano A, Alvarez J, Hawtin R, Janetzki S, Kirsch I, et al. Validation of biomarkers to predict response to immunotherapy in cancer: volume II – clinical validation and regulatory considerations. *J Immunother Cancer* (2016) 4:77. doi:10.1186/s40425-016-0179-0
21. Masucci GV, Cesano A, Hawtin R, Janetzki S, Zhang J, Kirsch I, et al. Validation of biomarkers to predict response to immunotherapy in cancer: volume I – pre-analytical and analytical validation. *J Immunother Cancer* (2016) 4:76. doi:10.1186/s40425-016-0178-1
22. Brierley JD, Gospodarowicz MK, Wittekind C. *TNM Classification of Malignant Tumours*. 8th ed. Oxford, UK: Wiley Blackwell (2017).
23. Weide B, Martens A, Hassel JC, Berking C, Postow MA, Bisschop K, et al. Baseline biomarkers for outcome of melanoma patients treated with pembrolizumab. *Clin Cancer Res* (2016) 22:5487–96. doi:10.1158/1078-0432.CCR-16-0127
24. Nosrati A, Tsai KK, Goldinger SM, Tumeh P, Grimes B, Loo K, et al. Evaluation of clinicopathological factors in PD-1 response: derivation and validation of a prediction scale for response to PD-1 monotherapy. *Br J Cancer* (2017) 116:1141–7. doi:10.1038/bjc.2017.70
25. Tumeh PC, Hellmann MD, Hamid O, Tsai KK, Loo KL, Gubens MA, et al. Liver metastasis and treatment outcome with anti-PD-1 monoclonal antibody in patients with melanoma and NSCLC. *Cancer Immunol Res* (2017) 5:417–24. doi:10.1158/2326-6066.CIR-16-0325
26. Joseph RW, Elassaiss-Schaap J, Kefford RF, Hwu WJ, Wolchok JD, Joshua AM, et al. Baseline tumor size is an independent prognostic factor for overall survival in patients with melanoma treated with pembrolizumab. *Clin Cancer Res* (2018). doi:10.1158/1078-0432.CCR-17-2386
27. Long GV, Atkinson V, Lo S, Sandhu S, Guminski AD, Brown MP, et al. Combination nivolumab and ipilimumab or nivolumab alone in melanoma brain metastases: a multicentre randomised phase 2 study. *Lancet Oncol* (2018) 19:672–81. doi:10.1016/S1470-2045(18)30139-6
28. Kluger HM, Zito CR, Barr ML, Baine MK, Chiang VL, Sznol M, et al. Characterization of PD-L1 expression and associated T-cell infiltrates in metastatic melanoma samples from variable anatomic sites. *Clin Cancer Res* (2015) 21:3052–60. doi:10.1158/1078-0432.CCR-14-3073
29. Tawbi HA-H, Forsyth PAJ, Algazi AP, Hamid O, Hodi FS, Moschos SJ, et al. Efficacy and safety of nivolumab (NIVO) plus ipilimumab (IPI) in patients with melanoma (MEL) metastatic to the brain: results of the phase II study CheckMate 204. *J Clin Oncol* (2017) 35:9507. doi:10.1200/JCO.2017.35.15_suppl.9507
30. Nakamura Y, Kitano S, Takahashi A, Tsutsumida A, Namikawa K, Tanese K, et al. Nivolumab for advanced melanoma: pretreatment prognostic factors and early outcome markers during therapy. *Oncotarget* (2016) 7:77404–15. doi:10.18632/oncotarget.12677
31. Dick J, Lang N, Slynko A, Kopp-Schneider A, Schulz C, Dimitrakopoulou-Strauss A, et al. Use of LDH and autoimmune side effects to predict response to ipilimumab treatment. *Immunotherapy* (2016) 8:1033–44. doi:10.2217/imt-2016-0083
32. Weber JS, Hodi FS, Wolchok JD, Topalian SL, Schadendorf D, Larkin J, et al. Safety profile of nivolumab monotherapy: a pooled analysis of patients with advanced melanoma. *J Clin Oncol* (2017) 35:785–92. doi:10.1200/JCO.2015.66.1389
33. Faje AT, Sullivan R, Lawrence D, Tritos NA, Fadden R, Klibanski A, et al. Ipilimumab-induced hypophysitis: a detailed longitudinal analysis in a large cohort of patients with metastatic melanoma. *J Clin Endocrinol Metab* (2014) 99:4078–85. doi:10.1210/jc.2014-2306
34. Hua C, Boussemart L, Mateus C, Routier E, Boutros C, Cazenave H, et al. Association of vitiligo with tumor response in patients with metastatic melanoma treated with pembrolizumab. *JAMA Dermatol* (2016) 152:45–51. doi:10.1001/jamadermatol.2015.2707

35. Freeman-Keller M, Kim Y, Cronin H, Richards A, Gibney G, Weber JS. Nivolumab in resected and unresectable metastatic melanoma: characteristics of immune-related adverse events and association with outcomes. *Clin Cancer Res* (2016) 22:886–94. doi:10.1158/1078-0432.CCR-15-1136
36. Buder-Bakhaya K, Benesova K, Schulz C, Anwar H, Dimitrakopoulou-Strauss A, Weber TF, et al. Characterization of arthralgia induced by PD-1 antibody treatment in patients with metastasized cutaneous malignancies. *Cancer Immunol Immunother* (2018) 67:175–82. doi:10.1007/s00262-017-2069-9
37. Ascierto PA, Simeone E, Sileni VC, Pigozzo J, Maio M, Altomonte M, et al. Clinical experience with ipilimumab 3 mg/kg: real-world efficacy and safety data from an expanded access programme cohort. *J Transl Med* (2014) 12:116. doi:10.1186/1479-5876-12-116
38. Horvat TZ, Adel NG, Dang TO, Momtaz P, Postow MA, Callahan MK, et al. Immune-related adverse events, need for systemic immunosuppression, and effects on survival and time to treatment failure in patients with melanoma treated with ipilimumab at memorial Sloan Kettering Cancer Center. *J Clin Oncol* (2015) 33:3193–8. doi:10.1200/JCO.2015.60.8448
39. Kelderman S, Heemskerk B, Van Tinteren H, Van Den Brom RR, Hospers GA, Van Den Eertwegh AJ, et al. Lactate dehydrogenase as a selection criterion for ipilimumab treatment in metastatic melanoma. *Cancer Immunol Immunother* (2014) 63:449–58. doi:10.1007/s00262-014-1528-9
40. Valpione S, Martinoli C, Fava P, Mocellin S, Campana LG, Quaglino P, et al. Personalised medicine: development and external validation of a prognostic model for metastatic melanoma patients treated with ipilimumab. *Eur J Cancer* (2015) 51:2086–94. doi:10.1016/j.ejca.2015.06.130
41. Martens A, Wistuba-Hamprecht K, Geukes Foppen M, Yuan J, Postow MA, Wong P, et al. Baseline peripheral blood biomarkers associated with clinical outcome of advanced melanoma patients treated with ipilimumab. *Clin Cancer Res* (2016) 22:2908–18. doi:10.1158/1078-0432.CCR-15-2412
42. Diem S, Kasenda B, Spain L, Martin-Liberal J, Marconcini R, Gore M, et al. Serum lactate dehydrogenase as an early marker for outcome in patients treated with anti-PD-1 therapy in metastatic melanoma. *Br J Cancer* (2016) 114:256–61. doi:10.1038/bjc.2015.467
43. Krajsova I, Arenberger P, Lakomy R, Kubala E, Brezinova I, Poprach A, et al. Long-term survival with ipilimumab: experience from a national expanded access program for patients with melanoma. *Anticancer Res* (2015) 35:6303–10.
44. Maccalli C, Giannarelli D, Chiarucci C, Cutaia O, Giacobini G, Hendrickx W, et al. Soluble NKG2D ligands are biomarkers associated with the clinical outcome to immune checkpoint blockade therapy of metastatic melanoma patients. *Oncoimmunology* (2017) 6:e1323618. doi:10.1080/2162402X.2017.1323618
45. Simeone E, Gentilcore G, Giannarelli D, Grimaldi AM, Caraco C, Curvietto M, et al. Immunological and biological changes during ipilimumab treatment and their potential correlation with clinical response and survival in patients with advanced melanoma. *Cancer Immunol Immunother* (2014) 63:675–83. doi:10.1007/s00262-014-1545-8
46. Ferrucci PF, Ascierto PA, Pigozzo J, Del Vecchio M, Maio M, Antonini Cappellini GC, et al. Baseline neutrophils and derived neutrophil-to-lymphocyte ratio: prognostic relevance in metastatic melanoma patients receiving ipilimumab. *Ann Oncol* (2016) 27:732–8. doi:10.1093/annonc/mdw016
47. Martens A, Wistuba-Hamprecht K, Yuan J, Postow MA, Wong P, Capone M, et al. Increases in absolute lymphocytes and circulating CD4+ and CD8+ T cells are associated with positive clinical outcome of melanoma patients treated with ipilimumab. *Clin Cancer Res* (2016) 22:4848–58. doi:10.1158/1078-0432.CCR-16-0249
48. Zaragoza J, Caille A, Beneton N, Bens G, Christiann F, Maillard H, et al. High neutrophil to lymphocyte ratio measured before starting ipilimumab treatment is associated with reduced overall survival in patients with melanoma. *Br J Dermatol* (2016) 174:146–51. doi:10.1111/bjd.14155
49. Chasseuil E, Saint-Jean M, Chasseuil H, Peuvrel L, Quereux G, Nguyen JM, et al. Blood predictive biomarkers for nivolumab in advanced melanoma. *Acta Derm Venereol* (2017) 98(4):406–10. doi:10.2340/00015555-2872
50. Fujisawa Y, Yoshino K, Otsuka A, Funakoshi T, Fujimura T, Yamamoto Y, et al. Baseline neutrophil to lymphocyte ratio combined with serum LDH level associated with outcome of nivolumab immunotherapy in a Japanese advanced melanoma population. *Br J Dermatol* (2018). doi:10.1111/bjd.16427
51. Gebhardt C, Sevko A, Jiang H, Lichtenberger R, Reith M, Tarnanidis K, et al. Myeloid cells and related chronic inflammatory factors as novel predictive markers in melanoma treatment with ipilimumab. *Clin Cancer Res* (2015) 21:5453–9. doi:10.1158/1078-0432.CCR-15-0676
52. Weber J, Gibney G, Kudchadkar R, Yu B, Cheng P, Martinez AJ, et al. Phase I/II study of metastatic melanoma patients treated with nivolumab who had progressed after ipilimumab. *Cancer Immunol Res* (2016) 4:345–53. doi:10.1158/2326-6066.CIR-15-0193
53. Krieg C, Nowicka M, Guglietta S, Schindler S, Hartmann FJ, Weber LM, et al. High-dimensional single-cell analysis predicts response to anti-PD-1 immunotherapy. *Nat Med* (2018) 24:144–53. doi:10.1038/nm.4466
54. Subrahmanyam PB, Dong Z, Gusenleitner D, Giobbie-Hurder A, Severgnini M, Zhou J, et al. Distinct predictive biomarker candidates for response to anti-CTLA-4 and anti-PD-1 immunotherapy in melanoma patients. *J Immunother Cancer* (2018) 6:18. doi:10.1186/s40425-018-0328-8
55. Jacquelot N, Roberti MP, Enot DP, Rusakiewicz S, Ternes N, Jegou S, et al. Predictors of responses to immune checkpoint blockade in advanced melanoma. *Nat Commun* (2017) 8:592. doi:10.1038/s41467-017-00608-2
56. Chowell D, Morris LGT, Grigg CM, Weber JK, Samstein RM, Makarov V, et al. Patient HLA class I genotype effects cancer response to checkpoint blockade immunotherapy. *Science* (2018) 359:582–7. doi:10.1126/science.aao4572
57. Postow MA, Manuel M, Wong P, Yuan J, Dong Z, Liu C, et al. Peripheral T cell receptor diversity is associated with clinical outcomes following ipilimumab treatment in metastatic melanoma. *J Immunother Cancer* (2015) 3:23. doi:10.1186/s40425-015-0070-4
58. Leung AM, Lee AF, Ozao-Choy J, Ramos RI, Hamid O, O'Day SJ, et al. Clinical benefit from ipilimumab therapy in melanoma patients may be associated with serum CTLA4 levels. *Front Oncol* (2014) 4:110. doi:10.3389/fonc.2014.00110
59. Zhou J, Mahoney KM, Giobbie-Hurder A, Zhao F, Lee S, Liao X, et al. Soluble PD-L1 as a biomarker in malignant melanoma treated with checkpoint blockade. *Cancer Immunol Res* (2017) 5:480–92. doi:10.1158/2326-6066.CIR-16-0329
60. Hannani D, Vetizou M, Enot D, Rusakiewicz S, Chaput N, Klatzmann D, et al. Anticancer immunotherapy by CTLA-4 blockade: obligatory contribution of IL-2 receptors and negative prognostic impact of soluble CD25. *Cell Res* (2015) 25:208–24. doi:10.1038/cr.2015.3
61. Koguchi Y, Hoen HM, Bambina SA, Rynning MD, Fuerstenberg RK, Curti BD, et al. Serum immunoregulatory proteins as predictors of overall survival of metastatic melanoma patients treated with ipilimumab. *Cancer Res* (2015) 75:5084–92. doi:10.1158/0008-5472.CAN-15-2303
62. Yamazaki N, Kiyohara Y, Uhara H, Iizuka H, Uehara J, Otsuka F, et al. Cytokine biomarkers to predict antitumor responses to nivolumab suggested in a phase 2 study for advanced melanoma. *Cancer Sci* (2017) 108:1022–31. doi:10.1111/cas.13226
63. Weber JS, Sznol M, Sullivan RJ, Blackmon S, Boland G, Kluger HM, et al. A serum protein signature associated with outcome after anti-PD-1 therapy in metastatic melanoma. *Cancer Immunol Res* (2018) 6:79–86. doi:10.1158/2326-6066.CIR-17-0412
64. Hong X, Sullivan RJ, Kalinich M, Kwan TT, Giobbie-Hurder A, Pan S, et al. Molecular signatures of circulating melanoma cells for monitoring early response to immune checkpoint therapy. *Proc Natl Acad Sci U S A* (2018) 115:2467–72. doi:10.1073/pnas.1719264115
65. Gray ES, Reid AL, Bowyer S, Calapre L, Siew K, Pearce R, et al. Circulating melanoma cell subpopulations: their heterogeneity and differential responses to treatment. *J Invest Dermatol* (2015) 135:2040–8. doi:10.1038/jid.2015.127
66. Chaput N, Lepage P, Coutzac C, Soularue E, Le Roux K, Monot C, et al. Baseline gut microbiota predicts clinical response and colitis in metastatic melanoma patients treated with ipilimumab. *Ann Oncol* (2017) 28:1368–79. doi:10.1093/annonc/mdx108
67. Gopalakrishnan V, Spencer CN, Nezi L, Reuben A, Andrews MC, Karpinets TV, et al. Gut microbiome modulates response to anti-PD-1 immunotherapy in melanoma patients. *Science* (2018) 359:97–103. doi:10.1126/science.aan4236
68. Frankel AE, Coughlin LA, Kim J, Froehlich TW, Xie Y, Frenkel EP, et al. Metagenomic shotgun sequencing and unbiased metabolomic profiling identify specific human gut microbiota and metabolites associated with

immune checkpoint therapy efficacy in melanoma patients. *Neoplasia* (2017) 19:848–55. doi:10.1016/j.neo.2017.08.004

69. Matson V, Fessler J, Bao R, Chongsuwat T, Zha Y, Alegre ML, et al. The commensal microbiome is associated with anti-PD-1 efficacy in metastatic melanoma patients. *Science* (2018) 359:104–8. doi:10.1126/science.aao3290
70. Hassel JC, Buder-Bakhaya K, Bender C, Zimmer L, Weide B, Loquai C, et al. Progression patterns under BRAF inhibitor treatment and treatment beyond progression in patients with metastatic melanoma. *Cancer Med* (2018) 7:95–104. doi:10.1002/cam4.1267
71. Bagley SJ, Kothari S, Aggarwal C, Bauml JM, Alley EW, Evans TL, et al. Pretreatment neutrophil-to-lymphocyte ratio as a marker of outcomes in nivolumab-treated patients with advanced non-small-cell lung cancer. *Lung Cancer* (2017) 106:1–7. doi:10.1016/j.lungcan.2017.01.013
72. Gershenwald JE, Scolyer RA, Hess KR, Sondak VK, Long GV, Ross MI, et al. Melanoma staging: evidence-based changes in the American Joint Committee on Cancer eighth edition cancer staging manual. *CA Cancer J Clin* (2017) 67:472–92. doi:10.3322/caac.21409
73. Manola J, Atkins M, Ibrahim J, Kirkwood J. Prognostic factors in metastatic melanoma: a pooled analysis of Eastern Cooperative Oncology Group trials. *J Clin Oncol* (2000) 18:3782–93. doi:10.1200/JCO.2000.18.22.3782
74. Long GV, Grob JJ, Nathan P, Ribas A, Robert C, Schadendorf D, et al. Factors predictive of response, disease progression, and overall survival after dabrafenib and trametinib combination treatment: a pooled analysis of individual patient data from randomised trials. *Lancet Oncol* (2016) 17:1743–54. doi:10.1016/S1470-2045(16)30578-2
75. Fang S, Wang Y, Sui D, Liu H, Ross MI, Gershenwald JE, et al. C-reactive protein as a marker of melanoma progression. *J Clin Oncol* (2015) 33:1389–96. doi:10.1200/JCO.2014.58.0209
76. Shrotriya S, Walsh D, Bennani-Baiti N, Thomas S, Lorton C. C-reactive protein is an important biomarker for prognosis tumor recurrence and treatment response in adult solid tumors: a systematic review. *PLoS One* (2015) 10:e0143080. doi:10.1371/journal.pone.0143080
77. Oya Y, Yoshida T, Kuroda H, Mikubo M, Kondo C, Shimizu J, et al. Predictive clinical parameters for the response of nivolumab in pretreated advanced non-small-cell lung cancer. *Oncotarget* (2017) 8:103117–28. doi:10.18632/oncotarget.21602
78. Rosales C. Neutrophil: a cell with many roles in inflammation or several cell types? *Front Physiol* (2018) 9:113. doi:10.3389/fphys.2018.00113
79. Bigot F, Castanon E, Baldini C, Hollebecque A, Carmona A, Postel-Vinay S, et al. Prospective validation of a prognostic score for patients in immunotherapy phase I trials: the gustave roussy immune score (GRIm-score). *Eur J Cancer* (2017) 84:212–8. doi:10.1016/j.ejca.2017.07.027
80. Diem S, Schmid S, Krapf M, Flatz L, Born D, Jochum W, et al. Neutrophil-to-lymphocyte ratio (NLR) and platelet-to-lymphocyte ratio (PLR) as prognostic markers in patients with non-small cell lung cancer (NSCLC) treated with nivolumab. *Lung Cancer* (2017) 111:176–81. doi:10.1016/j.lungcan.2017.07.024
81. Jeyakumar G, Kim S, Bumma N, Landry C, Silski C, Suisham S, et al. Neutrophil lymphocyte ratio and duration of prior anti-angiogenic therapy as biomarkers in metastatic RCC receiving immune checkpoint inhibitor therapy. *J Immunother Cancer* (2017) 5:82. doi:10.1186/s40425-017-0287-5
82. Finon A, Zaragoza J, Maillard H, Beneton N, Bens G, Samimi M, et al. A high neutrophil to lymphocyte ratio prior to BRAF inhibitor treatment is a predictor of poor progression-free survival in patients with metastatic melanoma. *Eur J Dermatol* (2018) 28:38–43. doi:10.1684/ejd.2017.3167
83. Kvistborg P, Philips D, Kelderman S, Hageman L, Ottensmeier C, Joseph-Pietras D, et al. Anti-CTLA-4 therapy broadens the melanoma-reactive CD8+ T cell response. *Sci Transl Med* (2014) 6:254ra128. doi:10.1126/scitranslmed.3008918
84. Arrieta O, Montes-Servín E, Hernandez-Martinez JM, Cardona AF, Casas-Ruiz E, Crispin JC, et al. Expression of PD-1/PD-L1 and PD-L2 in peripheral T-cells from non-small cell lung cancer patients. *Oncotarget* (2017) 8:101994–2005. doi:10.18632/oncotarget.22025
85. Snyder A, Nathanson T, Funt SA, Ahuja A, Buros Novik J, Hellmann MD, et al. Contribution of systemic and somatic factors to clinical response and resistance to PD-L1 blockade in urothelial cancer: an exploratory multi-omic analysis. *PLoS Med* (2017) 14:e1002309. doi:10.1371/journal.pmed.1002309
86. Wistuba-Hamprecht K, Di Benedetto S, Schilling B, Sucker A, Schadendorf D, Garbe C, et al. Phenotypic characterization and prognostic impact of circulating gammadelta and alphabeta T-cells in metastatic malignant melanoma. *Int J Cancer* (2016) 138:698–704. doi:10.1002/ijc.29818
87. Ward FJ, Dahal LN, Wijesekera SK, Abdul-Jawad SK, Kaewarpai T, Xu H, et al. The soluble isoform of CTLA-4 as a regulator of T-cell responses. *Eur J Immunol* (2013) 43:1274–85. doi:10.1002/eji.201242529
88. Okuma Y, Hosomi Y, Nakahara Y, Watanabe K, Sagawa Y, Homma S. High plasma levels of soluble programmed cell death ligand 1 are prognostic for reduced survival in advanced lung cancer. *Lung Cancer* (2017) 104:1–6. doi:10.1016/j.lungcan.2016.11.023
89. Zhu X, Lang J. Soluble PD-1 and PD-L1: predictive and prognostic significance in cancer. *Oncotarget* (2017) 8:97671–82. doi:10.18632/oncotarget.18311
90. Finkelmeier F, Canli O, Tal A, Pleli T, Trojan J, Schmidt M, et al. High levels of the soluble programmed death-ligand (sPD-L1) identify hepatocellular carcinoma patients with a poor prognosis. *Eur J Cancer* (2016) 59:152–9. doi:10.1016/j.ejca.2016.03.002
91. Shrikant P, Khoruts A, Mescher MF. CTLA-4 blockade reverses CD8+ T cell tolerance to tumor by a CD4+ T cell- and IL-2-dependent mechanism. *Immunity* (1999) 11:483–93. doi:10.1016/S1074-7613(00)80123-5
92. Ugurel S, Rappl G, Tilgen W, Reinhold U. Increased serum concentration of angiogenic factors in malignant melanoma patients correlates with tumor progression and survival. *J Clin Oncol* (2001) 19:577–83. doi:10.1200/JCO.2001.19.2.577
93. Van Raemdonck K, Van Den Steen PE, Liekens S, Van Damme J, Struyf S. CXCR3 ligands in disease and therapy. *Cytokine Growth Factor Rev* (2015) 26:311–27. doi:10.1016/j.cytogfr.2014.11.009
94. Buder-Bakhaya K, Machiraju D, Hassel JC. Liquid biopsy: value for melanoma therapy. *Oncol Res Treat* (2017) 40:430–4. doi:10.1159/000478893
95. Bao H, Bai T, Takata K, Yokobori T, Ohnaga T, Hisada T, et al. High expression of carcinoembryonic antigen and telomerase reverse transcriptase in circulating tumor cells is associated with poor clinical response to the immune checkpoint inhibitor nivolumab. *Oncol Lett* (2018) 15:3061–7. doi:10.3892/ol.2017.7671
96. Anantharaman A, Friedlander T, Lu D, Krupa R, Premasekharan G, Hough J, et al. Programmed death-ligand 1 (PD-L1) characterization of circulating tumor cells (CTCs) in muscle invasive and metastatic bladder cancer patients. *BMC Cancer* (2016) 16:744. doi:10.1186/s12885-016-2758-3
97. Strati A, Koutsodontis G, Papaxoinis G, Angelidis I, Zavridou M, Economopoulou P, et al. Prognostic significance of PD-L1 expression on circulating tumor cells in patients with head and neck squamous cell carcinoma. *Ann Oncol* (2017) 28:1923–33. doi:10.1093/annonc/mdx206
98. Cabel L, Riva F, Servois V, Livartowski A, Daniel C, Rampanou A, et al. Circulating tumor DNA changes for early monitoring of anti-PD1 immunotherapy: a proof-of-concept study. *Ann Oncol* (2017) 28:1996–2001. doi:10.1093/annonc/mdx212
99. Khagi Y, Goodman AM, Daniels GA, Patel SP, Sacco AG, Randall JM, et al. Hypermutated circulating tumor DNA: correlation with response to checkpoint inhibitor-based immunotherapy. *Clin Cancer Res* (2017) 23:5729–36. doi:10.1158/1078-0432.CCR-17-1439
100. Saenger Y, Magidson J, Liaw B, De Moll E, Harcharik S, Fu Y, et al. Blood mRNA expression profiling predicts survival in patients treated with tremelimumab. *Clin Cancer Res* (2014) 20:3310–8. doi:10.1158/1078-0432.CCR-13-2906
101. Bullman S, Pedamallu CS, Sicinska E, Clancy TE, Zhang X, Cai D, et al. Analysis of *Fusobacterium* persistence and antibiotic response in colorectal cancer. *Science* (2017) 358:1443–8. doi:10.1126/science.aal5240
102. Vetizou M, Pitt JM, Daillere R, Lepage P, Waldschmitt N, Flament C, et al. Anticancer immunotherapy by CTLA-4 blockade relies on the gut microbiota. *Science* (2015) 350:1079–84. doi:10.1126/science.aad1329
103. Sivan A, Corrales L, Hubert N, Williams JB, Aquino-Michaels K, Earley ZM, et al. Commensal *Bifidobacterium* promotes antitumor immunity and facilitates anti-PD-L1 efficacy. *Science* (2015) 350:1084–9. doi:10.1126/science.aac4255
104. Routy B, Le Chatelier E, Derosa L, Duong CPM, Alou MT, Daillere R, et al. Gut microbiome effects efficacy of PD-1-based immunotherapy against epithelial tumors. *Science* (2018) 359:91–7. doi:10.1126/science.aan3706
105. Topalian SL, Hodi FS, Brahmer JR, Gettinger SN, Smith DC, Mcdermott DF, et al. Safety, activity, and immune correlates of anti-PD-1 antibody in cancer. *N Engl J Med* (2012) 366:2443–54. doi:10.1056/NEJMoa1200690

106. Taube JM, Klein A, Brahmer JR, Xu H, Pan X, Kim JH, et al. Association of PD-1, PD-1 ligands, and other features of the tumor immune microenvironment with response to anti-PD-1 therapy. *Clin Cancer Res* (2014) 20:5064–74. doi:10.1158/1078-0432.CCR-13-3271
107. Herbst RS, Baas P, Kim DW, Felip E, Perez-Gracia JL, Han JY, et al. Pembrolizumab versus docetaxel for previously treated, PD-L1-positive, advanced non-small-cell lung cancer (KEYNOTE-010): a randomised controlled trial. *Lancet* (2016) 387:1540–50. doi:10.1016/S0140-6736(15)01281-7
108. Reck M, Rodriguez-Abreu D, Robinson AG, Hui R, Csoszi T, Fulop A, et al. Pembrolizumab versus chemotherapy for PD-L1-positive non-small-cell lung cancer. *N Engl J Med* (2016) 375:1823–33. doi:10.1056/NEJMoa1606774
109. Carbone DP, Reck M, Paz-Ares L, Creelan B, Horn L, Steins M, et al. First-line nivolumab in stage IV or recurrent non-small-cell lung cancer. *N Engl J Med* (2017) 376:2415–26. doi:10.1056/NEJMoa1613493
110. Borghaei H, Brahmer J, Horn L, Ready N, Steins M, Felip E, et al. P2.35: nivolumab vs docetaxel in advanced NSCLC: CheckMate 017/057 2-Y update and exploratory cytokine profile analysis: track: immunotherapy. *J Thorac Oncol* (2016) 11:S237–8. doi:10.1016/j.jtho.2016.08.106
111. Sharma P, Retz M, Siefker-Radtke A, Baron A, Necchi A, Bedke J, et al. Nivolumab in metastatic urothelial carcinoma after platinum therapy (CheckMate 275): a multicentre, single-arm, phase 2 trial. *Lancet Oncol* (2017) 18:312–22. doi:10.1016/S1470-2045(17)30065-7
112. Chow LQM, Haddad R, Gupta S, Mahipal A, Mehra R, Tahara M, et al. Antitumor activity of pembrolizumab in biomarker-unselected patients with recurrent and/or metastatic head and neck squamous cell carcinoma: results from the phase Ib KEYNOTE-012 expansion cohort. *J Clin Oncol* (2016) 34:3838–45. doi:10.1200/JCO.2016.68.1478
113. Herbst RS, Soria JC, Kowanetz M, Fine GD, Hamid O, Gordon MS, et al. Predictive correlates of response to the anti-PD-L1 antibody MPDL3280A in cancer patients. *Nature* (2014) 515:563–7. doi:10.1038/nature14011
114. Wolchok JD, Chiarion-Sileni V, Gonzalez R, Rutkowski P, Grob JJ, Cowey CL, et al. Overall survival with combined nivolumab and ipilimumab in advanced melanoma. *N Engl J Med* (2017) 377:1345–56. doi:10.1056/NEJMoa1709684
115. Hamid O, Schmidt H, Nissan A, Ridolfi L, Aamdal S, Hansson J, et al. A prospective phase II trial exploring the association between tumor microenvironment biomarkers and clinical activity of ipilimumab in advanced melanoma. *J Transl Med* (2011) 9:204. doi:10.1186/1479-5876-9-204
116. Daud AI, Loo K, Pauli ML, Sanchez-Rodriguez R, Sandoval PM, Taravati K, et al. Tumor immune profiling predicts response to anti-PD-1 therapy in human melanoma. *J Clin Invest* (2016) 126:3447–52. doi:10.1172/JCI87324
117. Tumeh PC, Harview CL, Yearley JH, Shintaku IP, Taylor EJ, Robert L, et al. PD-1 blockade induces responses by inhibiting adaptive immune resistance. *Nature* (2014) 515:568–71. doi:10.1038/nature13954
118. Johnson DB, Estrada MV, Salgado R, Sanchez V, Doxie DB, Opalenik SR, et al. Melanoma-specific MHC-II expression represents a tumour-autonomous phenotype and predicts response to anti-PD-1/PD-L1 therapy. *Nat Commun* (2016) 7:10582. doi:10.1038/ncomms10582
119. Johnson DB, Frampton GM, Rioth MJ, Yusko E, Xu Y, Guo X, et al. Targeted next generation sequencing identifies markers of response to PD-1 blockade. *Cancer Immunol Res* (2016) 4:959–67. doi:10.1158/2326-6066.CIR-16-0143
120. Snyder A, Wolchok JD, Chan TA. Genetic basis for clinical response to CTLA-4 blockade. *N Engl J Med* (2015) 372:783. doi:10.1056/NEJMc1415938
121. Van Allen EM, Miao D, Schilling B, Shukla SA, Blank C, Zimmer L, et al. Genomic correlates of response to CTLA-4 blockade in metastatic melanoma. *Science* (2015) 350:207–11. doi:10.1126/science.aad0095
122. Hugo W, Zaretsky JM, Sun L, Song C, Moreno BH, Hu-Lieskovan S, et al. Genomic and transcriptomic features of response to anti-PD-1 therapy in metastatic melanoma. *Cell* (2016) 165:35–44. doi:10.1016/j.cell.2016.02.065
123. McGranahan N, Furness AJ, Rosenthal R, Ramskov S, Lyngaa R, Saini SK, et al. Clonal neoantigens elicit T cell immunoreactivity and sensitivity to immune checkpoint blockade. *Science* (2016) 351:1463–9. doi:10.1126/science.aaf1490
124. Turajlic S, Litchfield K, Xu H, Rosenthal R, Mcgranahan N, Reading JL, et al. Insertion-and-deletion-derived tumour-specific neoantigens and the immunogenic phenotype: a pan-cancer analysis. *Lancet Oncol* (2017) 18:1009–21. doi:10.1016/S1470-2045(17)30516-8
125. Riaz N, Havel JJ, Makarov V, Desrichard A, Urba WJ, Sims JS, et al. Tumor and microenvironment evolution during immunotherapy with nivolumab. *Cell* (2017) 171:934–49.e915. doi:10.1016/j.cell.2017.09.028
126. Johnson DB, Lovly CM, Flavin M, Panageas KS, Ayers GD, Zhao Z, et al. Impact of NRAS mutations for patients with advanced melanoma treated with immune therapies. *Cancer Immunol Res* (2015) 3:288–95. doi:10.1158/2326-6066.CIR-14-0207
127. Eroglu Z, Zaretsky JM, Hu-Lieskovan S, Kim DW, Algazi A, Johnson DB, et al. High response rate to PD-1 blockade in desmoplastic melanomas. *Nature* (2018) 553:347–50. doi:10.1038/nature25187
128. Ji RR, Chasalow SD, Wang L, Hamid O, Schmidt H, Cogswell J, et al. An immune-active tumor microenvironment favors clinical response to ipilimumab. *Cancer Immunol Immunother* (2012) 61:1019–31. doi:10.1007/s00262-011-1172-6
129. Karachaliou N, Gonzalez-Cao M, Crespo G, Drozdowskyj A, Aldeguer E, Gimenez-Capitan A, et al. Interferon gamma, an important marker of response to immune checkpoint blockade in non-small cell lung cancer and melanoma patients. *Ther Adv Med Oncol* (2018) 10:1758834017749748. doi:10.1177/1758834017749748
130. Sachpekidis C, Larribere L, Pan L, Haberkorn U, Dimitrakopoulou-Strauss A, Hassel JC. Predictive value of early 18F-FDG PET/CT studies for treatment response evaluation to ipilimumab in metastatic melanoma: preliminary results of an ongoing study. *Eur J Nucl Med Mol Imaging* (2015) 42:386–96. doi:10.1007/s00259-014-2944-y
131. Cho SY, Lipson EJ, Im HJ, Rowe SP, Gonzalez EM, Blackford A, et al. Prediction of response to immune checkpoint inhibitor therapy using early-time-point (18)F-FDG PET/CT imaging in patients with advanced melanoma. *J Nucl Med* (2017) 58:1421–8. doi:10.2967/jnumed.116.188839
132. Anwar H, Sachpekidis C, Winkler J, Kopp-Schneider A, Haberkorn U, Hassel JC, et al. Absolute number of new lesions on (18)F-FDG PET/CT is more predictive of clinical response than SUV changes in metastatic melanoma patients receiving ipilimumab. *Eur J Nucl Med Mol Imaging* (2018) 45:376–83. doi:10.1007/s00259-017-3870-6
133. Seith F, Forschner A, Schmidt H, Pfannenberg C, Guckel B, Nikolaou K, et al. 18F-FDG-PET detects complete response to PD1-therapy in melanoma patients two weeks after therapy start. *Eur J Nucl Med Mol Imaging* (2018) 45:95–101. doi:10.1007/s00259-017-3813-2
134. Zhang L, Conejo-Garcia JR, Katsaros D, Gimotty PA, Massobrio M, Regnani G, et al. Intratumoral T cells, recurrence, and survival in epithelial ovarian cancer. *N Engl J Med* (2003) 348:203–13. doi:10.1056/NEJMoa020177
135. Galon J, Costes A, Sanchez-Cabo F, Kirilovsky A, Mlecnik B, Lagorce-Pages C, et al. Type, density, and location of immune cells within human colorectal tumors predict clinical outcome. *Science* (2006) 313:1960–4. doi:10.1126/science.1129139
136. Thomas NE, Busam KJ, From L, Kricker A, Armstrong BK, Anton-Culver H, et al. Tumor-infiltrating lymphocyte grade in primary melanomas is independently associated with melanoma-specific survival in the population-based genes, environment and melanoma study. *J Clin Oncol* (2013) 31:4252–9. doi:10.1200/JCO.2013.51.3002
137. Gibney GT, Weiner LM, Atkins MB. Predictive biomarkers for checkpoint inhibitor-based immunotherapy. *Lancet Oncol* (2016) 17:e542–51. doi:10.1016/S1470-2045(16)30406-5
138. Budczies J, Bockmayr M, Klauschen F, Endris V, Frohling S, Schirmacher P, et al. Mutation patterns in genes encoding interferon signaling and antigen presentation: a pan-cancer survey with implications for the use of immune checkpoint inhibitors. *Genes Chromosomes Cancer* (2017) 56:651–9. doi:10.1002/gcc.22468
139. Zaretsky JM, Garcia-Diaz A, Shin DS, Escuin-Ordinas H, Hugo W, Hu-Lieskovan S, et al. Mutations associated with acquired resistance to PD-1 blockade in melanoma. *N Engl J Med* (2016) 375:819–29. doi:10.1056/NEJMoa1604958
140. Shin DS, Zaretsky JM, Escuin-Ordinas H, Garcia-Diaz A, Hu-Lieskovan S, Kalbasi A, et al. Primary resistance to PD-1 blockade mediated by JAK1/2 mutations. *Cancer Discov* (2017) 7:188–201. doi:10.1158/2159-8290.CD-16-1223
141. Liu W, Ye H, Liu YF, Xu CQ, Zhong YX, Tian T, et al. Transcriptome-derived stromal and immune scores infer clinical outcomes of patients with cancer. *Oncol Lett* (2018) 15:4351–7. doi:10.3892/ol.2018.7855
142. Lawrence MS, Stojanov P, Mermel CH, Robinson JT, Garraway LA, Golub TR, et al. Discovery and saturation analysis of cancer genes across 21 tumour types. *Nature* (2014) 505:495–501. doi:10.1038/nature12912
143. Van Allen EM, Wagle N, Sucker A, Treacy DJ, Johannessen CM, Goetz EM, et al. The genetic landscape of clinical resistance to RAF inhibition in

metastatic melanoma. *Cancer Discov* (2014) 4:94–109. doi:10.1158/2159-8290.CD-13-0617
144. Rizvi NA, Hellmann MD, Snyder A, Kvistborg P, Makarov V, Havel JJ, et al. Cancer immunology. Mutational landscape determines sensitivity to PD-1 blockade in non-small cell lung cancer. *Science* (2015) 348:124–8. doi:10.1126/science.aaa1348
145. Balar AV, Galsky MD, Rosenberg JE, Powles T, Petrylak DP, Bellmunt J, et al. Atezolizumab as first-line treatment in cisplatin-ineligible patients with locally advanced and metastatic urothelial carcinoma: a single-arm, multicentre, phase 2 trial. *Lancet* (2017) 389:67–76. doi:10.1016/S0140-6736(16)32455-2
146. Le DT, Uram JN, Wang H, Bartlett BR, Kemberling H, Eyring AD, et al. PD-1 blockade in tumors with mismatch-repair deficiency. *N Engl J Med* (2015) 372:2509–20. doi:10.1056/NEJMoa1500596
147. Kim ST, Klempner SJ, Park SH, Park JO, Park YS, Lim HY, et al. Correlating programmed death ligand 1 (PD-L1) expression, mismatch repair deficiency, and outcomes across tumor types: implications for immunotherapy. *Oncotarget* (2017) 8:77415–23. doi:10.18632/oncotarget.20492
148. Teo MY, Seier K, Ostrovnaya I, Regazzi AM, Kania BE, Moran MM, et al. Alterations in DNA damage response and repair genes as potential marker of clinical benefit from PD-1/PD-L1 blockade in advanced urothelial cancers. *J Clin Oncol* (2018) 36(17):1685–94. doi:10.1200/JCO.2017.75.7740
149. Colli LM, Machiela MJ, Myers TA, Jessop L, Yu K, Chanock SJ. Burden of nonsynonymous mutations among TCGA cancers and candidate immune checkpoint inhibitor responses. *Cancer Res* (2016) 76:3767–72. doi:10.1158/0008-5472.CAN-16-0170
150. Beaver JA, Hazarika M, Mulkey F, Mushti S, Chen H, He K, et al. Patients with melanoma treated with an anti-PD-1 antibody beyond RECIST progression: a US Food and Drug Administration pooled analysis. *Lancet Oncol* (2018) 19:229–39. doi:10.1016/S1470-2045(17)30846-X
151. Balachandran VP, Luksza M, Zhao JN, Makarov V, Moral JA, Remark R, et al. Identification of unique neoantigen qualities in long-term survivors of pancreatic cancer. *Nature* (2017) 551:512–6. doi:10.1038/nature24462
152. Luksza M, Riaz N, Makarov V, Balachandran VP, Hellmann MD, Solovyov A, et al. A neoantigen fitness model predicts tumour response to checkpoint blockade immunotherapy. *Nature* (2017) 551:517–20. doi:10.1038/nature24473
153. Nathanson T, Ahuja A, Rubinsteyn A, Aksoy BA, Hellmann MD, Miao D, et al. Somatic mutations and neoepitope homology in melanomas treated with CTLA-4 blockade. *Cancer Immunol Res* (2017) 5:84–91. doi:10.1158/2326-6066.CIR-16-0019
154. Shahabi V, Whitney G, Hamid O, Schmidt H, Chasalow SD, Alaparthy S, et al. Assessment of association between BRAF-V600E mutation status in melanomas and clinical response to ipilimumab. *Cancer Immunol Immunother* (2012) 61:733–7. doi:10.1007/s00262-012-1227-3
155. Larkin J, Lao CD, Urba WJ, Mcdermott DF, Horak C, Jiang J, et al. Efficacy and safety of nivolumab in patients with BRAF V600 mutant and BRAF wild-type advanced melanoma: a pooled analysis of 4 clinical trials. *JAMA Oncol* (2015) 1:433–40. doi:10.1001/jamaoncol.2015.1184
156. Ribas A, Puzanov I, Dummer R, Schadendorf D, Hamid O, Robert C, et al. Pembrolizumab versus investigator-choice chemotherapy for ipilimumab-refractory melanoma (KEYNOTE-002): a randomised, controlled, phase 2 trial. *Lancet Oncol* (2015) 16:908–18. doi:10.1016/S1470-2045(15)00083-2
157. Robert C, Schachter J, Long GV, Arance A, Grob JJ, Mortier L, et al. Pembrolizumab versus ipilimumab in advanced melanoma. *N Engl J Med* (2015) 372:2521–32. doi:10.1056/NEJMoa1503093
158. Jakob JA, Bassett RL Jr, Ng CS, Curry JL, Joseph RW, Alvarado GC, et al. NRAS mutation status is an independent prognostic factor in metastatic melanoma. *Cancer* (2012) 118:4014–23. doi:10.1002/cncr.26724
159. Lee WC, Diao L, Wang J, Zhang J, Roarty EB, Varghese S, et al. Multiregion gene expression profiling reveals heterogeneity in molecular subtypes and immunotherapy response signatures in lung cancer. *Mod Pathol* (2018) 31(6):947–55. doi:10.1038/s41379-018-0029-3
160. Spigel D, Betzig-Schrock A, Fabrizio D, Frampton GM, Sun J, He J. Total mutation burden in lung cancer and relationship with response to PD-1/PD-L1 targeted therapies. *J Clin Oncol* (2016) 34:9017. doi:10.1200/JCO.2016.34.15_suppl.9017
161. Eisenhauer EA, Therasse P, Bogaerts J, Schwartz LH, Sargent D, Ford R, et al. New response evaluation criteria in solid tumours: revised RECIST guideline (version 1.1). *Eur J Cancer* (2009) 45:228–47. doi:10.1016/j.ejca.2008.10.026
162. Joseph RW, Elassaiss-Schaap J, Wolchok JD, Joshua AM, Ribas A, Hodi FS, et al. Baseline tumor size as an independent prognostic factor for overall survival in patients with metastatic melanoma treated with the anti-PD-1 monoclonal antibody MK-3475. *J Clin Oncol* (2014) 32:3015. doi:10.1200/jco.2014.32.15_suppl.3015
163. Wolchok JD, Hoos A, O'Day S, Weber JS, Hamid O, Lebbe C, et al. Guidelines for the evaluation of immune therapy activity in solid tumors: immune-related response criteria. *Clin Cancer Res* (2009) 15:7412–20. doi:10.1158/1078-0432.CCR-09-1624
164. Young H, Baum R, Cremerius U, Herholz K, Hoekstra O, Lammertsma AA, et al. Measurement of clinical and subclinical tumour response using [18F]-fluorodeoxyglucose and positron emission tomography: review and 1999 EORTC recommendations. European Organization for Research and Treatment of Cancer (EORTC) PET study group. *Eur J Cancer* (1999) 35: 1773–82. doi:10.1016/S0959-8049(99)00229-4
165. Wahl RL, Jacene H, Kasamon Y, Lodge MA. From RECIST to PERCIST: evolving considerations for PET response criteria in solid tumors. *J Nucl Med* (2009) 50(Suppl 1):122S–50S. doi:10.2967/jnumed.108.057307
166. Gilardi L, Grana CM, Paganelli G. Evaluation of response to immunotherapy: new challenges and opportunities for PET imaging. *Eur J Nucl Med Mol Imaging* (2014) 41:2090–2. doi:10.1007/s00259-014-2848-x
167. Kaira K, Higuchi T, Naruse I, Arisaka Y, Tokue A, Altan B, et al. Metabolic activity by (18)F-FDG-PET/CT is predictive of early response after nivolumab in previously treated NSCLC. *Eur J Nucl Med Mol Imaging* (2018) 45:56–66. doi:10.1007/s00259-017-3806-1
168. Herrmann K, Buck AK. Proliferation imaging with (1)(8)F-fluorothymidine PET/computed tomography: physiologic uptake, variants, and pitfalls. *PET Clin* (2014) 9:331–8. doi:10.1016/j.cpet.2014.03.005
169. Enslow MS, Zollinger LV, Morton KA, Butterfield RI, Kadrmas DJ, Christian PE, et al. Comparison of 18F-fluorodeoxyglucose and 18F-fluorothymidine PET in differentiating radiation necrosis from recurrent glioma. *Clin Nucl Med* (2012) 37:854–61. doi:10.1097/RLU.0b013e318262c76a
170. Wieder H, Beer AJ, Siveke J, Schuster T, Buck AK, Herrmann K, et al. (18) F-fluorothymidine PET for predicting survival in patients with resectable pancreatic cancer. *Oncotarget* (2018) 9:10128–34. doi:10.18632/oncotarget.24176
171. Mogensen MB, Loft A, Aznar M, Axelsen T, Vainer B, Osterlind K, et al. FLT-PET for early response evaluation of colorectal cancer patients with liver metastases: a prospective study. *EJNMMI Res* (2017) 7:56. doi:10.1186/s13550-017-0302-3
172. Nguyen NC, Yee MK, Tuchayi AM, Kirkwood JM, Tawbi H, Mountz JM. Targeted therapy and immunotherapy response assessment with F-18 fluorothymidine positron-emission tomography/magnetic resonance imaging in melanoma brain metastasis: a pilot study. *Front Oncol* (2018) 8:18. doi:10.3389/fonc.2018.00018
173. Poulsen SH, Urup T, Grunnet K, Christensen IJ, Larsen VA, Jensen ML, et al. The prognostic value of FET PET at radiotherapy planning in newly diagnosed glioblastoma. *Eur J Nucl Med Mol Imaging* (2017) 44:373–81. doi:10.1007/s00259-016-3494-2
174. Unterrainer M, Galldiks N, Suchorska B, Kowalew LC, Wenter V, Schmid-Tannwald C, et al. (18)F-FET PET uptake characteristics in patients with newly diagnosed and untreated brain metastasis. *J Nucl Med* (2017) 58:584–9. doi:10.2967/jnumed.116.180075
175. Sanghera B, Wong WL, Sonoda LI, Beynon G, Makris A, Woolf D, et al. FLT PET-CT in evaluation of treatment response. *Indian J Nucl Med* (2014) 29:65–73. doi:10.4103/0972-3919.130274
176. Kebir S, Rauschenbach L, Galldiks N, Schlaak M, Hattingen E, Landsberg J, et al. Dynamic O-(2-[18F]fluoroethyl)-L-tyrosine PET imaging for the detection of checkpoint inhibitor-related pseudoprogression in melanoma brain metastases. *Neuro Oncol* (2016) 18:1462–4. doi:10.1093/neuonc/now154
177. Little RA, Barjat H, Hare JI, Jenner M, Watson Y, Cheung S, et al. Evaluation of dynamic contrast-enhanced MRI biomarkers for stratified cancer medicine: how do permeability and perfusion vary between human tumours? *Magn Reson Imaging* (2018) 46:98–105. doi:10.1016/j.mri.2017.11.008
178. Lee M, Baek SE, Moon J, Roh YH, Lim JS, Park MS, et al. Dynamic contrast-enhanced MRI coupled with a subtraction technique is useful for treatment response evaluation of malignant melanoma hepatic metastasis. *Oncotarget* (2016) 7:38513–22. doi:10.18632/oncotarget.9567

179. Ahrens ET, Bulte JW. Tracking immune cells in vivo using magnetic resonance imaging. *Nat Rev Immunol* (2013) 13:755–63. doi:10.1038/nri3531
180. Rashidian M, Ingram JR, Dougan M, Dongre A, Whang KA, Legall C, et al. Predicting the response to CTLA-4 blockade by longitudinal noninvasive monitoring of CD8 T cells. *J Exp Med* (2017) 214:2243–55. doi:10.1084/jem.20161950
181. Tavare R, Escuin-Ordinas H, Mok S, Mccracken MN, Zettlitz KA, Salazar FB, et al. An effective immuno-PET imaging method to monitor CD8-dependent responses to immunotherapy. *Cancer Res* (2016) 76:73–82. doi:10.1158/0008-5472.CAN-15-1707
182. Natarajan A, Mayer AT, Reeves RE, Nagamine CM, Gambhir SS. Development of novel ImmunoPET tracers to image human PD-1 checkpoint expression on tumor-infiltrating lymphocytes in a humanized mouse model. *Mol Imaging Biol* (2017) 19:903–14. doi:10.1007/s11307-017-1060-3
183. Lesniak WG, Chatterjee S, Gabrielson M, Lisok A, Wharram B, Pomper MG, et al. PD-L1 detection in tumors using [(64)Cu]atezolizumab with PET. *Bioconjug Chem* (2016) 27:2103–10. doi:10.1021/acs.bioconjchem.6b00348
184. Kikuchi M, Clump DA, Srivastava RM, Sun L, Zeng D, Diaz-Perez JA, et al. Preclinical immunoPET/CT imaging using Zr-89-labeled anti-PD-L1 monoclonal antibody for assessing radiation-induced PD-L1 upregulation in head and neck cancer and melanoma. *Oncoimmunology* (2017) 6:e1329071. doi:10.1080/2162402X.2017.1329071
185. Truillet C, Oh HLJ, Yeo SP, Lee CY, Huynh LT, Wei J, et al. Imaging PD-L1 expression with ImmunoPET. *Bioconjug Chem* (2018) 29:96–103. doi:10.1021/acs.bioconjchem.7b00631

5

Metabolic Checkpoints: Novel Avenues for Immunotherapy of Cancer

Ivan Shevchenko[1] and Alexandr V. Bazhin[2,3]*

[1] Institute for Immunology, Ludwig-Maximilians University, Munich, Germany, [2] Department of General, Visceral and Transplantation Surgery, Ludwig-Maximilians University, Munich, Germany, [3] German Cancer Consortium (DKTK), Partner Site Munich, Munich, Germany

Edited by:
Salem Chouaib,
Institut Gustave Roussy, France

Reviewed by:
Zong Sheng Guo,
University of Pittsburgh,
United States
Carlos Alfaro,
NavarraBiomed, Spain
Abhishek D. Garg,
KU Leuven, Belgium

***Correspondence:**
Ivan Shevchenko
ivshevch87@gmail.com

Novel therapies targeting immune checkpoint molecules have redefined the treatment of cancer at advanced stages and brought hope to millions of patients worldwide. Monoclonal antibodies targeting immune-inhibitory receptors often lead to complete and objective responses as well as to durable progression-free survival where all other therapeutic approaches fail. Yet, many tumors show significant resistance to checkpoint blockade through mechanisms that are only starting to come to light. An alluring alternative strategy to reinvigorate anticancer immune responses comes from the emerging field of immuno-metabolism. Over the past few years, numerous studies revealed that many well-known metabolic playmakers also serve as critical checkpoints in immune homeostasis and immunity against tumors. Here, we survey recent insights into the intimate and intertwining links between T cell metabolic programs and environmental cues in the tumor milieu. Transferring these new findings from the bench to the bedside may soon entirely re-shape the field of cancer immunotherapy and significantly improve the lives of patients.

Keywords: metabolic checkpoints, immune checkpoints, cancer immunotherapy, PD-1, checkpoint blockade, mammalian target of rapamycin pathway

INTRODUCTION

Immunotherapy has become a paradigm-shifting approach showing unmatched efficacy in patients with advanced malignancies. Targeting immune regulatory receptors, such as CTLA-4, PD-1, and PD-1 ligand (PD-L1), leads to spectacular clinical responses (1). Unfortunately, the success of these treatments is often limited to minor cohorts of patients. This calls for the development of alternative strategies for reinvigorating anticancer immunity. Recently, research into immuno-metabolism has emerged as an extraordinarily vibrant and productive area of study that is likely to become a launch-pad for novel therapeutic approaches (2, 3). Over the past few years, the immunological community has witnessed a veritable Cambrian explosion of remarkable studies identifying the critical metabolic programs and checkpoints in the activation, differentiation, and migration of immune cells (2, 4). This research has illuminated the metabolic requirements for successful T cell-mediated effector responses and memory T cell generation in cancer. Furthermore, several groups have revealed the complex effects of multiple micro-environmental factors on T cell functionality in the tumor (5, 6). For instance, the pleiotropic roles of oxygen tension in the regulation of anticancer immunity are now coming to light.

Importantly, pathways controlling T cell responses to external challenges often converge on the same limited set of enzymes, transcription factors, and signaling complexes serving as metabolic checkpoints (7, 8). This highlights the elegant simplicity and dazzling complexity of T cell biology.

Untangling these immuno-metabolic nodes will be essential for the rational design of future therapies for cancer.

IMMUNO-METABOLIC CHECKPOINTS IN T CELL DIFFERENTIATION AND FUNCTION

Metabolic changes occur throughout the lifespan of a T cell and provide the essential energetic currency and building blocks to help the T cell meet the emerging needs (4). Effective T cell responses against tumors strongly depend on the differentiation pathways taken up by individual CD4+ and CD8+ T cells upon their interaction with tumor antigens (9). The lineage commitment of stimulated T cells depends on the integration of the plethora of environmental cues and cell-intrinsic signals during activation, initial proliferation rounds, development of effector functions, and until final differentiation steps (2, 10).

Throughout their developmental path, T cells must strike a balance between increasing energy demands and a growing need for substrates to maintain their functionality and proliferation (2). Naive or quiescent T cells rely mainly on oxidative phosphorylation (OXPHOS), a highly efficient pathway for generating ATP from glucose. Upon activation, however, a switch to aerobic glycolysis takes place. In this rather inefficient process, only two ATP molecules are produced per each molecule of glucose. Switching to aerobic glycolysis might appear very inefficient, due to the low ATP/glucose ratio. Yet, at the same time, aerobic glycolysis yields a higher number of building blocks for anabolism. Importantly, the glycolytic switch is also essential for T cells to acquire diverse effector functions (e.g., production of IL-2, IFN-γ, etc.), since it relieves the blockade of IFN-γ mRNA translation by the glycolytic enzyme GAPDH (11).

The metabolic switch upon T cell activation is governed by a plethora of transcription factors and signaling pathways. Together, TCR engagement, costimulation, and cytokine signaling boost glycolysis by upregulating the expression of nutrient transporters (such as the Glut1 glucose importer) and activating the central metabolic regulator mammalian target of rapamycin (mTOR) complex (12–14). mTOR drives the development of all the effector T cell subsets but hampers peripheral Treg induction. This can be accounted for the requirement of intensified glycolysis during effector T cell expansion, while Treg cells primarily deploy OXPHOS and oxidation of fatty acids. mTOR comprises two distinct complexes, mTORC1 and mTORC2, and orchestrates cellular responses to changes in nutrient levels and energy status (15). Costimulation *via* CD28 activates PI3K recruiting 3-phosphoinositide-dependent protein kinase-1 and Akt, which, in turn, activates mTOR. This pathway leads to the quick upregulation of Glut1 expression and to its increased transport to the plasma membrane. The rapid intensification of glucose import is critical for efficient T cell activation, clonal expansion, and survival.

Of note, a study by Macintyre et al. (16) suggested that Glut1 is only indispensable for the differentiation of Th1, Th2, and Th17 cells, but not CD8+ T cells or Tregs. A plausible explanation might be coming from recent proteomic studies indicating that Glut1 and Glut3 protein levels are comparable in CD8+ T cells (17). Therefore, glucose transporters can act in a somewhat redundant fashion to meet the demands of T cells for glucose.

The multifaceted role of glucose uptake in Treg biology has recently been further elucidated in a study by Rathmell and colleagues who identified toll-like receptor (TLR) signals that drive Treg cell proliferation *via* PI(3)K–Akt–mTORC1 signaling, which intensifies glycolysis and glucose import by Glut1 (18). Conversely, TLR-induced mTORC1 signaling also diminished the ability of Tregs to suppress effector T cell proliferation. In line with previous studies, the transcription factor Foxp3 dampened the effects of PI(3)K–Akt–mTORC1 signaling to hamper glycolysis and anabolism while boosting OXPHOS and catabolic pathways. Likewise, although Glut1 expression promoted Treg expansion, it also reduced their suppressive activity and Foxp3 expression. This indicates that Treg cells might occasionally switch to aerobic glycolysis and expand when they receive inflammatory signals, and subsequently switch back to FAO and OXPHOS to achieve maximal suppressive potency. These findings further highlight glycolysis as a critical metabolic axis in maintaining the immunological balance. Therefore, glycolytic enzymes and nutrient transporters represent attractive targets for future immuno-metabolic therapies of cancer. Specifically, administration of glucose uptake inhibitors or Glut knockdown in adoptively transferred cells could be instrumental for pushing antitumor T cell differentiation toward long-lived memory cell lineage for the generation of enduring antitumor immunity (9, 19).

Migration of activated Treg cells to the site of inflammation is crucial for their immune-inhibitory function (20). Kishore et al. (21) have studied the metabolic needs for migratory Treg. They demonstrated that glycolysis strongly promotes Treg migration and is triggered by a PI3K–mTORC2-mediated pathway driving the activation of the enzyme glucokinase. These findings also suggest a new attractive strategy to avert Treg infiltration into tumors by manipulating their metabolic programs.

The transcription factors c-Myc and hypoxia-inducible factor-1α (HIF-1α) coordinately activate the genes required for the vigorous proliferation of effector T cells during clonal expansion (22, 23). Importantly, both Myc and HIF-1α are under the control of the mTOR complex. C-Myc promotes the expression of enzymes involved in aerobic glycolysis and glutaminolysis and fine-tunes these metabolic pathways to the biosynthesis of lipids, amino acids, and nucleic acids. HIF-1α mediates T cell responses to oxygen levels and also promotes glucose uptake and breakdown (24). Thus, the same transcription master regulators that control such fundamental processes as cell proliferation and cellular response to oxygen tension are also responsible for adjusting T cell metabolism to emerging needs. This underscores the startling universality and efficiency of these most fundamental mechanisms of epigenetic regulation and indicates that a robust reprogramming of antitumor T cell metabolism might be achieved by only targeting a few select molecules.

The dichotomy between glycolysis versus OXPHOS and FAO is not only central to the control of T cell activation and effector function but is also decisive in the fate of differentiating T cells. Most importantly, in precursors of long-lived memory cells, OXPHOS and FAO are engaged to balance out the effects of aerobic glycolysis (25). A pivotal role for mitochondria (26) in these cells is manifest in the dynamics of their ultrastructure. In memory T cells, mitochondrial cristae fuse into elaborate networks, while mitochondria in effector T cells exhibit extensive fission. The functionality of mature memory cells is also sustained by the higher biomass and spare respiratory capacity of their mitochondria through IL-15-driven upregulation of carnitine palmitoyl-transferase. This enzyme drives FAO and engenders stronger and more protracted OXPHOS and glycolysis upon restimulation.

Importantly, a wealth of recent evidence illuminates the possibilities to improve clinical responses to immune checkpoint inhibitors by combining these therapies with modulation of metabolic pathways. For instance, a series of elegant studies by Chi and colleagues (7, 27, 28) have demonstrated the intimate interplay between immune and metabolic checkpoints in T cell differentiation. Specifically, mTORC1 signaling was established as a key "rheostat" in Treg cell function (28). Treg-intrinsic disruption of mTORC1 led to a drastic slump in Treg suppressive activity and launched a deadly early-onset inflammatory disease. Raptor/ mTORC1 signaling in Tregs boosted the metabolism of cholesterol and lipids, while the mevalonate pathway proved essential for orchestrating Treg proliferation and upregulated expression of the checkpoint molecules CTLA4 and ICOS. Another study by the same group highlighted the role of autophagy in the lineage stability and survival of Treg cells (29). Treg cell-specific deficiency in Atg7 or Atg5, two pivotal genes in autophagy, resulted in a diminished Treg compartment, improved antitumor immunity, and development of inflammatory disorders. Autophagy kept in check mTORC1, c-Myc, and glycolytic enzymes, thereby coupling environmental signals to metabolic homeostasis.

METABOLIC COMPETITION IN THE TUMOR MICROENVIRONMENT

Recent studies have directly linked T cell metabolism, T cell exhaustion, and antitumor immunity. In the tumor, the scarcity of nutrients can profoundly affect cell proliferation, survival, and functionality. T cell-infiltrating tumors become enmeshed into teeming metabolic networks established within the hostile microenvironment and are forced to face ruthless competition for nutrients. Cancer cells can express various enzymes that deprive T cells of critical substrates and produce immune-inhibitory metabolites (**Figure 1**). For instance, many tumors contain large amounts of indoleamine 2,3-dioxygenase (IDO), an enzyme that eliminates tryptophan from the microenvironment and hampers T cell proliferation (30). Of note, despite the significant efficacy of IDO inhibitors in mouse models of cancer, these compounds have shown no measurable antitumor efficacy in clinical settings (31). The potential advantages and pitfalls of therapeutically exploiting the metabolic differences between normal and malignant cells have recently been comprehensively surveyed by Martinez-Outschoorn and coauthors (32).

In two pioneering studies, published side by side in *Cell* (5, 6), the groups of Susan Kaech and Erika Pearce reported that tumor cells outcompete T cells for glucose, thereby dampening their effector function and evading immune destruction. Ho et al. (5) demonstrated that unperturbed glucose metabolism in T cells is critical for TCR-induced Ca^{2+} flux. Extracellular glucose promoted accumulation of phosphoenolpyruvate, a glycolytic metabolite that inhibited sequestering of Ca^{2+} from the cytoplasm into the ER, thereby sustaining activation-induced Ca^{2+} flux and T cell effector function. Conversely, increased expression of the glycolysis gatekeeper hexokinase 2 in tumor cells facilitated tumor escape from $CD4^+$ T cell-mediated immune surveillance, further corroborating the importance of metabolic competition between tumor-infiltrating lymphocytes (TILs) and tumor cells.

In the other study, Chang et al. (6) demonstrated that signaling through PD-L1 in tumor cells promotes glycolysis *via* activation of the AKT/mTOR pathway. Therapeutic blockade of PD-L1 decreased glycolysis rate by triggering PD-L1 internalization, restored glucose levels in the microenvironment, and hindered tumor progression. These data provided a breakthrough in our understanding of the deeply intertwined metabolic and immune checkpoint signaling pathways and underscore the potential of future immune-metabolic therapies.

Conversely, rather than targeting the metabolism of tumor cells, Ho et al. (5) put forward an alternative strategy to reinforce T cell function by artificially increasing PEP levels in adoptively transferred tumor-reactive T cells. PEP carboxykinase (PCK1) catalyzes conversion of oxaloacetate into PEP. Overexpression of PCK1 in transferred T cells allowed the authors to restore TCR-driven Ca^{2+} flux and anticancer T cell activity, thus overriding the effects of low glucose levels in the tumor microenvironment. Overall, these reports provided inspiring examples of reprogramming T cell metabolism to enhance the efficacy of adoptive cell therapies for cancer and spawned many further studies exploring T cell metabolic dysfunction in the tumor.

For instance, the latest works by Delgoffe and colleagues shed new light on various aspects of T cell metabolism in cancer. For example, Scharping et al. (33) reported a continuous loss of mitochondrial mass and functionality in tumor-infiltrating T cells, which proved restricted to the tumor milieu and was not a mere consequence of activation. Due to chronic Akt signaling, TILs showed dwindling expression of PPAR-gamma coactivator 1α (PGC1α), a vital factor in mitochondrial biogenesis. Reprogramming TILs through forced expression of PGC1α reinvigorated their metabolic and effector function. Interestingly, in a study by Wherry and colleagues (34), PD-1 was shown to inhibit PGC1α and thereby serve as a dominant-negative regulator of glycolysis in activated T cells.

More recently, it has been reported that T cell activation leads to a rapid glycolytic switch independently of transcription, translation, costimulation through CD28, or Akt signaling and without an increase in glucose uptake or in the activity of glycolytic enzymes (35). Instead, TCR engagement enhances activation of pyruvate dehydrogenase kinase 1 (PDHK1), thereby hampering import of pyruvate into mitochondria and promoting its cleavage into lactate. Intriguingly, inhibiting PDHK1 revealed that the early glycolytic switch is required for immediate cytokine production but not for cytotoxicity. Recently, Menk et al. (36) demonstrated that ligation of 4-1BB (a costimulatory molecule highly expressed

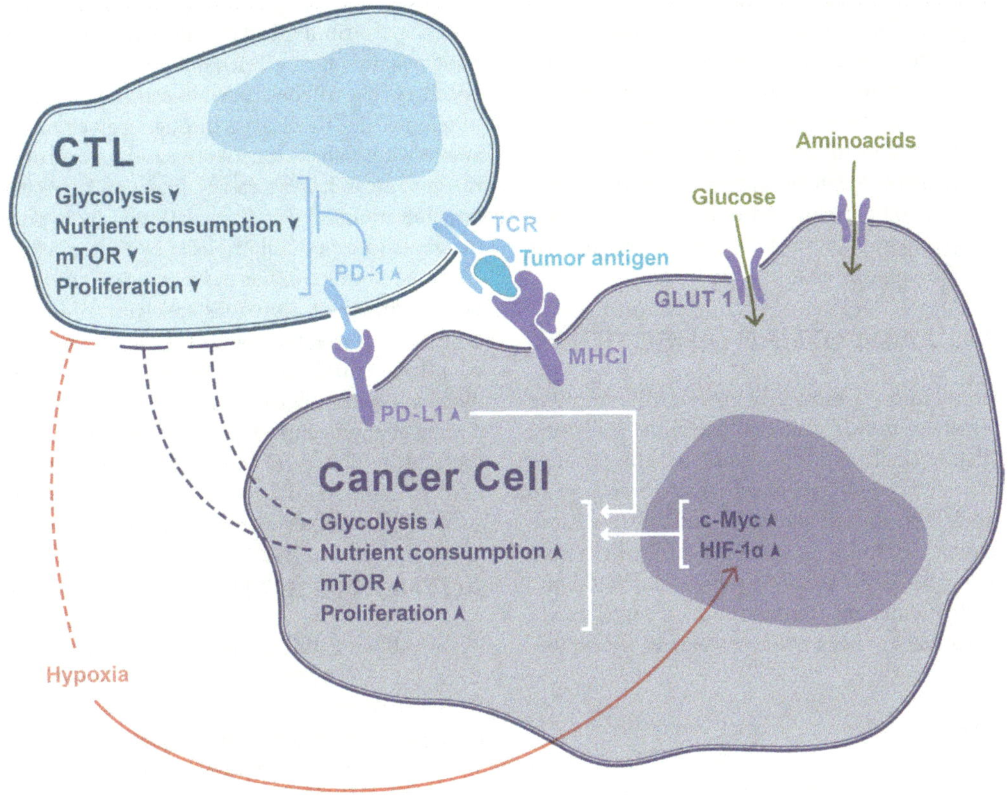

FIGURE 1 | Rapidly proliferating tumor cells avidly consume nutrients from the microenvironment, thereby outcompeting T cells in a contest for metabolic fitness. Increased activity of hypoxia-inducible factor-1α (HIF-1α) driven by tumor hypoxia further intensifies glycolysis and exacerbates the paucity of glucose in the milieu. This results in T cell deprivation of essential fuel for their effector function, resulting in a thwarted antitumor immune response. PD-1 signaling in T cells dampens their glycolytic activity and proliferation, while PD-1 ligand (PD-L1) ligation leads to opposite effects in cancer cells.

on exhausted T cells) provides metabolic support to tumor-infiltrating T cells by enhancing their mitochondrial capacity and engaging PGC1α-mediated pathways. Remarkably, 4-1BB stimulation combined with PD-1 blockade resulted in robust antitumor immunity. This study further highlights the potential of combinatorial strategies targeting immune-metabolic checkpoints for reshaping the immune-inhibitory tumor milieu.

OXYGEN SENSING

The transcription factor HIF-1α is a critical driver of effector T cell responses, which is particularly important for the differentiation of $CD4^+$ Th17 cells (37), $CD8^+$ T cell effector function (22), and interferon IFN-γ production by T regulatory cells. Besides governing the glycolytic switch in Th17 cells, HIF-1α also transactivates the gene encoding the Th17 master transcription factor RORγt (37). It has been demonstrated that HIF-1α-mediated T cell response to hypoxia upregulates the expression of Glut1, as well as glycolytic enzymes, and therefore strongly affects T cell differentiation and function. For instance, Cretenet et al. (38) demonstrated that hypoxia significantly enhances Glut1 upregulation in response to TCR stimulation. Furthermore, $Glut1^{hi}$ T lymphocytes displayed more pronounced Th1 effector phenotype and higher proliferation rate than their $Glut1^{lo}$ counterparts, both under normoxic and hypoxic conditions. Therefore, enhancing glucose uptake in adoptively transferred T cells might allow for efficiently countering hypoxia-driven immune suppression.

The activity of HIF-1a is tightly controlled by the oxygen-sensing prolyl-hydroxylase (PHD) proteins. Under normoxia, PHDs hydroxylate HIF-1α and HIF-2α, thereby targeting them for degradation. In their recent study, Restifo and colleagues (39) found that expression of PHDs in T cells ensures local tolerance for harmless antigens in the lung but markedly facilitates the seeding of circulating tumor cells. In line with their role as HIF-1α inhibitors, PHDs limited pulmonary Th1 responses, promoted Treg cell induction, and dampened $CD8^+$ T cell function. Importantly, it was shown that the effects of the PHD enzymes are primarily mediated by the repression of HIF-driven glycolytic metabolism.

Specifically, T cells stimulated in TGF-β-containing media exhibited a PHD-dependent reduction of glycolytic activity. On the other hand, PHD-deficient $CD4^+$ T cells exhibited accelerated uptake of glucose and switched to an anaerobic metabolic program. PHD proteins also restrained glycolysis in $CD8^+$ T cells. Remarkably, targeting mTOR-driven glycolytic metabolism with rapamycin and 2-deoxyglucose completely blocked spontaneous Th1 development and partially restored iTreg cell differentiation in PHD-deficient T cells. Hence, oxygen sensing appears to coordinate transcriptional and metabolic programs driving the differentiation of Th1 and iTreg cells. Recent clinical studies have demonstrated the efficacy and overall safety of PHD inhibitors in patients with anemia and other hypoxia-driven pathologies (40). However, the complexity and the near-universal nature of the HIF pathways necessitate thorough evaluation of adverse effects. Collectively, targeting PHD proteins and other links in oxygen sensing is an alluring strategy to tilt the balance between immune activation and immune suppression in the tumor.

CONCLUSION AND FUTURE DIRECTIONS

Metabolism is integral to every biological process. The immune system largely consists of mobile cells that patrol the body and need to adapt to diverse challenging environments. This requires tight and sophisticated coordination of their bioenergetic machinery with their homeostatic pathways and effector functions. Here, we summarized the latest studies shedding light onto the specific roles of particular substrates, enzymes, and metabolic regulators in T cell differentiation and antitumor activity. Despite the startling progress that has been made in the field within just a few years, several critical questions remain unanswered. For instance, the timing and the mutual causality of the major metabolic switches during T cell differentiation remain largely elusive. Specifically, it will be crucial to capture the exact moments when differentiating T cells pass through a given metabolic checkpoint and how this affects the identity and the fate of a T cell. Likewise, further research is necessary to gain a more integrative view of how intratumoral T cells are affected by hypoxia and relentless metabolic competition imposed by cancer cells.

In the same vein, there is a pressing need to assess the therapeutic efficacy of a broader spectrum of genetic modifications targeting diverse metabolic regulators and oxygen sensors in adoptively transferred T cells. Importantly, the ubiquity of many metabolic pathways calls for careful target selection and cautious design of therapeutic regimens based on highly specific small molecule inhibitors. Overall, future immune-metabolic therapies have all the potential to make a critical difference for patients suffering from otherwise untreatable cancers.

AUTHOR CONTRIBUTIONS

IS and AB wrote this manuscript. IS generated the figures.

REFERENCES

1. Ribas A, Wolchok JD. Cancer immunotherapy using checkpoint blockade. *Science* (2018) 359(6382):1350–5. doi:10.1126/science.aar4060
2. Buck MD, Sowell RT, Kaech SM, Pearce EL. Metabolic instruction of immunity. *Cell* (2017) 169(4):570–86. doi:10.1016/j.cell.2017.04.004
3. Chang CH, Pearce EL. Emerging concepts of T cell metabolism as a target of immunotherapy. *Nat Immunol* (2016) 17(4):364–8. doi:10.1038/ni.3415
4. Geltink RIK, Kyle RL, Pearce EL. Unraveling the complex interplay between T cell metabolism and function. *Annu Rev Immunol* (2018) 36:461–88. doi:10.1146/annurev-immunol-042617-053019
5. Ho PC, Bihuniak JD, MacIntyre AN, Staron M, Liu X, Amezquita R, et al. Phosphoenolpyruvate is a metabolic checkpoint of anti-tumor T cell responses. *Cell* (2015) 162(6):1217–28. doi:10.1016/j.cell.2015.08.012
6. Chang CH, Qiu J, O'Sullivan D, Buck MD, Noguchi T, Curtis JD, et al. Metabolic competition in the tumor microenvironment is a driver of cancer progression. *Cell* (2015) 162(6):1229–41. doi:10.1016/j.cell.2015.08.016
7. Zeng H, Chi H. mTOR signaling in the differentiation and function of regulatory and effector T cells. *Curr Opin Immunol* (2017) 46:103–11. doi:10.1016/j.coi.2017.04.005
8. Hough KP, Chisolm DA, Weinmann AS. Transcriptional regulation of T cell metabolism. *Mol Immunol* (2015) 68(2 Pt C):520–6. doi:10.1016/j.molimm.2015.07.038
9. Kishton RJ, Sukumar M, Restifo NP. Metabolic regulation of T cell longevity and function in tumor immunotherapy. *Cell Metab* (2017) 26(1):94–109. doi:10.1016/j.cmet.2017.06.016
10. Roychoudhuri R, Eil RL, Restifo NP. The interplay of effector and regulatory T cells in cancer. *Curr Opin Immunol* (2015) 33:101–11. doi:10.1016/j.coi.2015.02.003
11. Chang C-H, Curtis JD, Maggi LB, Faubert B, Villarino AV, O'Sullivan D, et al. Posttranscriptional control of T cell effector function by aerobic glycolysis. *Cell* (2013) 153(6):1239–51. doi:10.1016/j.cell.2013.05.016
12. Frauwirth KA, Riley JL, Harris MH, Parry RV, Rathmell JC, Plas DR, et al. The CD28 signaling pathway regulates glucose metabolism. *Immunity* (2002) 16(6):769–77. doi:10.1016/S1074-7613(02)00323-0
13. Wieman HL, Wofford JA, Rathmell JC. Cytokine stimulation promotes glucose uptake via phosphatidylinositol-3 kinase/Akt regulation of Glut1 activity and trafficking. *Mol Biol Cell* (2007) 18(4):1437–46. doi:10.1091/mbc.e06-07-0593
14. Kolev M, Markiewski MM. Targeting complement-mediated immunoregulation for cancer immunotherapy. *Semin Immunol* (2018) 37:85–97. doi:10.1016/j.smim.2018.02.003
15. Laplante M, Sabatini DM. mTOR signaling in growth control and disease. *Cell* (2012) 149(2):274–93. doi:10.1016/j.cell.2012.03.017
16. Macintyre AN, Gerriets VA, Nichols AG, Michalek RD, Rudolph MC, Deoliveira D, et al. The glucose transporter Glut1 is selectively essential for CD4 T cell activation and effector function. *Cell Metab* (2014) 20(1):61–72. doi:10.1016/j.cmet.2014.05.004
17. Sanin DE, Pearce EJ. The cell identity of cytotoxic T lymphocytes. *Nat Immunol* (2016) 17(1):45–6. doi:10.1038/ni.3350
18. Gerriets VA, Kishton RJ, Johnson MO, Cohen S, Siska PJ, Nichols AG, et al. Foxp3 and toll-like receptor signaling balance Treg cell anabolic metabolism for suppression. *Nat Immunol* (2016) 17(12):1459–66. doi:10.1038/ni.3577
19. Sukumar M, Kishton RJ, Restifo NP. Metabolic reprograming of anti-tumor immunity. *Curr Opin Immunol* (2017) 46:14–22. doi:10.1016/j.coi.2017.03.011
20. Campbell DJ. Control of regulatory T cell migration, function, and homeostasis. *J Immunol* (2015) 195(6):2507–13. doi:10.4049/jimmunol.1500801
21. Kishore M, Cheung KCP, Fu H, Bonacina F, Wang G, Coe D, et al. Regulatory T cell migration is dependent on glucokinase-mediated glycolysis. *Immunity* (2017) 47(5):875–89.e10. doi:10.1016/j.immuni.2017.10.017
22. Doedens AL, Phan AT, Stradner MH, Fujimoto JK, Nguyen JV, Yang E, et al. Hypoxia-inducible factors enhance the effector responses of CD8 + T cells to persistent antigen. *Nat Immunol* (2013) 14(11):1173–82. doi:10.1038/ni.2714
23. Wang R, Dillon CP, Shi LZ, Milasta S, Carter R, Finkelstein D, et al. The transcription factor Myc controls metabolic reprogramming upon T lymphocyte activation. *Immunity* (2011) 35(6):871–82. doi:10.1016/j.immuni.2011.09.021
24. Phan AT, Doedens AL, Palazon A, Tyrakis PA, Cheung KP, Johnson RS, et al. Constitutive glycolytic metabolism supports CD8+ T cell effector memory differentiation during viral infection. *Immunity* (2016) 45(5):1024–37. doi:10.1016/j.immuni.2016.10.017
25. O'Sullivan D, vanderWindt GWJ, Huang SCC, Curtis JD, Chang CH, Buck MDL, et al. Memory CD8^{+} T cells use cell-intrinsic lipolysis to support the metabolic programming necessary for development. *Immunity* (2014) 41(1):75–88. doi:10.1016/j.immuni.2014.06.005
26. van der Windt GJ, Everts B, Chang CH, Curtis JD, Freitas TC, Amiel E, et al. Mitochondrial respiratory capacity is a critical regulator of CD8+ T cell memory development. *Immunity* (2012) 36(1):68–78. doi:10.1016/j.immuni.2011.12.007

27. Yang K, Blanco DB, Neale G, Vogel P, Avila J, Clish CB, et al. Homeostatic control of metabolic and functional fitness of Treg cells by LKB1 signalling. *Nature* (2017) 548(7669):602–6. doi:10.1038/nature23665
28. Zeng H, Cohen S, Guy C, Shrestha S, Neale G, Brown SA, et al. mTORC1 and mTORC2 kinase signaling and glucose metabolism drive follicular helper T cell differentiation. *Immunity* (2016) 45(3):540–54. doi:10.1016/j.immuni.2016.08.017
29. Wei J, Long L, Yang K, Guy C, Shrestha S, Chen Z, et al. Autophagy enforces functional integrity of regulatory T cells by coupling environmental cues and metabolic homeostasis. *Nat Immunol* (2016) 17(3):277–85. doi:10.1038/ni.3365
30. Munn DH, Mellor AL. Indoleamine 2,3 dioxygenase and metabolic control of immune responses. *Trends Immunol* (2013) 34(3):137–43. doi:10.1016/j.it.2012.10.001
31. Garber K. A new cancer immunotherapy suffers a setback. *Science* (2018) 360(6389):588. doi:10.1126/science.360.6389.588
32. Martinez-Outschoorn UE, Peiris-Pagés M, Pestell RG, Sotgia F, Lisanti MP. Cancer metabolism: a therapeutic perspective. *Nat Rev Clin Oncol* (2017) 14(1):11–31. doi:10.1038/nrclinonc.2016.60
33. Scharping NE, Menk AV, Moreci RS, Whetstone RD, Dadey RE, Watkins SC, et al. The tumor microenvironment represses T cell mitochondrial biogenesis to drive intratumoral T cell metabolic insufficiency and dysfunction. *Immunity* (2016) 45(2):374–88. doi:10.1016/j.immuni.2016.07.009
34. Bengsch B, Johnson AL, Kurachi M, Odorizzi PM, Pauken KE, Attanasio J, et al. Bioenergetic insufficiencies due to metabolic alterations regulated by the inhibitory receptor PD-1 are an early driver of CD8+T cell exhaustion. *Immunity* (2016) 45(2):358–73. doi:10.1016/j.immuni.2016.07.008
35. Menk AV, Scharping NE, Moreci RS, Zeng X, Guy C, Salvatore S, et al. Early TCR signaling induces rapid aerobic glycolysis enabling distinct acute T cell effector functions. *Cell Rep* (2018) 22(6):1509–21. doi:10.1016/j.celrep.2018.01.040
36. Menk AV, Scharping NE, Rivadeneira DB, Calderon MJ, Watson MJ, Dunstane D, et al. 4-1BB costimulation induces T cell mitochondrial function and biogenesis enabling cancer immunotherapeutic responses. *J Exp Med* (2018) 215(4):1091–100. doi:10.1084/jem.20171068
37. Dang EV, Barbi J, Yang HY, Jinasena D, Yu H, Zheng Y, et al. Control of TH17/Treg balance by hypoxia-inducible factor 1. *Cell* (2011) 146(5):772–84. doi:10.1016/j.cell.2011.07.033
38. Cretenet G, Clerc I, Matias M, Loisel S, Craveiro M, Oburoglu L, et al. Cell surface Glut1 levels distinguish human CD4 and CD8 T lymphocyte subsets with distinct effector functions. *Sci Rep* (2016) 6:24129. doi:10.1038/srep24129
39. Clever D, Roychoudhuri R, Constantinides MG, Askenase MH, Sukumar M, Klebanoff CA, et al. Oxygen sensing by T cells establishes an immunologically tolerant metastatic niche. *Cell* (2016) 166(5):1117–31.e14. doi:10.1016/j.cell.2016.07.032
40. Chan MC, Holt-Martyn JP, Schofield CJ, Ratcliffe PJ. Pharmacological targeting of the HIF hydroxylases – a new field in medicine development. *Mol Aspects Med* (2016) 47–48:54–75. doi:10.1016/j.mam.2016.01.001

6

Myeloid-Derived Suppressor Cells Hinder the Anti-Cancer Activity of Immune Checkpoint Inhibitors

*Rebekka Weber[1,2,3], Viktor Fleming[1,2,3], Xiaoying Hu[1,2], Vasyl Nagibin[1,2], Christopher Groth[1,2], Peter Altevogt[1,2], Jochen Utikal[1,2] and Viktor Umansky[1,2]**

[1] Skin Cancer Unit, German Cancer Research Center (DKFZ), Heidelberg, Germany, [2] Department of Dermatology, Venereology and Allergology, University Medical Center Mannheim, Ruprecht-Karl University of Heidelberg, Mannheim, Germany, [3] Faculty of Biosciences, Ruprecht-Karl University of Heidelberg, Heidelberg, Germany

Edited by:
Amedeo Amedei, Università degli Studi di Firenze, Italy

Reviewed by:
Rodabe N. Amaria, University of Texas MD Anderson Cancer Center, United States
Ekaterina Jordanova, Center for Gynecologic Oncology Amsterdam, Netherlands

***Correspondence:**
Viktor Umansky
v.umansky@dkfz.de

Immune checkpoint inhibitors (ICI) used for cancer immunotherapy were shown to boost the existing anti-tumor immune response by preventing the inhibition of T cells by tumor cells. Antibodies targeting two negative immune checkpoint pathways, namely cytotoxic T-lymphocyte-associated protein 4 (CTLA-4), programmed cell death protein 1 (PD-1), and programmed cell death-ligand 1 (PD-L1), have been approved first for patients with melanoma, squamous non-small cell lung cancer (NSCLC), and renal cell carcinoma. Clinical trials are ongoing to verify the efficiency of these antibodies for other cancer types and to evaluate strategies to block other checkpoint molecules. However, a number of patients do not respond to this treatment possibly due to profound immunosuppression, which is mediated partly by myeloid-derived suppressor cells (MDSC). This heterogeneous population of immature myeloid cells can strongly inhibit anti-tumor activities of T and NK cells and stimulate regulatory T cells (Treg), leading to tumor progression. Moreover, MDSC can contribute to patient resistance to immune checkpoint inhibition. Accumulating evidence demonstrates that the frequency and immunosuppressive function of MDSC in cancer patients can be used as a predictive marker for therapy response. This review focuses on the role of MDSC in immune checkpoint inhibition and provides an analysis of combination strategies for MDSC targeting together with ICI to improve their therapeutic efficiency in cancer patients.

Keywords: myeloid-derived suppressor cells, immunosuppression, cancer immunotherapy, immune checkpoint inhibition, combination therapy

---

Abbreviations: ATRA, all-trans retinoic acid; ARG-1, arginase-1; bFGF, basic fibroblast growth factor; CCR, C-C chemokine receptor; CCL, C-C motif chemokine ligand; CXCL, C-X-C motif chemokine ligand; CCRK, cell cycle-related kinase; CSF-1R, colony stimulating factor 1 receptor; CTLA-4, cytotoxic T-lymphocyte-associated protein 4; DAMP, damage-associated molecular pattern; DC, dendritic cells; GM-CSF, granulocyte-macrophage colony stimulating factor; ICI, immune checkpoint inhibitors; IDO, indoleamine 2,3-dioxygenase; iNOS, inducible nitric oxide synthase; IFN, interferon; IL, interleukin; JAK, Janus kinase; MMP, matrix metalloproteinases; MyD88, myeloid differentiation primary response 88, MDSC, myeloid-derived suppressor cells; NK, natural killer; NO, nitric oxide; NSCLC, non-small cell lung cancer; NF-κB, nuclear factor "kappa-light-chain-enhancer" of activated B-cells; NY-ESO-1, New York esophageal squamous cell carcinoma-1; PBMC, peripheral blood mononuclear cells; PI3K, phosphatidylinositol-4,5-bisphosphate 3-kinase; PDE5, phosphodiesterase-5; PD-1, programmed cell death protein 1, PD-L1, programmed cell death-ligand 1; ROS, reactive oxygen species; Treg, regulatory T cells; STAT, signal transducer and activator of transcription; TCR, T cell receptor; TLR, toll-like receptor; TGF, transforming growth factor; VEGF, vascular endothelial growth factor; VEGFR, VEGF receptor.

INTRODUCTION

Cancer immunotherapy has become a promising approach to treat patients over the past decade (1). Furthermore, new types of cancer immunotherapy that are currently under investigation will impact the treatment of cancer patients in the future. Among immunotherapeutic approaches, immune checkpoint inhibition is very promising. However, other types of immunotherapies such as monoclonal antibodies against tumor-associated antigens, cancer vaccines, cell therapy, and unspecific boosting of the immune system with interleukins (IL), interferons (IFN), or toll-like receptor (TLR) ligands are also used and/or under investigation (2).

Immune checkpoint pathways are important to restrict excessive immune responses (3). However, under cancer conditions, tumor cells can exploit these mechanisms to impair or prevent the tumor-targeted immune response. Signals transmitted to T cells either *via* programmed cell death protein 1 (PD-1) or cytotoxic T-lymphocyte-associated protein 4 (CTLA-4) promote T cell anergy and thereby switch off the immune response. Therefore, blockers of these immune checkpoint molecules have been shown to restore an immune response against cancer and increase patient survival (4, 5).

Ipilimumab (monoclonal antibody against CTLA-4) is used for the therapy of cutaneous melanoma. Nivolumab and pembrolizumab (monoclonal antibodies against PD-1) are approved for the therapy of cutaneous melanoma, non-small cell lung cancer (NSCLC), kidney cancer, bladder cancer, head and neck cancers, and Hodgkin lymphoma. Atezolizumab [monoclonal antibody against programmed cell death-ligand 1 (PD-L1)] is approved for the treatment of NSCLC and bladder cancer and avelumab (monoclonal antibody against PD-L1) is approved for gastric cancer and Merkel cell carcinoma therapy. Despite the fact that these immune checkpoint inhibitors (ICI) have proved to be effective, therapeutic resistance occurs in the majority of patients, leading to tumor progression (5, 6). This occurs due to the immunosuppressive tumor microenvironment represented by several immunosuppressive factors and cells, including myeloid-derived suppressor cells (MDSC) (7–10). Importantly, the efficacy of cancer immunotherapy has been reported to be negatively correlated with an increased MDSC frequency and function (11–15).

Myeloid-derived suppressor cells play a leading role in immunosuppression in various cancer types. Accumulating evidences in recent years have even highlighted them as a major driver of an immunosuppressive tumor microenvironment (7–10, 16). Therefore, MDSC could be a promising target in cancer immunotherapy especially in combination with ICI. In this review, we discuss the phenotypic and functional properties of MDSC as well as strategies for their therapeutic targeting. In particular, we address the role of MDSC in immune checkpoint inhibition and provide an analysis of the combination strategies for MDSC targeting together with ICI to improve their therapeutic efficiency in cancer patients.

PHENOTYPIC AND FUNCTIONAL PROPERTIES OF MDSC

Myeloid-derived suppressor cells represent a heterogeneous population of myeloid cells that fail to differentiate into granulocytes, macrophages, or dendritic cells (DC) but expand during cancer and chronic infection (17–20). They can strongly suppress the activity of T cells, natural killer (NK) cells, and some myeloid cells such as DC (8). MDSC have been identified to expand and play an important role in various cancer types, for example, in patients with melanoma (15, 21–24), multiple myeloma (25), hepatocellular carcinoma (26), NSCLC (27), renal cell carcinoma (28), breast cancer (29), prostate cancer (30), and colorectal cancer (31).

MDSC Phenotype

In mice, MDSC were characterized by the expression of CD11b and Gr1. However, the use of these markers is no longer sufficient, since MDSC can be divided into two subpopulations in mice: $CD11b^{+}Ly6G^{-}Ly6C^{high}$ monocytic MDSC (M-MDSC) and $CD11b^{+}Ly6G^{high}Ly6C^{low}$ polymorphonuclear MDSC (PMN-MDSC) (32). Human M-MDSC are defined as $Lin^{-}CD11b^{+}CD14^{+}CD15^{-}HLA\text{-}DR^{-/low}$ and PMN-MDSC as $Lin^{-}CD11b^{+}CD14^{-}CD15^{+}HLA\text{-}DR^{-}$ or $Lin^{-}CD11b^{+}CD14^{-}CD66b^{+}$ (32, 33). One-third subtype of human MDSC, containing more immature $HLA\text{-}DR^{-}CD33^{+}CD15^{-}CD14^{-}$ MDSC, has been recently proposed and was termed early stage MDSC (eMDSC) (32).

MDSC Expansion and Activation

Myeloid-derived suppressor cells are absent in the circulation under homeostatic conditions, but they can be accumulated under pathological conditions like chronic inflammation and cancer (34–39). The expansion and activation of MDSC are controlled by a complex network of soluble factors like IL-6, granulocyte-macrophage colony stimulating factor (GM-CSF), IL-10, M-CSF, G-CSF, and vascular endothelial growth factor (VEGF) as well as TLR ligands (8, 17, 20, 32, 40). The process of MDSC generation is supposed to be divided into two phases that include MDSC accumulation and activation (8, 18–20, 40). MDSC enrichment is mediated by the blockade of the terminal differentiation of immature myeloid cells into granulocytes, macrophages, and DC due to an alteration of the growth factor composition, where G-CSF, GM-CSF, and VEGF play a major role. MDSC activation is mediated by the long-term secretion of cytokines like IL-6, IL-10, IL-1β, and IFN-γ, as well as TLR ligands, such as damage-associated molecular pattern molecules produced under chronic inflammation (8, 18–20, 40).

The production of immunosuppressive factors is driven *via* the Janus kinase (JAK)/signal transducer and activator of transcription (STAT) and myeloid differentiation primary response 88/nuclear factor "kappa-light-chain-enhancer" of activated B-cells signal transduction cascades in MDSC (17, 40).

MDSC Function

Activated MDSC produce elevated levels of nitric oxide (NO) *via* inducible nitric oxide synthase (iNOS) and upregulate the expression of arginase-1 (ARG-1), both leading to cell cycle arrest in T cells *via* depletion of the amino acid L-arginine from the tumor microenvironment (41, 42) and to T cell anergy induced by the downregulation of T cell receptor (TCR) ζ-chain expression (16, 43). Moreover, NO and reactive oxygen species produced by MDSC can induce T cell apoptosis or TCR nitrosylation (44, 45). In addition, activated MDSC express high levels of PD-L1

(46, 47) that interacts with PD-1 on T cells and causes their exhaustion (48). MDSC also express elevated levels of indoleamine 2,3-dioxygenase (IDO), an enzyme degrading L-tryptophan into N-formylkynurenine (49). The starvation from the amino acid L-tryptophan can lead to T cell arrest and anergy (50). Furthermore, it has been shown to drive the differentiation of $CD4^+$ T cells into immunosuppressive regulatory T cells (Tregs) (51). MDSC can also induce Treg expansion and reduction of the anti-tumor activity of effector T cells *via* the expression of CD40 (52) and the secretion of transforming growth factor-β and IL-10 (53–55). Furthermore, MDSC impair the Fc receptor-mediated functions of NK cells by the production of NO (56).

In addition to their immunosuppressive properties, MDSC can have other tumor promoting effects. In particular, they stimulate tumor angiogenesis by secreting VEGF and basic fibroblast growth factor (57, 58). By secreting matrix metalloproteinases (MMP), especially MMP9, they mediate a lower integrity of the extracellular matrix and the basal membrane, which enables tumor cells to enter the blood stream and form metastasis (59, 60). MDSC were also shown to play an important role in the formation of the pre-metastatic niche, a microenvironment in a secondary organ, facilitating metastasis (61).

MDSC AS A PREDICTIVE MARKER IN IMMUNE CHECKPOINT INHIBITION FOR CANCER THERAPY

Myeloid-derived suppressor cells have been reported to be an important prognostic marker for ICI treatment. Interestingly, MDSC levels could be used to predict therapy response or resistance to ipilimumab treatment in metastatic melanoma patients (62). Clinical responders to ipilimumab therapy showed a significantly lower percentage of $Lin^-CD14^+HLA\text{-}DR^-$ M-MDSC in the peripheral blood as compared to non-responders. This finding suggests the use of circulating M-MDSC frequency as a marker of response, since low frequencies identified patients who could benefit from ipilimumab treatment (62). These data are in agreement with the results from another study, showing that a higher M-MDSC frequency prevented ipilimumab-induced activation and expansion of tumor-specific T cells resulting in the lower clinical response (23). It was shown by three more studies that a lower frequency of circulating MDSC at baseline can be used as a predictive marker for ipilimumab treatment of malignant melanoma patients (14, 15, 63). Moreover, in prostate cancer patients treated with a cancer vaccine in combination with ipilimumab, a lower frequency of circulating MDSC was found to correlate with an increased overall survival of patients (64).

STRATEGIES FOR MDSC THERAPEUTIC TARGETING TO OVERCOME RESISTANCE TO ICI

Due to important role of MDSC in tumor-induced immunosuppression, these cells could be a promising target for a combination therapy with ICI. There are three different approaches to target MDSC, namely the inhibition of (i) MDSC accumulation; (ii) MDSC trafficking; and (iii) MDSC-mediated immunosuppression.

Reduction of MDSC Frequency

To reduce MDSC frequency, the process of myelopoiesis has to be normalized and MDSC accumulation has to be blocked. Some chemotherapeutics were shown to affect MDSC in tumor-bearing hosts. Using the *RET* transgenic mouse model of malignant melanoma, it was demonstrated that ultra-low non-cytotoxic doses of paclitaxel induced a reduction of MDSC numbers and immunosuppressive activity, resulting in an increased survival of melanoma-bearing mice (65). Furthermore, the treatment of pancreatic cancer patients with gemcitabine led to a reduced number of PMN-MDSC (66). In colorectal cancer patients, the treatment with FOLFOX (folinic acid, 5-fluorouracil, and oxaliplatin) resulted in a reduced immunosuppression and a better clinical outcome that could be attributed to a decrease in MDSC frequency and restored anti-tumor immunity (67).

It has been described that the blockade of retinoic acid signal transduction by all-trans retinoic acid (ATRA) led to the differentiation of MDSC into macrophages and DC in murine and human cell samples (68). ATRA has been applied in two clinical trials, including patients with metastatic renal cell carcinoma and late stage small cell lung cancer, leading to a reduction of MDSC frequencies and an improvement of the patient survival (69, 70).

Blockade of MDSC Recruitment

To exhibit their immunosuppressive phenotype, MDSC have to be recruited to the tumor site. This process is mediated mainly by chemokines secreted in the tumor microenvironment and chemokine receptors expressed on MDSC (71, 72). The role of C-C motif chemokine ligand (CCL)2 and its receptors C-C chemokine receptor (CCR)2 and 4 in the recruitment of M-MDSC has been well-documented (71, 73). Moreover, it was recently found that CCR5 is expressed on MDSC in *RET* transgenic melanoma-bearing mice and melanoma patients, playing an important role in their recruitment to the tumor microenvironment *via* the CCR5 ligands (CCL3, CCL4, and CCL5) (74, 75). Interestingly, $CCR5^+$ MDSC were reported to display higher immunosuppressive potential than their $CCR5^-$ counterpart both in mice and patients (74). Moreover, the blockade of the interaction of CCR5 with its ligands by a mCCR5-Ig fusion protein significantly improved the survival of melanoma-bearing animals (74). In addition, in a prostate cancer mouse model, the recruitment of $CD11b^+Gr1^+$ MDSC could be blocked by a CXC chemokine receptor 2 antagonist, thereby potentiating the therapeutic effect of the chemotherapeutic drug docetaxel (76).

Inhibition of MDSC-Mediated Immunosuppression

Phosphodiesterase-5 inhibitors (sildenafil, tadalafil, and vardenafil) are currently in clinical use for non-tumor conditions (77). However, sildenafil was already shown in several transplantable tumor mouse models to downregulate ARG-1 and iNOS expression in MDSC reducing thereby their immunosuppressive capacity and leading to an enhanced intratumoral T cell infiltration and activation, a reduction of tumor growth, and an improvement of the anti-tumor efficacy of adoptive T cell therapy (78). In the *RET* transgenic melanoma mouse model, sildenafil could also prolong mouse survival that was associated with reduced levels and activity of MDSC in the tumor microenvironment and, therefore, with a restored $CD8^+$ T cell infiltration and function (79). Furthermore, in an inflammation-dependent murine colon cancer model, sildenafil prevented tumorigenesis by inhibiting tumor infiltration with MDSC (80).

In clinical trials, tadalafil was applied in patients with head and neck squamous cell carcinoma and metastatic melanoma (81–83). It improved clinical outcome and augmented the anti-tumor immune response of patients due to the reduction of peripheral and tumor-infiltrating MDSC, highlighting thereby its potential application in combined immunotherapy (81–83).

Another promising approach is targeting of STAT3, since it is a main regulator of MDSC immunosuppressive activity (8, 18–20, 40, 84). Systemic administration of the STAT3 antisense oligonucleotide inhibitor AZD9150 was already tested in a phase I clinical trial in patients with lung cancer and lymphoma (85). It has been recently developed a strategy aiming to target STAT3 decoy oligonucleotides specifically to myeloid cells by coupling them to the TLR9 ligand CpG, which led to a reduced ARG-1 expression and to the restoration of T cell functions in patients with acute myeloid leukemia (86).

COMBINATION OF ICI AND MDSC NEUTRALIZATION

In recent years, the combination of MDSC targeting with ICI treatment has been applied in preclinical tumor models and cancer patients. **Figure 1** illustrates the effect of combination of ICI and MDSC-targeted therapy to enable an anti-tumor immune response. Interestingly, it was shown that anti-PD-1

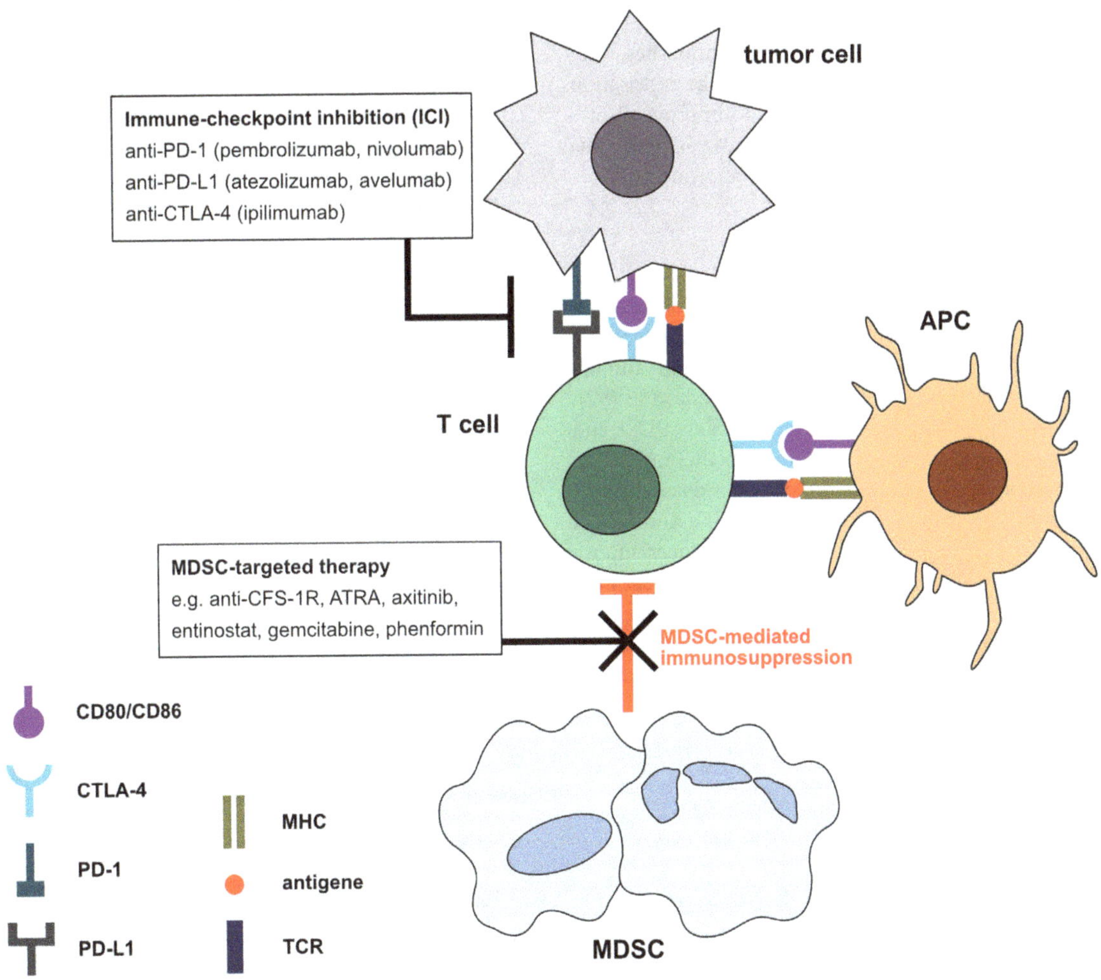

FIGURE 1 | Mechanism of immune checkpoint inhibitors (ICI) in combination with myeloid-derived suppressor cell (MDSC) neutralization. In the tumor microenvironment, tumor and antigen-presenting cells express the ligands for programmed cell death protein 1 and cytotoxic T-lymphocyte-associated protein 4 receptors on T cells. Signals transmitted *via* these receptors induce a T cell arrest and the termination of the anti-tumor immune response. Blockade of these negative checkpoint molecules can restore the anti-tumor activity of T cells. However, MDSC can induce T cell inhibition by mechanisms different from negative checkpoint molecules. The combination of MDSC inhibition with ICI could further increase T cell-mediated anti-tumor immune responses and the clinical outcome of cancer patients.

antibodies themselves seem to have a direct effect on peripheral blood mononuclear cells (PBMC) from cancer patients. It was reported that anti-PD-1 antibodies stimulated *in vitro* PBMC proliferation induced by anti-CD3 antibodies and inhibited the induction of MDSC in the same experimental settings (87).

ICI Plus Reduction of MDSC Frequency

In two different tumor mouse models, the reduction of MDSC by a histone-deacetylase inhibitor, entinostat, in combination with antibodies against CTLA-4 and PD-1 led to 80% tumor eradication although the application of these ICI alone failed to induce anti-tumor effects (88). In Lewis lung and renal cell carcinoma mouse models, MDSC blocking by entinostat in combination with PD-1 blockade resulted in a significantly increased survival in comparison to anti-PD-1 therapy alone (89). Furthermore, MDSC inhibition by phenformin, an antidiabetic drug from the biguanide class, was able to enhance the effect of PD-1 blockade reflected by an increased $CD8^+$ T cell infiltration in the BRAF V600E/PTEN-null melanoma mouse model (90).

In a murine oral cancer model, anti-Ly6G antibodies were applied to deplete PMN-MDSC that resulted in the restoration of antigen-specific T cell responses but failed to improve mouse survival (91). However, the combination of anti-Ly6G and anti-CTLA-4 antibodies induced a complete tumor rejection (91).

ICI Combined With an Alteration of MDSC Function

In a B16 melanoma mouse model expressing IDO, it has been shown that the blockade of colony stimulating factor 1 receptor (CSF-1R) by the kinase inhibitor PLX647 could inhibit tumor-infiltrating MDSC and enhance anti-tumor T cell responses (92). Moreover, this therapy sensitized the tumor for anti-PD-1 and anti-CTLA-4 antibodies, since the combination therapy led to an increased tumor regression and prolonged mouse survival as compared to the therapy with ICI alone (92). The same effect could be shown in CT26 colon and 4T1 breast cancer mouse models, where the combination of anti-CTLA-4 treatment with CSF-1/CSF-1R blockade enhanced the beneficial effect by reprogramming MDSC (93). Moreover, the expression of CSF-1 on tumor cells in melanoma and NSCLC patients correlated with the enrichment of MDSC that could be inhibited *in vitro* by the blockade of CSF-1/CSF-1R signaling (93). This observation was supported by another study, demonstrating that the blockade of M-CSF/CSF-1R interaction by BLZ945 could result in an improved efficacy of PD-1 blockade by inhibiting MDSC in mice with neuroblastoma (94).

The blockade of the VEGF receptor by axitinib in combination with anti-CTLA-4 antibodies increased survival of mice with subcutaneous melanoma and intracranial melanoma metastasis (95). This effect was due to an increased antigen-presenting capacity of DC and to a reduced suppressive capacity of M-MDSC, inducing the stimulation of $CD8^+$ and $CD4^+$ T cells (95).

Importantly, ICI treatment of head and neck cancer was reported to be noneffective due to the recruitment of MDSC (96). However, the treatment of mice bearing head and neck tumors with IPI-145, an inhibitor of phosphatidylinositol-4,5-bisphosphate 3-kinase (PI3K)δ and PI3Kγ isoforms, in combination with anti-PD-L1 antibodies resulted in the inhibition of MDSC activity associated with $CD8^+$ T cell-dependent delay of tumor growth and with an improved survival (97).

It has been demonstrated that cell cycle-related kinase (CCRK) from human hepatocytes stimulated an expansion of $CD11b^+CD33^+HLA\text{-}DR^-$ MDSC *via* an NFκB/IL-6-dependent mechanism (98). Similarly, in CCRK transgenic mice, PMN-MDSC frequency and activity were shown to be increased. Thus, upon inhibition of CCRK, PMN-MDSC numbers were decreased, an increased infiltration of $IFN\text{-}\gamma^+TNF\text{-}\alpha^+CD8^+$ T cells was observed, and tumor progression was impaired (98). The beneficial effect was even stronger upon the combination with anti-PD-L1 antibodies (98).

Ongoing Clinical Trials

Some strategies modulating MDSC frequency and immunosuppressive function are already used in various clinical trials in combination with ICI (**Table 1**). Thus, a combined therapy with the anti-PD-L1 antibody atezolizumab and the histone-deacetylase inhibitor entinostat is currently under investigation in a phase I/II clinical trial in renal cell carcinoma patients. Furthermore, ATRA was applied in combination with ipilimumab in a phase II clinical trial in melanoma patients, inducing an improvement of clinical outcome associated with increased tumor antigen-specific T cell

TABLE 1 | Clinical trials combining myeloid-derived suppressor cell (MDSC) targeting with immune checkpoint inhibitors (ICI) in cancer patients.

No	Title	Disease or conditions	Interventions	Trial number
1	Atezolizumab in combination with entinostat and bevacizumab in patients with advanced renal cell carcinoma	Advanced renal cell carcinoma	Atezolizumab, entinostat, bevacizumab	NCT03024437
2	Ipilimumab and all-trans retinoic acid (ATRA) combination treatment of stage IV melanoma	Melanoma	ATRA, ipilimumab	NCT02403778
3	Depletion of MDSC to enhance anti-programmed cell death protein 1 therapy	Non-small cell lung cancer	Nivolumab, gemcitabine	NCT03302247
4	SX-682 treatment in subjects with metastatic melanoma concurrently treated with pembrolizumab	Melanoma	SX-682, pembrolizumab	NCT03161431
5	RTA 408 capsules in patients with melanoma—REVEAL	Melanoma	Omaveloxolone, ipilimumab, nivolumab	NCT02259231
6	Antibody DS-8273a administered in combination with nivolumab in subjects with advanced colorectal cancer	Colorectal neoplasm	DS-8273a, nivolumab	NCT02991196

responses and decreased MDSC frequencies as compared to ipilimumab alone (99). Two other clinical trials in melanoma patients are utilizing the combination of ICI treatment with MDSC targeting by SX-682, a small-molecule dual-inhibitor of C-X-C motif chemokine ligand 1 and 2, or by the antioxidative and anti-inflammatory drug omaveloxolone (RTA 408). Since it was shown that gemcitabine induced a reduction in MDSC numbers in pancreatic cancer patients (66), potentially increasing thereby the efficacy of nivolumab treatment, the combination of these drugs is applied in a phase II clinical trial in NSCLC patients. Furthermore, the tumor necrosis factor-related apoptosis inducing ligand (TRAIL) receptor 2 blocking antibodies DS-8273a, targeting MDSC in cancer patients (100), were applied in a phase I clinical trial in colorectal cancer patients in combination with nivolumab.

CONCLUSION

Immune checkpoint inhibitors for cancer therapy are approved for the treatment of cutaneous melanoma, NSCLC, kidney cancer, bladder cancer, head and neck cancers, Merkel cell carcinoma, gastric cancer, and Hodgkin lymphoma and could significantly improve the clinical outcome of cancer patients. However, the resistance to ICI after initial response or total lack of response is still a problem. Resistance can be mediated by MDSC, which makes these cells a promising target for combination therapy.

In various preclinical tumor models, it has been reported that MDSC targeting potentiated the effect of ICI and led to a significantly increased survival and even to full tumor regression, which was not observed upon the treatment with ICI alone. However, only six early phase clinical trials are running to date to improve ICI outcome in cancer patients by reducing MDSC-mediated immunosuppression.

Therefore, more combinatorial trials are needed to use the strategies of MDSC neutralization to further improve the outcome of cancer immunotherapy by ICI.

AUTHOR CONTRIBUTIONS

RW: writing, review, and revision of the manuscript, preparation and revision of the figure and table. XH: preparation of the figure. VN: preparation of the table. VF, CG, PA, and JU: review and revision of the manuscript. VU: writing, review, and revision of the manuscript and revision of the table and figure.

REFERENCES

1. Farkona S, Diamandis EP, Blasutig IM. Cancer immunotherapy: the beginning of the end of cancer? *BMC Med* (2016) 14:73. doi:10.1186/s12916-016-0623-5
2. Emens LA, Ascierto PA, Darcy PK, Demaria S, Eggermont AMM, Redmond WL, et al. Cancer immunotherapy: opportunities and challenges in the rapidly evolving clinical landscape. *Eur J Cancer* (2017) 81:116–29. doi:10.1016/j.ejca.2017.01.035
3. Nirschl CJ, Drake CG. Molecular pathways: coexpression of immune checkpoint molecules: signaling pathways and implications for cancer immunotherapy. *Clin Cancer Res* (2013) 19:4917–24. doi:10.1158/1078-0432.CCR-12-1972
4. Wolchok JD, Saenger Y. The mechanism of anti-CTLA-4 activity and the negative regulation of T-cell activation. *Oncologist* (2008) 13(Suppl 4):2–9. doi:10.1634/theoncologist.13-S4-2
5. Hodi FS, O'Day SJ, McDermott DF, Weber RW, Sosman JA, Haanen JB, et al. Improved survival with ipilimumab in patients with metastatic melanoma. *N Engl J Med* (2010) 363:711–23. doi:10.1056/NEJMoa1003466
6. Robert C, Long GV, Brady B, Dutriaux C, Maio M, Mortier L, et al. Nivolumab in previously untreated melanoma without BRAF mutation. *N Engl J Med* (2015) 372:320–30. doi:10.1056/NEJMoa1412082
7. Umansky V, Sevko A. Melanoma-induced immunosuppression and its neutralization. *Semin Cancer Biol* (2012) 22:319–26. doi:10.1016/j.semcancer.2012.02.003
8. Kumar V, Patel S, Tcyganov E, Gabrilovich DI. The nature of myeloid-derived suppressor cells in the tumor microenvironment. *Trends Immunol* (2016) 37:208–20. doi:10.1016/j.it.2016.01.004
9. Ostrand-Rosenberg S, Fenselau C. Myeloid-derived suppressor cells: immune-suppressive cells that impair antitumor immunity and are sculpted by their environment. *J Immunol* (2018) 200:422–31. doi:10.4049/jimmunol.1701019
10. Tcyganov E, Mastio J, Chen E, Gabrilovich DI. Plasticity of myeloid-derived suppressor cells in cancer. *Curr Opin Immunol* (2018) 51:76–82. doi:10.1016/j.coi.2018.03.009
11. Hansen GL, Gaudernack G, Brunsvig PF, Cvancarova M, Kyte JA. Immunological factors influencing clinical outcome in lung cancer patients after telomerase peptide vaccination. *Cancer Immunol Immunother* (2015) 64:1609–21. doi:10.1007/s00262-015-1766-5
12. Limagne E, Euvrard R, Thibaudin M, Rébé C, Derangère V, Chevriaux A, et al. Accumulation of MDSC and Th17 cells in patients with metastatic colorectal cancer predicts the efficacy of a FOLFOX–bevacizumab drug treatment regimen. *Cancer Res* (2016) 76:5241–52. doi:10.1158/0008-5472.CAN-15-3164
13. Chesney JA, Mitchell RA, Yaddanapudi K. Myeloid-derived suppressor cells—a new therapeutic target to overcome resistance to cancer immunotherapy. *J Leukoc Biol* (2017) 102:727–40. doi:10.1189/jlb.5VMR1116-458RRR
14. Gebhardt C, Sevko A, Jiang H, Lichtenberger R, Reith M, Tarnanidis K, et al. Myeloid cells and related chronic inflammatory factors as novel predictive markers in melanoma treatment with ipilimumab. *Clin Cancer Res* (2015) 21:5453–9. doi:10.1158/1078-0432.CCR-15-0676
15. Martens A, Wistuba-Hamprecht K, Geukes Foppen M, Yuan J, Postow MA, Wong P, et al. Baseline peripheral blood biomarkers associated with clinical outcome of advanced melanoma patients treated with ipilimumab. *Clin Cancer Res* (2016) 22:2908–18. doi:10.1158/1078-0432.CCR-15-2412
16. Parker KH, Beury DW, Ostrand-Rosenberg S. Myeloid-derived suppressor cells: critical cells driving immune suppression in the tumor microenvironment. *Adv Cancer Res* (2015) 128:95–139. doi:10.1016/bs.acr.2015.04.002
17. Gabrilovich DI, Nagaraj S. Myeloid-derived suppressor cells as regulators of the immune system. *Nat Rev Immunol* (2009) 9:162–74. doi:10.1038/nri2506
18. Gabrilovich DI, Ostrand-Rosenberg S, Bronte V. Coordinated regulation of myeloid cells by tumours. *Nat Rev Immunol* (2012) 12:253–68. doi:10.1038/nri3175
19. Ostrand-Rosenberg S. Myeloid-derived suppressor cells: more mechanisms for inhibiting antitumor immunity. *Cancer Immunol Immunother* (2010) 59:1593–600. doi:10.1007/s00262-010-0855-8
20. Veglia F, Perego M, Gabrilovich D. Myeloid-derived suppressor cells coming of age. *Nat Immunol* (2018) 19:108–19. doi:10.1038/s41590-017-0022-x

21. Poschke I, Mougiakakos D, Hansson J, Masucci GV, Kiessling R. Immature immunosuppressive CD14+HLA-DR-/low cells in melanoma patients are Stat3hi and overexpress CD80, CD83, and DC-sign. *Cancer Res* (2010) 70:4335–45. doi:10.1158/0008-5472.CAN-09-3767
22. Jordan KR, Amaria RN, Ramirez O, Callihan EB, Gao D, Borakove M, et al. Myeloid-derived suppressor cells are associated with disease progression and decreased overall survival in advanced-stage melanoma patients. *Cancer Immunol Immunother* (2013) 62:1711–22. doi:10.1007/s00262-013-1475-x
23. Weide B, Martens A, Zelba H, Stutz C, Derhovanessian E, Di Giacomo AM, et al. Myeloid-derived suppressor cells predict survival of patients with advanced melanoma: comparison with regulatory T cells and NY-ESO-1- or melan-A-specific T cells. *Clin Cancer Res* (2014) 20:1601–9. doi:10.1158/1078-0432.CCR-13-2508
24. Jiang H, Gebhardt C, Umansky L, Beckhove P, Schulze TJ, Utikal J, et al. Elevated chronic inflammatory factors and myeloid-derived suppressor cells indicate poor prognosis in advanced melanoma patients. *Int J Cancer* (2015) 136:2352–60. doi:10.1002/ijc.29297
25. Brimnes MK, Vangsted AJ, Knudsen LM, Gimsing P, Gang AO, Johnsen HE, et al. Increased level of both CD4+FOXP3+ regulatory T cells and CD14+HLA-DR−/low myeloid-derived suppressor cells and decreased level of dendritic cells in patients with multiple myeloma. *Scand J Immunol* (2010) 72:540–7. doi:10.1111/j.1365-3083.2010.02463.x
26. Hoechst B, Ormandy LA, Ballmaier M, Lehner F, Krüger C, Manns MP, et al. New population of myeloid-derived suppressor cells in hepatocellular carcinoma patients induces CD4+CD25+Foxp3+ T cells. *Gastroenterology* (2008) 135:234–43. doi:10.1053/j.gastro.2008.03.020
27. Liu C-Y, Wang Y-M, Wang C-L, Feng P-H, Ko H-W, Liu Y-H, et al. Population alterations of L-arginase- and inducible nitric oxide synthase-expressed CD11b+/CD14−/CD15+/CD33+ myeloid-derived suppressor cells and CD8+ T lymphocytes in patients with advanced-stage non-small cell lung cancer. *J Cancer Res Clin Oncol* (2010) 136:35–45. doi:10.1007/s00432-009-0634-0
28. van Cruijsen H, van der Veldt AAM, Vroling L, Oosterhoff D, Broxterman HJ, Scheper RJ, et al. Sunitinib-induced myeloid lineage redistribution in renal cell cancer patients: CD1c+ dendritic cell frequency predicts progression-free survival. *Clin Cancer Res* (2008) 14:5884–92. doi:10.1158/1078-0432.CCR-08-0656
29. Danilin S, Merkel AR, Johnson JR, Johnson RW, Edwards JR, Sterling JA. Myeloid-derived suppressor cells expand during breast cancer progression and promote tumor-induced bone destruction. *Oncoimmunology* (2012) 1:1484–94. doi:10.4161/onci.21990
30. Vuk-Pavlović S, Bulur PA, Lin Y, Qin R, Szumlanski CL, Zhao X, et al. Immunosuppressive CD14 + HLA-DR low/− monocytes in prostate cancer. *Prostate* (2010) 70:443–55. doi:10.1002/pros.21078
31. Chun E, Lavoie S, Michaud M, Gallini CA, Kim J, Soucy G, et al. CCL2 promotes colorectal carcinogenesis by enhancing polymorphonuclear myeloid-derived suppressor cell population and function. *Cell Rep* (2015) 12:244–57. doi:10.1016/j.celrep.2015.06.024
32. Bronte V, Brandau S, Chen S-H, Colombo MP, Frey AB, Greten TF, et al. Recommendations for myeloid-derived suppressor cell nomenclature and characterization standards. *Nat Commun* (2016) 7:12150. doi:10.1038/ncomms12150
33. Solito S, Marigo I, Pinton L, Damuzzo V, Mandruzzato S, Bronte V. Myeloid-derived suppressor cell heterogeneity in human cancers. *Ann N Y Acad Sci* (2014) 1319:47–65. doi:10.1111/nyas.12469
34. Zhao F, Obermann S, von Wasielewski R, Haile L, Manns MP, Korangy F, et al. Increase in frequency of myeloid-derived suppressor cells in mice with spontaneous pancreatic carcinoma. *Immunology* (2009) 128:141–9. doi:10.1111/j.1365-2567.2009.03105.x
35. Gabitass RF, Annels NE, Stocken DD, Pandha HA, Middleton GW. Elevated myeloid-derived suppressor cells in pancreatic, esophageal and gastric cancer are an independent prognostic factor and are associated with significant elevation of the Th2 cytokine interleukin-13. *Cancer Immunol Immunother* (2011) 60:1419. doi:10.1007/s00262-011-1028-0
36. Ostrand-Rosenberg S, Sinha P. Myeloid-derived suppressor cells: linking inflammation and cancer. *J Immunol* (2009) 182:4499–506. doi:10.4049/jimmunol.0802740
37. Ostrand-Rosenberg S. Myeloid derived-suppressor cells: their role in cancer and obesity. *Curr Opin Immunol* (2018) 51:68–75. doi:10.1016/j.coi.2018.03.007
38. Umansky V, Sevko A. Overcoming immunosuppression in the melanoma microenvironment induced by chronic inflammation. *Cancer Immunol Immunother* (2012) 61:275–82. doi:10.1007/s00262-011-1164-6
39. Meirow Y, Kanterman J, Baniyash M. Paving the road to tumor development and spreading: myeloid-derived suppressor cells are ruling the fate. *Front Immunol* (2015) 6:523. doi:10.3389/fimmu.2015.00523
40. Condamine T, Gabrilovich DI. Molecular mechanisms regulating myeloid-derived suppressor cell differentiation and function. *Trends Immunol* (2011) 32:19–25. doi:10.1016/j.it.2010.10.002
41. Rodriguez PC, Quiceno DG, Zabaleta J, Ortiz B, Zea AH, Piazuelo MB, et al. Arginase I production in the tumor microenvironment by mature myeloid cells inhibits T-cell receptor expression and antigen-specific T-cell responses. *Cancer Res* (2004) 64:5839–49. doi:10.1158/0008-5472.CAN-04-0465
42. Rodriguez PC, Quiceno DG, Ochoa AC. L-arginine availability regulates T-lymphocyte cell-cycle progression. *Blood* (2007) 109:1568–73. doi:10.1182/blood-2006-06-031856
43. Baniyash MTCR. ζ-chain downregulation: curtailing an excessive inflammatory immune response. *Nat Rev Immunol* (2004) 4:675–87. doi:10.1038/nri1434
44. Nagaraj S, Gupta K, Pisarev V, Kinarsky L, Sherman S, Kang L, et al. Altered recognition of antigen is a mechanism of CD8+ T cell tolerance in cancer. *Nat Med* (2007) 13:828–35. doi:10.1038/nm1609
45. Bogdan C. Nitric oxide and the immune response. *Nat Immunol* (2001) 2:907–16. doi:10.1038/ni1001-907
46. Noman MZ, Desantis G, Janji B, Hasmim M, Karray S, Dessen P, et al. PD-L1 is a novel direct target of HIF-1α, and its blockade under hypoxia enhanced MDSC-mediated T cell activation. *J Exp Med* (2014) 211:781–90. doi:10.1084/jem.20131916
47. Ostrand-Rosenberg S, Horn LA, Haile ST. The programmed death-1 immune-suppressive pathway: barrier to antitumor immunity. *J Immunol* (2014) 193:3835–41. doi:10.4049/jimmunol.1401572
48. Dieterich LC, Ikenberg K, Cetintas T, Kapaklikaya K, Hutmacher C, Detmar M. Tumor-associated lymphatic vessels upregulate PDL1 to inhibit T-cell activation. *Front Immunol* (2017) 8:66. doi:10.3389/fimmu.2017.00066
49. Yu J, Du W, Yan F, Wang Y, Li H, Cao S, et al. Myeloid-derived suppressor cells suppress antitumor immune responses through IDO expression and correlate with lymph node metastasis in patients with breast cancer. *J Immunol* (2013) 190:3783–97. doi:10.4049/jimmunol.1201449
50. Platten M, Wick W, Van den Eynde BJ. Tryptophan catabolism in cancer: beyond IDO and tryptophan depletion. *Cancer Res* (2012) 72:5435–40. doi:10.1158/0008-5472.CAN-12-0569
51. Munn DH, Sharma MD, Baban B, Harding HP, Zhang Y, Ron D, et al. GCN2 kinase in T cells mediates proliferative arrest and anergy induction in response to indoleamine 2,3-dioxygenase. *Immunity* (2005) 22:633–42. doi:10.1016/j.immuni.2005.03.013
52. Pan P-Y, Ma G, Weber KJ, Ozao-Choy J, Wang G, Yin B, et al. Immune stimulatory receptor CD40 is required for T-cell suppression and T regulatory cell activation mediated by myeloid-derived suppressor cells in cancer. *Cancer Res* (2010) 70:99–108. doi:10.1158/0008-5472.CAN-09-1882
53. Pistoia V, Morandi F, Bianchi G, Pezzolo A, Prigione I, Raffaghello L. Immunosuppressive microenvironment in neuroblastoma. *Front Oncol* (2013) 3:167. doi:10.3389/fonc.2013.00167
54. Umemura N, Saio M, Suwa T, Kitoh Y, Bai J, Nonaka K, et al. Tumor-infiltrating myeloid-derived suppressor cells are pleiotropic-inflamed monocytes/macrophages that bear M1- and M2-type characteristics. *J Leukoc Biol* (2008) 83.1136–44. doi:10.1189/jlb.0907611
55. Sinha P, Clements VK, Bunt SK, Albelda SM, Ostrand-Rosenberg S. Cross-talk between myeloid-derived suppressor cells and macrophages subverts tumor immunity toward a Type 2 response. *J Immunol* (2007) 179:977–83. doi:10.4049/jimmunol.179.2.977
56. Stiff A, Trikha P, Mundy-Bosse B, McMichael E, Mace TA, Benner B, et al. Nitric oxide production by myeloid-derived suppressor cells plays a role in impairing Fc receptor-mediated natural killer cell function. *Clin Cancer Res* (2018) 24:1891–904. doi:10.1158/1078-0432.CCR-17-0691

57. Shen P, Wang A, He M, Wang Q, Zheng S. Increased circulating Lin(-/low) CD33(+) HLA-DR(-) myeloid-derived suppressor cells in hepatocellular carcinoma patients. *Hepatol Res* (2014) 44:639–50. doi:10.1111/hepr.12167
58. Schmid MC, Varner JA. Myeloid cells in tumor inflammation. *Vasc Cell* (2012) 4:14. doi:10.1186/2045-824X-4-14
59. Baniyash M. Myeloid-derived suppressor cells as intruders and targets: clinical implications in cancer therapy. *Cancer Immunol Immunother* (2016) 65:857–67. doi:10.1007/s00262-016-1849-y
60. Jacob A, Prekeris R. The regulation of MMP targeting to invadopodia during cancer metastasis. *Front Cell Dev Biol* (2015) 3:4. doi:10.3389/fcell.2015.00004
61. Sceneay J, Parker BS, Smyth MJ, Möller A. Hypoxia-driven immunosuppression contributes to the pre-metastatic niche. *Oncoimmunology* (2013) 2:e22355. doi:10.4161/onci.22355
62. Meyer C, Cagnon L, Costa-Nunes CM, Baumgaertner P, Montandon N, Leyvraz L, et al. Frequencies of circulating MDSC correlate with clinical outcome of melanoma patients treated with ipilimumab. *Cancer Immunol Immunother* (2014) 63:247–57. doi:10.1007/s00262-013-1508-5
63. Sade-Feldman M, Kanterman J, Klieger Y, Ish-Shalom E, Olga M, Saragovi A, et al. Clinical significance of circulating CD33+CD11b+HLA-DR- myeloid cells in patients with Stage IV melanoma treated with ipilimumab. *Clin Cancer Res* (2016) 22:5661–72. doi:10.1158/1078-0432.CCR-15-3104
64. Santegoets SJ, Stam AG, Lougheed SM, Gall H, Jooss K, Sacks N, et al. Myeloid derived suppressor and dendritic cell subsets are related to clinical outcome in prostate cancer patients treated with prostate GVAX and ipilimumab. *J Immunother Cancer* (2014) 2:31. doi:10.1186/s40425-014-0031-3
65. Sevko A, Michels T, Vrohlings M, Umansky L, Beckhove P, Kato M, et al. Antitumor effect of paclitaxel is mediated by inhibition of myeloid-derived suppressor cells and chronic inflammation in the spontaneous melanoma model. *J Immunol* (2013) 190:2464–71. doi:10.4049/jimmunol.1202781
66. Eriksson E, Wenthe J, Irenaeus S, Loskog A, Ullenhag G. Gemcitabine reduces MDSCs, tregs and TGFβ-1 while restoring the teff/treg ratio in patients with pancreatic cancer. *J Transl Med* (2016) 14:282. doi:10.1186/s12967-016-1037-z
67. Kanterman J, Sade-Feldman M, Biton M, Ish-Shalom E, Lasry A, Goldshtein A, et al. Adverse immunoregulatory effects of 5FU and CPT11 chemotherapy on myeloid-derived suppressor cells and colorectal cancer outcomes. *Cancer Res* (2014) 74:6022–35. doi:10.1158/0008-5472.CAN-14-0657
68. Nefedova Y, Fishman M, Sherman S, Wang X, Beg AA, Gabrilovich DI. Mechanism of all-trans retinoic acid effect on tumor-associated myeloid-derived suppressor cells. *Cancer Res* (2007) 67:11021–8. doi:10.1158/0008-5472.CAN-07-2593
69. Mirza N, Fishman M, Fricke I, Dunn M, Neuger AM, Frost TJ, et al. All-trans-retinoic acid improves differentiation of myeloid cells and immune response in cancer patients. *Cancer Res* (2006) 66:9299–307. doi:10.1158/0008-5472.CAN-06-1690
70. Iclozan C, Antonia S, Chiappori A, Chen D-T, Gabrilovich D. Therapeutic regulation of myeloid-derived suppressor cells and immune response to cancer vaccine in patients with extensive stage small cell lung cancer. *Cancer Immunol Immunother* (2013) 62:909–18. doi:10.1007/s00262-013-1396-8
71. Lesokhin AM, Hohl TM, Kitano S, Cortez C, Hirschhorn-Cymerman D, Avogadri F, et al. Monocytic CCR2(+) myeloid-derived suppressor cells promote immune escape by limiting activated CD8 T-cell infiltration into the tumor microenvironment. *Cancer Res* (2012) 72:876–86. doi:10.1158/0008-5472.CAN-11-1792
72. Umansky V, Blattner C, Gebhardt C, Utikal J. CCR5 in recruitment and activation of myeloid-derived suppressor cells in melanoma. *Cancer Immunol Immunother* (2017) 66:1015–23. doi:10.1007/s00262-017-1988-9
73. Zhang J, Patel L, Pienta KJ. CC chemokine ligand 2 (CCL2) promotes prostate cancer tumorigenesis and metastasis. *Cytokine Growth Factor Rev* (2010) 21:41–8. doi:10.1016/j.cytogfr.2009.11.009
74. Blattner C, Fleming V, Weber R, Himmelhan B, Altevogt P, Gebhardt C, et al. CCR5 + myeloid-derived suppressor cells are enriched and activated in melanoma lesions. *Cancer Res* (2018) 78:157–67. doi:10.1158/0008-5472.CAN-17-0348
75. Hawila E, Razon H, Wildbaum G, Blattner C, Sapir Y, Shaked Y, et al. CCR5 directs the mobilization of CD11b+Gr1+Ly6clowpolymorphonuclear myeloid cells from the bone marrow to the blood to support tumor development. *Cell Rep* (2017) 21:2212–22. doi:10.1016/j.celrep.2017.10.104
76. Di Mitri D, Toso A, Chen JJ, Sarti M, Pinton S, Jost TR, et al. Tumour-infiltrating Gr-1+ myeloid cells antagonize senescence in cancer. *Nature* (2014) 515:134–7. doi:10.1038/nature13638
77. Giovannoni MP, Vergelli C, Graziano A, Dal Piaz V. PDE5 inhibitors and their applications. *Curr Med Chem* (2010) 17:2564–87. doi:10.2174/092986710791859360
78. Serafini P, Meckel K, Kelso M, Noonan K, Califano J, Koch W, et al. Phosphodiesterase-5 inhibition augments endogenous antitumor immunity by reducing myeloid-derived suppressor cell function. *J Exp Med* (2006) 203:2691–702. doi:10.1084/jem.20061104
79. Meyer C, Sevko A, Ramacher M, Bazhin AV, Falk CS, Osen W, et al. Chronic inflammation promotes myeloid-derived suppressor cell activation blocking antitumor immunity in transgenic mouse melanoma model. *Proc Natl Acad Sci U S A* (2011) 108:17111–6. doi:10.1073/pnas.1108121108
80. Lin S, Wang J, Wang L, Wen J, Guo Y, Qiao W, et al. Phosphodiesterase-5 inhibition suppresses colonic inflammation-induced tumorigenesis via blocking the recruitment of MDSC. *Am J Cancer Res* (2017) 7:41–52.
81. Califano JA, Khan Z, Noonan KA, Rudraraju L, Zhang Z, Wang H, et al. Tadalafil augments tumor specific immunity in patients with head and neck squamous cell carcinoma. *Clin Cancer Res* (2015) 21:30–8. doi:10.1158/1078-0432.CCR-14-1716
82. Weed DT, Vella JL, Reis IM, De la Fuente AC, Gomez C, Sargi Z, et al. Tadalafil reduces myeloid-derived suppressor cells and regulatory T cells and promotes tumor immunity in patients with head and neck squamous cell carcinoma. *Clin Cancer Res* (2015) 21:39–48. doi:10.1158/1078-0432.CCR-14-1711
83. Hassel JC, Jiang H, Bender C, Winkler J, Sevko A, Shevchenko I, et al. Tadalafil has biologic activity in human melanoma. Results of a pilot trial with tadalafil in patients with metastatic melanoma (TaMe). *Oncoimmunology* (2017) 6:e1326440. doi:10.1080/2162402X.2017.1326440
84. Vasquez-Dunddel D, Pan F, Zeng Q, Gorbounov M, Albesiano E, Fu J, et al. STAT3 regulates arginase-I in myeloid-derived suppressor cells from cancer patients. *J Clin Invest* (2013) 123:1580–9. doi:10.1172/JCI60083
85. Hong D, Kurzrock R, Kim Y, Woessner R, Younes A, Nemunaitis J, et al. AZD9150, a next-generation antisense oligonucleotide inhibitor of STAT3 with early evidence of clinical activity in lymphoma and lung cancer. *Sci Transl Med* (2015) 7:314ra185. doi:10.1126/scitranslmed.aac5272
86. Zhang Q, Hossain DMS, Duttagupta P, Moreira D, Zhao X, Won H, et al. Serum-resistant CpG-STAT3 decoy for targeting survival and immune checkpoint signaling in acute myeloid leukemia. *Blood* (2016) 127:1687–700. doi:10.1182/blood-2015-08-665604
87. Akiyama Y, Nonomura C, Kondou R, Miyata H, Ashizawa T, Maeda C, et al. Immunological effects of the anti-programmed death-1 antibody on human peripheral blood mononuclear cells. *Int J Oncol* (2016) 49:1099–107. doi:10.3892/ijo.2016.3586
88. Kim K, Skora AD, Li Z, Liu Q, Tam AJ, Blosser RL, et al. Eradication of metastatic mouse cancers resistant to immune checkpoint blockade by suppression of myeloid-derived cells. *Proc Natl Acad Sci U S A* (2014) 111:11774–9. doi:10.1073/pnas.1410626111
89. Orillion A, Hashimoto A, Damayanti N, Shen L, Adelaiye-Ogala R, Arisa S, et al. Entinostat neutralizes myeloid-derived suppressor cells and enhances the antitumor effect of PD-1 inhibition in murine models of lung and renal cell carcinoma. *Clin Cancer Res* (2017) 23:5187–201. doi:10.1158/1078-0432.CCR-17-0741
90. Kim SH, Li M, Trousil S, Zhang Y, Pasca di Magliano M, Swanson KD, et al. Phenformin inhibits myeloid-derived suppressor cells and enhances the anti-tumor activity of PD-1 blockade in melanoma. *J Invest Dermatol* (2017) 137(8):1740–8. doi:10.1016/j.jid.2017.03.033
91. Clavijo PE, Moore EC, Chen J, Davis RJ, Friedman J, Kim Y, et al. Resistance to CTLA-4 checkpoint inhibition reversed through selective elimination of granulocytic myeloid cells. *Oncotarget* (2017) 8:55804–20. doi:10.18632/oncotarget.18437
92. Holmgaard RB, Zamarin D, Lesokhin A, Merghoub T, Wolchok JD. Targeting myeloid-derived suppressor cells with colony stimulating factor-1 receptor blockade can reverse immune resistance to immunotherapy in indoleamine 2,3-dioxygenase-expressing tumors. *EBioMedicine* (2016) 6:50–8. doi:10.1016/j.ebiom.2016.02.024

93. Holmgaard RB, Brachfeld A, Gasmi B, Jones DR, Mattar M, Doman T, et al. Timing of CSF-1/CSF-1R signaling blockade is critical to improving responses to CTLA-4 based immunotherapy. *Oncoimmunology* (2016) 5:e1151595. doi:10.1080/2162402X.2016.1151595
94. Mao Y, Eissler N, Blanc KL, Johnsen JI, Kogner P, Kiessling R. Targeting suppressive myeloid cells potentiates checkpoint inhibitors to control spontaneous neuroblastoma. *Clin Cancer Res* (2016) 22:3849–59. doi:10.1158/1078-0432.CCR-15-1912
95. Du Four S, Maenhout SK, Niclou SP, Thielemans K, Neyns B, Aerts JL. Combined VEGFR and CTLA-4 blockade increases the antigen-presenting function of intratumoral DCs and reduces the suppressive capacity of intratumoral MDSCs. *Am J Cancer Res* (2016) 6:2514–31.
96. Höchst B, Knolle PA. Checkpoint inhibition in head and neck cancer: immune therapeutic options, limitations, and beyond. *ORL J Otorhinolaryngol Relat Spec* (2017) 79:24–33. doi:10.1159/000455810
97. Davis RJ, Moore EC, Clavijo PE, Friedman J, Cash H, Chen Z, et al. Anti-PD-L1 efficacy can be enhanced by inhibition of myeloid-derived suppressor cells with a selective inhibitor of PI3Kδ/γ. *Cancer Res* (2017) 77:2607–19. doi:10.1158/0008-5472.CAN-16-2534
98. Zhou J, Liu M, Sun H, Feng Y, Xu L, Chan AWH, et al. Hepatoma-intrinsic CCRK inhibition diminishes myeloid-derived suppressor cell immunosuppression and enhances immune-checkpoint blockade efficacy. *Gut* (2017) 67(5):931–44. doi:10.1136/gutjnl-2017-314032
99. Tobin RP, Davis D, Jordan KR, McCarter MD. The clinical evidence for targeting human myeloid-derived suppressor cells in cancer patients. *J Leukoc Biol* (2017) 102:381–91. doi:10.1189/jlb.5VMR1016-449R
100. Dominguez GA, Condamine T, Mony S, Hashimoto A, Wang F, Liu Q, et al. Selective targeting of myeloid-derived suppressor cells in cancer patients using DS-8273a, an agonistic TRAIL-R2 antibody. *Clin Cancer Res* (2017) 23:2942–50. doi:10.1158/1078-0432.CCR-16-1784

7

Checkpoint Blockade Rescues the Repressive Effect of Histone Deacetylases Inhibitors on γδ T Cell Function

*Sajad A. Bhat[1,2], Disha Mohan Vedpathak[1,2] and Shubhada V. Chiplunkar[1,2]**

[1] Chiplunkar Laboratory, Advanced Centre for Treatment, Research and Education in Cancer (ACTREC), Tata Memorial Centre, Navi Mumbai, India, [2] HomiBhabha National Institute, Mumbai, India

Edited by:
Amedeo Amedei,
Università degli Studi di Firenze, Italy

Reviewed by:
Cara Haymaker,
University of Texas MD Anderson Cancer Center, United States
Zong Sheng Guo,
University of Pittsburgh, United States
Alessandro Poggi,
Ospedale Policlinico San Martino, Italy
Daniel Olive,
Aix Marseille Université, France

***Correspondence:**
Shubhada V. Chiplunkar
schiplunkar@actrec.gov.in

Histone deacetylases (HDAC) are one of the key epigenetic modifiers that control chromatin accessibility and gene expression. Their role in tumorigenesis is well established and HDAC inhibitors have emerged as an effective treatment modality. HDAC inhibitors have been investigated for their specific antitumor activities and also clinically evaluated in treatment of various malignancies. In the present study, we have investigated the effect of HDAC inhibitors on the effector functions of human γδ T cells. HDAC inhibitors inhibit the antigen-specific proliferative response of γδ T cells and cell cycle progression. In antigen-activated γδ T cells, the expression of transcription factors (Eomes and Tbet) and effector molecules (perforin and granzyme B) were decreased upon treatment with HDAC inhibitors. Treatment with HDAC inhibitors attenuated the antitumor cytotoxic potential of γδ T cells, which correlated with the enhanced expression of immune checkpoints programmed death-1 (PD-1) and programmed death ligand-1 in γδ T cells. Interestingly, PD-1 blockade improves the antitumor effector functions of HDAC inhibitor-treated γδ T cells, which is reflected in the increased expression of Granzyme B and Lamp-1. This study provides a rationale for designing HDAC inhibitor and immune check point blockade as a combinatorial treatment modality for cancer.

Keywords: gamma delta (γδ) T cells, phosphoantigen, histone deacetylases inhibitors, effector functions, programmed death-1, programmed death ligand-1

INTRODUCTION

Gamma delta T cells, the enigmatic brethren of alpha beta (αβ) T cells were discovered coincidently during cloning the αβ T-cell receptor (TCR) locus (1). This small subset of T cells, γδ T cells constitute about 5–10% of the circulating T cell population, which express the variant form of TCR heterodimer (2). γδ T cells manifest the features of both innate and adaptive immunity (3). TheVγ9Vδ2 T cell subset of γδ T cells predominates in peripheral blood, and these cells play an important role in the defense against microbial pathogens, stressed cells, and tumor cells of various origin (4, 5). γδ T cells differ from αβ T cells by their TCR gene usage, tissue tropism, and MHC-independent antigen recognition (6, 7). γδ T-cells display broad functional plasticity, like regulatory potential, antigen-presenting capacity, B-cell helper activity, and have the potential for diverse cytokine production (8). γδ T cells recognize non-peptide phosphoantigens such as isopentenyl pyrophosphate (IPP) or 4-hydroxy-3-methyl-but-2-eneyl pyrophosphate (HMBPP), which are produced through the mevalonate pathway in mammalian cells or non-mevalonate/Rohmer pathway in non-mammalian cells, respectively (9). γδ T cells are also activated indirectly by aminobisphosphonates such as Zoledronate. Aminobisphosphonates inhibit the key enzyme of mevalonate pathway, farnesyl pyrophosphate synthase and lead to accumulation of IPP. Tumor cells treated with aminobisphophonates show increase in the intracellular level of IPP and, therefore, are easily targeted by γδ Tcells (10, 11).

Activated γδ T cells are known to produce large amounts of the pro-inflammatory cytokines interferon-γ (IFN-γ) and tumor necrosis factor-α (TNF-α) as well as the chemokines MIP-1 (macrophage inflammatory protein) and RANTES (regulated on activation, normal T cell expressed, and secreted) (12). In addition, cytolytic mediators such as granzyme B and perforin are produced to induce specific lysis of cells with elevated phosphoantigen levels (13). Transcription factors like Eomes and Tbet are known to be expressed upon activation by γδ T cells and are essential for antitumor effector functions (14).

Nucleosome is the basic structure of eukaryotic chromatin, composed of histones and DNA. Each nucleosome comprises 146 bp of DNA wrapped around an octamer of core histones (two H2A–H2B dimers and a H3–H4 tetramer) (15). Histone proteins are rich in basic amino acids lysine and arginine. It is through interaction with these histone proteins that massive DNA is packed inside the nucleus. The tails of histone proteins undergo different complex and coordinated posttranslational modifications like histone acetylation, methylation, phosphorylation, and ubiquitination. According to histone code hypothesis, these modifications are read by specific factors, which ultimately lead to downstream events (16). Histone modifications are reversible in nature and influence many fundamental biological processes. Histone acetylation are directed by histone modifying enzymes, histone acetyl transferases (HAT), and histone deacetylases (HDAC), which participate in potential cross-talk between different modifications (15). Normal physiological functions require a balance between HAT and HDAC. Abrupt alterations that skew this balance can give rise to different pathophysiological conditions like cancer (17, 18).

Histone deacetylases inhibitors, including Trichostatin-A (TSA) and sodium valproate (VPA), can alter the acetylation of histones in chromatin and enhance gene transcription. In the recent decades HDAC inhibitors have received attention as antineoplastic treatment. Extensive evidence suggests that HDAC inhibitors play a role in antitumor immunity (19). HDAC inhibitors lead to growth arrest, induction of apoptosis, and differentiation in tumors. Pan HDAC inhibitors like VPA, TSA, and suberoylanilidehydroxamic acid (SAHA) target Class I (HDAC 1, 2, 3, and 8), Class II (HDAC 4, 5, 7, 9, 6, and 10) HDACs. Hence, their anticancer activities are pleotropic in nature, mediated by altering the expression of various genes that are regulated by class I and II HDACs. Additionally, they also target several non-histone proteins such as transcription factors (p53, E2f1) and cytoplasmic proteins (tubulin, hsp, β-catenin). Hyperacetylation of these histone and non-histone proteins brought about by HDAC inhibiton culminate in induction of cell-death pathways in cancer cells. Several studies have established effective tumor reduction *in vitro* as well as *in vivo* upon HDAC inhibitor treatment (20).

Moreover, HDAC inhibitors inhibit angiogenesis and increase the tumor cell antigenicity (21, 22). HDAC inhibitors mediate elevated expression of antigens on tumor cells so that they can be easily targeted by immune cells (23, 24). Due to these promising antitumor functions, HDAC inhibitors are now assessed in clinical trials and some of them have been approved for treatment (25, 26). Recent reports have demonstrated that HDAC inhibitors enhance response to immune checkpoint blockade in triple negative breast cancer, lung adenocarcinoma, melanoma, and multiple myeloma (27–30).

Although the impact of HDAC inhibitors on tumor cells is well studied, their effect on immune cells has recently surfaced. HDAC inhibitors have been shown to have a dual effect on immune cells, either enhancing their activation in cases of CD4 T cell and Tregs whereas dampening the effector functions of NK cells and CD8 T cells. HDAC inhibitors are also known to inhibit the cytotoxic potential of NK cells. HDAC inhibitors are also reported to downregulate the co-stimulatory molecules and cytokine signals in antigen-presenting cells (31). Previous studies have shown that HDAC inhibitor treated tumor cells are easily targeted by γδ T cells (32), but the impact of HDAC inhibitors on the functional responses of human γδ T cells are not well understood.

For successful immunotherapy, T cell responses are essential. Besides the TCR signal, co-stimulatory signal also determines the functional response of T cells. Co-stimulatory signal may be of positive or negative. Negative co stimulatory signals may be from different receptors like programmed death-1 (PD-1) and PD ligand-1 (PD-L1) interaction. PD-1 and PD-L1 are the members of immunoglobin family like that of CD28. Interaction of PD-1 and PD-L1 leads to functional impairment in T cells (33). It is well-known fact that tumors use this mechanism to escape the immune attack. Blocking antibodies for these immune check points can enhance antitumor responses, and these immune-modulating antibodies have achieved clinical success with FDA approved treatments for several malignancies (34). It has been shown that γδ T cells express PD-1 and PD-L1 and blocking of this signaling lead to increase in the antitumor potential of γδ T cells (35).

The present study focuses on investigating the direct impact of HDAC inhibitors on human γδ T cells. We have studied the effect of three different HDAC inhibitors, TSA, SAHA, and VPA on γδ T cells. We observed that HDAC inhibitors suppress the antigen-specific proliferative responses of γδ T cells and their antitumor effector functions by increasing the expression of immune checkpoints (PD-1 and PD-L1). The study further demonstrates that blocking of immune checkpoints on γδ T cells is capable of augmenting their antitumor cytotoxic potential. The present study will open new avenues in the field of cancer immunotherapy using HDAC inhibitors.

MATERIALS AND METHODS

γδ T Cell Separation

Heparinized peripheral blood was collected from healthy individuals. Peripheral blood mononuclear cells (PBMCs) were isolated by differential density gradient centrifugation using Ficoll Hypaque (Sigma-Aldrich, St. Louis, MO, USA). The study was approved by the Institutional Ethics Committee (TMC-IECIII Project no. 166) and written informed consent was obtained from the donors prior to collection of blood samples. The experimental conditions and procedures for handling blood samples were performed as per the biosafety guidelines of the Institute Biosafety Committee. In short, blood samples were handled in biosafety cabinets and personnel handling blood samples were vaccinated against Hepatitis B. γδ T cells were purified from PBMCs using immunomagnetic MicroBeads (Miltenyi Biotech, Bergish Gladbach, Germany) by positive selection, as per manufacturer's instructions. The purity of separated γδ T cells was >95% as confirmed by flow cytometry (FACS Aria, BD Biosciences, USA). Isolated γδ T cells were cultured in RPMI 1640 supplemented with 10% heat inactivated AB serum, 2 mM glutamine, and antibiotics.

Cell Viability Assay

The viability of γδ T cells upon treatment with HDAC inhibitors was evaluated with MTT assay and Annexin V and 7-AAD staining. Briefly, 0.1 × 10^6 γδ T cells, seeded in 96-well flat bottom plates (Nunc), were treated with the following HDAC inhibitors for the given concentration range: VPA (4–0.25 mM; Sigma-Aldrich), TSA (200–25 nM; Sigma-Aldrich), and SAHA (4–0.25 μM; Sigma-Aldrich) along with HDMAPP (1 nM; Echelon) and rIL-2 (50 IU/ml; Peprotech) for 72 h. γδ T cells treated only with HDMAPP (1 nM) and rIL-2 (50 IU/ml) were used as control. DMSO was used as vehicle control. Following 72 h of treatment, MTT (5 mg/ml) was added and incubated for 4 h at 37°C. After incubation, the spent medium was discarded, the formazan crystals were dissolved in DMSO, and the absorbance was measured at 570 nm by microplate reader (TECAN, Switzerland). Untreated γδ T cells were used as reference for calculating the viability. Concentrations of HDAC inhibitors, which had no impact on viability of γδ T cells were further validated by Annexin V and 7-AAD staining. The concentration of HDAC inhibitors showing viability more or equal to 90% in γδ T cells were used for all the further experimental procedures.

Quantitative Real-Time PCR (qPCR)

The purified γδ T cells, activated with HDMAPP (1 nM) and rIL-2 (50 IU/ml) were treated in the presence or absence of HDAC inhibitors at the given concentrations VPA (2, 1, 0.5 mM), TSA (100, 50, 25 nM), and SAHA (1, 0.5, 0.25 μM) for 72 h. DMSO was used as vehicle control. Total cellular RNA was isolated by using Trizol reagent (Invitrogen Life Technologies, NY, USA) in accordance with the company's instructions and cDNA was synthesized by High-Capacity cDNA Reverse transcription kit (Applied Biosystems) according to manufacturer's instructions. The gene expression of T-bet, Eomes, perforin, granzyme B, IFN-γ, and TNF-α was evaluated by Quantstudio 15k Flex system (Applied Biosystems) using Power SYBR Green reagents (Applied Biosystems) as per manufacture's procedure. All samples were analyzed with the following sequence specific primers: Perforin forward and reverse primer 5′-GACACACAAAGGTTCCTGCG-3′and5′-GACTTTGGCCCTGGTTACAT-3′, respectively, Granzyme B forward and reverse primer 5′-CAACCAATCCTGCTTCTGCT-3′ and 5′-GTCGTCTCGTATCAGGAAGC-3′, respectively, Eomes forward and reverse primer 5′-ATTCCACCGCCACCAAAC TG-3′ and 5′-GCACCACCTCTACGAACAC-3′, respectively, Tbet forward and reverse primer 5′-GTGACCCAGATGATTGTG CT-3′ and 5′-ATGCGTGTTGGAAGCGTTGC-3′, respectively, IFN-γ forward and reverse primer5′-GCATCGTTTTGGGTT CTCTTG-3′ and 5′-AGTTCCATTATCCGCTACATCTG-3′, respectively, TNF-α forward and reverse primer 5′-ACTTTG GAGTGATCGGCC-3′ and 5′-GCTTGAGGGTTTGCTACA AC-3′, respectively, and 18S rRNA forward and reverse primer 5′-AACGGCTACCACATCCAA-3′ and 5′-TTCCAATTACACG GCCTC-3′, respectively. The gene expression was determined by threshold cycle (C_T) method by applying $2^{-\Delta\Delta Ct}$. All the values were normalized to the expression of 18S rRNA as endogenous control.

Western Blot Analysis

1 × 10^6 freshly isolated γδ T cells were cultured with HDMAPP (1 nM), rIL-2 (50 IU/ml), and with or without HDAC inhibitors at the given concentrations VPA (2, 1, 0.5 mM), TSA (100, 50, 25 nM), and SAHA (1, 0.5, 0.25 μM) at 37°C. After 72 h of treatment, cells were harvested and whole cell lysates were prepared with SDS lysis buffer (1 M Tris–HCl pH 6.8, 10%w/v SDS, glycerol, β-mercaptoethanol, 1M DTT, and bromophenol blue). 10% Polyacrylamide gels were used to resolve the protein samples and transferred to Hybond-ECL nitrocellulose membrane (Amersham Pharmacia Biotech, Piscataway, NJ, USA). The primary antibodies to T-bet (1:1,000) (Cell Signalling Technology), p21 (1:1,000) (Abcam), Eomes (1:1,000) (Abcam), p53 (1:500) (Santa Cruz), NF-κB (1:1,000) (Abcam), total H3 (Abcam) (1:1,000), total H4 (Abcam) (1:1,000), acetyl H3 (Abcam) (1:1,000), acetyl H4 (Abcam) (1:1,000), and β-actin (1:4,000) (Sigma-Aldrich) as loading control were added at different dilution. Immunostaining was performed using appropriate secondary antibody at a dilution of 1:10,000 and developed with ECL plus Western blot detection system (Amersham Pharmacia).

Immunostaining and Cell Cycle Analysis

The magnetically sorted γδ T cells were kept overnight in RPMI supplemented with 10% FBS and were stained for various cell surface markers such as Vδ2 TCR, CD14, CD19, and CD56. Briefly, the cells were harvested from culture, washed with ice cold PBS, and fixed with 1% paraformaldehyde at 4°C for 15 min. The cells were washed with FACS buffer and then labeled with fluorophore tagged antibodies Vδ2-PE, CD3-PECy7, CD14-PerCP, CD19-FITC, and CD56 PerCP Cy5.5 (BD Biosciences, USA) for 30 min at 4°C. Further, the cells were washed and acquired on FACS Aria (BD Biosciences, San Jose, CA, USA). γδT cells treated with or without HDAC inhibitors for 72 h as described earlier were stained with live–dead (LD) fixable dead cell stain kit (Thermo Fischer) as per manufacturer's protocol. After staining with LD dye, the cells were fixed with paraformaldehyde and permeabilized with 1% saponin. Cells were washed and stained with γδ TCR-PE, CD25-PerCPCy5.5, CD69-APC (BD Biosciences, USA), Perforin-BV421, Granzyme B-PECF594, PD-1-PECF594, and PD-L1-PerCP Cy5.5 (BioLegend, San Diego, CA, USA), NKG2D-APC, CD16-BV421, KIRD2L2/3-PE (Miltenyi Biotech,

Bergish Gladbach, Germany). For determination of degranulation marker, Lamp-1 (CD107a) and effector molecule Granzyme B release, purified γδ T cells were activated with rIL2 (50 IU/ml) and HDMAPP (1 nM) in the presence and absence of TSA (100 nM), SAHA (1 μM), and VPA (2 mM) for 72 h at 37°C. Additionally, for PD-1 blockade, anti-PD1 antibody (3 μg/ml; BioLegend, San Diego, CA, USA) was added along with HDAC inhibitors. These effectors were then cocultured with zoledronate treated tumor targets (AW13516 Oral cancer cell line, COLO-205 Colon cancer cell line and Raji B lymphoblastic cell line) for 4 h in polypropylene tubes (BD Biosciences, USA) at effector target ratio of 4:1 in presence of monensin (5 mg/ml; Sigma-Aldrich) as described previously (36). Anti CD107a APC Ab (BioLegend, San Diego, CA, USA) was added at the start of coculture assay. After 4 h, cells were washed, fixed, and stained with anti-human TCR γδ PE and Granzyme B-PECF-594 (BD Biosciences, USA). Cells were acquired on FACS Aria (BD Biosciences, USA) and analysis was done by using FlowJo software (Tree Star, Ashland, OR, USA). The expression of various cell surface markers and intracellular proteins were analyzed on the γδ TCR$^+$ cells gated populations.

For cell cycle analysis, 1×10^6 γδ T cells treated with HDAC inhibitors VPA (0.5, 1, 2 mM), TSA (25, 50, 100 nM), and SAHA (0.25, 0.5, 1 μM) for 72 h or kept untreated, were harvested, and fixed by adding chilled 70% ethanol. Next day, cells were washed with PBS and stained with DNA intercalating dye propidium iodide (PI) along with RNAse A at a concentration of 40 and 10 μg/ml, respectively. Cells were incubated at room temperature for 30 min. The samples were acquired on FACS Calibur (BD Biosciences, USA) and analyzed using ModFit software.

Proliferation Assay

Proliferation of γδ T cells was analyzed using ^{3}H-Thymidine (3HTdR) incorporation assay. A total of 5×10^4 γδ T cells were treated in the presence or absence of HDAC inhibitors VPA (0.5, 1, 2 mM), TSA (25, 50, 100 nM), and SAHA (0.25, 0.5, 1 μM) along with HDMAPP (1 nM) and rIL2 (50 IU/ml) for 72 h in 96-well tissue culture plates. The cultures were pulsed with 1 μCi [^{3}H] thymidine (Board of Radiation and Isotope Technology, Mumbai) 18 h prior to termination of the assay. Following the incubation, cells were transferred upon glass-wool filters using cell harvester (Perkin Elmer, UK). The radioactivity incorporated into the DNA was measured in a liquid beta scintillation counter (Packard, Meriden, CT, USA). Data were expressed as counts per minute (cpm).

Cytokine ELISA

For cytokine ELISA, supernatants were collected from γδ T cells treated in the presence of different concentrations of HDAC inhibitors VPA (0.5, 1, 2 mM), TSA (25, 50, 100 nM), and SAHA (0.25, 0.5, 1 μM) along with HDMAPP (1 nM) and rIL2 (50 IU/ml) for 24 h. The concentration of secreted cytokines IFNγ and TNFα was measured by human IFN-γ and TNF-α ELISA kit, respectively (BD Biosciences, USA) as per manufacture's procedure.

Cytotoxicity Assay

Cytotoxic potential of γδ T cells against panel of tumor cell lines, oral tumor cell line (AW13516), colon tumor cell line (COLO-205), and B lymphoblastic cell line (Raji) was performed using lactate dehydrogenase (LDH) release assay as described previously (37). Tumor cell lines were treated for 18 h with zoledronate (100 μM; Sigma-Aldrich). γδ T cells were treated with HDMAPP (1 nM) and rIL-2 (50 IU/ml) in presence and absence of HDAC inhibitors, VPA (2 mM), TSA (100 nM), and SAHA (1 μM) for 72 h at 37°C were used as effectors. Additionally, for PD-1 blockade, anti-PD1 antibody (3 μg/ml) was added to HDAC inhibitor treated γδ T cells for 72 h at 37°C and were also used as effectors. Briefly, tumor cell lines were cocultured with effectors at 40:1 effector target (E/T) ratio for 4 h at 37°C in 96-well plates (Nunc, Denmark). After 4 h of coculture, an aliquot of 50 μl of media was used in LDH cytotoxic assay using the LDH cytotoxic assay kit (Thermo Fisher Scientific, USA) according to manufactures protocol. γδ T cell cytotoxicity was defined as % specific lysis = Experimental value - Effector cells spontaneous control – Target cells spontaneous control/Target Cell Maximum Control – Target cells spontaneous control.

Chromatin Immunoprecipitation (ChIP) qPCR Assays

Chromatin Immunoprecipitation assays were performed using MAGnify TM Chromatin Immunoprecipitation System (Thermo Fisher Scientific, USA) according to the manufacturer's instructions. Specific anti-acetyl histone H3 (Abcam) and anti-acetyl histone H4 (Abcam) were used to determine the promoter acetylation of perforin and granzyme-B. Normal rabbit IgG was used as negative control. DNA was extracted and analyzed by quantitative real time PCR (qPCR) with specific primers for perforin (region I forward:5′-GATGAGGGCTGAGGACAG-3′; region I reverse:5′-TCTTCACCGAGGCTCCTG-3′; region II forward:5′-CTGCTGGCCTGTTCATCAAC-3′; region II reverse: 5′-CTGTCCTCAGCCCTCATC-3′) and granzyme B (region I forward: 5′-GGGTGGGCAGCATTTACAG-3′; region I reverse: 5′-TTCTCAGGAAGGCTGCCC-3′; region II forward: 5′-CACT TCATAGGCTTGGGTTCC-3′; region II reverse: 5′-CCTCTGG TTTTGTGGTGTCTC-3′). 1% of starting chromatin was used as input. Relative data quantification was performed using $2^{-\Delta\Delta Ct}$ method, using formula: % Input = 2 (Ct Input – Ct ChIP) × Input dilution factor × 100 and expressed in the form of % input as described earlier (38).

Statistical Analysis

Data analysis was done by Student's *t*-test using GraphPad Prism software (GraphPad Software Inc., CA, USA). The comparative CT method was applied in the quantitative real time RT-PCR according to $2^{-(\Delta\Delta Ct)}$ method. Results were indicated as means ± SE and considered significant at $p < 0.05$.

RESULTS

Effect of HDAC Inhibitors on Viability of γδ T Cells

We first studied effects of HDAC inhibitors VPA (0.25–4 mM), TSA (25—200 nM), and SAHA (0.25–4 μM) on the viability of γδ T cells. Magnetically sorted γδ T cells from peripheral blood of healthy individuals were activated with HDMAPP (1 nM) and rIL2 (50 IU/ml) in presence and absence of above mentioned HDAC inhibitor concentrations for 72 h. HDMAPP is a synthetic analog of IPP and potent activator of γδ T cells. Immunomagnetically sorted γδ T cells were positive for γδ TCR (90%), CD56 (53%), and negative for αβ TCR, CD14, and CD 19 (Figure S2A in Supplementary Material). Viability of γδ T cells was assessed by MTT assay. It was observed that higher concentrations of HDAC inhibitors were toxic to γδ T cells. γδ T cells showed least viability at VPA (3–4 mM); TSA (150–200 nM), and SAHA (3–4 μM). At lower concentrations, these HDAC inhibitors were not toxic and γδ T cell were viable (>90%) (Figure S1 in Supplementary Material). For further validation of viability, γδ T cells activated with HDMAPP and rIL2 in the presence or absence of HDAC inhibitorsVPA (0.5–2 mM), TSA (25–100 nM), and SAHA (0.25–1 μM) were stained with Annexin V and 7-AAD. We observed that at these concentrations HDAC inhibitors did not induce any significant apoptosis. Since HDAC inhibitor concentrations, VPA (0.5–2 mM), TSA (25–100 nM), and SAHA (0.25–1 μM) showed least effect on the viability of γδ T cells (Figures S2B,C in Supplementary Material), these were selected in further experiments.

HDAC Inhibitors Inhibit the Antigen-Driven Proliferation and Cell Cycle Progression of γδ T Cells

γδ T cell show robust proliferation when stimulated with phosphoantigen (HDMAPP) in presence of rIL2. In order to investigate the effect of HDAC inhibitors on proliferation of γδ T cells, γδ T cells were stimulated with phosphoantigen HDMAPP and rIL2 in the presence or absence of different concentration of HDAC inhibitors (VPA; 0.5–2 mM, TSA; 25–100 nM, and SAHA; 0.25–1 μM) and proliferation was monitored using ^{3}H thymidine incorporation assay. γδ T cells showed robust proliferative responses to phosphoantigen HDMAPP in presence of rIL-2, compared to unstimulated γδ T cells. However, in the presence of various concentrations of VPA, TSA, and SAHA, the proliferative responses of γδ T cells were significantly reduced in a concentration-dependent manner (Figure S3A in Supplementary Material), with maximum decrease in proliferation of γδ T cells observed at higher concentration of HDAC inhibitors, VPA 2 mM, TSA 100 nM, and SAHA 1 μM, respectively. Further, we also evaluated the role of HDAC inhibitors on cell cycle progression of γδ T cells. Freshly isolated γδ T cells were stimulated with HDMAPP and rIL2 in presence or absence of different concentrations of HDAC inhibitors. Upon stimulation with HDMAPP and rIL2, significant number of γδ T cells were in S phase and G2/M phase. However, upon treatment of HDAC inhibitors, γδ T cells were arrested in G0/G1 phase (Figures S3B,C in Supplementary Material). This inhibition of cell cycle progression in γδ T cells upon HDAC inhibitor treatment was reflected in the increased expression of p53 and its downstream target p21, suggesting that HDAC inhibitors impede the G0/G1-S phase transition in γδ T cells in p53-dependent manner (**Figures 1A–C**) and (**Figures 1D–I**).

HDAC Inhibitors Regulate Cytokine Production and Activation in γδ T Cells

γδ T cells upon activation secrete copious amount of cytokines such as IFN-γ and TNF-α (36). We examined the effect of HDAC inhibitors on expression of these cytokines in γδ T cells. Marked increase in the expression of cytokines IFN-γ and TNF-α was observed upon stimulation of γδ T cells with HDMAPP and rIL2 compared to unstimulated γδ T cells. Expression of IFN-γ (**Figures 2A,B**) and TNF-α (**Figures 2C,D**) was decreased significantly when treated with HDAC inhibitors TSA, SAHA, and VPA. This inhibition was observed both at mRNA and protein levels. It was observed that inhibition of cytokine expression was concentration dependent for HDAC inhibitors. We also evaluated the effect of HDAC inhibitors on the expression of early activation marker CD69 and late activation marker CD25 on γδ T cells. Treatment of γδ T cells with HDAC inhibitors led to decrease in the expression of early activation (**Figures 3A,B**) and late activation marker on γδ T cells (**Figures 3C,D**). The expression of these activation markers on γδ T cells were significantly reduced in a concentration-dependent manner, with maximum decrease at VPA 2 mM, TSA 100 nM, and SAHA 1 μM, respectively. Percentage of γδ T cells positive for these markers was also less in HDAC inhibitor treated γδ T cells as compared to untreated γδ T cells. To investigate the role of HDAC inhibitors on the expression of other activating receptors like NKG2D, CD16, and inhibitory receptors like KIR2DL2/3 (CD158b), γδ T cells were treated with HDAC inhibitors VPA 2 mM, TSA 100 nM, and SAHA 1 μM for 72 h. We found that HDAC inhibitor-treated γδ T cells show decreased expression of NKG2D (Figure S4A in Supplementary Material) as compared to untreated γδ T cells. On the contrary, γδ T cells treated with HDAC inhibitors VPA 2 mM, TSA 100 nM, and SAHA 1 μM show increase in the expression of inhibitory receptor KIR2DL2/3 (CD158b) (Figure S4B in Supplementary Material). However, we did not observe any change in CD16 expression (Figure S4C in Supplementary Material). Collectively, the data advocate the role of HDAC inhibitors in abating the expression of activation markers (CD69, CD25, NKG2D) and cytokine (IFN-γ, TNF-α) production in γδ T cells.

HDAC Inhibitors Suppress the Expression of Transcription Factors Eomes and Tbet in γδ T Cells

Eomes and Tbet are two main T-box transcription factors expressed in T cells. They are the main transcription factors, which regulate the effector functions of CD8 T cells through the expression of effector genes perforin and granzyme B (39, 40). Besides CD8 T cells, γδ T cells also express Eomes and Tbet (41). Upon activation with phosphoantigen (HDMAPP) and rIL2, γδ T cells show increased expression of these two transcription factors. We hypothesized that HDAC inhibitors may have an impact on the expression of these two transcription factors in γδ T cells. Therefore, the role of HDAC inhibitors was analyzed in regulating expression of Eomes and Tbet in γδ T cells activated with phosphoantigen (HDMAPP) and rIL2. γδ T cells treated with HDAC inhibitors showed decrease in the expression of Eomes and Tbet at both mRNA (**Figures 4A,B**) and protein level (**Figure 4C**).

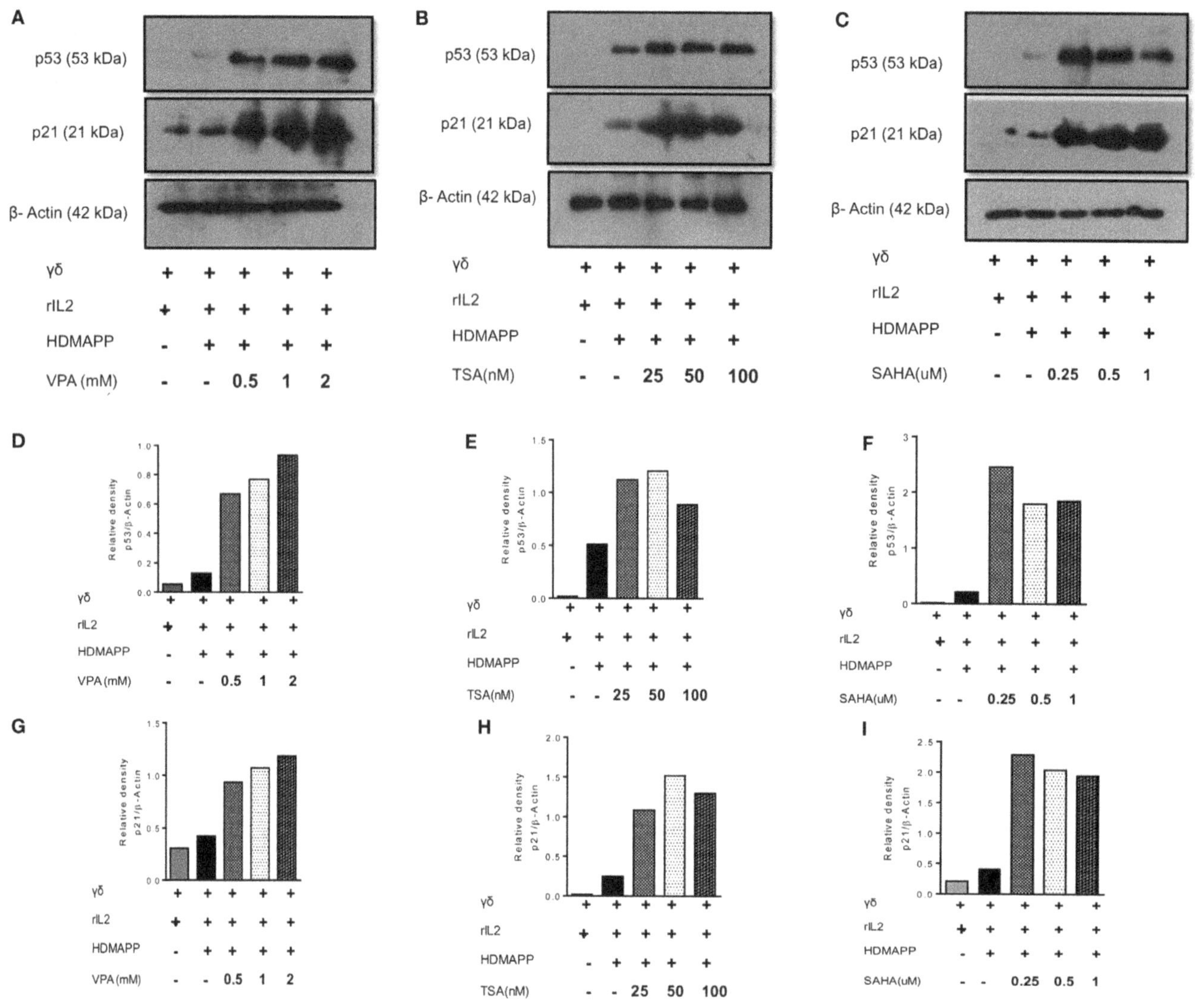

FIGURE 1 | Histone deacetylases (HDAC) inhibitors increase the expression of cell cycle checkpoint proteins p53 and p21. Protein expression of p53 and p21 by γδ T cells upon treatment with **(A)** sodium valproate (VPA), **(B)** Trichostatin-A (TSA), and **(C)** suberoylanilidehydroxamic acid (SAHA) as detected by western blotting. Cell lysates of γδ T cells, stimulated with HDMAPP after treatment with HDAC inhibitors at different concentrations for 72 h were prepared and p53, p21 proteins were detected. β-actin was used as loading control. Densitometry quantification of p53 **(D–F)** and p21 **(G–I)** expression in γδ T cells upon treatment with VPA, TSA, and SAHA, relative to β-actin.

In addition to Eomes and Tbet transcriptional factors, γδ T cells treated with HDAC inhibitors also show decreased expression of NF-κB (Figures S4D–F in Supplementary Material) as compared to untreated γδ T cells. Inhibition of Eomes, Tbet, and NF-κB by HDAC inhibitors clearly demonstrates that HDAC inhibitors regulate the effector functions of γδ T cells.

HDAC Inhibitors Inhibit the Antitumor Cytotoxic Potential of γδ T Cells

To evaluate the role of HDAC inhibitors in modulation of antitumor potential of γδ T cells, we analyzed the expression of effector molecules Perforin and Granzyme B in γδ T cells at mRNA and protein level. Perforin and Granzyme B are the effector molecules, which are responsible for the antitumor functions of CD8 and γδ T cells (42, 43). Freshly isolated γδ T cells activated with phosphoantigen HDMAPP and rIL2 show increased expression of these two effector genes; however, γδ T cells activated in presence of HDAC inhibitors showed decrease in the expression of perforin (**Figures 5A–C**) and granzyme B. (**Figures 5D–F**). Maximum effect on the expression of perforin and granzyme B was observed with VPA 2 mM, TSA 100 nM, and SAHA 1 μM. These concentrations of HDAC inhibitors were used in further cytotoxicity experiments. We next evaluated whether decrease in expression of effector molecules perforin and granzyme B are regulated by histone modifications in γδ T cells. To investigate this, we checked the total histone H3 and H4 acetylation in γδ T cells treated with HDAC inhibitors VPA 2 mM, TSA 100 nM, and SAHA 1 μM. We observed that the total level of H3 acetylation and H4 acetylation increases in γδ T cells after treatment of

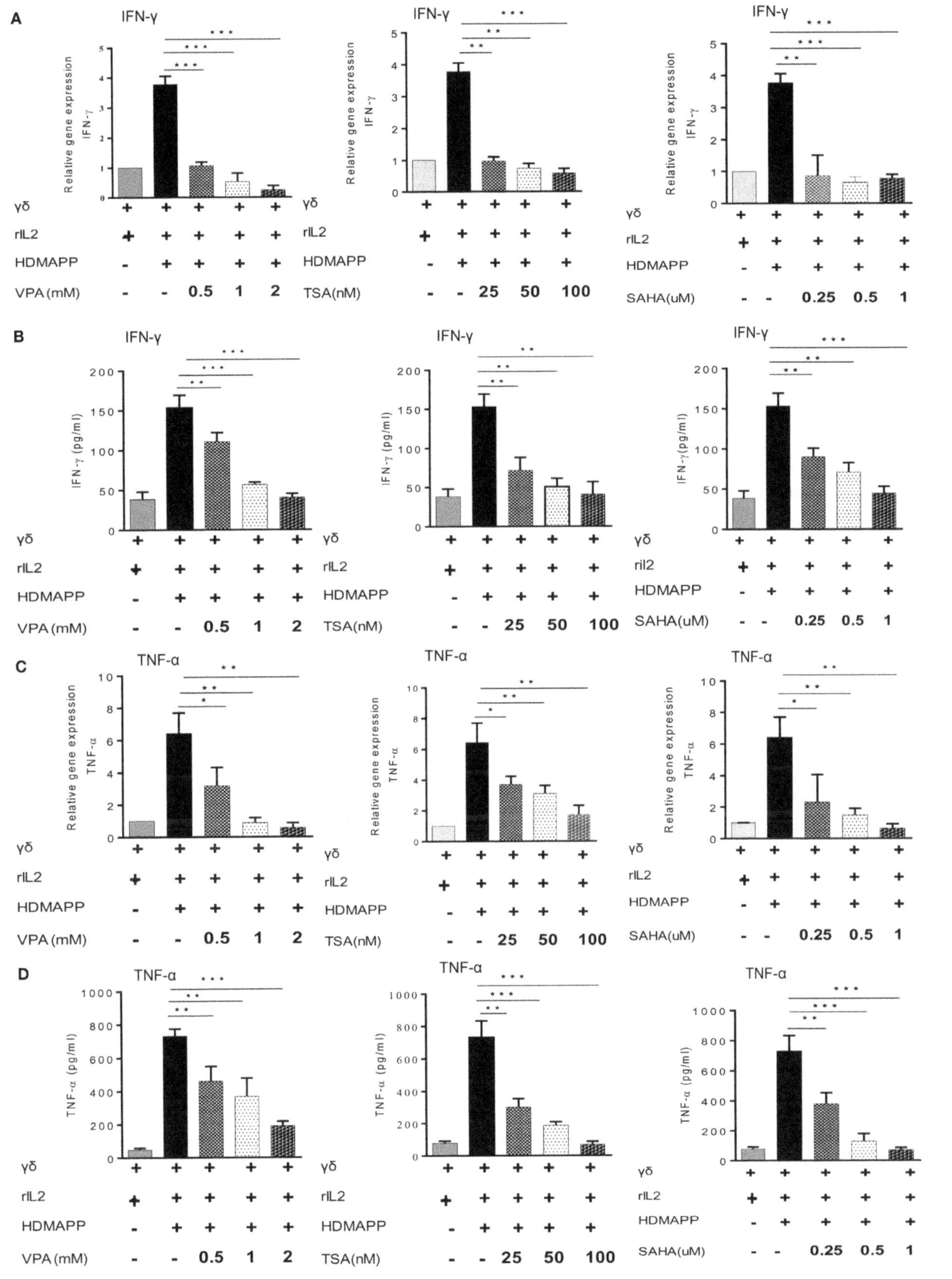

FIGURE 2 | Continued

FIGURE 2 | Histone deacetylases (HDAC) inhibitors regulate cytokine production. Expressions of IFN-γ and TNF-α were detected by quantitative real-time PCR and sandwich ELISA. **(A,B)** IFN-γ expression by γδ T cells stimulated with HDMAPP, treated with or without HDAC inhibitors sodium valproate (VPA), Trichostatin-A (TSA), and suberoylanilidehydroxamic acid (SAHA) at different concentrations at mRNA and protein levels, respectively. **(C,D)** Expression of TNF-α in the supernatants collected from HDMAPP stimulated γδ T cells in the presence or absence of HDAC inhibitors VPA, TSA, and SAHA at different concentrations at mRNA and protein levels, respectively. The expression of different m-RNA transcripts was normalized to 18S r-RNA. All the results indicated are mean ± SEM of three independent experiments, where $^{*}p < 0.05$, $^{**}p < 0.005$, $^{***}p < 0.0005$.

HDAC inhibitors as compared to untreated γδ T cells (Figure S5A in Supplementary Material). However, HDAC inhibitor-treated γδ T cells show less histone H3 acetylation and H4 acetylation on promoters of perforin and granzyme B compared to untreated γδ T cells determined by ChIP qPCR assay. Histone acetylation is positively correlated with transcriptional activity. Thus, our data show that epigenetic changes on promoters of effector molecules perforin and granzyme B control the expression of these molecules in HDAC inhibitor treated γδ T cells (Figures S5B,C in Supplementary Material). The cytotoxic potential of HDAC inhibitor treated γδ T cells was evaluated against panel of zoledronate-treated tumor cells lines (AW13516, COLO-205, and Raji). At different E/T ratios starting from 5:1 to 40:1, HDMAPP-activated γδ T cells in the presence of IL-2 efficiently lysed zoledronate-treated tumor cells lines (AW13516, COLO-205, and Raji). Maximum cytotoxicity of γδ T cells was observed at E/T ratio of 40:1 (**Figures 6A–C**). This ratio of E: T was used in further experiments, to assess the effect of HDAC inhibitors TSA, VPA, and SAHA on cytolytic ability of γδ T cells. γδ T cells stimulated with HDMAPP and rIL2 in presence of HDAC inhibitors VPA (2 mM), TSA (100 nM), and SAHA (1 μM) for 72 h were used as effector against zoledronate-treated tumor cell lines (AW13516, COLO205 and Raji) as targets at E/T ratio of 40:1. Zoledronate, an aminobisphonate drug, inhibits the enzyme farnesyl pyrophosphate synthase in the mevalonate pathway leading to accumulation of IPP, which stimulates γδ T cell activation *via* TCR signaling. γδ T cells treated with different HDAC inhibitors showed significant decrease in their cytotoxic potential against zoledronate treated tumor targets (AW13516, COLO 205, and Raji) (**Figures 6D–F**). It was observed that all the three HDAC inhibitors (VPA, TSA, and SAHA) significantly inhibited the ability of γδ T cells to kill zoledronate treated tumor cell lines.

HDAC Inhibitors Abrogate the Effector Functions of γδ T Cells by Upregulating the Immune Checkpoint Proteins PD-1 and PD-L1

Programmed death-1 receptor and its ligand PD-L1 are commonly expressed on immune cells. PD-1 and PD-L1 belong to the family of immune checkpoint proteins that act as co-inhibitory signaling inducers. Upon activation, T cells show enhanced expression of immune check point PD-1. Interaction between PD-1 and PD-L1 halt the T cell activation, thus maintaining the immune homeostasis. Tumor cells exploit this pathway to evade immune response. The effect of HDAC inhibitors on the expression of PD-1 and PD-L1 on γδ T cells was studied. γδ T cells were treated with different concentrations of HDAC inhibitors and expression of PD-1 and PD-L1 was analyzed by flow cytometry. Upon activation with antigen HDMAPP and rIL-2, expression of PD-1 and PD-L1 increases on γδ T cells. However, the expression of PD-1 and PD-L1 on γδ T cells substantially increased upon treatment with HDAC inhibitors. Maximum increase in the expression of PD-1 (**Figures 7A,B**) and PD-L1 (**Figures 7C,D**) on HDMAPP and rIL-2 activated γδ T cells was observed after treatment with VPA (2 mM), TSA (100 nm), and SAHA (1 μM). To assess the role of PD1/PD-L1 signaling in HDAC inhibitor treated γδ T cells, γδ T cells were activated with HDMAPP and rIL2, treated or untreated with HDAC inhibitors for 72 h. PD-1 blocking antibody was added at the start of culture. After 72 h, these γδ T cells were cultured with zoledronate-treated tumor cell lines AW13516, COLO-205, and Raji for 4 h at E/T ratio of 4:1. Blockade of PD-1 in HDAC inhibitor treated HDMAPP activated γδ T cells rescued the expression of effector molecules Lamp-1 (CD107a) (**Figure 8A**) and granzyme B (**Figure 8B**) as compared to only HDAC inhibitor treated γδ T cells. To further evaluate the role of HDAC inhibitors on the PD1/PD-L1 signaling axis in γδ T cells, we did the similar experiment by coculturing the effectors and above mentioned tumor targets to analyze the cytotoxic potential by LDH release assay at a ratio of 40:1 for 4 h. Blocking of PD-1 in HDMAPP-activated γδ T cells treated with HDAC inhibitorsVPA (2 mM), TSA (100 nM), and SAHA (1 μM) improves the cytolytic potential of γδ T cells as compared to γδ T cells treated with HDAC inhibitor only (**Figure 8C**). Thus, the results shows that blockade of PD-1 and PD-L1 signaling in HDAC inhibitor treated γδ T cells rescue their effector functions.

DISCUSSION

γδ T cell immunotherapy has become the emerging lead in the landscape of cancer immunotherapies due to their distinctive immune features and potent antitumor effector functions. They have been extensively targeted against diverse tumors such as melanoma, renal cell carcinoma, as well as B cell malignancies and have shown promising results in clinical settings (44). While these therapies have encountered modest clinical success, they have to overcome certain challenges such as limited availability of γδ T cells and rapid exhaustion upon repeated *in vitro* activation. Hence, combinational approaches have been envisaged with chemotherapeutics, monoclonal antibodies, small molecule inhibitors, etc. Newer treatment modality may include combining γδ T cell immunotherapy with antitumor drugs and other immune-modulating antibodies.

Epigenetic dysregulation is one of the hallmarks of cancer. Hence, epigenetic modifiers such as HDAC inhibitors are being comprehensively explored for their anticancer potential. Besides anticancer properties, HDAC inhibitors have also shown promising results in controlling the other pathological conditions such as neurological disorders and viral infections and are well tolerated

(45, 46). Currently, VPA along with other short-chain fatty acids HDAC inhibitors are being clinically evaluated as anticancer drugs (47). HDAC inhibitors employ wide range of antitumor mechanisms such as induction of apoptosis, senescence, differentiation, or inhibition of cell cycle (48, 49). Vorinostat (SAHA), is among the first HDAC inhibitor to be approved by United

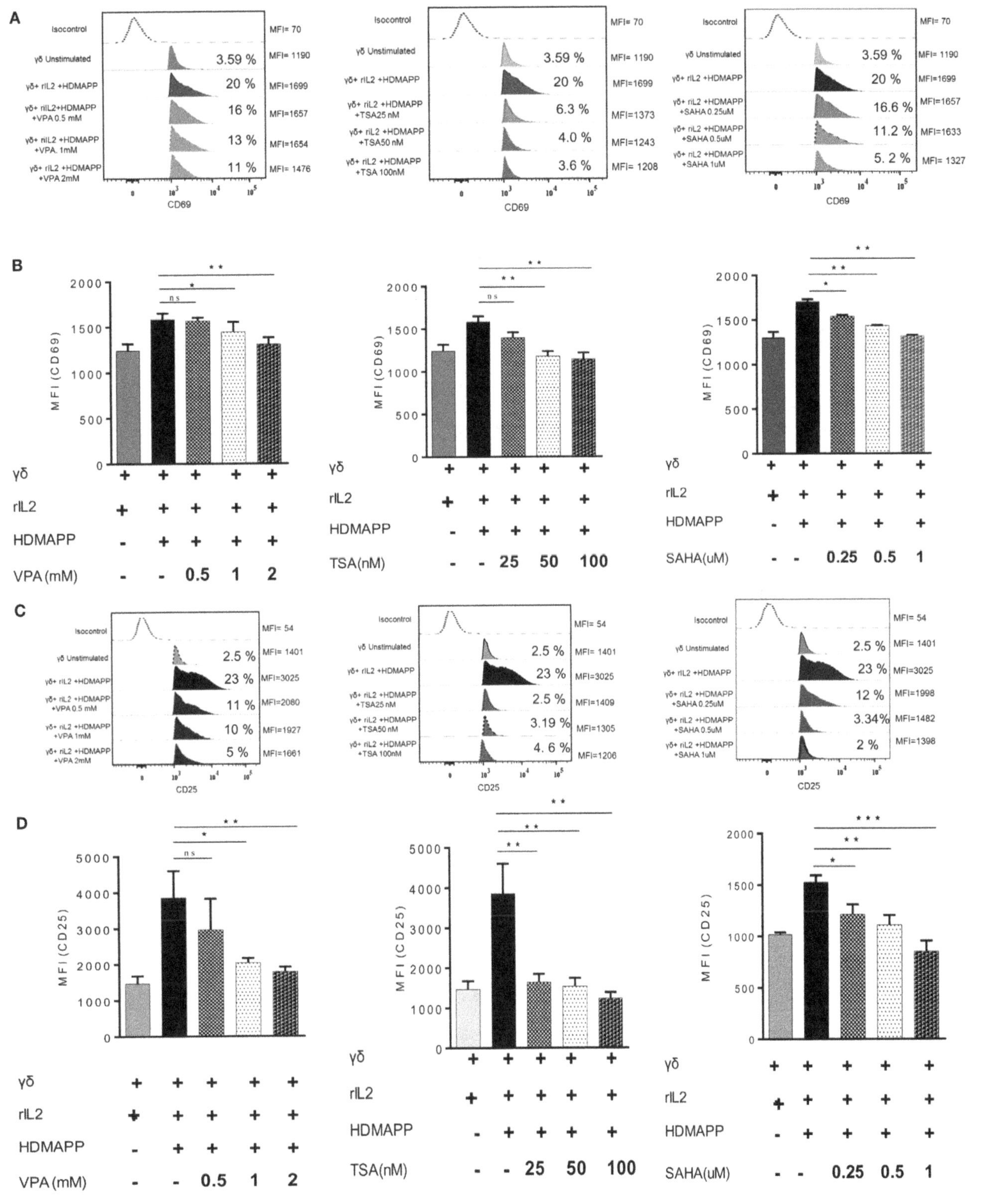

FIGURE 3 | Continued

FIGURE 3 | Histone deacetylases (HDAC) inhibitors affect the activation markers on γδ T cells. **(A)** The expression of early activation marker (CD69) on unstimulated γδ T cells and HDMAPP and rIL-2 stimulated γδ T cells with or without HDAC inhibitor treatment was analyzed by multi-color flow cytometry. Values on right side indicate the median fluorescence intensity (MFI) of CD69, while the values inside the histogram represent the percent CD69-positive γδ T cells. The histograms shown are representative of three independent experiments. **(B)** The cumulative MFI of CD69 expression on γδ T cells is represented as bar graphs. Data shown are representative of three independent experiments where $^*p < 0.05$, $^{**}p < 0.005$, $^{***}p < 0.0005$. **(C)** The effect of HDAC inhibitors on expression of late activation marker CD25 was assessed by flow cytometry. Unstimulated γδ T cells and HDMAPP stimulated γδ T cells with or without HDAC inhibitors at different concentrations, after 72 h were stained with the flurophore-tagged antibody and acquired on FACS Aria. Values on right side indicate the MFI of CD25, while the values inside the histogram represent the percent CD25-positive γδ T cells. The histograms depicted are representative of three independent experiments. **(D)** The results shown are cumulative MFI of CD25 expression on γδ T cells. HDAC inhibition decreases expression of CD25. Data shown are representative of three independent experiments where $^*p < 0.05$, $^{**}p < 0.005$, $^{***}p < 0.0005$.

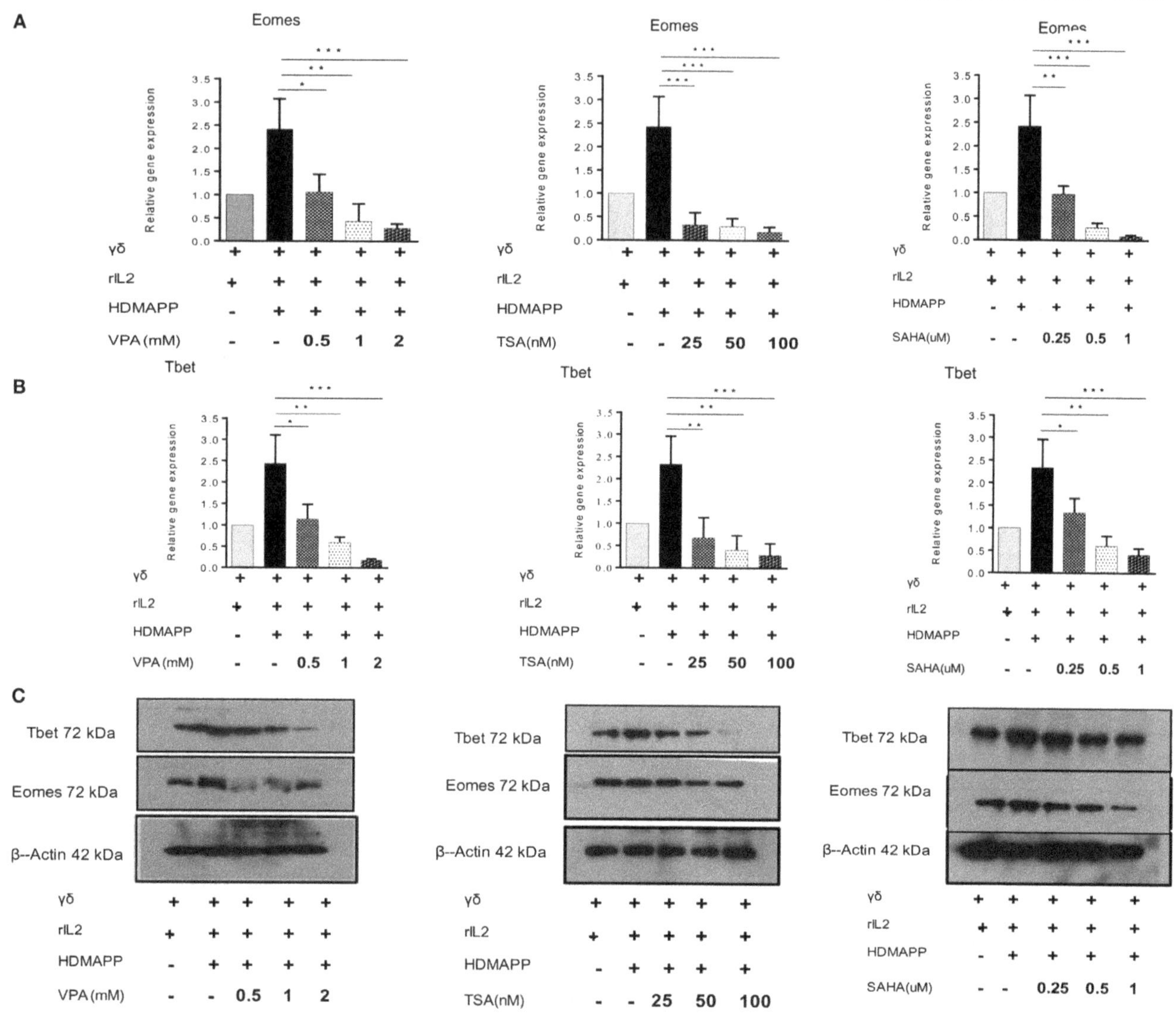

FIGURE 4 | Histone deacetylases (HDAC) inhibition abrogates expression of transcription factors regulating effector functions of γδ T cells. The m-RNA expression of Eomes **(A)** and T bet **(B)** in γδ T cells activated with HDMAPP, in the presence or absence of HDAC inhibitors sodium valproate, Trichostatin-A, and suberoylanilidehydroxamic acid at different concentrations was quantified by quantitative real-time PCR. The results indicated are cumulative mean of relative gene expression normalized to 18S r-RNA where $^*p < 0.05$, $^{**}p < 0.005$, $^{***}p < 0.0005$, compared with γδ T cells activated with HDMAPP. The data shown are representative of three independent experiments. **(C)** The protein level expression of T bet and Eomes was detected by western blotting. HDAC inhibitor treatment decreases the expression of T-bet and Eomes. β-actin was maintained as loading control. The blots shown are representative of three experiments.

States Food and Drug Administration (FDA) for the treatment of relapsed and refractory cutaneous T-cell lymphoma (50). Although HDAC inhibitors are approved for hematological malignancies, but clear proof-of-concept data for the clinical efficacy of HDAC inhibitors in solid tumors remains to be established (51). Recent studies have demonstrated that HDAC inhibitors exhibit higher

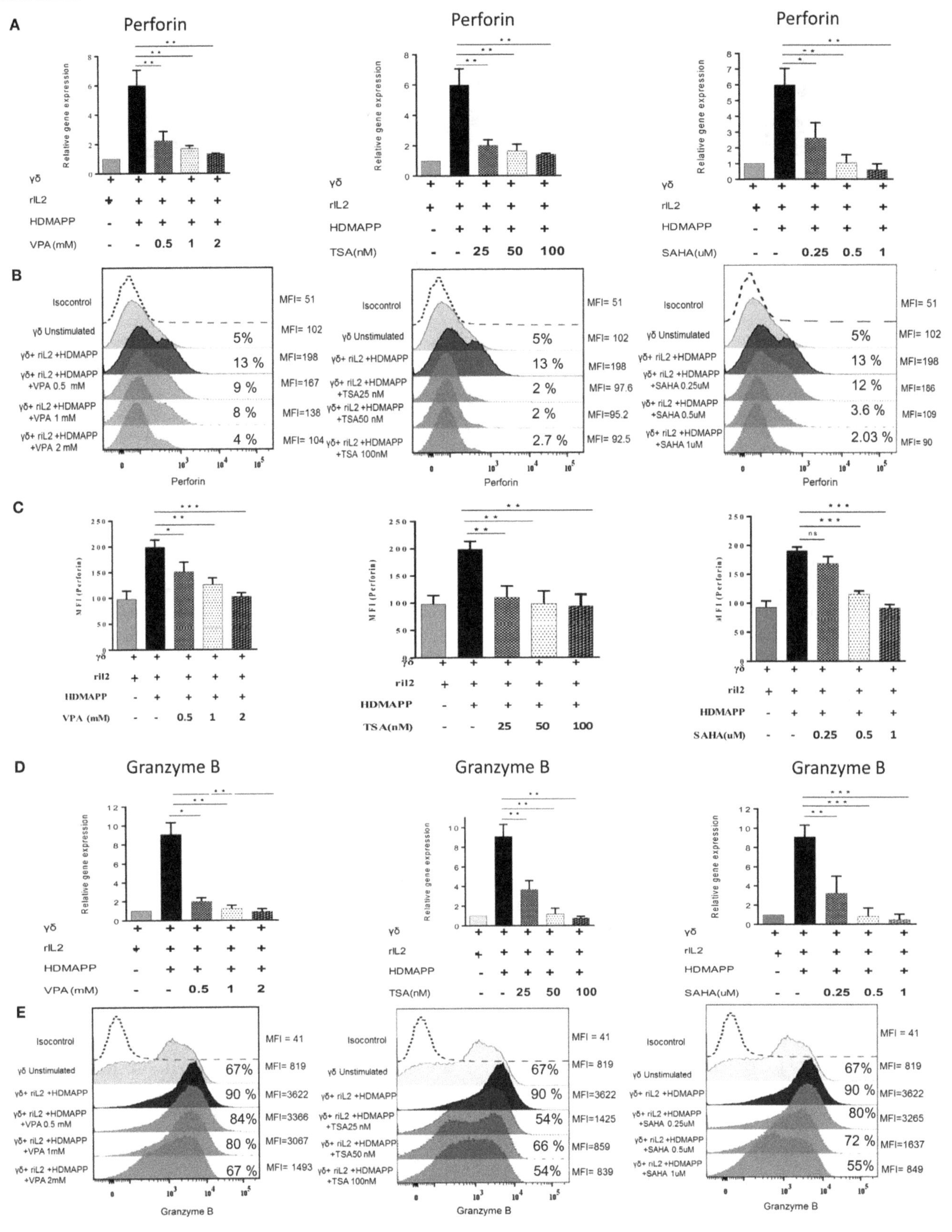

FIGURE 5 | Continued

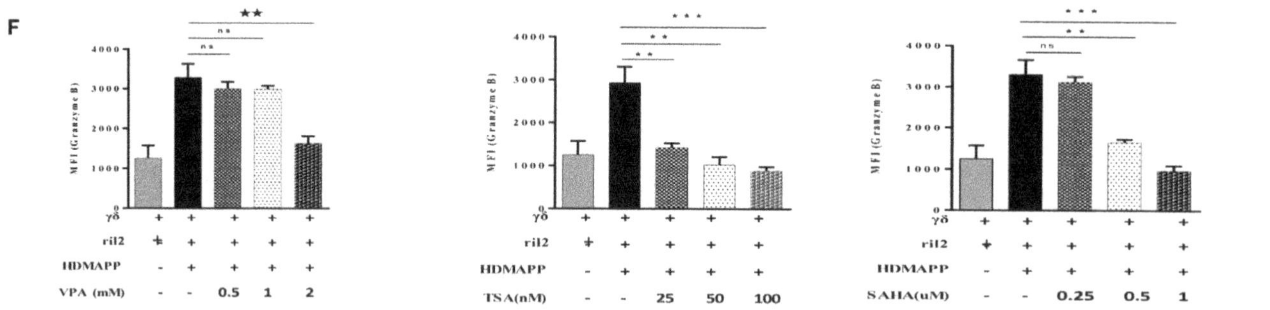

FIGURE 5 | Histone deacetylases (HDAC) inhibitor treatment abrogates the antitumor potential of γδ T cells. Expression of perforin and granzyme was studied at mRNA and protein levels using quantitative real-time PCR and flow cytometry, respectively. The gene expression of **(A)** perforin and **(D)** granzyme B by HDMAPP-stimulated γδ T cells with or without HDAC inhibitor treatment was quantified by quantitative real-time PCR. The results shown are cumulative means of relative gene expression, normalized to 18S r-RNA, and representative of three independent experiments. **(B)** γδ T cells activated by HDMAPP with or without sodium valproate, Trichostatin-A, and suberoylanilidehydroxamic acid at different concentrations were stained after 72 h with corresponding flurophore tagged antibody and expression of perforin was analyzed by flow cytometry. The values on right side of histograms indicate median fluorescence intensity (MFI) of perforin, while the values inside the histogram represent the percent positive γδ T for perforin. **(C)** Bar graphs represent cumulative MFI values where *$p < 0.05$, **$p < 0.005$, ***$p < 0.0005$, compared with γδ T cells activated with HDMAPP. **(E)** Expression of granzyme B by unstimulated γδ T cells and HDMAPP activated γδ T cells with or without HDAC inhibitor treatment was assessed by flow cytometric analysis. The values on right side of histograms indicate MFI of granzyme B, while the values inside the histogram represent the percent positive γδ T for granzyme B. The histograms are representative of three independent experiments. **(F)** The graphs represent MFI values of granzyme B where *$p < 0.05$, **$p < 0.005$, ***$p < 0.0005$.

therapeutic efficiency when combined with other antineoplastic agents (52). Hence, there is growing interest in exploring other combined therapeutic strategies with HDAC inhibitors.

Emerging evidence suggest that HDAC play a crucial role in T cell differentiation and effector functions. A number of studies have demonstrated that HDAC inhibitors suppress the immune response of T cells in severe inflammatory conditions and induce tolerance in organ transplantation (53). Specifically, HDAC inhibitors have shown to induce the regulatory T cell (Tregs) generation or stabilization of Tregs in inflammatory microenvironment due to which they have shown promising responses in experimental colitis (54). HDAC inhibitors increase the immunogenicity of tumors by increasing the expression of tumor antigens recognized by the immune cells. The antitumor responses of cytotoxic T lymphocytes like γδ T cells are mediated through recognition of stress molecules (ULBP, HSPs) or danger signals like MICA/B expressed on tumor cells by class of activating receptors known as NKG2D (55–57). Studies have demonstrated that HDAC inhibitors upregulate the NKG2D ligands on tumor cells, thereby sensitizing tumor cells to cytotoxicity mediated by γδ T cells in bladder cancer as well as NK cells in other malignancies such as osteosarcoma, pancreatic cancer, and multiple myeloma (32, 58–60). However, the causal effect of HDAC inhibitors on immune scenario is not well investigated and is contradictory. Several studies have shown that HDAC inhibitors affect each immune subset distinctly either leading to activation as in the case of CD4 T cells and CD8 T cells or by abrogating the effector functions of cells such as NK cell (61–63). Furthermore, for a particular immune cell type, the nature of immune regulation differs based on the type of HDAC inhibitor (64, 65). A recent study demonstrated that NKG2D expression in NK cells is inhibited by VPA (66).

Most of the studies have focused on investigating the impact of HDAC inhibitors on tumor cell lines and immune cells other than γδ T cells. Report by Suzuki et al. demonstrated that the antitumor effect of γδ T cells on bladder cancer was enhanced by treatment with VPA (32). The study focuses only on the impact of HDAC inhibitor, VPA on bladder cancer cell line. VPA leads to increase in the expression of MICA and MICB, which are recognized by NKG2D receptor on γδ T cells. The study does not explain the direct effect of HDAC inhibitors on γδ T cells. Earlier study by Kabelitz et al. reported that HDAC inhibitor VPA induces differential modulation of cell surface markers on γδ T cells compared to αβ T cells (67). Although the study shows the direct effect of VPA on γδ T cells, the functional responses of γδ T cells were not investigated in detail. In the present study, we have used three different HDAC inhibitors to delineate their effect on the functional responses of pure and sorted population of γδ T cells. We used clinically relevant concentrations of VPA, TSA, and SAHA in our study, which have been used in *in vitro* studies by other investigators (68, 69). We showed that three different HDAC inhibitors used suppressed the antitumor effector functions of γδ T cells.

We observed that γδ T cells activated with the phosphoantigen, HDMAPP in the presence of HDAC inhibitors showed decreased proliferative potential. One of the mechanism by which HDAC inhibitors exhibit their anticancer properties is through induction of cell differentiation and cell cycle arrest at G1 phase (48, 49). Besides affecting histone proteins, these inhibitors also have several non-histone protein substrates like p53, p21, Rb, and E2F1 in tumors (70, 71). On the other hand, it was demonstrated that downmodulation of p53 in T cells enhances their antigen-specific proliferative response and also augments antitumor cytotoxic functions (72, 73). Studies from our lab have shown that CD3-activated T cells upon activation show robust proliferative capacity and decreased expression of p53 and its downstream target p21 (74). Thus, the decrease in the antigen-specific proliferative response of γδ T cells in presence of HDAC inhibitors incited us to look for effect of HDAC inhibitors on cell cycle

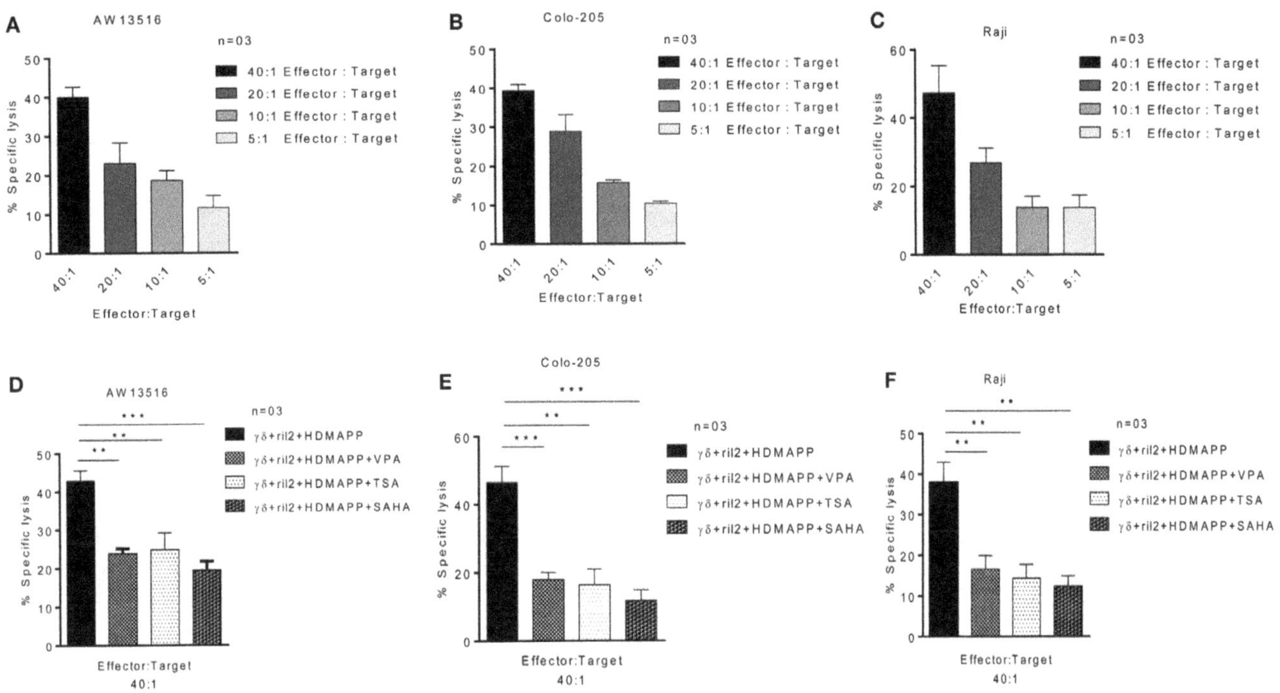

FIGURE 6 | Histone deacetylases inhibitors decrease the cytotoxic effector functions of γδ T cells. Cytotoxic effector function of γδ T cells was assessed against three tumor cell lines **(A)** AW13516, **(B)** COLO205, and **(C)** Raji. Zoledronate-treated tumor targets were cocultured with γδ T cells for 4 h and cytotoxicity was assessed by lactate dehydrogenase (LDH) assay. The results indicated are mean percent specific lysis at different effector:target ratio. Data are representative of three individual experiments. Cytotoxic potential of γδ T cells activated with HDMAPP in the presence of rIL-2 with or without treatment with sodium valproate (2 mM), suberoylanilidehydroxamic acid (1 μM), and Trichostatin-A (100 nM) was assessed against three zoledronate-treated tumor targets AW13516 **(D)**, COLO-205 **(E)**, and Raji **(F)** by LDH cytotoxicity assay. The results indicated are percent specific lysis at the effector to target ratio of 40:1 where $^{**}p < 0.005$ and $^{***}p < 0.0005$ when compared with γδ T cells activated with HDMAPP in the presence of rIL-2 ($n = 3$).

progression and expression of cell cycle regulators p53 and its downstream target p21. Decrease in the proliferation of γδ T cells in presence of HDAC inhibitors was associated with the increase in the expression of p53 and its downstream target p21. γδ T cells show increased expression of activation markers CD69 and CD25 when activated with phosphoantigens (36, 75). We observed that HDAC inhibitors inhibit the expression of CD69 and CD25 activation markers. CD25 is the high-affinity IL-2 receptor subunit and IL-2 signaling is necessary for the proliferation of T cells. It would be logical to conclude that HDAC inhibitors abrogate the IL-2 signaling and thus inhibit the proliferation of γδ T cells. We have used three different HDAC inhibitors VPA, TSA, and SAHA at different concentrations and they showed varied effects on expression of all the γδ T cell markers we studied. The likely explanation for the differences observed in their effects could be their structural diversity and also the biological activities they exert may be cell-type dependent.

Activated γδ T cells express Tbet and eomesodermin (Eomes) transcription factors. The T-box transcription factors T-bet and Eomes are important for acquisition of effector functions in cytotoxic T cells including γδ T cells (41, 76). Eomes and T-bet are highly homologous transcription factors and have cooperative and redundant functions in regulating the expression of different genes involved in the effector functions of CD8 T cells and activated natural killer cells. T-bet and Eomes regulate the expression of perforin, Granzyme-B, and IFN-γ by binding to promoter regions of these effector genes (14, 39). Knowing that HDAC inhibitors decrease the activation and proliferation of γδ T cells, we further hypothesized that HDAC inhibitors may modulate the effector functions of γδ T cells by affecting the expression of transcription factors Eomes and T-bet. We observed that treatment of γδ T cells with HDAC inhibitors lead to decrease in the expression of Eomes and T-bet. To further establish impact of HDAC inhibitors on the antitumor cytotoxic function of γδ T cell, we used panel of tumor cell lines (AW13516, COLO-205, and Raji) treated with zoledronate as target cell line in cytotoxicity assay. Previous work from our laboratory and others has demonstrated that tumor cells treated with zoledronate are aggressively killed by γδ T cells (10, 77). Our data demonstrate that treatment of HDAC inhibitors retard the ability of γδ T cells to kill zoledronate-treated tumor targets. Further, we proved that this inhibition of cytotoxic potential of γδ T cells was due to decrease in the expression of perforin and granzyme-B in these cells.

The activation of T cells initiated through T cell receptor is regulated by balance between co-stimulatory and inhibitory signals (immune checkpoints). Imbalance between these signals lead to different pathological conditions like tumor. Majority of the tumors use these immune checkpoints such as PD-1 or its ligand PD-L1 to escape from the immune surveillance. Immune check point inhibitors have revolutionized the field

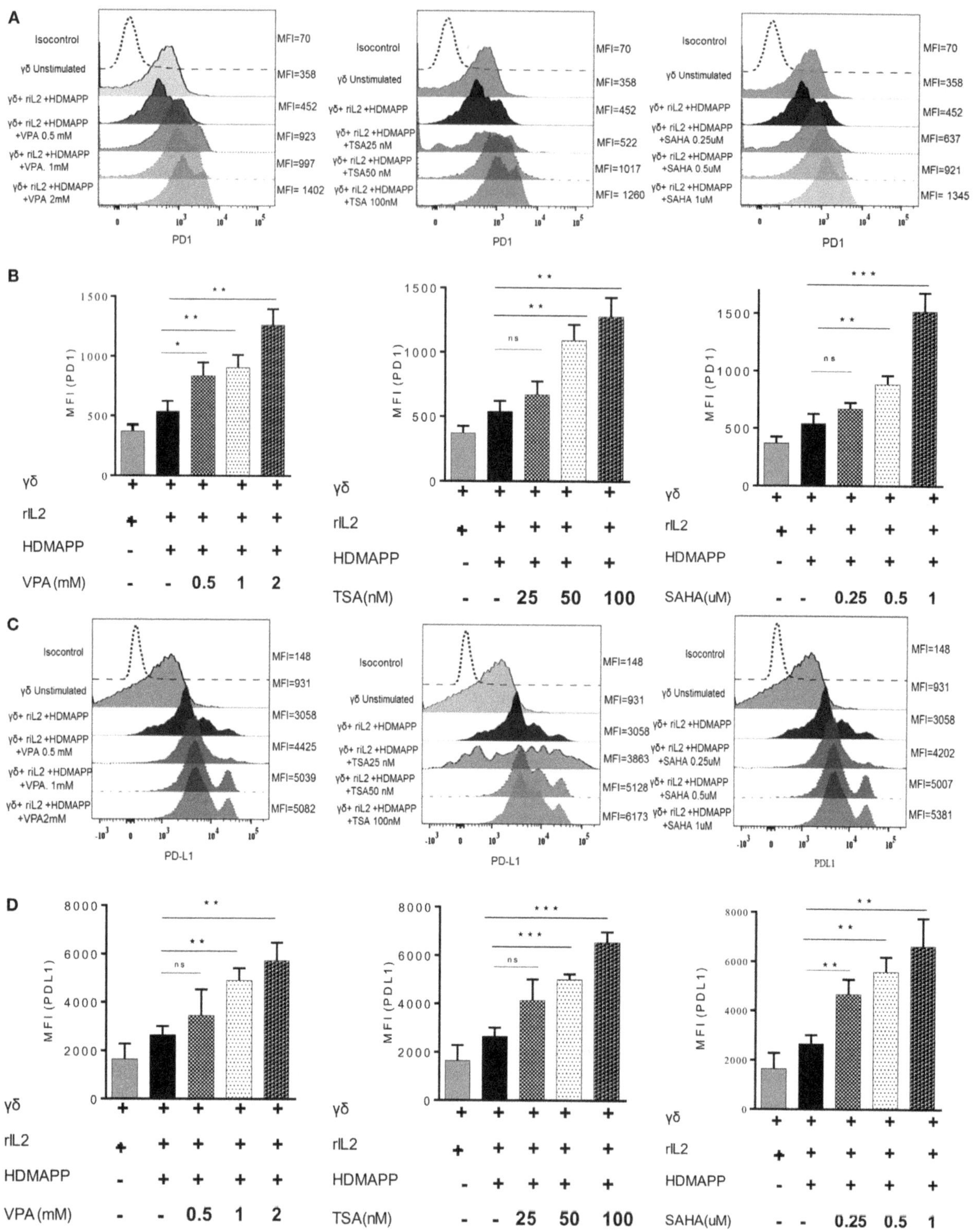

FIGURE 7 | Histone deacetylases (HDAC) inhibitors upregulate the expression of immune checkpoints on γδ T cells. **(A)** The expression of programmed death-1 by HDAC inhibitor-treated γδ T cells at their respective concentration. Histograms are representative of three individual experiments. The values on right side of histograms indicate median fluorescence intensity (MFI) of PD1. **(B)** MFI of PD1 expression as bar graphs where $^{*}p < 0.05$, $^{**}p < 0.005$, $^{***}p < 0.0005$ and ns, not significant when compared with γδ T cells activated with HDMAPP in the presence of rIL-2. **(C)** The expression of programmed death ligand-1 (PD-L1) by γδ T cells treated with HDAC inhibitors sodium valproate, Trichostatin-A, and suberoylanilidehydroxamic acid at their respective concentration was analyzed by immunostaining. Histograms shown are representative of three individual experiments. The values on right side of histograms indicate MFI of PD-L1. The results indicated in **(D)** are MFI of PD-L1 expression where $^{*}p < 0.05$, $^{**}p < 0.005$, $^{***}p < 0.0005$ and ns, not significant when compared with γδ T cells activated with HDMAPP.

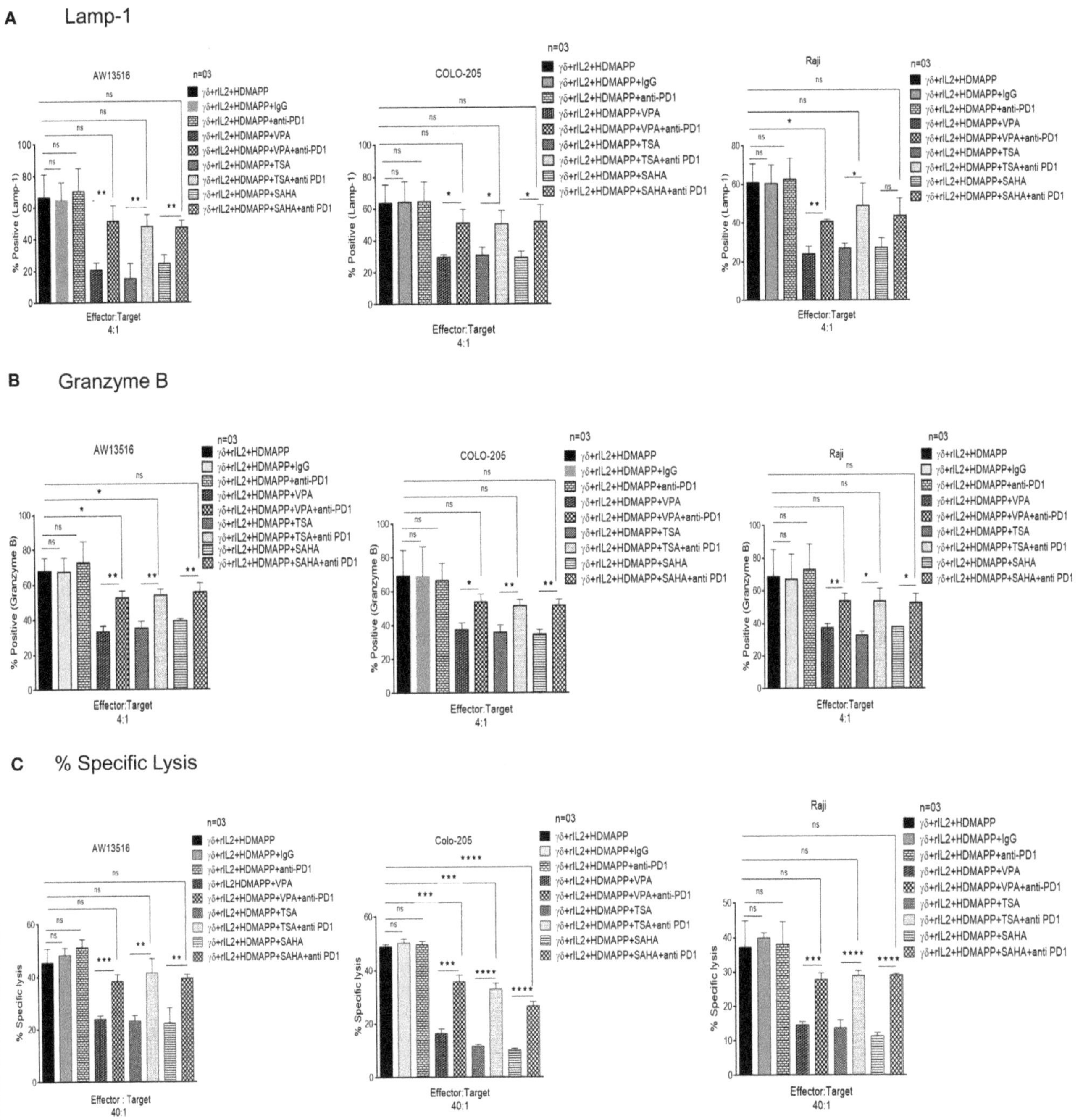

FIGURE 8 | Histone deacetylases (HDAC) inhibitors abrogate effector functions of γδ T cells *via* programmed death-1 (PD-1) upregulation. Expression of of **(A)** degranulation marker CD107a and **(B)** granzyme B by γδ T cells was assessed by flow cytometric analysis. HDMAPP activated γδ T cells upon treatment with sodium valproate (VPA) (2 mM), Trichostatin-A (TSA) (100 nM), and suberoylanilidehydroxamic acid (SAHA) (1 μM) in the presence or absence of PD1 blocking antibody were cocultured with three zoledronate treated tumor targets (AW 13516, Raji, COLO205) cells for 4 h at effector to target ratio of 4:1. The data represent consolidated median fluorescence intensity values of granzyme B and CD 107a expressing cells, indicative of three independent experiments (**$p < 0.005$, *$p < 0.05$, and ns, not significant). **(C)** The cytotoxic ability of γδ T cells treated with HDAC inhibitors TSA, SAHA, and VPA in the presence or absence of PD-1 blocking antibody was assessed against three zoledronate treated tumor targets (AW 13516, Raji, COLO205) by lactate dehydrogenase cytotoxicity assay. HDAC inhibitor treated γδ T cells show increased cytotoxic potential in the presence of PD-1 blocking antibody. The results indicate percent cytotoxicity where **$p < 0.005$, ***$p < 0.0005$, and ns, not significant, when compared with HDMAPP-activated γδ T cells treated with the respective HDAC inhibitor. Data represent three independent experiments.

of tumor immunotherapy (34). Besides surgery, radiation, and chemotherapy, immune check point inhibitors have surfaced as an important immunotherapeutic approach for cancer treatment. Due to their promising antitumor effects in experimental animal models, preclinical studies and successful clinical trials, immune check point inhibitors have been now approved by the U.S Food and Drug Administration (FDA) for treatment of different malignancies. PD-1/PD-L1 blocking strategy has led to tumor regression in patients with melanoma, renal cell carcinoma, non-small cell lung cancer, and bladder cancer (78–82).

Recent reports have shown that tumors associated with PD-1 expressing NK cells show poor survival (83). PD-1/PD-L1 signaling axis along with NKG2D signaling axis determine effector response of NK cells. Blockade of PD1/PD-L1 signaling cascade in NK cells along with other antitumor drugs have shown promising responses in cancer patients (84). This study supports our observation that HDAC inhibitors modulate the effector functions of human γδ T cells against tumors *via* PD1/PD-L1 signaling axis. We observed that γδ T cells show increased expression of immune check points PD1 and PD-L1 upon HDAC inhibitor treatment.

A report by Garcia-Diaz et al. have shown that induction of PD-L1 and PD-L2 on tumor cells is regulated *via* IFN-γ (85). In the present study, we have demonstrated that HDAC inhibitors decrease the expression of IFN-γ and TNF-α in antigen-activated γδ T cells. It has been demonstrated that Tbet transcription factor binds to PD-1 promoter and mediates the suppression of PD-1 expression (86). In the present study, we have shown that upon HDAC inhibitor treatment of γδ T cells, Tbet protein and mRNA is decreased significantly indicating that less Tbet may be available to bind PD-1 promoter to suppress PD-1 expression. This mechanism may explain the IFN-γ independent mechanism of PD-1 expression on γδ T cells.

Activated γδ T cells are known to express PD-1, which was investigated by Iwaski et al., on expanded γδ T cells population. They found that γδ T cells express PD-1 rapidly from day 3 of induction and PD-1$^+$ γδ T cells exhibit attenuated effector functions and decreased cytotoxicity against PD-L1 expressing tumors. However, they observed that zoledronate treatment to tumor cells, which induces IPP release along with PD-L1 blockade, rescued the γδ T cell cytotoxicity (35). While our study also confirms that blocking of PD-1 in γδ T cells increases the antitumor cytotoxic potential, our study reports on the effect of HDAC inhibitors on the freshly isolated γδ T cells activated with antigen for 72 h, whereas Iwaski group used γδ T cells already in activation state for their experimental purposes. Another interesting study by Castella et al. explores the multifunctional role of zoledronate in augmenting γδ T cells responses against multiple myeloma. In this study, zoledronate-treated autologous DCs were found to efficiently activate γδ T cells and enhance their cytotoxic functions against myeloma cells. Additionally, zoledronate was also shown to promote antitumor immunity *via* suppression of regulatory T cell function, downregulation of PD-L1 expression on DCs, and increased proliferation of tumor antigen-specific CD8 T cells. Although, their study has effectively demonstrated role of zoledronate in enhancing antitumor responses γδ T cells, it is specific only to multiple myeloma and uses zoledronate expanded γδ T cells from patient PBMNCs (87). Converse to our observation, they found that DC-activated γδ T cells did not express PD-1, this might be due to the immune modulation by zoledronate, which needs further exploration.

We observed that blockade of PD1/PD-L1 signaling partially restores the antitumor cytotoxic function of γδ T cells in the presence of HDAC inhibitors, which reflected in increased expression of effector molecules granzyme B and Lamp-1. Wei et al. have demonstrated that PD-1 ligation dramatically shifts the dose–response curve, making CD8+ Tcells much less sensitive to TCR generated signals (88). Although, this was shown in CD8+ αβ T cells, it may also apply to γδ T cells. Thus, PD-1 ligation affects TCR signaling and thereby reduces the cytotoxic function of γδ T cells. The role of other activating receptors such as NKG2D interacting with MICA/B and inhibitory receptors KIR2DL2/3 (CD158b) cannot be ignored and it explains the incomplete restoration of cytotoxic effector function γδ T cells upon PD-1 blocking.

Our results implicate that HDAC inhibitors along with the immune checkpoint modulating antibodies could be developed as combination immunotherapy to treat different malignancies. Thus, in future, this strategy may be applied for overcoming the limitations of HDAC inhibitor-based cancer therapies. The underlying mechanistic link of PD-1/PD-L1 may be targeted in developing more efficacious combination γδ T cell-based therapies in the future.

ETHICS STATEMENT

The study was approved by the Institutional Ethics Committee of ACTREC-TMC. All subjects gave written informed consent in accordance with the Declaration of Institutional Ethics Committee, ACTREC-TMC.

AUTHOR CONTRIBUTIONS

SC supervised, contributed conceptionally, and helped to write the manuscript. SB conducted experiments and wrote the manuscript. DV helped in conducting experiments. All authors contributed in final approval of manuscript.

ACKNOWLEDGMENTS

We acknowledge Department of Biotechnology, India for providing fellowships to SB. This work was supported by Department of Biotechnology Unit of Excellence, India grant BT/MED/30/SP11288/2015 to SC.

SUPPLEMENTARY MATERIAL

FIGURE S1 | Histone deacetylases (HDAC) inhibitors and viability of γδ T cells. HDAC inhibitors affect viability of γδ T cells only beyond specific concentrations. γδ T cells stimulated with HDMAPP in the presence of rIL-2 were treated with HDAC inhibitors sodium valproate (4, 3, 2, 1, and 0.5 mM), Trichostatin-A (250,

150, 100, 50, and 25 nM), and suberoylanilidehydroxamic acid (4, 3, 2, 1, 0.5 μM) for 72 h. The viability of γδ T cells was assessed by MTT assay. The results indicated are mean ± SE percent viability of γδ T cells and are representative of three experiments.

FIGURE S2 | The effect of histone deacetylases (HDAC) inhibitors on γδ T cells viability. **(A)** Purity of sorted γδ T cells. γδ T cells were positively sorted from peripheral blood mononuclear cells and were positive for γδ T-cell receptor (TCR) (90.8%), CD56 (53.2%), and negative for αβTCR, CD14, CD19. **(B)** Effect of HDAC inhibitor treatment on viability of γδ T cells. γδ T cells were activated with HDMAPP and rIL-2. HDAC inhibitors sodium valproate (2, 1, and 0.5 mM), Trichostatin-A (100, 50, and 25 nM), and suberoylanilidehydroxamic acid (1, 0.5, and 0.25 μM) were added to the culture and apoptosis was measured after 72 h with Annexin V and 7-AAD staining. Data shown are representative of three independent experiments. **(C)** The graphs show consolidated γδ T cell viability post HDAC inhibitor treatment ($n = 3$). Data represent mean ± SE.

FIGURE S3 | Histone deacetylases (HDAC) inhibitors impede proliferation of γδ T cells in a dose-dependent manner and leads to cell cycle arrest in G0–G1 phase. **(A)** The proliferative response of γδ T cells was assessed by thymidine incorporation assay. Sorted γδ T cells were stimulated with phosphoantigen HDMAPP, with or without treatment with HDAC inhibitors sodium valproate, Trichostatin-A, and suberoylanilidehydroxamic acid at different concentrations for 72 h. The graphs illustrate the cumulative mean cpm and are representative of three independent experiments where $^{*}p < 0.05$, $^{**}p < 0.005$, $^{***}p < 0.0005$. **(B)** Cell cycle analysis of γδ T cells upon HDAC inhibitor treatment. Freshly isolated γδ T cells were activated with HDMAPP with or without HDAC inhibitors for 72 h, and cell cycle progression was analyzed with propidium iodide (PI) staining using FACS calibur. The histograms are representative of three independent experiments. **(C)** The graphs indicate cumulative mean percentage of PI-positive cells in each phase of cell cycle. The graphs are representative of three independent experiments where $^{*}p < 0.05$, $^{**}p < 0.005$, $^{***}p < 0.0005$.

FIGURE S4 | Histone deacetylases (HDAC) inhibitors differentially affects the expression of activating and inhibitory receptors in γδ T cells. The expression of **(A)** NKG2D, **(B)** KIR2D2L2/3, and **(C)** CD16 by γδ T cells in the presence and absence of HDAC inhibitors after 72 h was analyzed by flow cytometry. The histograms are representative of three individual experiments. The values on right side of histograms indicate median fluorescence intensity. HDAC inhibitors reduce NFκB expression in γδ T cells. Protein expression of NFκB by γδ T cells upon treatment with **(C)** sodium valproate, **(D)** Trichostatin-A, and **(E)** suberoylanilidehydroxamic acid as detected by western blotting. Cell lysates of γδ T cells, stimulated with HDMAPP after treatment with HDAC inhibitors at different concentrations for 72 h were probed with NFκB antibody, β-actin was used as loading control. The blots shown are representative of three experiments.

FIGURE S5 | Histone deacetylases (HDAC) inhibitors decrease the acetylation on promoters of perforin and granzyme B in γδ T cells. **(A)** γδ T cells treated with HDAC inhibitors sodium valproate (VPA), Trichostatin-A (TSA), and suberoylanilidehydroxamic acid (SAHA) show increased acetylation of H3 and H4. Expression of acetyl Histone 3 and acetyl histone 4 in γδ T cells was detected by western blotting and total H3 and total H4 were used as loading control. The blots shown are representative of three experiments. Chromatin immunoprecipitation qPCR was used to analyze the histone H3 acetylation **(B)** and histone H4 acetylation **(C)** on perforin region I (−103 to +27 bp), perforin region II (−309 to −130 bp); granzyme B region I (−130 to +11 bp), and granzyme B region II (−263 to −77 bp) from the transcription start site (TSS) of perforin and granzyme B in γδ T cells treated with or without HDAC inhibitors VPA (2 mM), TSA (100 nM), and SAHA (1 μM) for 72 h. Enrichment of promoter regions of Perforin and Granzyme B was quantified by qPCR and expressed as percentage of input DNA. The images above the graphs are schematic representation of Perforin and granzyme B promoter regions including the TSS. All results indicated are mean + SEM where $^{*}p < 0.05$, $^{**}p < 0.005$, $^{***}p < 0.0005$.

REFERENCES

1. Heilig JS, Tonegawa S. Diversity of murine gamma genes and expression in fetal and adult T lymphocytes. *Nature* (1986) 322(6082):836–40. doi:10.1038/322836a0
2. Du SH, Li Z, Chen C, Tan WK, Chi Z, Kwang TW, et al. Co-expansion of cytokine-induced killer cells and Vγ9Vδ2 T cells for CAR T-cell therapy. *PLoS One* (2016) 11(9):e0161820. doi:10.1371/journal.pone.0161820
3. Kadivar M, Petersson J, Svensson L, Marsal J. CD8αβ+ γδ T cells: a novel T cell subset with a potential role in inflammatory bowel disease. *J Immunol* (2016) 197(12):4584–92. doi:10.4049/jimmunol.1601146
4. Bouet-Toussaint F, Cabillic F, Toutirais O, Le Gallo M, Thomas de la Pintière C, Daniel P, et al. Vgamma9Vdelta2 T cell-mediated recognition of human solid tumors. Potential for immunotherapy of hepatocellular and colorectal carcinomas. *Cancer Immunol Immunother* (2008) 57(4):531–9. doi:10.1007/s00262-007-0391-3
5. Fowler DW, Bodman-Smith MD. Harnessing the power of Vdelta2 cells in cancer immunotherapy. *Clin Exp Immunol* (2015) 180(1):1–10. doi:10.1111/cei.12564
6. Chiplunkar S, Dhar S, Wesch D, Kabelitz D. gammadelta T cells in cancer immunotherapy: current status and future prospects. *Immunotherapy* (2009) 1(4):663–78. doi:10.2217/imt.09.27
7. Hayday AC. [gamma][delta] cells: a right time and a right place for a conserved third way of protection. *Annu Rev Immunol* (2000) 18:975–1026. doi:10.1146/annurev.immunol.18.1.975
8. Kabelitz D, He W. The multifunctionality of human Vgamma9Vdelta2 gammadelta T cells: clonal plasticity or distinct subsets? *Scand J Immunol* (2012) 76(3):213–22. doi:10.1111/j.1365-3083.2012.02727.x
9. Morita CT, Jin C, Sarikonda G, Wang H. Nonpeptide antigens, presentation mechanisms, and immunological memory of human Vgamma2Vdelta2 T cells: discriminating friend from foe through the recognition of prenyl pyrophosphate antigens. *Immunol Rev* (2007) 215:59–76. doi:10.1111/j.1600-065X.2006.00479.x
10. Dhar S, Chiplunkar SV. Lysis of aminobisphosphonate-sensitized MCF-7 breast tumor cells by Vgamma9Vdelta2 T cells. *Cancer Immun* (2010) 10:10.
11. Das H, Wang L, Kamath A, Bukowski JF. Vgamma2Vdelta2 T-cell receptor-mediated recognition of aminobisphosphonates. *Blood* (2001) 98(5):1616–8. doi:10.1182/blood.V98.5.1616
12. Chen ZW, Letvin NL. Vgamma2Vdelta2+ T cells and anti-microbial immune responses. *Microbes Infect* (2003) 5(6):491–8. doi:10.1016/S1286-4579(03)00074-1
13. Caccamo N, Dieli F, Meraviglia S, Guggino G, Salerno A. Gammadelta T cell modulation in anticancer treatment. *Curr Cancer Drug Targets* (2010) 10(1):27–36. doi:10.2174/156800910790980188
14. Sullivan BM, Juedes A, Szabo SJ, von Herrath M, Glimcher LH. Antigen-driven effector CD8 T cell function regulated by T-bet. *Proc Natl Acad Sci U S A* (2003) 100(26):15818–23. doi:10.1073/pnas.2636938100
15. Kouzarides T. Chromatin modifications and their function. *Cell* (2007) 128(4):693–705. doi:10.1016/j.cell.2007.02.005
16. Strahl BD, Allis CD. The language of covalent histone modifications. *Nature* (2000) 403(6765):41–5. doi:10.1038/47412
17. Zhu P, Martin E, Mengwasser J, Schlag P, Janssen KP, Göttlicher M. Induction of HDAC2 expression upon loss of APC in colorectal tumorigenesis. *Cancer Cell* (2004) 5(5):455–63. doi:10.1016/S1535-6108(04)00114-X
18. Minucci S, Nervi C, Lo Coco F, Pelicci PG. Histone deacetylases: a common molecular target for differentiation treatment of acute myeloid leukemias? *Oncogene* (2001) 20(24):3110–5. doi:10.1038/sj.onc.1204336
19. Wang HF, Ning F, Liu ZC, Wu L, Li ZQ, Qi YF, et al. Histone deacetylase inhibitors deplete myeloid-derived suppressor cells induced by 4T1 mammary tumors in vivo and in vitro. *Cancer Immunol Immunother* (2017) 66(3):355–66. doi:10.1007/s00262-016-1935-1
20. Bolden JE, Peart MJ, Johnstone RW. Anticancer activities of histone deacetylase inhibitors. *Nat Rev Drug Discov* (2006) 5(9):769–84. doi:10.1038/nrd2133
21. Kim MS, Kwon HJ, Lee YM, Baek JH, Jang JE, Lee SW, et al. Histone deacetylases induce angiogenesis by negative regulation of tumor suppressor genes. *Nat Med* (2001) 7(4):437–43. doi:10.1038/86507
22. Osuka S, Takano S, Watanabe S, Ishikawa E, Yamamoto T, Matsumura A. Valproic acid inhibits angiogenesis in vitro and glioma angiogenesis in vivo in the brain. *Neurol Med Chir (Tokyo)* (2012) 52(4):186–93. doi:10.2176/nmc.52.186

23. McCaw TR, Randall TD, Forero A, Buchsbaum DJ. Modulation of antitumor immunity with histone deacetylase inhibitors. *Immunotherapy* (2017) 9(16):1359–72. doi:10.2217/imt-2017-0134
24. Gameiro SR, Malamas AS, Tsang KY, Ferrone S, Hodge JW. Inhibitors of histone deacetylase 1 reverse the immune evasion phenotype to enhance T-cell mediated lysis of prostate and breast carcinoma cells. *Oncotarget* (2016) 7(7):7390–402. doi:10.18632/oncotarget.7180
25. Minucci S, Pelicci PG. Histone deacetylase inhibitors and the promise of epigenetic (and more) treatments for cancer. *Nat Rev Cancer* (2006) 6(1):38–51. doi:10.1038/nrc1779
26. Halsall JA, Turner BM. Histone deacetylase inhibitors for cancer therapy: an evolutionarily ancient resistance response may explain their limited success. *Bioessays* (2016) 38(11):1102–10. doi:10.1002/bies.201600070
27. Terranova-Barberio M, Thomas S, Ali N, Pawlowska N, Park J, Krings G, et al. HDAC inhibition potentiates immunotherapy in triple negative breast cancer. *Oncotarget* (2017) 8(69):114156–72. doi:10.18632/oncotarget.23169
28. Zheng H, Zhao W, Yan C, Watson CC, Massengill M, Xie M, et al. HDAC inhibitors enhance T-cell chemokine expression and augment response to PD-1 immunotherapy in lung adenocarcinoma. *Clin Cancer Res* (2016) 22(16):4119–32. doi:10.1158/1078-0432.CCR-15-2584
29. Whitehill GD, Chivers A, Danielson B, Tessier JS, Hernandez Duran G, Bender GL, et al. Immunomodulatory effects of HDACi in combination with checkpoint blockade and lenalidomide in the immunosuppressive multiple myeloma bone marrow microenvironment. *Blood* (2017) 130(Suppl 1):4422.
30. Woods DM, Sodré AL, Villagra A, Sarnaik A, Sotomayor EM, Weber J. HDAC inhibition upregulates PD-1 ligands in melanoma and augments immunotherapy with PD-1 blockade. *Cancer Immunol Res* (2015) 3(12):1375–85. doi:10.1158/2326-6066.CIR-15-0077-T
31. Kroesen M, Gielen P, Brok IC, Armandari I, Hoogerbrugge PM, Adema GJ. HDAC inhibitors and immunotherapy; a double edged sword? *Oncotarget* (2014) 5(16):6558–72. doi:10.18632/oncotarget.2289
32. Suzuki T, Terao S, Acharya B, Naoe M, Yamamoto S, Okamura H, et al. The antitumour effect of {gamma}{delta} T-cells is enhanced by valproic acid-induced up-regulation of NKG2D ligands. *Anticancer Res* (2010) 30(11):4509–13.
33. Liechtenstein T, Dufait I, Lanna A, Breckpot K, Escors D. Modulating costimulation during antigen presentation to enhance cancer immunotherapy. *Immunol Endocr Metab Agents Med Chem* (2012) 12(3):224–35. doi:10.2174/187152212802001875
34. Gong J, Chehrazi-Raffle A, Reddi S, Salgia R. Development of PD-1 and PD-L1 inhibitors as a form of cancer immunotherapy: a comprehensive review of registration trials and future considerations. *J Immunother Cancer* (2018) 6(1):8. doi:10.1186/s40425-018-0316-z
35. Iwasaki M, Tanaka Y, Kobayashi H, Murata-Hirai K, Miyabe H, Sugie T, et al. Expression and function of PD-1 in human γδ T cells that recognize phosphoantigens. *Eur J Immunol* (2011) 41(2):345–55. doi:10.1002/eji.201040959
36. Gogoi D, Dar AA, Chiplunkar SV. Involvement of Notch in activation and effector functions of gammadelta T cells. *J Immunol* (2014) 192(5):2054–62. doi:10.4049/jimmunol.1300369
37. Lertworapreecha M, Patumraj S, Niruthisard S, Hansasuta P, Bhattarakosol P. Cytotoxic function of gamma delta (gamma/delta) T cells against pamidronate-treated cervical cancer cells. *Indian J Exp Biol* (2013) 51(8):597–605.
38. Lai Q, Du W, Wu J, Wang X, Li X, Qu X, et al. H3K9ac and HDAC2 activity are involved in the expression of monocarboxylate transporter 1 in oligodendrocyte. *Front Mol Neurosci* (2017) 10:376. doi:10.3389/fnmol.2017.00376
39. Pearce EL, Mullen AC, Martins GA, Krawczyk CM, Hutchins AS, Zediak VP, et al. Control of effector CD8+ T cell function by the transcription factor eomesodermin. *Science* (2003) 302(5647):1041–3. doi:10.1126/science.1090148
40. Cho OH, Shin HM, Miele L, Golde TE, Fauq A, Minter LM, et al. Notch regulates cytolytic effector function in CD8+ T cells. *J Immunol* (2009) 182(6):3380–9. doi:10.4049/jimmunol.0802598
41. Chen L, He W, Kim ST, Tao J, Gao Y, Chi H, et al. Epigenetic and transcriptional programs lead to default IFN-gamma production by gammadelta T cells. *J Immunol* (2007) 178(5):2730–6. doi:10.4049/jimmunol.178.5.2730
42. Alexander AA, Maniar A, Cummings JS, Hebbeler AM, Schulze DH, Gastman BR, et al. Isopentenyl pyrophosphate-activated CD56+ {gamma}{delta} T lymphocytes display potent antitumor activity toward human squamous cell carcinoma. *Clin Cancer Res* (2008) 14(13):4232–40. doi:10.1158/1078-0432.CCR-07-4912
43. Salti SM, Hammelev EM, Grewal JL, Reddy ST, Zemple SJ, Grossman WJ, et al. Granzyme B regulates antiviral CD8+ T cell responses. *J Immunol* (2011) 187(12):6301–9. doi:10.4049/jimmunol.1100891
44. Lamb LS Jr, Lopez RD. gammadelta T cells: a new frontier for immunotherapy? *Biol Blood Marrow Transplant* (2005) 11(3):161–8. doi:10.1016/j.bbmt.2004.11.015
45. Phiel CJ, Zhang F, Huang EY, Guenther MG, Lazar MA, Klein PS. Histone deacetylase is a direct target of valproic acid, a potent anticonvulsant, mood stabilizer, and teratogen. *J Biol Chem* (2001) 276(39):36734–41. doi:10.1074/jbc.M101287200
46. Archin NM, Eron JJ, Palmer S, Hartmann-Duff A, Martinson JA, Wiegand A, et al. Valproic acid without intensified antiviral therapy has limited impact on persistent HIV infection of resting CD4+ T cells. *AIDS* (2008) 22(10):1131–5. doi:10.1097/QAD.0b013e3282fd6df4
47. Mottamal M, Zheng S, Huang TL, Wang G. Histone deacetylase inhibitors in clinical studies as templates for new anticancer agents. *Molecules* (2015) 20(3):3898–941. doi:10.3390/molecules20033898
48. Borbone E, Berlingieri MT, De Bellis F, Nebbioso A, Chiappetta G, Mai A, et al. Histone deacetylase inhibitors induce thyroid cancer-specific apoptosis through proteasome-dependent inhibition of TRAIL degradation. *Oncogene* (2010) 29(1):105–16. doi:10.1038/onc.2009.306
49. Nebbioso A, Clarke N, Voltz E, Germain E, Ambrosino C, Bontempo P, et al. Tumor-selective action of HDAC inhibitors involves TRAIL induction in acute myeloid leukemia cells. *Nat Med* (2005) 11(1):77–84. doi:10.1038/nm1161
50. Duvic M, Talpur R, Ni X, Zhang C, Hazarika P, Kelly C, et al. Phase 2 trial of oral vorinostat (suberoylanilide hydroxamic acid, SAHA) for refractory cutaneous T-cell lymphoma (CTCL). *Blood* (2007) 109(1):31–9. doi:10.1182/blood-2006-06-025999
51. Lin KT, Wang YW, Chen CT, Ho CM, Su WH, Jou YS. HDAC inhibitors augmented cell migration and metastasis through induction of PKCs leading to identification of low toxicity modalities for combination cancer therapy. *Clin Cancer Res* (2012) 18(17):4691–701. doi:10.1158/1078-0432.CCR-12-0633
52. Kuendgen A, Schmid M, Schlenk R, Knipp S, Hildebrandt B, Steidl C, et al. The histone deacetylase (HDAC) inhibitor valproic acid as monotherapy or in combination with all-trans retinoic acid in patients with acute myeloid leukemia. *Cancer* (2006) 106(1):112–9. doi:10.1002/cncr.21552
53. Choi SW, Gatza E, Hou G, Sun Y, Whitfield J, Song Y, et al. Histone deacetylase inhibition regulates inflammation and enhances Tregs after allogeneic hematopoietic cell transplantation in humans. *Blood* (2015) 125(5):815–9. doi:10.1182/blood-2014-10-605238
54. Glauben R, Batra A, Fedke I, Zeitz M, Lehr HA, Leoni F, et al. Histone hyperacetylation is associated with amelioration of experimental colitis in mice. *J Immunol* (2006) 176(8):5015–22. doi:10.4049/jimmunol.176.8.5015
55. Nausch N, Cerwenka A. NKG2D ligands in tumor immunity. *Oncogene* (2008) 27(45):5944–58. doi:10.1038/onc.2008.272
56. Rincon-Orozco B, Kunzmann V, Wrobel P, Kabelitz D, Steinle A, Herrmann T. Activation of Vγ9Vδ2 T cells by NKG2D. *J Immunol* (2005) 175(4):2144–51. doi:10.4049/jimmunol.175.4.2144
57. Corvaisier M, Moreau-Aubry A, Diez E, Bennouna J, Mosnier J-F, Scotet E, et al. Vγ9Vδ2 T cell response to colon carcinoma cells. *J Immunol* (2005) 175(8):5481–8. doi:10.4049/jimmunol.175.8.5481
58. Yamanegi K, Yamane J, Kobayashi K, Kato-Kogoe N, Ohyama H, Nakasho K, et al. Sodium valproate, a histone deacetylase inhibitor, augments the expression of cell-surface NKG2D ligands, MICA/B, without increasing their soluble forms to enhance susceptibility of human osteosarcoma cells to NK cell-mediated cytotoxicity. *Oncol Rep* (2010) 24(6):1621–7. doi:10.3892/or_00001026
59. Shi P, Yin T, Zhou F, Cui P, Gou S, Wang C. Valproic acid sensitizes pancreatic cancer cells to natural killer cell-mediated lysis by upregulating MICA and MICB via the PI3K/Akt signaling pathway. *BMC Cancer* (2014) 14:370. doi:10.1186/1471-2407-14-370
60. Wu X, Tao Y, Hou J, Meng X, Shi J. Valproic acid upregulates NKG2D ligand expression through an ERK-dependent mechanism and potentially enhances NK cell-mediated lysis of myeloma. *Neoplasia* (2012) 14(12):1178–89. doi:10.1593/neo.121236
61. Setiadi AF, Omilusik K, David MD, Seipp RP, Hartikainen J, Gopaul R, et al. Epigenetic enhancement of antigen processing and presentation

promotes immune recognition of tumors. *Cancer Res* (2008) 68(23):9601–7. doi:10.1158/0008-5472.CAN-07-5270
62. Murakami T, Sato A, Chun NA, Hara M, Naito Y, Kobayashi Y, et al. Transcriptional modulation using HDACi depsipeptide promotes immune cell-mediated tumor destruction of murine B16 melanoma. *J Invest Dermatol* (2008) 128(6):1506–16. doi:10.1038/sj.jid.5701216
63. Turner TB, Meza-Perez S, Londoño A, Katre A, Peabody JE, Smith HJ, et al. Epigenetic modifiers upregulate MHC II and impede ovarian cancer tumor growth. *Oncotarget* (2017) 8(27):44159–70. doi:10.18632/oncotarget.17395
64. Pace M, Williams J, Kurioka A, Gerry AB, Jakobsen B, Klenerman P, et al. Histone deacetylase inhibitors enhance CD4 T cell susceptibility to NK cell killing but reduce NK cell function. *PLoS Pathog* (2016) 12(8):e1005782. doi:10.1371/journal.ppat.1005782
65. Bridle BW, Chen L, Lemay CG, Diallo JS, Pol J, Nguyen A, et al. HDAC inhibition suppresses primary immune responses, enhances secondary immune responses, and abrogates autoimmunity during tumor immunotherapy. *Mol Ther* (2013) 21(4):887–94. doi:10.1038/mt.2012.265
66. Ni L, Wang L, Yao C, Ni Z, Liu F, Gong C, et al. The histone deacetylase inhibitor valproic acid inhibits NKG2D expression in natural killer cells through suppression of STAT3 and HDAC3. *Sci Rep* (2017) 7:45266. doi:10.1038/srep45266
67. Bhat J, Oberg HH, Kabelitz D. Modulation of human gamma/delta T-cell activation and phenotype by histone deacetylase inhibitors. *Cell Immunol* (2015) 296(1):50–6. doi:10.1016/j.cellimm.2015.01.019
68. Blaheta RA, Michaelis M, Driever PH, Cinatl J Jr. Evolving anticancer drug valproic acid: insights into the mechanism and clinical studies. *Med Res Rev* (2005) 25(4):383–97. doi:10.1002/med.20027
69. Kelly WK, Marks PA. Drug insight: histone deacetylase inhibitors – development of the new targeted anticancer agent suberoylanilide hydroxamic acid. *Nat Clin Pract Oncol* (2005) 2(3):150–7. doi:10.1038/ncponc0106
70. Zhao Y, Tan J, Zhuang L, Jiang X, Liu ET, Yu Q. Inhibitors of histone deacetylases target the Rb-E2F1 pathway for apoptosis induction through activation of proapoptotic protein Bim. *Proc Natl Acad Sci U S A* (2005) 102(44):16090–5. doi:10.1073/pnas.0505585102
71. Condorelli F, Gnemmi I, Vallario A, Genazzani AA, Canonico PL. Inhibitors of histone deacetylase (HDAC) restore the p53 pathway in neuroblastoma cells. *Br J Pharmacol* (2008) 153(4):657–68. doi:10.1038/sj.bjp.0707608
72. Banerjee A, Thyagarajan K, Chatterjee S, Chakraborty P, Kesarwani P, Soloshchenko M, et al. Lack of p53 augments antitumor functions in cytolytic T cells. *Cancer Res* (2016) 76(18):5229–40. doi:10.1158/0008-5472.CAN-15-1798
73. Watanabe M, Moon KD, Vacchio MS, Hathcock KS, Hodes RJ. Downmodulation of tumor suppressor p53 by T cell receptor signaling is critical for antigen-specific CD4(+) T cell responses. *Immunity* (2014) 40(5):681–91. doi:10.1016/j.immuni.2014.04.006
74. Dar AA, Bhat SA, Gogoi D, Gokhale A, Chiplunkar SV. Inhibition of Notch signalling has ability to alter the proximal and distal TCR signalling events in human CD3(+) αβ T-cells. *Mol Immunol* (2017) 92:116–24. doi:10.1016/j.molimm.2017.10.013
75. Kjeldsen-Kragh J, Quayle AJ, Skålhegg BS, Sioud M, Førre O. Selective activation of resting human gamma delta T lymphocytes by interleukin-2. *Eur J Immunol* (1993) 23(9):2092–9. doi:10.1002/eji.1830230908
76. Dimova T, Brouwer M, Gosselin F, Tassignon J, Leo O, Donner C, et al. Effector Vγ9Vδ2 T cells dominate the human fetal γδ T-cell repertoire. *Proc Natl Acad Sci U S A* (2015) 112(6):E556–65. doi:10.1073/pnas.1412058112
77. Nussbaumer O, Gruenbacher G, Gander H, Komuczki J, Rahm A, Thurnher M. Essential requirements of zoledronate-induced cytokine and γδ T cell proliferative responses. *J Immunol* (2013) 191(3):1346–55. doi:10.4049/jimmunol.1300603
78. Hamid O, Robert C, Daud A, Hodi FS, Hwu WJ, Kefford R, et al. Safety and tumor responses with lambrolizumab (anti-PD-1) in melanoma. *N Engl J Med* (2013) 369(2):134–44. doi:10.1056/NEJMoa1305133
79. Kim J. Immune checkpoint blockade therapy for bladder cancer treatment. *Investig Clin Urol* (2016) 57(Suppl 1):S98–105. doi:10.4111/icu.2016.57.S1.S98
80. Chang K, Qu Y, Dai B, Zhao JY, Gan H, Shi G, et al. PD-L1 expression in Xp11.2 translocation renal cell carcinoma: indicator of tumor aggressiveness. *Sci Rep* (2017) 7(1):2074. doi:10.1038/s41598-017-02005-7
81. Inman BA, Longo TA, Ramalingam S, Harrison MR. Atezolizumab: a PD-L1-blocking antibody for bladder cancer. *Clin Cancer Res* (2017) 23(8):1886–90. doi:10.1158/1078-0432.CCR-16-1417
82. Kazandjian D, Khozin S, Blumenthal G, Zhang L, Tang S, Libeg M, et al. Benefit-risk summary of nivolumab for patients with metastatic squamous cell lung cancer after platinum-based chemotherapy: a report from the us food and drug administration. *JAMA Oncol* (2016) 2(1):118–22. doi:10.1001/jamaoncol.2015.3934
83. Liu Y, Cheng Y, Xu Y, Wang Z, Du X, Li C, et al. Increased expression of programmed cell death protein 1 on NK cells inhibits NK-cell-mediated anti-tumor function and indicates poor prognosis in digestive cancers. *Oncogene* (2017) 36(44):6143–53. doi:10.1038/onc.2017.209
84. Yang L, Shen M, Xu LJ, Yang X, Tsai Y, Keng PC, et al. Enhancing NK cell-mediated cytotoxicity to cisplatin-resistant lung cancer cells via MEK/Erk signaling inhibition. *Sci Rep* (2017) 7(1):7958. doi:10.1038/s41598-017-08483-z
85. Garcia-Diaz A, Shin DS, Moreno BH, Saco J, Escuin-Ordinas H, Rodriguez GA, et al. Interferon receptor signaling pathways regulating PD-L1 and PD-L2 expression. *Cell Rep* (2017) 19(6):1189–201. doi:10.1016/j.celrep.2017.04.031
86. Taylor A, Harker JA, Chanthong K, Stevenson PG, Zuniga EI, Rudd CE. Glycogen synthase kinase 3 inactivation drives T-bet-mediated downregulation of co-receptor PD-1 to enhance CD8(+) cytolytic T cell responses. *Immunity* (2016) 44(2):274–86. doi:10.1016/j.immuni.2016.01.018
87. Castella B, Riganti C, Fiore F, Pantaleoni F, Canepari ME, Peola S, et al. Immune modulation by zoledronic acid in human myeloma: an advantageous cross-talk between Vγ9Vδ2 T cells, alphabeta CD8+ T cells, regulatory T cells, and dendritic cells. *J Immunol* (2011) 187(4):1578–90. doi:10.4049/jimmunol.1002514
88. Wei F, Zhong S, Ma Z, Kong H, Medvec A, Ahmed R, et al. Strength of PD-1 signaling differentially affects T-cell effector functions. *Proc Natl Acad Sci U S A* (2013) 110(27):E2480–9. doi:10.1073/pnas.1305394110

8

Interferon-α Up-Regulates the Expression of PD-L1 Molecules on Immune Cells through STAT3 and p38 Signaling

Alexandr V. Bazhin[1,2], Katharina von Ahn[3], Jasmin Fritz[3], Jens Werner[1,2] and Svetlana Karakhanova[3,4]*

[1] Department of General, Visceral, and Transplant Surgery, Ludwig-Maximilians-University Munich, Munich, Germany, [2] German Cancer Consortium (DKTK), Partner Site Munich, Munich, Germany, [3] Department of General, Visceral and Transplantation Surgery, University of Heidelberg, Heidelberg, Germany, [4] Section Surgical Research, University of Heidelberg, Heidelberg, Germany

Edited by:
Giovanna Schiavoni, Istituto Superiore di Sanità (ISS), Italy

Reviewed by:
Marina Cella, Washington University in St. Louis, United States
Abhishek D. Garg, KU Leuven, Belgium

***Correspondence:**
Svetlana Karakhanova
s.karakhanova@gmx.de

Interferon-α (IFNα) has one of the longest histories of use amongst cytokines in clinical oncology and has been applied for the treatment of many types of cancers. Due to its immune-activating properties, IFNα is also an attractive candidate for combinatory anti-cancer therapies. Despite its extensive use in animal tumor models as well as in several clinical trials, the different mechanisms underlying patient responses and affecting desirable clinical benefits are still under investigation. Here we show that in addition to its immune-activating properties, IFNα induces the expression of a key negative regulator, immunosuppressive PD-L1 molecule, in the majority of the specific immune cell populations, particularly in the dendritic cells (DC). DC can modulate immune responses by a variety of mechanisms, including expression of T-cell regulatory molecules and cytokines. Our results showed that treatment of DC with IFNα-2b led to pronounced up-regulation of surface expression of PD-L1 molecules, increased IL-6 and decreased IL-12 production. Moreover, we present evidence that IFNα-treated DC exhibited a reduced capacity to stimulate interferon-γ production in T cells compared to control DC. This T-cell response after treatment of DC with IFNα was recovered by a pre-treatment with an anti-PD-L1 blocking antibody. Further analyses revealed that IFNα regulated PD-L1 expression through the STAT3 and p38 signaling pathways, since blocking of STAT3 and p38 activation with specific inhibitors prevented PD-L1 up-regulation. Our findings underline the important roles of p38 and STAT3 in the regulation of PD-L1 expression and prove that IFNα induces STAT3/p38-mediated expression of PD-L1 and thereby a reduced stimulatory ability of DC. The augmentation of PD-L1 expression in immune cells through IFNα treatment should be considered by use of IFNα in an anti-cancer therapy.

Keywords: PD-L1 (B7-H1), immunosuppression, IFNα, cancer immunotherapy, dendritic cell, STAT3 signaling

INTRODUCTION

The cytokine interferon-α (IFNα) has been used for a long time for treatment of many types of cancers, such as renal cell carcinoma, malignant melanoma or chronic myeloid leukemia (1, 2). However, the molecular mechanisms affecting patient responses and clinical outcome of IFNα therapy are still under investigation. IFNα is a member of the type I interferon family and is produced by various cell types, including monocytes, macrophages, lymphoblastoid cells, fibroblasts and plasmacytoid dendritic cells (3). Initially utilized as an anti-viral agent and meant for use in tumors where a viral origin was suspected, IFNα initiated a variety of biological activities that warranted further investigation. Indeed, this cytokine manifests direct suppressive effects on tumor cell growth *in vitro* and *in vivo* (4) and enhances tumor recognition by the increase in MHC-1 expression. Additionally, radio- and chemo-sensitizing capacities, as well as anti-angiogenic properties, have been described for IFNα (5, 6). Furthermore, Essers and colleagues have showed that the cytokine activated dormant hematopoietic stem cells *in vivo* (7). We have confirmed this phenomenon in pancreatic cancer, where we found that IFNα exhibited the ability to activate stem cell markers (8). Meanwhile, the immunostimulatory characteristics of IFNα have gained special attention since they can affect the differentiation of DC, survival of T cells, generation of $CD8^+$ memory cells, macrophage activities and activation of natural killer (NK) cells (9). A lot of tumor entities, like pancreatic cancer, are characterized by reduced immunological defense (10, 11). A combination of chemotherapy with immune stimulation could improve therapy efficacy and provide an optimal cancer treatment (12). Armed with its attributes, IFNα could be an attractive candidate for combinatory therapies. Indeed, IFNα-2b (trade name Intron-A), a well-known IFN-based therapeutic (13) that is approved for the treatment of various infectious diseases as well as for many types of cancer including leukemia, lymphoma, multiple myeloma and malignant melanoma, is also actively used in multiple clinical trials (http://www.druglib.com/druginfo/intron-a/trials/).

However, it has become increasingly clear in the last few years that certain cytokines originally described as immunostimulatory and pro-inflammatory, could also up-regulate immunosuppressive molecules. Such molecules are key elements of immune inhibitory pathways, so-called immunological checkpoints, which are crucial for maintaining self-tolerance and modulating the strength of immune responses. The most prominent of them is the PD-L1 (Programmed death-ligand 1, CD274, B7-H1)–PD-1 axis. PD-L1 is a type 1 transmembrane glycoprotein and one of two ligands for the CD28 homolog programmed death-1 receptor (PD-1) (14). The protein expression of PD-L1 can be found on immune cells as well as on non-immune endothelial and epithelial cells and can be up-regulated by different agents, such as cytokines and TLR (toll-like receptor) ligands (15–19). The PD-L1 molecule plays an important role in controlling immune reactions by inhibiting T-cell response and by influencing several other cell types. It is implicated in a number of human and mouse disorders as well as in transplant rejection and pregnancy complications (14, 20, 21). Additionally, it is responsible for the chronification of viral and bacterial infections (22). The expression of this molecule contributes as well to tumor immune evasion and correlates with a poor prognosis for the cancer patient (23–26). This makes PD-L1 and its regulation an important target for on-going investigations that aim to develop new anti-cancer treatment strategies. Interferons have been shown to be able to regulate PD-L1 expression not only on tumor (25) but as well on several non-tumor cell types: IFNγ increases PD-L1 in dermal fibroblasts (15), hepatic stellate cells (27) and DC (28, 29); the up-regulation of PD-L1 in DC by IFNβ contributes to immunomodulatory effects of this cytokine in multiple sclerosis and in lipopolysaccharide-induced immune paralysis (30, 31) and the expression of PD-L1 in hepatocytes and in myeloid cells *in vitro* can be augmented by IFNα (29, 32).

The stimulation of PD-L1 expression by IFNα could make a substantial negative contribution in patient responses and clinical outcomes of IFNα therapy through increased immunosuppression. Therefore, in this work we investigated the mechanisms of regulation of PD-L1 expression in specific immune cell populations by IFNα.

MATERIALS AND METHODS

Antibodies and Reagents

Anti-mouse monoclonal antibodies directly conjugated to fluorophores against the following targets of interest were used: F4/80, PD-L1, and Foxp3 (eBioscience, Germany); CD4, CD3e, CD44, CD8a, CD62L, CD45R, CD11b, CD11c, Gr-1, NK1.1, CD25, Ly6C, and PD-1 (BD Bioscience, Germany). Fc receptor binding inhibitor (anti-mouse CD16/CD32) was purchased from eBioscience (Germany). Anti-human antibodies included anti-PD-L1-PE and purified anti-PD-L1 blocking antibody (both from eBioscience, Germany). For western blot, anti-phospho-ERK42/44, anti-phospho-p38 and anti-phospho STAT3 along with their reference antibodies, anti-ERK42/44, anti-p38, and anti-STAT3 antibody (all from Cell Signaling Technology, USA), were used. Signal transduction inhibitors: UO126 (MEK1/2 inhibitor, Cell Signaling Technology, USA), SB203580 (p38 MAPK inhibitor, Cell Signaling Technology, USA), LY294002 (PI3K inhibitor), CAS457081-03-7 (Jak inhibitor 1, Calbiochem, Germany) and Cucurbitacin/JSI-124 (STAT3 inhibitor, Calbiochem, Germany). Cytokines used included IL-4, GM-CSF, TNF-α, IL-6, IL-1β, PGE2 (Promokine, Immunotools, Strathmann, Germany) and IFNα (R&D; IntronA, Interferon alfa-2b, Schering-Plough; Germany).

Mice

C57BL/6 mice were purchased from Charles River (Germany) and bred and maintained under specific pathogen-free conditions in the animal facility of the University of Heidelberg (IBF, Heidelberg). Animal experiments were carried out after approval by the Karlsruhe regional government council (Regierungspraesidium Karlsruhe, 35-9185.81/G-184/11). The following experimental groups have been used: (1) control group (vehicle injection) and (2) treatment group (injection of IFNα). Healthy mice were intraperitoneally injected three times within 1 week with 50 μl of IFNα (2×10^5 U/ml) or an equivalent volume of vehicle control with subsequent examination of the mouse splenocytes by flow cytometry.

Generation of Human DC

Buffy coats for research purposes were provided by blood donor service BSD Mannheim. Human peripheral blood myeloid DC (mDC) were isolated from freshly-prepared PBMCs from whole blood using MACS isolation kit (Miltenyi, Germany) as described elsewhere (19), according to the manufacturer's protocol. Human monocyte-derived DC (MoDC) were generated as described previously (19). Briefly, PBMCs were prepared from whole blood by Biocoll gradient centrifugation (Biochrom AG, Germany). Isolated plastic-adherent monocytes were cultured in *X-vivo* 15 medium (Bio-Whittaker, Belgium) supplemented with 1.5% human plasma in the presence of the cytokines GM-CSF and IL-4 for 5–6 days.

Cytokine Treatment

The following cytokine concentrations were used for the treatment of DC: standard cytokine cocktail for maturation (10 ng/ml TNF-α, 1,000 U/ml IL-6, 10 ng/ml IL-1β, 1 μg/ml PGE) and 500–6,000 U IFNα for generating the dose-dependent curve. For other experiments, DC were treated with 1,000 U/ml IFNα for 24 h and subjected to FACS analysis, western blot or DC-T-cell co-cultures.

DC-T-Cell Co-cultures

DC and T-cells were co-cultured as described previously (19). Generated or freshly isolated DC were pretreated with 1,000 U/ml IFNα for 24 h and then washed twice with medium. $CD4^+$ cells were isolated from freshly-prepared PBMCs using MACS beads (Miltenyi, Germany). $CD4^+$ cells and DC were cultured together in 96-well round-bottom plates for 5 days, after which the production of cytokines in supernatants was determined in triplicates using Luminex assay.

Immunocytochemistry

Immunocytochemistry was performed as described elsewhere (8). Briefly, cells were immobilized on microscope slides using a cytocentrifuge, fixed with 3.7% formaldehyde, pre-absorbed and incubated with anti-PD-L1 or control antibody. After incubation with secondary biotin-coupled antibodies followed by streptavidin-phosphatase complexes, PD-L1 was detected through the formation of a colored reaction product from the hydrolysis of substrate by alkaline phosphatase. Hematoxylin was used for counterstaining nuclei.

Western Blot Analysis

DC treated with 1,000 U/ml IFNα for the indicated periods of time were harvested, lysed in 2× sample buffer (100 mM Tris, pH 6.8, 4% SDS, 16% glycerol, 0.57 M β-mercaptoethanol, 0.01% bromophenol blue) and heated to 95°C for 5 min. SDS-PAGE was carried out after loading the proteins onto a 10% polyacrylamide gel. After transfer to PVDF membranes, the blots were sequentially blocked for 2 h using 5% milk in TBST solution (10 mM Tris, pH 8.0, 150 mM NaCl, 0.1% Tween-20), incubated overnight with primary antibodies in TBST containing 5% BSA, washed three times in TBST and incubated with HRP-conjugated secondary antibodies. Subsequently, the proteins of interest were detected by chemiluminescence produced by HRP-catalyzed oxidation of ECL substrate (Lumigen TMA6, UK).

Flow Cytometry Analysis

Cells were collected, washed and incubated for 15 min at 4°C in FACS buffer containing antibodies directly conjugated to fluorophores. The fluorescence was evaluated using a FACSCanto II flow cytometer (BD Biosciences, Germany) and data were analyzed with Diva and FlowJo Software (BD Biosciences, Germany). All isotype controls had fluorescence values that remained below a threshold of 1×10^3. For analysis of murine leukocytes, a freshly-isolated splenocyte cell suspension was prepared as described previously (33), resuspended in the stain buffer (PBS supplemented with 1% mouse serum and 1 mM EDTA), counted and adjusted to a concentration of 4×10^7 cells/mL. Cells were blocked with anti-mouse CD16/CD32 antibodies at 4°C in the dark for 10 min and then incubated with stain buffer containing various combinations of previously titrated monoclonal antibodies at 4°C in the dark for 15 min. After two washing steps with the stain buffer, the cells were used for flow cytometry analysis. For intracellular staining, Foxp3 buffer set was used according to the manufacturer's instruction. All the gates were set according to the corresponding fluorescence minus one (FMO) controls. For the gating strategy see **Figure S1** and the manuscript from Fritz et al. (33).

Luminex Assay

Analyses of human cytokines IL-6, IL-12(p40), IFNγ, IL-1b,−4,−5,−10,−12(p70), and−17 as well as TNF-α in culture supernatants were performed as described elsewhere (34) using a MILLIPLEX® MAP Kit (Millipore GmbH, Schwalbach/TS, Germany) according to the manufacturer's instructions. The measurements were performed in triplicates using a Luminex® 100/200 System.

Statistical Analysis

The data were analyzed with unpaired Student's *t*-test or one-way ANOVA using GraphPad PRISM 5.0. Values with $p < 0.05$ were considered significant. Quantitative data are expressed as mean ± SEM.

RESULTS

Expression of PD-L1 and PD-1 on Various Populations of Murine Immune Cells

Our first aim was to determine the distribution of PD-L1 and PD-1 expression on extracellular surfaces of different specific immune cell populations. For this purpose, splenocytes from BL6 mice were subjected to a deep FACS analyses (**Figure S1**) to obtain the results summarized in **Table 1**. Expression of PD-L1 was found on all immune cells tested with higher percentages of PD-L1$^+$ cells (more than 80%) in conventional myeloid DC (cDC, $CD11c^{high}CD11b^+$), macrophage ($CD11b^+Gr\text{-}1^-F4/80^+$), naïve CD8 cell ($CD62L^+CD44^-$), effector memory (em) CD4 cell ($CD62L^-CD44^+$) and regulatory T cell (Treg,

TABLE 1 | Distribution of PD-1 and PD-L1 expression on immune cell subpopulations.

	PD-1		PD-L1	
	Cell frequency, %	**MFI**	**Cell frequency, %**	**MFI**
$CD3^{-}NK1.1^{+}CD4^{-}$	4.02 (±1.35)	992.6 (±407.4)	n.d. (not detected)	n.d.
$CD3^{+}NK1.1^{+}CD4^{+}$	22.55 (±12.98)	2,308 (±298.2)	n.d.	n.d.
$CD11c^{high}CD11b^{+}$	n.d.	n.d.	91.73 (±4.44)	22,500 (±25.5)
$CD11c^{int}CD45R^{+}$	n.d.	n.d.	58.3 (±14.79)	5,913 (±233.3)
$CD11b^{+}Gr\text{-}1^{-}F4/80^{+}$	n.d.	n.d.	82.3 (±0.63)	9,223 (±70)
$CD11b^{+}Gr\text{-}1^{+}$	n.d.	n.d.	21.58 (±11.69)	7,669 (±2,250)
$CD11b^{+}Gr\text{-}1^{high}Ly\text{-}6C^{int}$	n.d.	n.d.	15.27 (±6.99)	4,040 (±2,329)
$CD11b^{+}Gr\text{-}1^{int}Ly\text{-}6C^{high}$	n.d.	n.d.	44 (±10.52)	6,772 (±1,539)
$CD8^{+}CD3^{+}$	11.16 (±6.72)	1,103 (±437.7)	81 (±26.73)	683 (±49.5)
$CD62L^{-}CD44^{+}CD8^{+}$	n.d.	n.d.	1.34 (±0.26)	993 (±162.6)
$CD62L^{+}CD44^{+}CD8^{+}$	n.d.	n.d.	64.65 (±0.26)	876 (±86.3)
$CD62L^{+}CD44^{-}CD8^{+}$	n.d.	n.d.	83.35 (±0.26)	554 (±22.6)
$CD62L^{-}CD44^{-}CD8^{+}$	n.d.	n.d.	1.47 (±0.26)	671 (±166.9)
$CD4^{+}CD3^{+}$	14. 54 (±4.88)	1,468 (±429.3)	57.87 (±27.65)	1,568 (±1,686)
$CD62L^{-}CD44^{+}CD4^{+}$	n.d.	n.d.	85.8 (±6.79)	1,490 (±16.3)
$CD62L^{+}CD44^{+}CD4^{+}$	n.d.	n.d.	44.05 (±7.99)	1,688 (±359.9)
$CD62L^{+}CD44^{-}CD4^{+}$	n.d.	n.d.	48.75 (±40.94)	801 (±14.1)
$CD62L^{-}CD44^{-}CD4^{+}$	n.d.	n.d.	41.9 (±40.94)	1,494 (±304.1)
$CD25^{dim}FoxP3^{+}CD4^{+}$	39.18 (±9.83)	2,226 (±343.5)	54.3 (±40.94)	3,156 (±2,771)
$CD25^{+}FoxP3^{+}CD4^{+}$	24.15 (±6.65)	2,213 (±355.8)	84.45 (±9.12)	3,223 (±2,785)
$CD25^{+}FoxP3^{-}CD4^{+}$	18.68 (±7.59)	1,654 (±266.4)	4.2 (±5.06)	2,632 (±2,722)
$CD25^{-}FoxP3^{-}CD4^{+}$	77.07 (±2.74)	1,400 (±187.3)	70.25 (±0.64)	2,583 (±2,786)

$CD4^{+}CD25^{+}FoxP3^{+}$) populations. The lowest percentages of PD-L1^{+} cells (lower than 5% positive cells) were found in em cells ($CD62L^{-}CD44^{+}$) and naïve $CD8^{+}$ cells as well as in activated conventional (con) T cells (Tcon, $CD4^{+}CD25^{+}FoxP3^{-}$). Expression of PD-1 was also found on all lymphoid cell populations analyzed (**Table 1**). Thus, PD-L1 and its receptor are commonly present on various murine immune cells.

IFNα Up-Regulates *ex vivo* and *in vivo* Expression of PD-L1 on Mouse Leukocytes

In the next step, isolated splenocytes were treated for 24 h with 1,000 U/ml IFNα and PD-L1 expression on splenocytes was detected with flow cytometry. IFNα treatment led to increased percentages of cells expressing PD-L1 in plasmacytoid DC (pDC), macrophage and $CD11b^{+}Gr^{-}1^{+}$ cell populations, but not in cDC in the myeloid leukocyte population (**Figure 1**). The reason is that cDC are already PD-L1 positive to a high percentage (**Table 1**). However, the level of PD-L1 expression (measured in MFI, mean fluorescent intensity) was positively affected in both DC subpopulations of $CD11b^{+}$ cell (**Figure 1**).

In the lymphocyte population, IFNα treatment increased a number of PD-L1^{+} cells and up-regulated the expression of PD-L1 in both $CD4^{+}$ and $CD8^{+}$ cells (**Figure 2**). In specific subpopulations of $CD4^{+}$ cells, the percentage of cells expressing PD-L1^{+} was increased in eff, em and cm ($CD62L^{+}CD44^{+}$) cells and the level of PD-L1 expression was higher after IFNα treatment in all subpopulations (**Figure 2**). Interferon-α was observed to exert a similar effect in Treg (**Figure 2**). For the gated $CD8^{+}$ cells, an increased number of PD-L1^{+} cells was found in eff, em and cm populations (**Figure 2**). The level of PD-L1 expression measured in MFI was higher after treatment with IFNα in all subpopulations except eff $CD8^{+}$ cells (**Figure 2**). Thus, IFNα is capable of up-regulating PD-L1 expression in different murine immune cells.

Since the highest initial percentage of PD-L1^{+} cells and up-regulation of PD-L1 after IFNα treatment was observed in DC in *ex vivo* splenocytes cultures, the *in vivo* regulation of PD-L1 expression by IFNα was examined and we verified a similar up-regulation in mouse DC (**Figure 3**) as well as in other myeloid cells (data not shown).

IFNα Up-Regulates the Expression of PD-L1, Increases the Production of IL-6 and Decreases the Production of IL-12 by Human DC

To increase the clinical relevance of our study, we extended our research to investigate PD-L1 regulation in human DC facilitated through the use of IFN-based therapeutic IFNα-2b (Intron A). Myeloid DC were isolated from buffy coats of healthy human subjects and cultivated with different concentrations of IFNα as indicated in **Figure 4**. The treatment induced dose-dependent up-regulation of PD-L1 expression in the cells (**Figure 4A**). Similarly, PD-L1 expression was up-regulated in MoDC obtained from buffy coats of human healthy donors

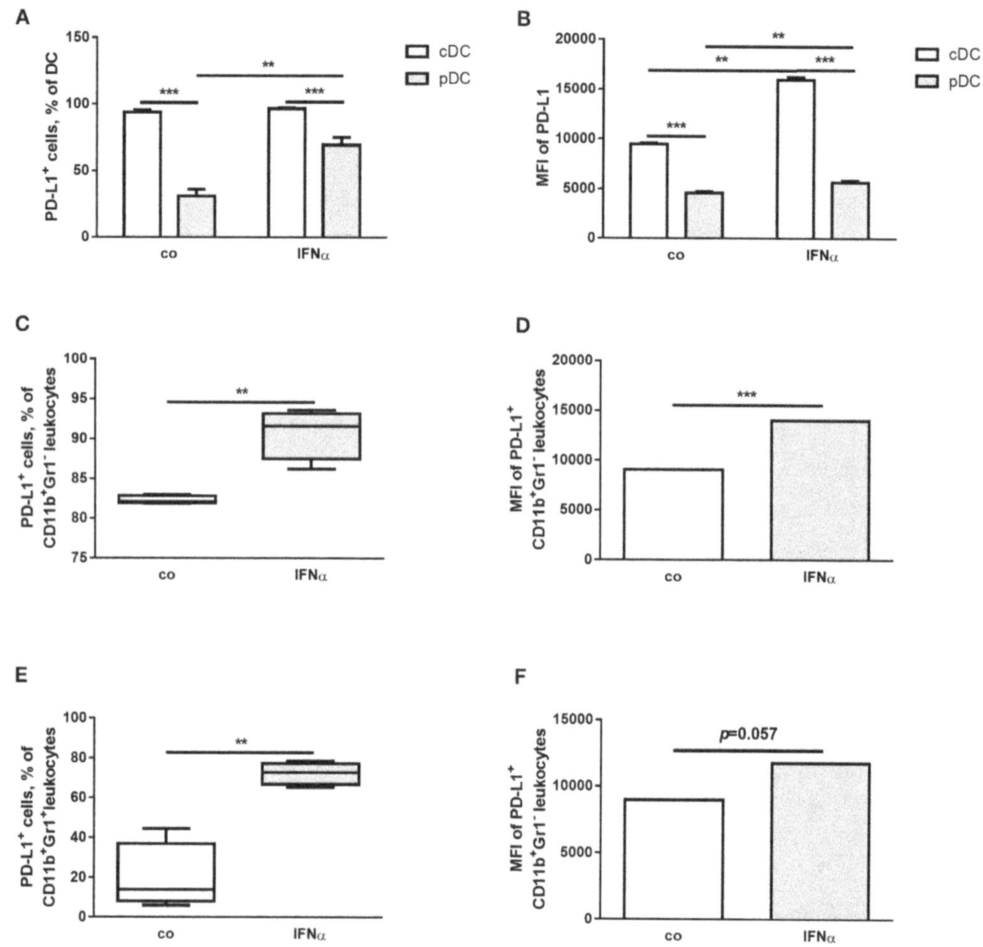

FIGURE 1 | IFNα up-regulates PD-L1 expression on different myeloid immune cell populations *ex vivo*. FACS analysis of PD-L1 expression on the surface of different myeloid immune cells from splenocytes of healthy mice. Splenocytes were isolated, treated for 24 h with 1,000 U/ml IFNα and investigated by flow cytometry. The results are presented as interleaved bars **(A,B)**, as box and whiskers plots **(C,E)** or column bar graphs **(D,F)** and statistically analyzed using two-way ANOVA **(A,B)** or unpaired *T*-tests **(C–F)**, $n = 4$, $^{**}p < 0.01$, and $^{***}p < 0.001$.

(**Figure 4B**). Remarkably, an increased PD-L1 expression was still induced when mDC and MoDC were pulsed with IFNα after incubation with a classical maturation cytokine cocktail (**Figure S2**). Therefore, IFNα can specifically induce PD-L1 overexpression in human DC.

Produced cytokines are important indicators of DC functionality. After the treatment of DC with IFNα, 10 human cytokines were measured in cell culture supernatants using the Luminex platform. We found an increased concentration of IL-6 and a decreased concentration of IL-12(p40) and IL-12(p70) in the supernatants (**Figure 4C**) after IFNα treatment. However, the production of IFNγ, IL-1β,−4,−5,−10, and−17 as well as TNF-α was not affected (data not shown).

Blocking PD-L1 Leads to Recovery of IFNγ Production by CD4+ Lymphocytes Cultivated With IFNα-Treated mDC

The expression of PD-L1 on DC negatively modulates their ability to activate CD4+ lymphocytes and subsequent IFNγ production (19). Based on our findings above indicating that IFNα treatment affects IFNγ production by co-cultured CD4+ lymphocytes but not DC, we aimed to investigate whether the blocking of PD-L1 protein with antibodies [anti (α)-PD-L1] could influence IFNγ production in our co-culture experiments. In order to achieve the above aim, we co-cultivated CD4+ cells with mDC pretreated with IFNα, anti-PD-L1 or both IFNα and anti-PD-L1. As expected, the co-cultivation of CD4+ cells with untreated mDC led to an increase in the amount of IFNγ in the supernatants and addition of anti-PD-L1 antibody further improved the cytokine release (**Figure 5**). Treatment of CD4+ cells with anti-PD-L1 but without mDC did not induce IFNγ production. Pre-incubation of mDC with IFNα resulted in a decrease in the amount of IFNγ in the supernatants of co-cultivated CD4+ cells (**Figure 5**), which could be explained by the up-regulation of PD-L1 expression on mDC. Indeed, blocking of IFNα-induced PD-L1 on DC led to higher IFNγ production from co-cultivated CD4+ cells compared to the co-cultures containing IFNα-DC without an

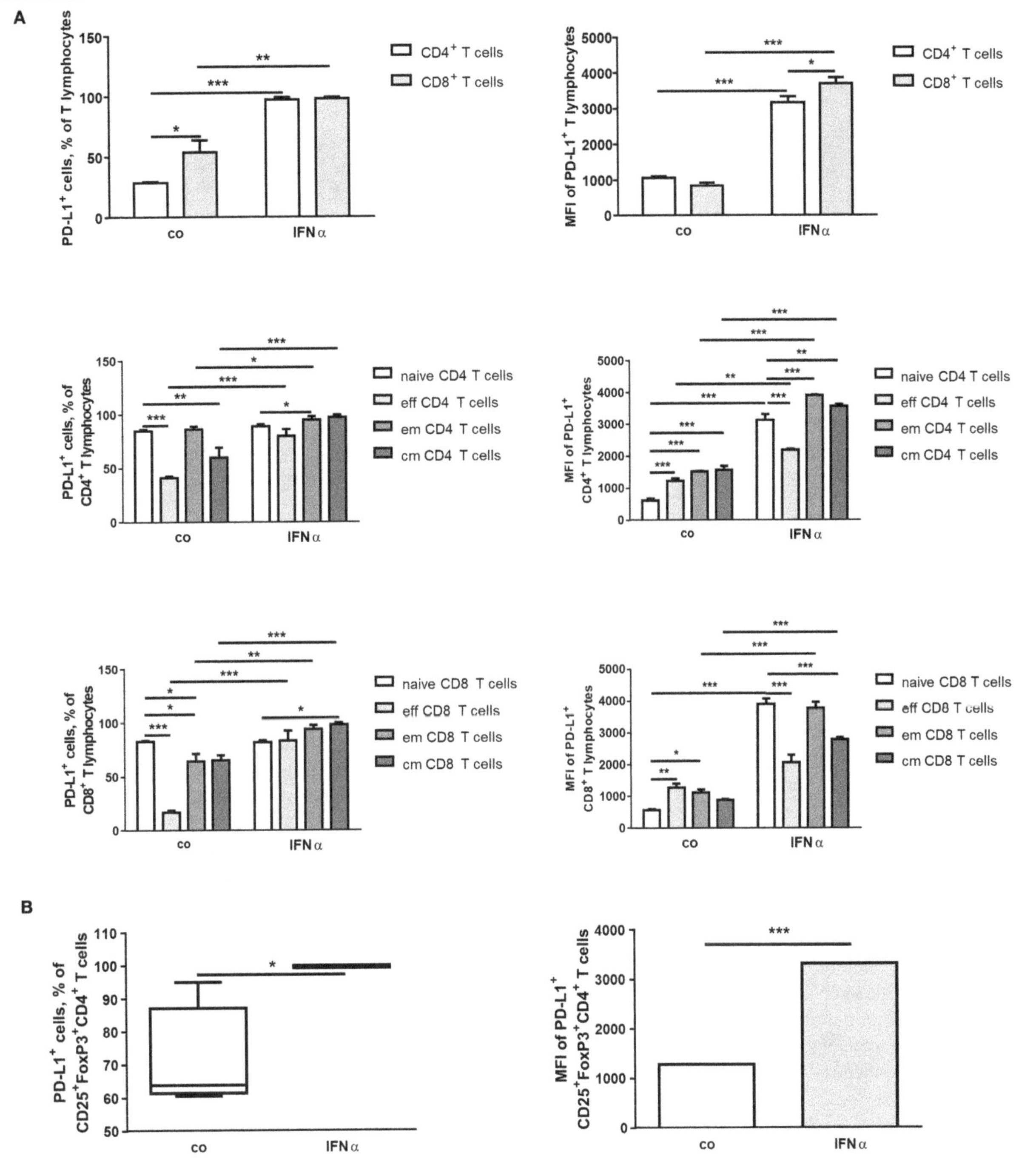

FIGURE 2 | IFNα up-regulates PD-L1 expression on different T-cell populations *ex vivo*. FACS analysis of PD-L1 expression on the surface of different lymphoid immune cells from spleens of healthy mice. Splenocytes were isolated, treated for 24 h with 1,000 U/ml IFNα and investigated by flow cytometry. The results are presented as interleaved bars **(A)** or as box and whiskers plot or column bar graph **(B)** and statistically analyzed using two-way ANOVA or unpaired *T*-tests, $n = 4$, $^{*}p < 0.05$, $^{**}p < 0.01$, and $^{***}p < 0.001$.

αPD-L1 antibody blockade. The restoration of IFNγ production, resulted in the same amount of the cytokine released into the supernatant as in the samples that were co-cultivated with mDC without any pre-treatment (**Figure 5**). Thus, blocking PD-L1 leads to the recovery of IFNγ production by $CD4^{+}$ lymphocytes activated with IFNα-treated mDC. The same results were observed when MoDC were used instead of mDC (data not shown).

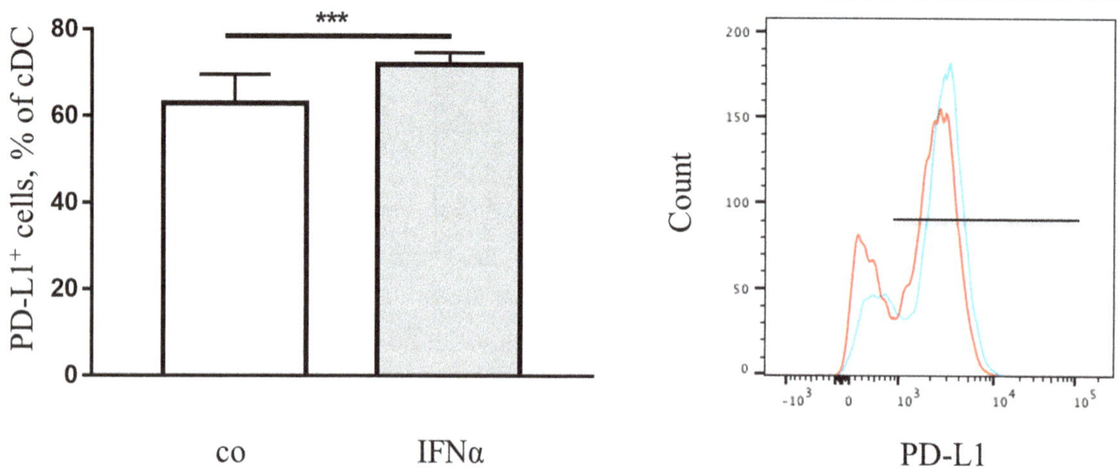

FIGURE 3 | IFNα up-regulates PD-L1 expression on DC *in vivo*. FACS analysis of PD-L1 expression on the surface of DC from spleens of healthy mice with or without treatment with IFNα. Splenocytes were isolated and examined using flow cytometry. The results are presented as percent of positive cells in a column bar graph and statistically analyzed using unpaired *T*-test, $n = 10$, $^{***}p < 0.001$. A representative FACS histogram (red-control, blue-IFNα) is shown.

Inhibitors of STAT3, p38 and Jak Down-Regulate the Expression of PD-L1 Induced by IFNα, Whilst PI3K or ERK Inhibitors Do Not Exert This Effect

Finally, we wanted to identify the molecular mechanisms by which IFNα up-regulates PD-L1 expression. We treated human mDC obtained from buffy coats with inhibitors of different signaling proteins as indicated in **Figure 6**. We found that IFNα-induced PD-L1 expression was down-regulated by inhibitors of p38, Jak and STAT3 but not by inhibitors of PI3K or ERK (**Figure 6A**). However, combinations of two different inhibitors did not show additive inhibitory effects (**Figure 6B**). In line with these observations, IFNα could increase the phosphorylation of p38 and STAT3 as shown by western blot (**Figure 6C**). In addition, we did not observe any effect on PD-L1 expression when NF-kB or STAT1/STAT5 were blocked with specific inhibitors (data not shown). Therefore, we concluded that signaling cascades including Jak/STAT3 and p38 could be involved in the regulation of PD-L1 expression.

DISCUSSION

In this study, we showed for the first time that PD-L1 molecule was expressed and could be up-regulated in the majority of specific immune cell populations by IFNα.

Programmed death-ligand 1, expressed on different immune cells, such as MDSC (35, 36), T cells (37), DC (19, 38), macrophages (39), pDC (40), is able to cause immunosuppression. Taking into account the ubiquitous expression of PD-L1 receptor (PD-1) on non-myeloid specific immune cells (CD8, CD4 and Treg), our results indicate that immunotherapy with IFNα could lead to an undesirable side effect of general immunosuppression and consequently to increased tumor immune evasion or chronification of infection. Our data could also explain the insufficiency of IFNα therapy observed in several models, despite its promising *in vitro* and immunomonitoring results (41–44). We propose that the combination of IFNα with checkpoint inhibitors like PD-L1 blocking antibody, could repress this immunosuppressive path and improve the efficiency of IFNα therapy by uncoiling the immune costimulatory potential of IFNα. While the majority of the DC are already positive for PD-L1, the intensity of this expression could be strongly up-regulated in our study by IFNα *in vivo*, *ex vivo*, and *in vitro*. DC play a crucial role in the control of adaptive tolerance and immunity and modulate immune responses by multiple mechanisms, including the production of cytokines and expression of T-cell regulatory molecules. Their final stimulatory capacity depends on the balance between stimulatory and suppressive pathways, whereby PD-L1 provides one of the most decisive suppressive signals and leads to unfavorable outcomes due to decreased anti-tumor immunity. This becomes particularly evident by documentation of reduced DC functions in several types of cancer and chronic infections (45–53). In cases utilizing vaccination as immunotherapeutic approaches against tumor and viral antigens, it is important that the produced DC display their full activation capacity (54, 55). Therefore, many therapies aim to activate DC to increase their stimulatory potential. IFNα was suggested as one of potential candidates for non-specific immune stimulation or as a replacement of IL-4 in the process of Mo-DC production (56–59). In accordance with our data, the MoDC produced from the monocytes treated with GM-CSF and IFNα (IFNα/GM-CSF MoDC) had a higher expression of PD-L1 molecules compared to those treated with IL-4/GM-CSF (60). In this case, the therapeutic efficacy of DC produced or activated with IFNα

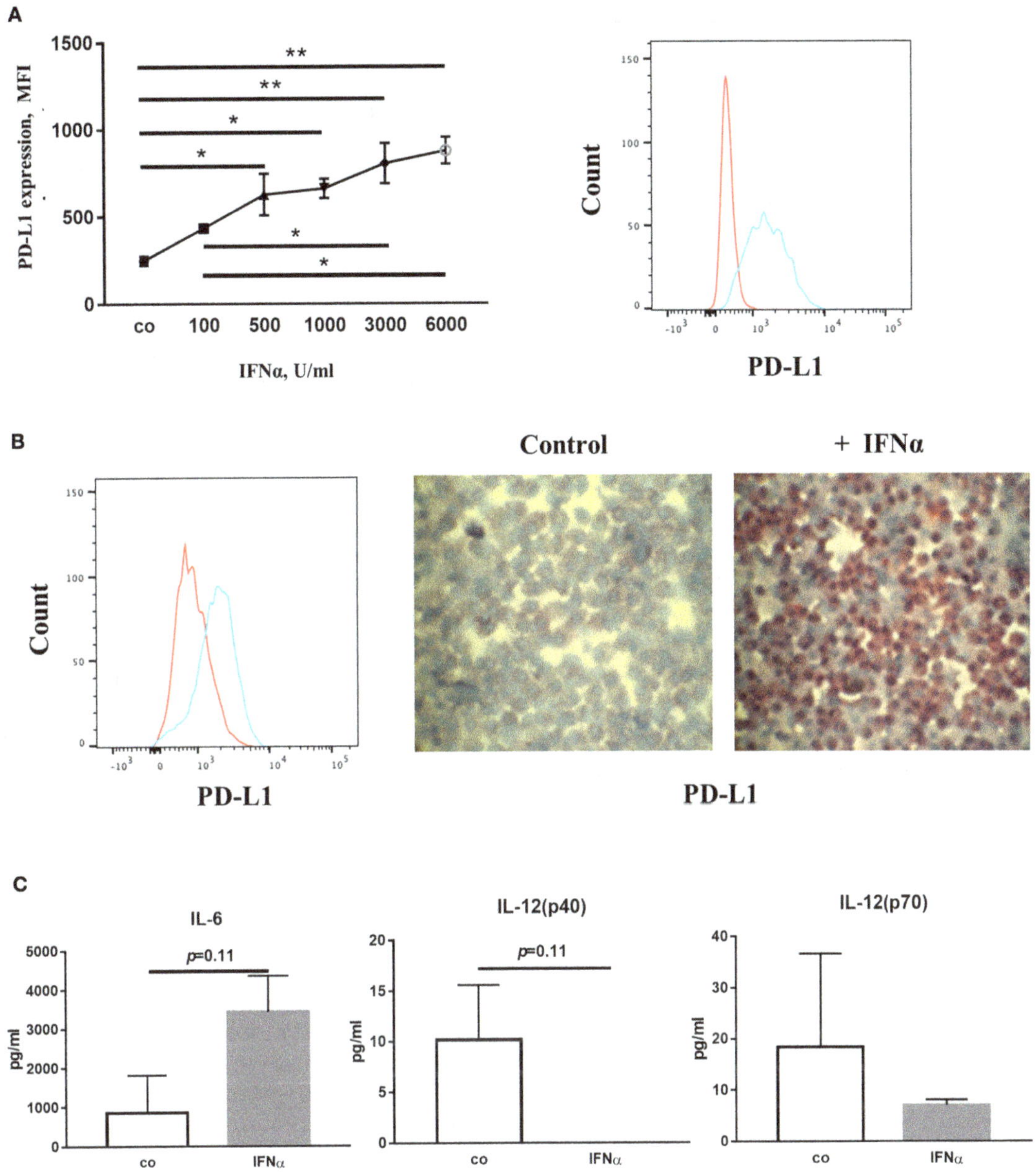

FIGURE 4 | IFNα up-regulates PD-L1 expression on human dendritic cells. **(A)** FACS analysis of PD-L1 expression on the surface of mDC. Myeloid DC were isolated, treated for 24 h with IFNα and analyzed with flow cytometry. The results are presented as column mean, error bars and mean connected and statistically analyzed using ordinary one-way ANOVA with the Tukey's multiple comparisons post-test, $n = 2$, $^{*}p < 0.05$ and $^{**}p < 0.01$. **(B)** FACS analysis and Immunocytochemistry (ICH) of PD-L1 expression on the surface of MoDC. MoDC were treated for 24 h with 1,000 U/ml IFNα and analyzed with flow cytometry. Alternatively, cytospin slides were produced and ICH was performed using an anti-PD-L1 primary antibody followed by a biotinylated secondary antibody. FACS histograms (red-control, blue-IFNα) and ICH pictures are representative for independent experiments. **(C)** Cytokines in the supernatant of the IFNα-treated DC analyzed with Luminex assays. The results are presented as column bar graphs and statistically analyzed using unpaired *T*-test, $n = 2$.

could be improved by the simultaneous reduction of PD-L1 expression.

The IFNα-treated DC demonstrated increased IL-6 and decreased IL-12 production. This is in line with the observation that TLR-antigen presenting cells, which express a high amount of PD-L1 and fail to induce T-cell proliferation, also exhibited increased IL-6 production (61). IFNα can inhibit IL-12 production in mouse splenocytes (62) and IL-12p40 production in human MoDC (57, 63). However, IL-6 has been shown to down-regulate IL-12 production by human MoDC (64). In our model, the cause of decreased IL-12 production, whether directly through IFNα treatment or partially caused as an

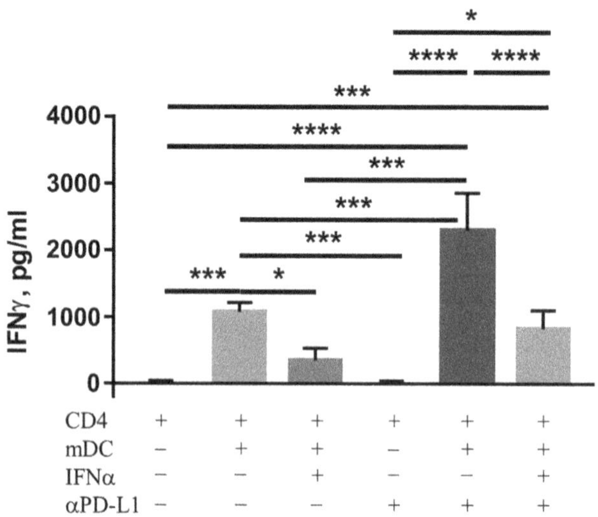

FIGURE 5 | PD-L1 controls IFNγ release from CD4 T cells stimulated by DC. Allogeneic CD4 cells were isolated and cocultured with DC in the presence or the absence of anti-PD-L1 blocking antibody or vehicle control. The level of IFNγ in supernatants was determined by Luminex assay. The results are presented as column bar graphs and statistically analyzed using ordinary one-way ANOVA with the Tukey's multiple comparisons post-test, $n = 3–6$, $^{*}p < 0.05$, $^{***}p < 0.001$, and $^{****}p < 0.0001$.

effect of IL-6, remains to be clarified. Moreover, we reported previously that IL-6 is able to induce PD-L1 in DC *per se* (18), thus PD-L1 expression could be boosted additionally by this loop.

In accordance with the findings of other researchers, we have shown previously that specific up-regulation of PD-L1 regulatory molecules on DC surfaces affect the capacity of DC to induce T-cell cytokine production (19, 30). In line with these previous results, we found that IFNα-treated DC strongly down-regulated IFNγ production by T cells. However, IL-12, produced by antigen-presenting cells including DC, can also control the production of IFNγ by T cells (65) and this is as well-evident when IFNγ release by co-cultured CD4 T cells decreased in response to diminished IL-12p70 production by IL-6 treated DC (64). In our study, the decrease in IL-12 production might not have an important role in stimulating IFNγ release in the co-cultures, since blocking PD-L1 on IFNα-treated DC could almost completely restore IFNγ release. Thus, in our experimental settings, the inhibitory ability of IFNα is directly linked to increased PD-L1 expression on DC. Given that IFNγ induces the expression of PD-L1 in DC (28, 29), repression of IFNγ production by T cells by IFNα could negatively regulate de novo expression of PD-L1 on the surface of DC during immune response *in vivo*.

The decisive role held by PD-L1 molecule in controlling immune response and anti-tumor immunity urges the investigation of signaling events controlling its up-regulation. Elucidation of the PD-L1 regulation on DC is an emerging field, as these cells govern the decision between tolerance and immunity. By canonical way, ligand engagement of the IFNα receptor (IFNAR, composed of the IFNAR1 and IFNAR2 subunits) activates Jak1 and tyrosine kinase 2 (TYK2) and can result in the recruitment of STATs as well as MAPKs, PI3K, Akt, NF-kB and PRMT1 (66). There are three predominant STAT complexes that might be formed in response to IFNs: (i) The interferon-stimulated gene factor 3 (ISGF3) complex [STAT1/STAT2 and IFN-regulatory factor 9 (IRF9)], which binds to IFN-stimulated response element (ISRE) sequences and activate antiviral genes, (ii) STAT1 homodimers, which bind to gamma-activated sequences (GASs) and initiate pro-inflammatory genes, and (iii) STAT3 homodimers which indirectly suppress pro-inflammatory gene expression. Our experiments revealed that IFNα regulates PD-L1 expression in a Jak-, STAT3-, and p38-dependent manner. Whether other downstream effectors of IFN1 signaling might be involved in the modulation of PD-L1 expression needs further investigations. Similarly, in mouse IL-27-treated pDC, STAT3-dependent enhancement of PD-L1 was described (40). The TLR-agonist-induced PD-L1 expression was modulated in a MAPK/STAT3-dependent way, whereby STAT3 was rapidly recruited to the PD-L1 promoter and in agreement with our findings, blocking of STAT3 activation prevented PD-L1 expression (61). We showed previously that IL-27-induced specific up-regulation of the PD-L1 regulatory molecule on DC was accompanied by the phosphorylation of another STAT family member, STAT1 protein (19), but we did not observe STAT1 involvement in the IFNα-induced PD-L1 expression.

Furthermore, in several tumor cell types, the role of Jaks/STATs in PD-L1 regulation was highlighted recently. Attenuation of IFNγ-induced PD-L1 expression in melanoma cells was proven to happen via down-regulation of the Jak/STAT/IRF-1 signaling pathway (67, 68), while activation of Jaks led to PD-L1 up-regulation in hematopoietic tumor cell lines and primary tumor cells (69). In contrast to our previous observations, neither PI3K nor ERK activation was essential for IFNα-induced PD-L1 expression (18). Thus, our findings underline the important roles of STATs in the regulation of PD-L1 expression and are in agreement with Barton et al. who states that the stimulatory ability of APCs depends on the degree of STAT3 activation (70). We can also speculate that therapies that target p38 and STAT3 pathways could potentially produce a desirable secondary effect on PD-L1 expression.

Another type I IFN, IFNβ, is also used as an immunomodulatory cytokine in the treatment of multiple sclerosis (71) and in anti-cancer therapies, for example against nasopharyngeal carcinoma (72). Since other type I IFNs bind the same IFNR1/2 receptor complexes and have a similar mode of action (73), one could assume that the effects found in our IFNα study might be valid for them as well and so more attention needs to be paid to these IFNs in future studies. Giving further evidence to support this hypothesis, IFNβ-dependent facilitated increase in PD-L1 expression in DC was documented in multiple sclerosis and in immune paralysis (30, 31).

Our findings underline the important roles of p38 and STAT3 in the regulation of PD-L1 expression and showed that IFNα-2b, which is clinically used for a wide range of indications including cancers, induced STAT3/p38-mediated expression of

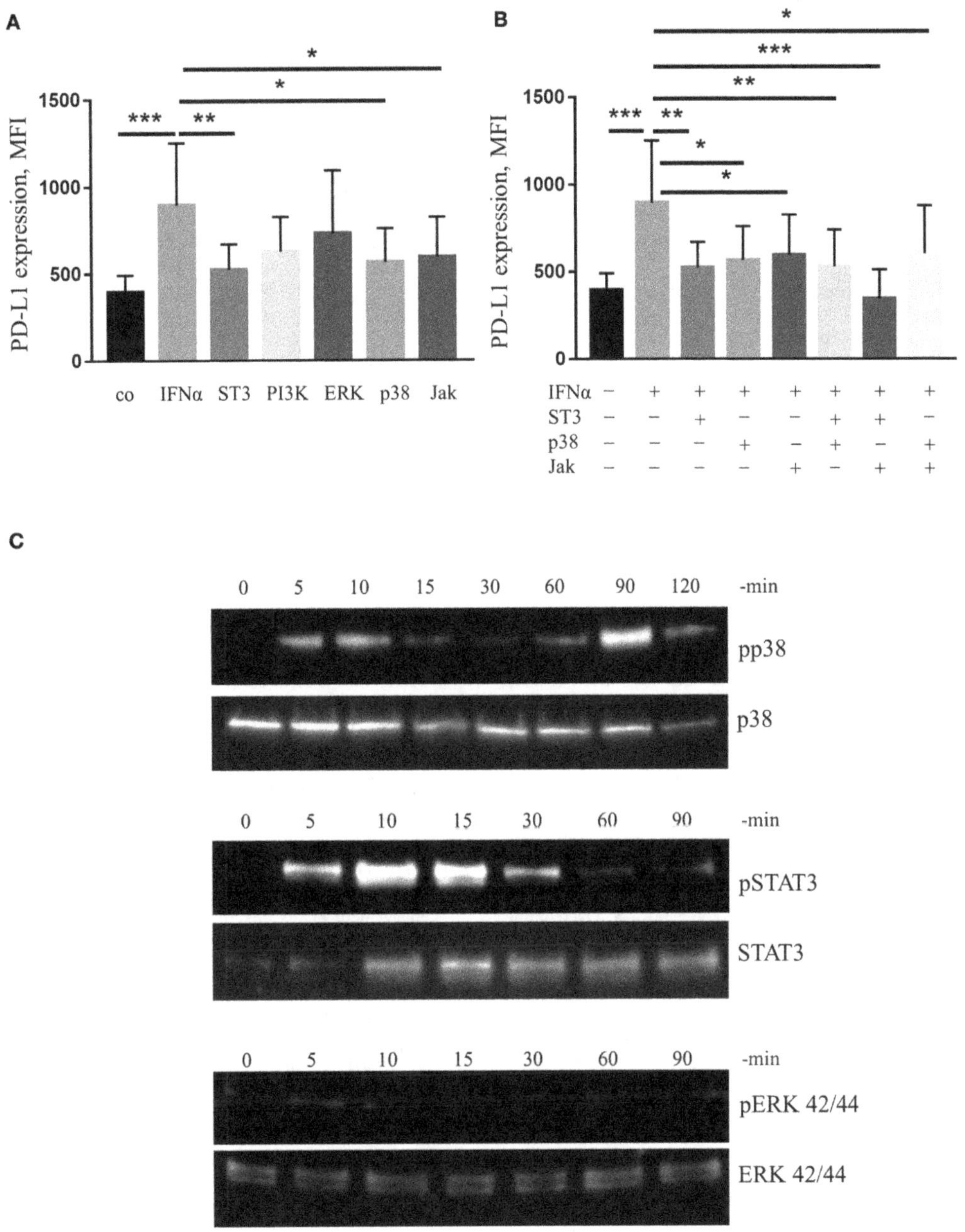

FIGURE 6 | IFNα up-regulates PD-L1 expression in mDC in p38/STAT3-dependent manner. **(A,B)** FACS analysis of PD-L1 expression on mDC activated for 24 h with 1,000 U/ml IFNα with or without 1 h pre-incubation with signal transduction inhibitors of p38, STAT3 (ST3), PI3K, ERK, p38, and Jak. The results are presented as column bar graphs and statistically analyzed using ordinary one-way ANOVA with the Dunnett's multiple comparisons post-test, $n = 8$–10, $^{*}p < 0.05$, $^{**}p < 0.01$, and $^{***}p < 0.001$. **(C)** Western blot analysis of p38, STAT3, and ERK phosphorylation (pp38, pERK, and pSTAT3 for phosphorylated form) in mDC before and after activation for indicated period of time with IFNα.

PD-L1, favoring a reduction in the stimulatory ability of DC. Particular consideration should be given to the enhanced PD-L1 expression in multiple immune cell types caused by the use of IFNα in anti-cancer therapy in the future.

The obtained results reveal a new avenue for the development of novel and optimization of existing therapeutic strategies with IFNα, in order to precisely modulate PD-L1 expression in DC and other target cells.

AUTHOR CONTRIBUTIONS

SK and AB participated in the research design; All authors participated in carrying out the research and analyzing the data; AB and SK participated in writing the manuscript and critical correction of the manuscript. AB, JW, and SK administered this work. All authors discussed the results and implications and gave constructive feedback on the manuscript at all stages.

ACKNOWLEDGMENTS

The authors thank Mr. Markus Herbst, Ms. Inna Schwarting and Ms. Tina Maxelon for their excellent technical assistance and Dr. Serene Lee for proofreading the manuscript.

REFERENCES

1. Belardelli F, Ferrantini M, Proietti E, Kirkwood JM. Interferon-alpha in tumor immunity and immunotherapy. *Cytokine Growth Factor Rev.* (2002) 13:119–34. doi: 10.1016/S1359-6101(01)00022-3
2. Kirkwood J. Cancer immunotherapy: the interferon-alpha experience. *Semin Oncol.* (2002) 29:18–26. doi: 10.1053/sonc.2002.33078
3. Gutterman JU. Cytokine therapeutics: lessons from interferon alpha. *Proc Natl Acad Sci USA.* (1994) 91:1198–205. doi: 10.1073/pnas.91.4.1198
4. Iacopino F, Ferrandina G, Scambia G, Benedetti-Panici P, Mancuso S, Sica G. Interferons inhibit EGF-stimulated cell growth and reduce EGF binding in human breast cancer cells. *Anticancer Res.* (1996) 16:1919–24.
5. Hoffmann K, Mehrle S, Schmidt J, Buchler MW, Marten A. Interferon-alpha restitutes the chemosensitivity in pancreatic cancer. *Anticancer Res.* (2008) 28:1499–507.
6. Zhu Y, Tibensky I, Schmidt J, Hackert T, Ryschich E, Jager D, et al. Interferon-alpha in combination with chemotherapy has potent antiangiogenic properties in an orthotopic mouse model for pancreatic adenocarcinoma. *J Immunother.* (2008) 31:28–33. doi: 10.1097/CJI.0b013e318157c682
7. Essers MA, Offner S, Blanco-Bose WE, Waibler Z, Kalinke U, Duchosal MA, et al. IFNalpha activates dormant haematopoietic stem cells *in vivo*. *Nature* (2009) 458:904–8. doi: 10.1038/nature07815
8. Zhu Y, Karakhanova S, Huang X, Deng SP, Werner J, Bazhin AV. Influence of interferon-alpha on the expression of the cancer stem cell markers in pancreatic carcinoma cells. *Exp Cell Res.* (2014) 324:146–56. doi: 10.1016/j.yexcr.2014.03.020
9. Pfeffer LM, Dinarello CA, Herberman RB, Williams BR, Borden EC, Bordens R, et al. Biological properties of recombinant alpha-interferons: 40th anniversary of the discovery of interferons. *Cancer Res.* (1998) 58:2489–99.
10. Bazhin AV, Bayry J, Umansky V, Werner J, Karakhanova S. Overcoming immunosuppression as a new immunotherapeutic approach against pancreatic cancer. *Oncoimmunology* (2013) 2:e25736. doi: 10.4161/onci.25736
11. Bazhin AV, Shevchenko I, Umansky V, Werner J, Karakhanova S. Two immune faces of pancreatic adenocarcinoma: possible implication for immunotherapy. *Cancer Immunol Immunother.* (2014) 63:59–65. doi: 10.1007/s00262-013-1485-8
12. Lake RA, Robinson BW. Immunotherapy and chemotherapy–a practical partnership. *Nat Rev Cancer* (2005) 5:397–405. doi: 10.1038/nrc1613
13. Nagata S, Taira H, Hall A, Johnsrud L, Streuli M, Ecsödi J, et al. Synthesis in *E. coli* of a polypeptide with human leukocyte interferon activity. *Nature* (1980) 284:316. doi: 10.1038/284316a0
14. Greenwald RJ, Freeman GJ, Sharpe AH. The B7 family revisited. *Annu Rev Immunol.* (2005) 23:515–48. doi: 10.1146/annurev.immunol.23.021704.115611
15. Lee SK, Seo SH, Kim BS, Kim CD, Lee JH, Kang JS, et al. IFN-gamma regulates the expression of B7-H1 in dermal fibroblast cells. *J Dermatol Sci.* (2005) 40:95–103. doi: 10.1016/j.jdermsci.2005.06.008
16. Liu J, Hamrouni A, Wolowiec D, Coiteux V, Kuliczkowski K, Hetuin D, et al. Plasma cells from multiple myeloma patients express B7-H1 (PD-L1) and increase expression after stimulation with IFN-{gamma} and TLR ligands via a MyD88-, TRAF6-, and MEK-dependent pathway. *Blood* (2007) 110:296–304. doi: 10.1182/blood-2006-10-051482
17. Qian Y, Deng J, Geng L, Xie H, Jiang G, Zhou L, et al. TLR4 signaling induces B7-H1 expression through MAPK pathways in bladder cancer cells. *Cancer Invest.* (2008) 1:816–21. doi: 10.1080/07357900801941852
18. Karakhanova S, Meisel S, Ring S, Mahnke K, Enk AH. ERK/p38 MAP-kinases and PI3K are involved in the differential regulation of B7-H1 expression in DC subsets. *Eur J Immunol.* (2010) 40:254–66. doi: 10.1002/eji.200939289
19. Karakhanova S, Bedke T, Enk AH, Mahnke K. IL-27 renders DC immunosuppressive by induction of B7-H1. *J Leukoc Biol.* (2011) 89:837–45. doi: 10.1189/jlb.1209788
20. Francisco LM, Sage PT, Sharpe AH. The PD-1 pathway in tolerance and autoimmunity. *Immunol Rev.* (2010) 236:219–42. doi: 10.1111/j.1600-065X.2010.00923.x
21. Greaves P, Gribben JG. The role of B7 family molecules in hematologic malignancy. *Blood* (2013) 121:734–44. doi: 10.1182/blood-2012-10-385591
22. Dong H, Chen X. Immunoregulatory role of B7-H1 in chronicity of inflammatory responses. *Cell Mol Immunol.* (2006) 3:179–187.
23. Thompson RH, Kuntz SM, Leibovich BC, Dong H, Lohse CM, Webster WS, et al. Tumor B7-H1 is associated with poor prognosis in renal cell carcinoma patients with long-term follow-up. *Cancer Res.* (2006) 66:3381–5. doi: 10.1158/0008-5472.CAN-05-4303
24. Hamanishi J, Mandai M, Iwasaki M, Okazaki T, Tanaka Y, Yamaguchi K, et al. Programmed cell death 1 ligand 1 and tumor-infiltrating CD8+ T lymphocytes are prognostic factors of human ovarian cancer. *Proc Natl Acad Sci USA.* (2007) 104:3360–5. doi: 10.1073/pnas.0611533104
25. Loos M, Giese NA, Kleeff J, Giese T, Gaida MM, Bergmann F, et al. Clinical significance and regulation of the costimulatory molecule B7-H1 in pancreatic cancer. *Cancer Lett.* (2008) 268:98–109. doi: 10.1016/j.canlet.2008.03.056
26. Hino R, Kabashima K, Kato Y, Yagi H, Nakamura M, Honjo T, et al. Tumor cell expression of programmed cell death-1 ligand 1 is a prognostic factor for malignant melanoma. *Cancer* (2010) 116:1757–66. doi: 10.1002/cncr.24899
27. Gu X, Wang Y, Xiang J, Chen Z, Wang L, Lu L, et al. Interferon-γ triggers hepatic stellate cell-mediated immune regulation through MEK/ERK signaling pathway. *Clin Dev Immunol.* (2013) 2013:6. doi: 10.1155/2013/389807
28. Freeman GJ, Long AJ, Iwai Y, Bourque K, Chernova T, Nishimura H, et al. Engagement of the Pd-1 immunoinhibitory receptor by a novel B7 family member leads to negative regulation of lymphocyte activation. *J Exp Med.* (2000) 192:1027–34. doi: 10.1084/jem.192.7.1027
29. Chen L, Zhang Z, Chen W, Zhang Z, Li Y, Shi M, et al. B7-H1 up-regulation on myeloid dendritic cells significantly suppresses T cell immune function in patients with chronic hepatitis B. *J Immunol.* (2007) 178:6634–41. doi: 10.4049/jimmunol.178.10.6634
30. Schreiner B, Mitsdoerffer M, Kieseier BC, Chen L, Hartung H-P, Weller M, et al. Interferon-β enhances monocyte and dendritic cell expression of B7-H1 (PD-L1), a strong inhibitor of autologous T-cell activation: relevance for the immune modulatory effect in multiple sclerosis. *J Neuroimmunol.* (2004) 155:172–82. doi: 10.1016/j.jneuroim.2004.06.013
31. Wang F, Wang YY, Li J, You X, Qiu XH, Wang YN, et al. Increased antigen presentation but impaired T cells priming after upregulation of interferon-beta induced by lipopolysaccharides is mediated by upregulation of B7H1 and GITRL. *PLoS ONE* (2014) 9:e105636. doi: 10.1371/journal.pone.0105636
32. Muhlbauer M, Fleck M, Schutz C, Weiss T, Froh M, Blank C, et al. PD-L1 is induced in hepatocytes by viral infection and by interferon-alpha and -gamma and mediates T cell apoptosis. *J Hepatol.* (2006) 45:520–8. doi: 10.1016/j.jhep.2006.05.007
33. Fritz J, Karakhanova S, Brecht R, Nachtigall I, Werner J, Bazhin AV. *In vitro* immunomodulatory properties of gemcitabine alone and in combination with interferon-alpha. *Immunol Lett.* (2015) 168:111–9. doi: 10.1016/j.imlet.2015.09.017
34. Karakhanova S, Oweira H, Steinmeyer B, Sachsenmaier M, Jung G, Elhadedy H, et al. Interferon-γ, interleukin-10 and interferon-inducible protein 10 (CXCL10) as serum biomarkers for the early allograft dysfunction after liver transplantation. *Transpl Immunol.* (2016) 34:14–24. doi: 10.1016/j.trim.2015.12.001

35. Liu Y, Zeng B, Zhang Z, Zhang Y, Yang R. B7-H1 on myeloid-derived suppressor cells in immune suppression by a mouse model of ovarian cancer. *Clin Immunol.* (2008) 129:471–81. doi: 10.1016/j.clim.2008.07.030
36. Chou H-S, Hsieh C-C, Charles R, Wang L, Wagner T, Fung JJ, et al. Myeloid-derived suppressor cells (MDSC) protect islet transplants via B7-H1 mediated enhancement of T regulatory cells. *Transplantation* (2012) 93:272–82. doi: 10.1097/TP.0b013e31823ffd39
37. Ghebeh H, Barhoush E, Tulbah A, Elkum N, Al-Tweigeri T, Dermime S. FOXP3(+)T(regs)and B7-H1(+)/PD-1(+)T lymphocytes co-infiltrate the tumor tissues of high-risk breast cancer patients: implication for immunotherapy. *BMC Cancer* (2008) 8:57–7. doi: 10.1186/1471-2407-8-57
38. Curiel TJ, Wei S, Dong H, Alvarez X, Cheng P, Mottram P, et al. Blockade of B7-H1 improves myeloid dendritic cell–mediated antitumor immunity. *Nat Med.* (2003) 9:562. doi: 10.1038/nm863
39. Wagner CJ, Huber S, Wirth S, Voehringer D. Chitin induces upregulation of B7-H1 on macrophages and inhibits T-cell proliferation. *Eur J Immunol.* (2010) 40:2882–90. doi: 10.1002/eji.201040422
40. Matta BM, Raimondi G, Rosborough BR, Sumpter TL, Thomson AW. IL-27 production and STAT3-dependent upregulation of B7-H1 mediate immune regulatory functions of liver plasmacytoid DC. *J Immunol.* (2012) 188:5227–37. doi: 10.4049/jimmunol.1103382
41. Nagano H, Obi S, Hatano E, Kaneko S, Kanai F, Omata M, et al. A multicenter, randomized, controlled trial of S-1 monotherapy versus S-1 and interferon-α combination therapy for hepatocellular carcinoma with extrahepatic metastases. *Hepatol Res.* (2018) 48:717–26. doi: 10.1111/hepr.13067
42. Schmidt J, Jäger D, Hoffmann K, Büchler MW, Märten A. Impact of interferon-α in combined chemoradioimmunotherapy for pancreatic adenocarcinoma (CapRI): first data from the immunomonitoring. *J Immunother.* (2007) 30:108–15. doi: 10.1097/01.cji.0000211317.15278.27
43. Schmidt J, Abel U, Debus J, Harig S, Hoffmann K, Herrmann T, et al. Open-label, multicenter, randomized phase III trial of adjuvant chemoradiation plus interferon alfa-2b versus fluorouracil and folinic acid for patients with resected pancreatic adenocarcinoma. *J Clin Oncol.* (2012) 30:4077–83. doi: 10.1200/jco.2011.38.2960
44. Karakhanova S, Mosl B, Harig S, von Ahn K, Fritz J, Schmidt J, et al. Influence of interferon-alpha combined with chemo (radio) therapy on immunological parameters in pancreatic adenocarcinoma. *Int J Mol Sci.* (2014) 15:4104–25. doi: 10.3390/ijms15034104
45. Ratta M, Fagnoni F, Curti A, Vescovini R, Sansoni P, Oliviero B, et al. Dendritic cells are functionally defective in multiple myeloma: the role of interleukin-6. *Blood* (2002) 100:230–7. doi: 10.1182/blood.V100.1.230
46. van der Molen RG, Sprengers D, Binda RS, de Jong EC, Niesters HGM, Kusters JG, et al., Functional impairment of myeloid and plasmacytoid dendritic cells of patients with chronic hepatitis B. *Hepatology* (2004) 40:738–46. doi: 10.1002/hep.20366
47. Della Bella S, Nicola S, Brambilla L, Riva A, Ferrucci S, Presicce P, et al. Quantitative and functional defects of dendritic cells in classic Kaposi's sarcoma. *Clin Immunol.* (2006) 119:317–29. https://doi.org/10.1016/j.clim.2006.01.011
48. Lee BN, Follen M, Rodriquez G, Shen DY, Malpica A, Shearer WT, et al. Deficiencies in myeloid antigen-presenting cells in women with cervical squamous intraepithelial lesions. *Cancer* (2006) 107:999–1007. doi: 10.1002/cncr.22092
49. Ormandy LA, Farber A, Cantz T, Petrykowska S, Wedemeyer H, Horning M, et al. Direct *ex vivo* analysis of dendritic cells in patients with hepatocellular carcinoma. *World J Gastroenterol.* (2006) 12:3275–82. doi: 10.3748/wjg.v12.i20.3275
50. Perrot I, Blanchard D, Freymond N, Isaac S, Guibert B, Pacheco Y, et al. Dendritic cells infiltrating human non-small cell lung cancer are blocked at immature stage. *J Immunol.* (2007) 178:2763–9. doi: 10.4049/jimmunol.178.5.2763
51. Pinzon-Charry A, Ho CS, Maxwell T, McGuckin MA, Schmidt C, Furnival C, et al. Numerical and functional defects of blood dendritic cells in early- and late-stage breast cancer. *Br J Cancer* (2007) 97:1251–9. doi: 10.1038/sj.bjc.6604018
52. Bellone G, Novarino A, Vizio B, Brondino G, Addeo A, Prati A, et al. Impact of surgery and chemotherapy on cellular immunity in pancreatic carcinoma patients in view of an integration of standard cancer treatment with immunotherapy. *Int J Oncol.* (2009) 34:1701–15. doi: 10.3892/ijo_00000301
53. Gabrilovich DI, Ostrand-Rosenberg S, Bronte V. Coordinated regulation of myeloid cells by tumours. *Nat Rev Immunol.* (2012) 12:253–68. doi: 10.1038/nri3175
54. Steinman RM, Dhodapkar M. Active immunization against cancer with dendritic cells: the near future. *Int J Cancer* (2001) 94:459–73. doi: 10.1002/ijc.1503
55. Lu W, Arraes LC, Ferreira WT, Andrieu J-M. Therapeutic dendritic-cell vaccine for chronic HIV-1 infection. *Nat Med.* (2004) 10:1359. doi: 10.1038/nm1147
56. Santini SM, Lapenta C, Logozzi M, Parlato S, Spada M, Di Pucchio T, et al. Type I interferon as a powerful adjuvant for monocyte-derived dendritic cell development and activity *in vitro* and in Hu-Pbl-Scid mice. *J Exp Med.* (2000) 191:1777–88. doi: 10.1084/jem.191.10.1777
57. Della Bella S, Nicola S, Riva A, Biasin M, Clerici M, Villa ML. Functional repertoire of dendritic cells generated in granulocyte macrophage-colony stimulating factor and interferon-α. *J Leukoc Biol.* (2004) 75:106–16. doi: 10.1189/jlb.0403154
58. Santini SM, Lapenta C, Belardelli F. Type I interferons as regulators of the differentiation/activation of human dendritic cells. In: Carr DJJ, editor. *Interferon Methods and Protocols*, Totowa, NJ: Humana Press (2005). p. 167–81.
59. Santini SM, Lapenta C, Santodonato L, D'Agostino G, Belardelli F, Ferrantini M. IFN-alpha in the generation of dendritic cells for cancer immunotherapy. In: Lombardi G, Riffo-Vasquez Y, editors. *Dendritic Cells*, Berlin; Heidelberg: Springer Berlin Heidelberg (2009). p. 295–317.
60. Leplina OY, Tyrinova TV, Tikhonova MA, Ostanin AA, Chernykh ER. Interferon alpha induces generation of semi-mature dendritic cells with high pro-inflammatory and cytotoxic potential. *Cytokine* (2015) 71:1–7. doi: 10.1016/j.cyto.2014.07.258
61. Wölfle SJ, Strebovsky J, Bartz H, Sähr A, Arnold C, Kaiser C, et al. PD-L1 expression on tolerogenic APCs is controlled by STAT-3. *Eur J Immunol.* (2011) 41:413–24. doi: 10.1002/eji.201040979
62. Cousens LP, Orange JS, Su HC, Biron CA. Interferon-α/β inhibition of interleukin 12 and interferon-γ production *in vitro* and endogenously during viral infection. *Proc Natl Acad Sci USA.* (1997) 94:634–9.
63. McRae BL, Semnani RT, Hayes MP, van Seventer GA. Type I IFNs inhibit human dendritic cell IL-12 production and Th1 cell development. *J Immunol.* (1998) 160:4298–304.
64. Ohno Y, Kitamura H, Takahashi N, Ohtake J, Kaneumi S, Sumida K, et al. IL-6 down-regulates HLA class II expression and IL-12 production of human dendritic cells to impair activation of antigen-specific $CD4^+$ T cells. *Cancer Immunol Immunother.* (2016) 65:193–204. doi: 10.1007/s00262-015-1791-4
65. Liu J, Cao S, Kim S, Chung EY, Homma Y, Guan X, et al. Interleukin-12: an update on its immunological activities, signaling and regulation of gene expression. *Curr Immunol Rev.* (2005) 1:119–37. doi: 10.2174/1573395054065115
66. A WN, Thao N. The interferons and their receptors—distribution and regulation. *Immunol Cell Biol.* (2012) 90:483–91. doi: 10.1038/icb.2012.9
67. Seo S-K, Seo D-I, Park WS, Jung W-K, Lee D-S, Park Ś-G, et al. Attenuation of IFN-γ-induced B7-H1 expression by 15-deoxy-delta12,14-prostaglandin J2 via downregulation of the Jak/STAT/IRF-1 signaling pathway. *Life Sci.* (2014) 112:82–9. doi: 10.1016/j.lfs.2014.07.021
68. Garcia-Diaz A, Shin DS, Moreno BH, Saco J, Escuin-Ordinas H, Rodriguez GA, et al. Interferon receptor signaling pathways regulating PD-L1 and PD-L2 expression. *Cell Rep.* (2017) 19:1189–201. doi: 10.1016/j.celrep.2017.04.031
69. Bellucci R, Martin A, Bommarito D, Wang K, Hansen SH, Freeman GJ, et al. Interferon-γ-induced activation of JAK1 and JAK2 suppresses tumor cell susceptibility to NK cells through upregulation of PD-L1 expression. *Oncoimmunology* (2015) 4:e1008824. doi: 10.1080/2162402X.2015.1008824
70. Barton BE. STAT3: a potential therapeutic target in dendritic cells for the induction of transplant tolerance. *Expert Opin Ther Targets* (2006) 10:459–70. doi: 10.1517/14728222.10.3.459

71. Paty DW, Li DKB. Interferon beta-1b is effective in relapsing-remitting multiple sclerosis. II. MRI analysis results of a multicenter, randomized, double-blind, placebo-controlled trial. *Neurology* (1993) 43:662–7. doi: 10.1212/wnl.43.4.662
72. Martina B, Michel ZC, Bernd G, Lisa L, Peter D, Peter V, et al. Multimodal treatment, including interferon beta, of nasopharyngeal carcinoma in children and young adults. *Cancer* (2012) 118:4892–900. doi: 10.1002/cncr.27395
73. Ivashkiv LB, Donlin LT. Regulation of type I interferon responses. *Nat Rev Immunol.* (2014) 14:36–49. doi: 10.1038/nri3581

9

Immune Checkpoint-Mediated Interactions Between Cancer and Immune Cells in Prostate Adenocarcinoma and Melanoma

*Angela Rita Elia, Sara Caputo and Matteo Bellone**

Cellular Immunology Unit, Department of Immunology, Transplantation and Infectious Diseases, San Raffaele Scientific Institute, Milan, Italy

Edited by:
*Amedeo Amedei,
Università degli Studi
di Firenze, Italy*

Reviewed by:
*Kawaljit Kaur,
University of California,
Los Angeles, United States
Alessandro Poggi,
Ospedale Policlinico
San Martino, Italy
Carlos Alfaro,
NavarraBiomed, Spain
Dennis O. Adeegbe,
Moffitt Cancer Center, United States
Giulio Cesare Spagnoli,
Universität Basel, Switzerland
Derre Laurent,
Centre Hospitalier Universitaire
Vaudois (CHUV), Switzerland*

***Correspondence:**
*Matteo Bellone
bellone.matteo@hsr.it*

Prostate adenocarcinoma (PCa) and melanoma are paradigmatic examples of tumors that are either poorly or highly sensitive to therapies based on monoclonal antibodies directed against regulatory pathways in T lymphocytes [i.e., immune checkpoint blockade (ICB)]. Yet, approximately 40% of melanoma patients are resistant or acquire resistance to ICB. What characterize the microenvironment of PCa and ICB-resistant melanoma are a scanty cytotoxic T cell infiltrate and a strong immune suppression, respectively. Here, we compare the tumor microenvironment in these two subgroups of cancer patients, focusing on some among the most represented immune checkpoint molecules: cytotoxic T lymphocyte-associated antigen-4, programmed death-1, lymphocyte activation gene-3, and T cell immunoglobulin and mucin-domain containing-3. We also report on several examples of crosstalk between cancer and immune cells that are mediated by inhibitory immune checkpoints and identify promising strategies aimed at overcoming ICB resistance both in PCa and melanoma.

Keywords: prostate cancer, melanoma, immunity, immune checkpoint, immunotherapy, cytotoxic T lymphocytes

INTRODUCTION

Activated T lymphocytes require mechanisms that timely and properly shut them down to prevent excessive damage at the inflammation site. Inhibitory immune checkpoint molecules, such as cytotoxic T lymphocyte-associated antigen-4 (CTLA-4), programmed death-1 (PD-1), lymphocyte activation gene-3 (LAG-3), and T cell immunoglobulin and mucin-domain containing-3 (TIM-3), are progressively upregulated on activated T cells, and, by interacting with their ligands, switch inhibitory pathways on in T cells (1). Interactions between immune checkpoint molecules on T cells and their ligands on target cells may also signal in the latters, thus generating a crosstalk between T lymphocytes and other cells (2–4). These mechanisms are crucial for self-tolerance, but also represent the Achilles' heel of cancer immunity, as ligands for inhibitory immune checkpoint molecules are expressed on neoplastic and other cells within the tumor microenvironment. In addition, a growing tumor may condition secondary lymphoid organs, thus limiting expansion of tumor-specific T cells (5).

Building on these evidences, monoclonal antibodies (mAbs) directed against regulatory pathways in T lymphocytes [i.e., immune checkpoint blockade (ICB) (6)] have been developed. Phase III clinical trials with anti-PD-1/programmed death-ligand 1 (PD-L1) or anti-CTLA-4 mAbs documented excellent efficacy, and ICB has been approved for the treatment of various solid and hematological malignancies (7). Because several inhibitory checkpoints act simultaneously, the combination of two or more mAbs can improve ICB therapeutic outcomes (8).

Although melanomas are generally sensitive to ICB, also because of their heavy cytotoxic T lymphocyte (CTL) infiltrate, approximately 40% of melanoma patients are resistant to ICB even when two mAbs are combined (9). ICB resistance was recently reviewed [e.g., Ref. (10, 11)]. Other tumors like prostate adenocarcinoma (PCa) are intrinsically resistant to ICB (12), and either anti-PD-1/PD-L1 or anti-CTLA-4 monotherapy did not impact PCa patients' overall survival (13, 14). ICB resistance in PCa is attributed to tumor cell intrinsic mechanisms and a scanty immune infiltrate (15) dominated by macrophages. In addition, soon after ICB, immune cells upregulate other inhibitory molecules such as V-domain Ig suppressor of T cell activation [VISTA; (16)], a phenomenon not limited to PCa (17). Interestingly, orally available small molecules targeting both PD-L1 and VISTA are investigated in patients affected by advanced tumors (ClinicalTrials.gov Identifier: NCT02812875).

Therefore, melanoma and PCa epitomize two classes of ICB-resistant tumors, in which tumor cell-intrinsic mechanisms of ICB resistance associate with heavy but immunosuppressed or modest immune infiltrates, respectively. Thus, while in the former the combination of two or more ICB mAbs should succeed, in the latter strategies to improve tumor infiltration by CTLs will be needed to improve ICB sensitivity. We will analyze differences and similarities in ICB-resistant melanoma and PCa, focusing on immune checkpoint-mediated interactions between tumor and immune cells. We will also highlight strategies that might improve sensitivity to ICB.

T CELL EXHAUSTION

Prolonged antigen exposure progressively impairs T cell proliferation and effector functions (18) through epigenetic mechanisms (19). In the early dysfunctional state, which is plastic and reprogrammable, $CD8^+$ T cells express PD-1 and LAG-3 and low TIM-3 levels. Later on, T cells enter fixed exhaustion characterized by TIM-3 upregulation, and the additional expression of high CD38 and CD101 and low CD5 levels. The latter cells are no longer reprogrammable by ICB (20). Partially exhausted $CD8^+$ T cells, expressing high levels of PD-1 and CTLA-4 predicted response to anti-PD-1 in metastatic melanoma patients (21). Because also activated T cells express PD-1, this molecule cannot be used as marker of exhaustion, which should instead be functionally defined (22). Additional exhaustion markers (e.g., 2B4 and TIGIT) cannot be discussed here because of space constraint.

Also $CD4^+$ T cells undergo exhaustion (23), loosing helper function and releasing IL-10 (24). CTLA-4 on $CD4^+$ Tregs is an additional mechanism of immune suppression in cancer (25).

CYTOTOXIC T LYMPHOCYTE-ASSOCIATED ANTIGEN-4

Cytotoxic T lymphocyte-associated antigen-4 has been the first immune checkpoint investigated in clinic. Because of higher affinity for CD80 and CD86 than CD28, CTLA-4 impairs T cell co-stimulation (26). Whereas CTLA-4 is expressed on activated effector T cells (27), it is constitutively expressed on Tregs and contributes to their immunosuppressive activity. Thus, anti-CTLA-4 mAbs mainly act in secondary lymphoid organs, also causing Treg depletion through antibody-dependent cellular toxicity (28).

IFN-γ signaling activates expression of CTLA-4 in melanoma cells, and after ipilimumab (anti-CTLA-4) treatment, human melanomas upregulated IFN-γ responsive genes, including CTLA-4, which associated with durable response (29). Thus, anti-CTLA-4 mAbs can directly affect melanoma cells (30). CTLA-4 on tumor cells might also act as local mechanism of immune escape. Of relevance, mutations in the IFN responsive genes associate with resistance to ICB (31). Restifo and collaborators found that also mutations in genes indirectly correlated to the IFN response (e.g., *APLNR*), profoundly affected *in vivo* sensitivity to both adoptive T cell therapy (ACT) and anti-CTLA-4 blockade (32). It is anticipated that investigations on such comprehensive lists of genes will identify new drugs overcoming ICB resistance.

An alternative strategy to increase sensitivity to ICB is to combine them with other therapeutic strategies, such as chemotherapy, hormonal therapy, vaccines, etc. (**Tables 1** and **2**). As an example, both in mice and humans, the combination of local chemotherapy and systemic ICB increased tumor infiltration by effector T cells, and clinical response rates (NCT01323517) (33). Others have shown that targeting myeloid-derived suppressor cells (MDSCs), which are relevant immunosuppressive populations in PCa (34, 35), with tyrosine kinase inhibitors increased sensitivity to ICB in castration-resistant PCa (36). Both in orthotopic melanoma and autochthonous PCa, even the combination of anti-CTLA-4 and anti-PD-1 exerted modest antitumor effects (37), and required the addition of fresh T cells (i.e., ACT) and minute amounts of TNF-α targeted to tumor-associated vessels to favor endothelial cell activation, tumor infiltration by fully effector T cells, and tumor debulking (38, 39). Interestingly, only this triple-combined treatment guaranteed a prolonged overall survival of the mice affected by autochthonous PCa, thus suggesting the treatment generated a potent tumor-specific memory response (37). Additional strategies can be implemented to favor access of both T cells and mAbs to the tumor (40).

Overall, these data support the concept that several therapeutic strategies need to be combined to overcome ICB resistance.

PD-1/PD-L1

Programmed death-1 is upregulated on T cells upon antigen recognition, and by interacting with either PD-L1 expressed on tumor, stromal and immune cells or PD-L2 expressed on myeloid cells, impairs T cell activation (41). An exhaustion-specific enhancer regulates PD-1 expression in T cells (42), and editing exhaustion-specific enhancers might improve the therapeutic efficacy of ACT. Similarly, blocking *de novo* DNA methylation in chronically stimulated $CD8^+$ T cells allowed retention of their effector functions (43).

Programmed death-1 blockade with nivolumab, lambrolizumab, or pembrolizumab has led to relevant clinical benefits

TABLE 1 | Clinical trials of immune checkpoint blockade (ICB) combined with other strategies in prostate adenocarcinoma (PCa).

Target	ICB drug	Partner drug	NCT number	Status
CTLA-4	Ipilimumab	Evofosfamide	NCT03098160	Recruiting
CTLA-4	Ipilimumab	Sipuleucel-T	NCT01804465	Recruiting
CTLA-4	Ipilimumab	Cryoimmunotherapy ciclophosphamide	NCT02423928	Recruiting
CTLA-4	Ipilimumab	PROSTVAC V/F	NCT02506114	Recruiting
PD-1	PDR001	NIS793[a]	NCT02947165	Recruiting
PD-1	M7824[b]	ALT-803[c]; NCB024360[d]	NCT03493945	Recruiting
PD-1	Nivolumab	PROSTVAC V/F	NCT02933255	Recruiting
PD-L1	MDI4736	Olaparib cedinarib	NCT02484404	Recruiting
CTLA-4 and PD-L1	Tremelimulab and durvalumab		NCT02788773	Recruiting
CTLA-4 and PD-L1	Tremelimulab and durvalumab	polyICLC[e]	NCT02643303	Recruiting
CTLA-4 and PD-1	Ipilimumab and nivolumab		NCT03061539	Recruiting
CTLA-4 and PD-1	Ipilimumab and REGN2810	Stereotactic body radiation	NCT03477864	Not yet recruiting
LAG-3 and PD-1	LAG525 and PDR001		NCT03365791	Recruiting

Selected clinical trials combining ICB and/or other therapies in PCa.
[a]Anti-TGF-β monoclonal antibody.
[b]Bifunctional fusion protein consisting of an anti-programmed death-ligand 1 (PD-L1) antibody and the extracellular domain of TGF-β receptor type 2.
[c]IL-15/IL-15Rα superagonist complex.
[d]IDO1 inhibitor.
[e]Toll-like receptor agonist.

TABLE 2 | Clinical trials of immune checkpoint blockade (ICB) combined with other strategies in melanoma.

Target	ICB drug	Partner drug	NCT number	Status
CTLA-4	Ipilimumab	Dabrafenib	NCT01940809	Recruiting
CTLA-4	Ipilimumab	6MHP[a] peptide vaccine	NCT02385669	Recruiting
PD-1		INT230-6[b]	NCT03058289	Recruiting
PD-1	Pembrolizumab	iMIQUIMOD[c]	NCT03276832	Recruiting
PD-1	Pembrolizumab	Dabrafenib; trametinib	NCT02130466	Recruiting
PD-1	Pembrolizumab	Navarixin[d]	NCT03473925	Recruiting
PD-1	Nivolumab	PD-L1/IDO peptide vaccine	NCT03047928	Recruiting
PD-1	Pembrolizumab	IMP321[e]	NCT02676869	Recruiting
PD-L1	Atzolizumab	RO719857[f]	NCT03289962	Recruiting
CTLA-4 and PD-1	Ipilimumab and nivolumab		NCT03354962	Not yet recruiting
CTLA-4 and PD-1	Ipilimumab and pembrolizumab	Aspirin®	NCT03396952	Recruiting
PD-1 and TIM-3	PDR001 and MBG453		NCT02608268	Recruiting
CTLA-4 and PDL-1	Durvalumab and tremelimumab	IMCgp100[g]	NCT02535078	Recruiting

Selected clinical trials combining ICB and/or other therapies in melanoma.
[a]High-dose IFN-α2b.
[b]Supermolecular complex of cisplatin, vinblastine, and an amphiphilic penetration enhancer.
[c]Synthetic agent with immune response modifying activity.
[d]CXCR2 antagonist.
[e]LAG-3Ig fusion protein.
[f]Messenger RNA based individually personalized cancer vaccine.
[g]Soluble gp100-specific T cell receptor with anti-CD3 single chain antibody fragment.

in cancer patients, mainly by rejuvenating cytotoxicity and cytokine secretion capability of T cells (44). However, as mentioned above, T cells undergoing fixed exhaustion are no longer reprogrammable by ICB. An interesting study compared the epigenetic regulation of tumor- or virus-specific T cells in melanoma-bearing mice. Only melanoma-infiltrating, tumor-specific T lymphocytes (TILs) upregulated PD-1, LAG-3, and TIM-3 and showed reduced TNF-α, IFN-γ, and IL-2 secretion ability when compared with virus-specific cells. Exhausted T cells displayed more accessible chromatin in proximity to PD-1 and LAG-3 gene promoters. Treatment with anti-PD-1 mAbs had a positive impact on effector functions of exhausted T cells and on tumor growth, but induced only limited changes in gene expression and chromatin accessibility (45). Similar findings have been reported in a transplantable model of PCa, in which tumor-specific $CD8^+$ T cells showed *de novo* methylation in *Tcf7*, *Ccr7*, *Myc*, and *IFN-γ* genes, and impaired proliferation and effector functions that could not be restored by ICB. Only combination of decitabine, inhibiting the DNA methyltransferase DNMT3A, and anti-PD-1 mAbs re-established proliferation capability of exhausted T cells, thus resulting in delayed tumor growth (43).

Clinical trials evaluating the efficacy of pembrolizumab in combination with epigenetic drugs are ongoing in advanced melanoma patients (NCT03278665, NCT02816021, and NCT02437136). Also in PCa, PD-1 blockade is clinically investigated in combination with ipilimumab (NCT02601014), anti-PD-L1 (NCT03170960, NCT03061539), and other therapies including hormone, vaccine, and cryosurgery (NCT02787005, NCT02499835, and NCT02489357).

Programmed death-1 can be found expressed also on tumor cells, and PD-1 triggering on melanoma cells increases three-dimensional growth capability with concomitant activation of the mTOR pathway (3). Interestingly, treatment with BRAF and MEK inhibitors associated with increased frequency of PD-1$^+$ tumor cells in melanoma patients, and PD-1 expression sensitized melanoma to PD-1 blockade in immunodeficient mice (46). The same authors also noticed a correlative expression of PD-1 and the stem cell marker Oct-4, thus linking PD-1 to cancer stem cells (46).

Also anti-PD-L1 mAbs may directly affect tumor cells by impacting tumor metabolism, reducing extracellular acidification, phosphorylation of mTOR, and glycolysis (4). *mTORC1* expression has been associated with PD-L1 expression in melanoma cells, and PD-L1^{low} cells showed decreased levels of *mTORC1*, and an altered autophagy pathway. Furthermore, treatment of immunodeficient mice with anti-PD-L1 mAbs delayed melanoma growth, reduced metastases, and prolonged animal survival (2). PD-L1 has also been found overexpressed in melanoma tumor-initiating cells, and the lack of PD-L1 significantly reduced the frequency of these cells in melanoma-bearing mice (47). Thus, interfering with the PD-1/PD-L1 axis may impact both tumor and immune cells.

LYMPHOCYTE ACTIVATION GENE-3

Lymphocyte activation gene-3 is closely related to CD4, is expressed on dysfunctional T cells (48), and TILs in melanoma patients express LAG-3 (49). Because LAG-3 binding to MHC class II molecules activates myeloid cells (50), and MHC class II can be expressed by melanoma cells (51), engagement of LAG-3 with MHC class II might provide a survival signal to tumor cells. LAG-3 also binds LSECtin and Galectin-3 (Gal-3) (49, 52) and associates with the CD3/TCR complex, thus impairs TCR signaling (18, 52). Conversely, LAG-3 binding on Tregs increases their immunosuppressive activity (53).

Lymphocyte activation gene-3 may synergize with other immune checkpoints, and the combination of anti-LAG-3 and anti-PD-1 resulted in more potent inhibition of murine tumor growth than single treatments (54). Anti-LAG-3 mAbs or LAG-3 fusion proteins are being tested in melanoma patients resistant to anti-PD-1/PD-L1 ICB as single agent (NCT01968109), or in combination to anti-PD-1 (NCT02676869).

Drake and collaborators originally reported that in PCa, tumor-specific CD4$^+$ and CD8$^+$ T cells rapidly upregulate LAG-3 upon *in vivo* antigen encounter. Treatment with anti-LAG-3 mAbs enhanced the number and effector function of tumor-specific CD8$^+$ T cells in TRAMP mice, and delayed tumor growth (55). Also Tregs in human PCa lesions upregulate both CTLA-4 and LAG-3 (56). The latter finding has been challenged by recent data showing low expression of LAG-3 in Tregs infiltrating PCa lesions (57). Further investigation is needed to better define the role of LAG-3 in T cell exhaustion and/or Treg function in PCa. One clinical trial is ongoing that investigates efficacy of anti-LAG-3 mAbs in combination with anti-PD-1 in castration-resistant PCa (NCT03365791).

T CELL IMMUNOGLOBULIN AND MUCIN-DOMAIN CONTAINING-3

Programmed death-1 expression in TILs is often associated with TIM-3, and its transient or persistent expression relates to short or chronic antigen stimulations, respectively (58). Indeed, PD-1$^+$TIM-3$^+$ T cells are functionally more exhausted than PD-1$^+$TIM-3$^{-/low}$ T cells (59), and TIM-3 can be considered a marker of terminally differentiated T cells.

T cell immunoglobulin and mucin-domain containing-3 is expressed on dysfunctional, tumor-specific CD8$^+$ T cells in melanoma (60) and PCa patients (61), and in ipilimumab-treated melanoma patients, increased expression and frequency of TIM-3 and PD-1 on both peripheral NK and T cells associated with poor prognosis (62). Correlative data on TIM-3 in PCa patients are conflicting. Whereas one report showed that high TIM-3 expression on PCa cells predicted short recurrence-free and progression-free survival in chemotherapy and radiotherapy naïve PCa patients (63), others found that negative TIM-3 expression was an independent prognostic factor of poor prognosis in advanced metastatic PCa (64). Outcome differences might be brought back to the different subpopulations of PCa patients analyzed in the two studies. The latter also showed that silencing TIM-3 in PCa cell lines reduced tumor cell proliferation and invasion *in vitro* (63), thus, suggesting that TIM-3 has a functional role in PCa cells. Interestingly, the combined targeting of TIM-3 and PD-1 pathways is more effective in controlling tumor growth than targeting either pathway alone (59).

Mechanistically, the interaction between TIM-3 on T cells and one of its ligands [i.e., Galectin-9 (Gal-9)] triggers cell death in effector T cells (65). Ceacam-1, an additional TIM-3 ligand, is co-expressed on exhausted T cells, can bind TIM-3 both in *cis* and *trans*, and both interactions drive the inhibitory function of TIM-3 (66). TIM-3 also enhances FoxP3$^+$ Tregs inhibitory functions (59), and is expressed and upregulated upon activation on human NK cells. In contrast to effector T cells, Gal-9-mediated TIM-3 triggering in NK cells induces IFN-γ production (67). Interestingly, it has been shown that MHC class I downregulation or deficiency in mouse tumors induces upregulation of PD-1 and TIM-3 on NK cells and their exhaustion. PD-1$^+$TIM-3$^+$ NK cells were also found in human melanoma samples, and correlated with low HLA expression (68). Because *in vitro*, TIM-3 blockade reversed NK cell exhaustion (69), it will be interesting to investigate the *in vivo* effects of mAbs against both PD-1 and TIM-3 on NK cells.

While TIM-3 is higher and more precociously upregulated on tumor-associated dendritic cells (DCs) than on CD8$^+$ T cells, its role in innate immunity is controversial (70). By interacting with phosphatidylserine, TIM-3 favors DC uptake of apoptotic cells and cross-presentation (71). Conversely, interaction of the alarmin high mobility group protein B1 with Tim-3 on DCs limits their release of pro-inflammatory cytokines, thus blunting type-1 immunity (72). TIM-3 is also expressed on tumor-associated macrophages (72), and TIM-3 negatively modulates the production of pro-inflammatory cytokines in human CD14$^+$ monocytes (73). Finally, TIM-3 can suppress the antitumor immunity by promoting induction of MDSCs (74).

Clinical trials are investigating safety and tolerability of anti-TIM-3 mAbs given either alone (NCT03489343) or in combination with anti-PD-1 (NCT02817633 and NCT02608268) or anti-PD-L1 (NCT03099109) in cancer patients.

GALECTINS

Apart from being ligands for LAG-3 and TIM-3, galectins also exert relevant pro-tumor functions (75). Increased expression of Gal-3 in melanoma lesions correlates with tumor progression (76), and Gal-3 activates NFAT1 (77), which also regulates IL-8 and MMP3 expression in melanoma cells, thus promoting a malignant phenotype (78). Gal-3 released by melanoma cells can also capture IFN-γ, thus reducing its antitumor activity (79). At odds, others reported that tumor cell expression of Gal-3 or myeloid cell expression of Gal-9 in melanoma lesions associated with a longer survival (80). The latter findings are counterintuitive and deserve further investigation.

Inhibiting Gal-3 together with anticancer vaccination restores the effector function of melanoma TILs (81). Therefore, Gal-3 not only contributes to melanoma tumor growth and metastasis but also dampens the antitumor immune response. Gal-3 inhibition is currently investigated in combination with ICB and vaccine in melanoma (NCT02575404, NCT02117362, and NCT01723813).

Galectin-3 is also expressed in PCa lesions, exerts direct pro-tumor and pro-metastatic functions, and correlates with biochemical recurrence (82). Indeed, administration of a Gal-3 inhibitor suppressed PCa lung metastasis (83).

Galectin-3 is a marker of cancer stem cells (84) and maintains stemness of carcinoma progenitor cells (85). In the TRAMP model, we found that PCa stem-like cells endowed with immunosuppressive activities express Gal-3 (86). We have also evidence that Gal-3 favors growth and metastasis of tumors generated by PCa stem-like cells (Caputo et al., manuscript in preparation). It will be interesting to investigate if Gal-3 also contributes to their immunosuppressive activity.

CONCLUDING REMARKS

Inhibitory immune checkpoint triggering in TILs cripples cancer immune surveillance. As consequence of local inflammation, immune checkpoints are also upregulated on cancer cells, supporting tumor growth and aggressiveness. Thus, the effect of ICB goes beyond rescuing of exhausted/dysfunctional TILs and may directly impact tumor cells.

To overcome TIL exhaustion, several promising combined approaches are envisioned among many others: coupling two or more mAbs against immune checkpoints; increase tumor immunogenicity by exploiting conventional chemotherapy and targeted anticancer agents (87); transiently modify the tumor vasculature to favor T cell infiltration (88–90); combine additional immunotherapeutic approaches such as vaccines and ACT (37); abolish additional mechanisms of local immune suppression (91). Several high throughput analyses (e.g., methylomics and metabolomics) and microbiota sequencing will likely define novel areas of therapeutic intervention in the field of ICB. Finally, it will be essential to focus on adverse events that increase along with therapeutic efficacy (92).

AUTHOR CONTRIBUTIONS

AE, SC, and MB wrote and reviewed the manuscript.

ACKNOWLEDGMENTS

We apologize with the many authors whose excellent work we could note cite due to space limitations.

REFERENCES

1. Pardoll DM. The blockade of immune checkpoints in cancer immunotherapy. *Nat Rev Cancer* (2012) 12(4):252–64. doi:10.1038/nrc3239
2. Clark CA, Gupta HB, Sareddy G, Pandeswara S, Lao S, Yuan B, et al. Tumor-intrinsic PD-L1 signals regulate cell growth, pathogenesis, and autophagy in ovarian cancer and melanoma. *Cancer Res* (2016) 76(23):6964–74. doi:10.1158/0008-5472.CAN-16-0258
3. Kleffel S, Posch C, Barthel SR, Mueller H, Schlapbach C, Guenova E, et al. Melanoma cell-intrinsic PD-1 receptor functions promote tumor growth. *Cell* (2015) 162(6):1242–56. doi:10.1016/j.cell.2015.08.052
4. Chang CH, Qiu J, O'Sullivan D, Buck MD, Noguchi T, Curtis JD, et al. Metabolic competition in the tumor microenvironment is a driver of cancer progression. *Cell* (2015) 162(6):1229–41. doi:10.1016/j.cell.2015.08.016
5. Chen DS, Mellman I. Oncology meets immunology: the cancer-immunity cycle. *Immunity* (2013) 39(1):1–10. doi:10.1016/j.immuni.2013.07.012
6. Callahan MK, Postow MA, Wolchok JD. Targeting T cell co-receptors for cancer therapy. *Immunity* (2016) 44(5):1069–78. doi:10.1016/j.immuni.2016.04.023
7. Melero I, Berman DM, Aznar MA, Korman AJ, Perez Gracia JL, Haanen J. Evolving synergistic combinations of targeted immunotherapies to combat cancer. *Nat Rev Cancer* (2015) 15(8):457–72. doi:10.1038/nrc3973
8. Jardim DL, de Melo Gagliato D, Giles FJ, Kurzrock R. Analysis of drug development paradigms for immune checkpoint inhibitors. *Clin Cancer Res* (2018) 24(8):1785–94. doi:10.1158/1078-0432.CCR-17-1970
9. Larkin J, Chiarion-Sileni V, Gonzalez R, Grob JJ, Cowey CL, Lao CD, et al. Combined nivolumab and ipilimumab or monotherapy in untreated melanoma. *N Engl J Med* (2015) 373(1):23–34. doi:10.1056/NEJMoa1504030
10. Restifo NP, Smyth MJ, Snyder A. Acquired resistance to immunotherapy and future challenges. *Nat Rev Cancer* (2016) 16(2):121–6. doi:10.1038/nrc.2016.2
11. Bellone M, Elia AR. Constitutive and acquired mechanisms of resistance to immune checkpoint blockade in human cancer. *Cytokine Growth Factor Rev* (2017) 36:17–24. doi:10.1016/j.cytogfr.2017.06.002
12. Sharma P, Hu-Lieskovan S, Wargo JA, Ribas A. Primary, adaptive, and acquired resistance to cancer immunotherapy. *Cell* (2017) 168(4):707–23. doi:10.1016/j.cell.2017.01.017
13. Beer TM, Kwon ED, Drake CG, Fizazi K, Logothetis C, Gravis G, et al. Randomized, double-blind, phase III trial of ipilimumab versus placebo in asymptomatic or minimally symptomatic patients with metastatic chemotherapy-naive castration-resistant prostate cancer. *J Clin Oncol* (2017) 35(1):40–7. doi:10.1200/JCO.2016.69.1584
14. Kwon ED, Drake CG, Scher HI, Fizazi K, Bossi A, van den Eertwegh AJ, et al. Ipilimumab versus placebo after radiotherapy in patients with metastatic castration-resistant prostate cancer that had progressed after

docetaxel chemotherapy (CA184-043): a multicentre, randomised, double-blind, phase 3 trial. *Lancet Oncol* (2014) 15(7):700–12. doi:10.1016/S1470-2045(14)70189-5
15. Petitprez F, Fossati N, Vano Y, Freschi M, Becht E, Luciano R, et al. PD-L1 expression and CD8+ T cell infiltrate are associated with clinical progression in patients with node positive prostate cancer. *Eur Urol Focus* (2017). doi:10.1016/j.euf.2017.05.013
16. Gao J, Ward JF, Pettaway CA, Shi LZ, Subudhi SK, Vence LM, et al. VISTA is an inhibitory immune checkpoint that is increased after ipilimumab therapy in patients with prostate cancer. *Nat Med* (2017) 23(5):551–5. doi:10.1038/nm.4308
17. Koyama S, Akbay EA, Li YY, Herter-Sprie GS, Buczkowski KA, Richards WG, et al. Adaptive resistance to therapeutic PD-1 blockade is associated with upregulation of alternative immune checkpoints. *Nat Commun* (2016) 7:10501. doi:10.1038/ncomms10501
18. Baitsch L, Baumgaertner P, Devevre E, Raghav SK, Legat A, Barba L, et al. Exhaustion of tumor-specific CD8(+) T cells in metastases from melanoma patients. *J Clin Invest* (2011) 121(6):2350–60. doi:10.1172/JCI46102
19. Schietinger A, Philip M, Krisnawan VE, Chiu EY, Delrow JJ, Basom RS, et al. Tumor-specific T cell dysfunction is a dynamic antigen-driven differentiation program initiated early during tumorigenesis. *Immunity* (2016) 45(2):389–401. doi:10.1016/j.immuni.2016.07.011
20. Philip M, Fairchild L, Sun L, Horste EL, Camara S, Shakiba M, et al. Chromatin states define tumour-specific T cell dysfunction and reprogramming. *Nature* (2017) 545(7655):452–6. doi:10.1038/nature22367
21. Daud AI, Loo K, Pauli ML, Sanchez-Rodriguez R, Sandoval PM, Taravati K, et al. Tumor immune profiling predicts response to anti-PD-1 therapy in human melanoma. *J Clin Invest* (2016) 126(9):3447–52. doi:10.1172/JCI87324
22. Singer M, Wang C, Cong L, Marjanovic ND, Kowalczyk MS, Zhang H, et al. A distinct gene module for dysfunction uncoupled from activation in tumor-infiltrating T cells. *Cell* (2016) 166(6):1500–11.e9. doi:10.1016/j.cell.2016.08.052
23. Severson JJ, Serracino HS, Mateescu V, Raeburn CD, McIntyre RC Jr, Sams SB, et al. PD-1+Tim-3+ CD8+ T lymphocytes display varied degrees of functional exhaustion in patients with regionally metastatic differentiated thyroid cancer. *Cancer Immunol Res* (2015) 3(6):620–30. doi:10.1158/2326-6066.CIR-14-0201
24. Parish IA, Marshall HD, Staron MM, Lang PA, Brustle A, Chen JH, et al. Chronic viral infection promotes sustained Th1-derived immunoregulatory IL-10 via BLIMP-1. *J Clin Invest* (2014) 124(8):3455–68. doi:10.1172/JCI66108
25. Greenwald RJ, Freeman GJ, Sharpe AH. The B7 family revisited. *Annu Rev Immunol* (2005) 23:515–48. doi:10.1146/annurev.immunol.23.021704.115611
26. Schildberg FA, Klein SR, Freeman GJ, Sharpe AH. Coinhibitory pathways in the B7-CD28 ligand-receptor family. *Immunity* (2016) 44(5):955–72. doi:10.1016/j.immuni.2016.05.002
27. Qureshi OS, Kaur S, Hou TZ, Jeffery LE, Poulter NS, Briggs Z, et al. Constitutive clathrin-mediated endocytosis of CTLA-4 persists during T cell activation. *J Biol Chem* (2012) 287(12):9429–40. doi:10.1074/jbc.M111.304329
28. Arce Vargas F, Furness AJS, Litchfield K, Joshi K, Rosenthal R, Ghorani E, et al. Fc effector function contributes to the activity of human anti-CTLA-4 antibodies. *Cancer Cell* (2018) 33(4):649–63.e4. doi:10.1016/j.ccell.2018.02.010
29. Mo X, Zhang H, Preston S, Martin K, Zhou B, Vadalia N, et al. Interferon-gamma signaling in melanocytes and melanoma cells regulates expression of CTLA-4. *Cancer Res* (2018) 78(2):436–50. doi:10.1158/0008-5472.CAN-17-1615
30. Laurent S, Queirolo P, Boero S, Salvi S, Piccioli P, Boccardo S, et al. The engagement of CTLA-4 on primary melanoma cell lines induces antibody-dependent cellular cytotoxicity and TNF-alpha production. *J Transl Med* (2013) 11:108. doi:10.1186/1479-5876-11-108
31. Gao J, Shi LZ, Zhao H, Chen J, Xiong L, He Q, et al. Loss of IFN-gamma pathway genes in tumor cells as a mechanism of resistance to anti-CTLA-4 therapy. *Cell* (2016) 167(2):397–404.e9. doi:10.1016/j.cell.2016.08.069
32. Patel SJ, Sanjana NE, Kishton RJ, Eidizadeh A, Vodnala SK, Cam M, et al. Identification of essential genes for cancer immunotherapy. *Nature* (2017) 548(7669):537–42. doi:10.1038/nature23477
33. Ariyan CE, Brady MS, Siegelbaum RH, Hu J, Bello DM, Rand J, et al. Robust antitumor responses result from local chemotherapy and CTLA-4 blockade. *Cancer Immunol Res* (2018) 6(2):189–200. doi:10.1158/2326-6066.CIR-17-0356
34. Rigamonti N, Bellone M. Prostate cancer, tumor immunity and a renewed sense of optimism in immunotherapy. *Cancer Immunol Immunother* (2012) 61(4):453–68. doi:10.1007/s00262-012-1216-6
35. Lopez-Bujanda Z, Drake CG. Myeloid-derived cells in prostate cancer progression: phenotype and prospective therapies. *J Leukoc Biol* (2017) 102(2):393–406. doi:10.1189/jlb.5VMR1116-491RR
36. Lu X, Horner JW, Paul E, Shang X, Troncoso P, Deng P, et al. Effective combinatorial immunotherapy for castration-resistant prostate cancer. *Nature* (2017) 543(7647):728–32. doi:10.1038/nature21676
37. Elia AR, Grioni M, Basso V, Curnis F, Freschi M, Corti A, et al. Targeting tumor vasculature with TNF leads effector T cells to the tumor and enhances therapeutic efficacy of immune checkpoint blockers in combination with adoptive cell therapy. *Clin Cancer Res* (2018) 24(9):2171–81. doi:10.1158/1078-0432.CCR-17-2210
38. Calcinotto A, Grioni M, Jachetti E, Curnis F, Mondino A, Parmiani G, et al. Targeting TNF-alpha to neoangiogenic vessels enhances lymphocyte infiltration in tumors and increases the therapeutic potential of immunotherapy. *J Immunol* (2012) 188(6):2687–94. doi:10.4049/jimmunol.1101877
39. Manzo T, Sturmheit T, Basso V, Petrozziello E, Hess Michelini R, Riba M, et al. T cells redirected to a minor histocompatibility antigen instruct intratumoral TNFalpha expression and empower adoptive cell therapy for solid tumors. *Cancer Res* (2017) 77(3):658–71. doi:10.1158/0008-5472.CAN-16-0725
40. Marcucci F, Bellone M, Rumio C, Corti A. Approaches to improve tumor accumulation and interactions between monoclonal antibodies and immune cells. *MAbs* (2013) 5(1):34–46. doi:10.4161/mabs.22775
41. Sharpe AH, Pauken KE. The diverse functions of the PD1 inhibitory pathway. *Nat Rev Immunol* (2018) 18(3):153–67. doi:10.1038/nri.2017.108
42. Sen DR, Kaminski J, Barnitz RA, Kurachi M, Gerdemann U, Yates KB, et al. The epigenetic landscape of T cell exhaustion. *Science* (2016) 354(6316):1165–9. doi:10.1126/science.aae0491
43. Ghoneim HE, Fan Y, Moustaki A, Abdelsamed HA, Dash P, Dogra P, et al. De novo epigenetic programs inhibit PD-1 blockade-mediated T cell rejuvenation. *Cell* (2017) 170(1):142–57.e19. doi:10.1016/j.cell.2017.06.007
44. Huang AC, Postow MA, Orlowski RJ, Mick R, Bengsch B, Manne S, et al. T-cell invigoration to tumour burden ratio associated with anti-PD-1 response. *Nature* (2017) 545(7652):60–5. doi:10.1038/nature22079
45. Mognol GP, Spreafico R, Wong V, Scott-Browne JP, Togher S, Hoffmann A, et al. Exhaustion-associated regulatory regions in CD8(+) tumor-infiltrating T cells. *Proc Natl Acad Sci U S A* (2017) 114(13):E2776–85. doi:10.1073/pnas.1620498114
46. Sanlorenzo M, Vujic I, Floris A, Novelli M, Gammaitoni L, Giraudo L, et al. BRAF and MEK inhibitors increase PD1-positive melanoma cells leading to a potential lymphocyte-independent synergism with anti-PD1 antibody. *Clin Cancer Res* (2018) 24(14):3377–85. doi:10.1158/1078-0432.CCR-17-1914
47. Gupta HB, Clark CA, Yuan B, Sareddy G, Pandeswara S, Padron AS, et al. Tumor cell-intrinsic PD-L1 promotes tumor-initiating cell generation and functions in melanoma and ovarian cancer. *Signal Transduct Target Ther* (2016) 1:16030. doi:10.1038/sigtrans.2016.30
48. Triebel F, Jitsukawa S, Baixeras E, Roman-Roman S, Genevee C, Viegas-Pequignot E, et al. LAG-3, a novel lymphocyte activation gene closely related to CD4. *J Exp Med* (1990) 171(5):1393–405. doi:10.1084/jem.171.5.1393
49. Xu F, Liu J, Liu D, Liu B, Wang M, Hu Z, et al. LSECtin expressed on melanoma cells promotes tumor progression by inhibiting antitumor T-cell responses. *Cancer Res* (2014) 74(13):3418–28. doi:10.1158/0008-5472.CAN-13-2690
50. Andreae S, Buisson S, Triebel F. MHC class II signal transduction in human dendritic cells induced by a natural ligand, the LAG-3 protein (CD223). *Blood* (2003) 102(6):2130–7. doi:10.1182/blood-2003-01-0273
51. Hemon P, Jean-Louis F, Ramgolam K, Brignone C, Viguier M, Bachelez H, et al. MHC class II engagement by its ligand LAG-3 (CD223) contributes to melanoma resistance to apoptosis. *J Immunol* (2011) 186(9):5173–83. doi:10.4049/jimmunol.1002050
52. Kouo T, Huang L, Pucsek AB, Cao M, Solt S, Armstrong T, et al. Galectin-3 shapes antitumor immune responses by suppressing CD8+ T cells via LAG-3 and inhibiting expansion of plasmacytoid dendritic cells. *Cancer Immunol Res* (2015) 3(4):412–23. doi:10.1158/2326-6066.CIR-14-0150

53. Hannier S, Tournier M, Bismuth G, Triebel F. CD3/TCR complex-associated lymphocyte activation gene-3 molecules inhibit CD3/TCR signaling. *J Immunol* (1998) 161(8):4058–65.
54. Woo SR, Turnis ME, Goldberg MV, Bankoti J, Selby M, Nirschl CJ, et al. Immune inhibitory molecules LAG-3 and PD-1 synergistically regulate T-cell function to promote tumoral immune escape. *Cancer Res* (2012) 72(4):917–27. doi:10.1158/0008-5472.CAN-11-1620
55. Grosso JF, Kelleher CC, Harris TJ, Maris CH, Hipkiss EL, De Marzo A, et al. LAG-3 regulates CD8+ T cell accumulation and effector function in murine self- and tumor-tolerance systems. *J Clin Invest* (2007) 117(11):3383–92. doi:10.1172/JCI31184
56. Sfanos KS, Bruno TC, Maris CH, Xu L, Thoburn CJ, DeMarzo AM, et al. Phenotypic analysis of prostate-infiltrating lymphocytes reveals TH17 and Treg skewing. *Clin Cancer Res* (2008) 14(11):3254–61. doi:10.1158/1078-0432.CCR-07-5164
57. Davidsson S, Andren O, Ohlson AL, Carlsson J, Andersson SO, Giunchi F, et al. FOXP3(+) regulatory T cells in normal prostate tissue, postatrophic hyperplasia, prostatic intraepithelial neoplasia, and tumor histological lesions in men with and without prostate cancer. *Prostate* (2018) 78(1):40–7. doi:10.1002/pros.23442
58. Sanchez-Fueyo A, Tian J, Picarella D, Domenig C, Zheng XX, Sabatos CA, et al. Tim-3 inhibits T helper type 1-mediated auto- and alloimmune responses and promotes immunological tolerance. *Nat Immunol* (2003) 4(11): 1093–101. doi:10.1038/ni987
59. Sakuishi K, Apetoh L, Sullivan JM, Blazar BR, Kuchroo VK, Anderson AC. Targeting Tim-3 and PD-1 pathways to reverse T cell exhaustion and restore anti-tumor immunity. *J Exp Med* (2010) 207(10):2187–94. doi:10.1084/jem.20100643
60. Fourcade J, Sun Z, Benallaoua M, Guillaume P, Luescher IF, Sander C, et al. Upregulation of Tim-3 and PD-1 expression is associated with tumor antigen-specific CD8+ T cell dysfunction in melanoma patients. *J Exp Med* (2010) 207(10):2175–86. doi:10.1084/jem.20100637
61. Japp AS, Kursunel MA, Meier S, Malzer JN, Li X, Rahman NA, et al. Dysfunction of PSA-specific CD8+ T cells in prostate cancer patients correlates with CD38 and Tim-3 expression. *Cancer Immunol Immunother* (2015) 64(11): 1487–94. doi:10.1007/s00262-015-1752-y
62. Tallerico R, Cristiani CM, Staaf E, Garofalo C, Sottile R, Capone M, et al. IL-15, TIM-3 and NK cells subsets predict responsiveness to anti-CTLA-4 treatment in melanoma patients. *Oncoimmunology* (2017) 6(2):e1261242. doi:10.1080/2162402X.2016.1261242
63. Piao YR, Piao LZ, Zhu LH, Jin ZH, Dong XZ. Prognostic value of T cell immunoglobulin mucin-3 in prostate cancer. *Asian Pac J Cancer Prev* (2013) 14(6):3897–901. doi:10.7314/APJCP.2013.14.6.3897
64. Wu J, Lin G, Zhu Y, Zhang H, Shi G, Shen Y, et al. Low TIM3 expression indicates poor prognosis of metastatic prostate cancer and acts as an independent predictor of castration resistant status. *Sci Rep* (2017) 7(1):8869. doi:10.1038/s41598-017-09484-8
65. Kang CW, Dutta A, Chang LY, Mahalingam J, Lin YC, Chiang JM, et al. Apoptosis of tumor infiltrating effector TIM-3+CD8+ T cells in colon cancer. *Sci Rep* (2015) 5:15659. doi:10.1038/srep15659
66. Huang YH, Zhu C, Kondo Y, Anderson AC, Gandhi A, Russell A, et al. CEACAM1 regulates TIM-3-mediated tolerance and exhaustion. *Nature* (2015) 517(7534):386–90. doi:10.1038/nature13848
67. Gleason MK, Lenvik TR, McCullar V, Felices M, O'Brien MS, Cooley SA, et al. Tim-3 is an inducible human natural killer cell receptor that enhances interferon gamma production in response to galectin-9. *Blood* (2012) 119(13):3064–72. doi:10.1182/blood-2011-06-360321
68. Seo H, Jeon I, Kim BS, Park M, Bae EA, Song B, et al. IL-21-mediated reversal of NK cell exhaustion facilitates anti-tumour immunity in MHC class I-deficient tumours. *Nat Commun* (2017) 8:15776. doi:10.1038/ncomms15776
69. da Silva IP, Gallois A, Jimenez-Baranda S, Khan S, Anderson AC, Kuchroo VK, et al. Reversal of NK-cell exhaustion in advanced melanoma by Tim-3 blockade. *Cancer Immunol Res* (2014) 2(5):410–22. doi:10.1158/2326-6066.CIR-13-0171
70. Han G, Chen G, Shen B, Li Y. Tim-3: an activation marker and activation limiter of innate immune cells. *Front Immunol* (2013) 4:449. doi:10.3389/fimmu.2013.00449
71. Nakayama M, Akiba H, Takeda K, Kojima Y, Hashiguchi M, Azuma M, et al. Tim-3 mediates phagocytosis of apoptotic cells and cross-presentation. *Blood* (2009) 113(16):3821–30. doi:10.1182/blood-2008-10-185884
72. Chiba S, Baghdadi M, Akiba H, Yoshiyama H, Kinoshita I, Dosaka-Akita H, et al. Tumor-infiltrating DCs suppress nucleic acid-mediated innate immune responses through interactions between the receptor TIM-3 and the alarmin HMGB1. *Nat Immunol* (2012) 13(9):832–42. doi:10.1038/ni.2376
73. Zhang Y, Ma CJ, Wang JM, Ji XJ, Wu XY, Moorman JP, et al. Tim-3 regulates pro- and anti-inflammatory cytokine expression in human CD14+ monocytes. *J Leukoc Biol* (2012) 91(2):189–96. doi:10.1189/jlb.1010591
74. Dardalhon V, Anderson AC, Karman J, Apetoh L, Chandwaskar R, Lee DH, et al. Tim-3/galectin-9 pathway: regulation of Th1 immunity through promotion of CD11b+Ly-6G+ myeloid cells. *J Immunol* (2010) 185(3):1383–92. doi:10.4049/jimmunol.0903275
75. Liu FT, Rabinovich GA. Galectins as modulators of tumour progression. *Nat Rev Cancer* (2005) 5(1):29–41. doi:10.1038/nrc1527
76. Prieto VG, Mourad-Zeidan AA, Melnikova V, Johnson MM, Lopez A, Diwan AH, et al. Galectin-3 expression is associated with tumor progression and pattern of sun exposure in melanoma. *Clin Cancer Res* (2006) 12(22):6709–15. doi:10.1158/1078-0432.CCR-06-0758
77. Braeuer RR, Zigler M, Kamiya T, Dobroff AS, Huang L, Choi W, et al. Galectin-3 contributes to melanoma growth and metastasis via regulation of NFAT1 and autotaxin. *Cancer Res* (2012) 72(22):5757–66. doi:10.1158/0008-5472.CAN-12-2424
78. Shoshan E, Braeuer RR, Kamiya T, Mobley AK, Huang L, Vasquez ME, et al. NFAT1 directly regulates IL8 and MMP3 to promote melanoma tumor growth and metastasis. *Cancer Res* (2016) 76(11):3145–55. doi:10.1158/0008-5472.CAN-15-2511
79. Gordon-Alonso M, Hirsch T, Wildmann C, van der Bruggen P. Galectin-3 captures interferon-gamma in the tumor matrix reducing chemokine gradient production and T-cell tumor infiltration. *Nat Commun* (2017) 8(1):793. doi:10.1038/s41467-017-00925-6
80. Melief SM, Visconti VV, Visser M, van Diepen M, Kapiteijn EH, van den Berg JH, et al. Long-term survival and clinical benefit from adoptive T-cell transfer in stage IV melanoma patients is determined by a four-parameter tumor immune signature. *Cancer Immunol Res* (2017) 5(2):170–9. doi:10.1158/2326-6066.CIR-16-0288
81. Demotte N, Wieers G, Van Der Smissen P, Moser M, Schmidt C, Thielemans K, et al. A galectin-3 ligand corrects the impaired function of human CD4 and CD8 tumor-infiltrating lymphocytes and favors tumor rejection in mice. *Cancer Res* (2010) 70(19):7476–88. doi:10.1158/0008-5472.CAN-10-0761
82. Knapp JS, Lokeshwar SD, Vogel U, Hennenlotter J, Schwentner C, Kramer MW, et al. Galectin-3 expression in prostate cancer and benign prostate tissues: correlation with biochemical recurrence. *World J Urol* (2013) 31(2):351–8. doi:10.1007/s00345-012-0925-y
83. Pienta KJ, Naik H, Akhtar A, Yamazaki K, Replogle TS, Lehr J, et al. Inhibition of spontaneous metastasis in a rat prostate cancer model by oral administration of modified citrus pectin. *J Natl Cancer Inst* (1995) 87(5):348–53. doi:10.1093/jnci/87.5.348
84. Ilmer M, Mazurek N, Byrd JC, Ramirez K, Hafley M, Alt E, et al. Cell surface galectin-3 defines a subset of chemoresistant gastrointestinal tumor-initiating cancer cells with heightened stem cell characteristics. *Cell Death Dis* (2016) 7(8):e2337. doi:10.1038/cddis.2016.239
85. Tummala KS, Brandt M, Teijeiro A, Grana O, Schwabe RF, Perna C, et al. Hepatocellular carcinomas originate predominantly from hepatocytes and benign lesions from hepatic progenitor cells. *Cell Rep* (2017) 19(3):584–600. doi:10.1016/j.celrep.2017.03.059
86. Jachetti E, Caputo S, Mazzoleni S, Brambillasca CS, Parigi SM, Grioni M, et al. Tenascin-C protects cancer stem-like cells from immune surveillance by arresting T-cell activation. *Cancer Res* (2015) 75(10):2095–108. doi:10.1158/0008-5472.CAN-14-2346
87. Galluzzi L, Buque A, Kepp O, Zitvogel L, Kroemer G. Immunological effects of conventional chemotherapy and targeted anticancer agents. *Cancer Cell* (2015) 28(6):690–714. doi:10.1016/j.ccell.2015.10.012
88. Bellone M, Calcinotto A. Ways to enhance lymphocyte trafficking into tumors and fitness of tumor infiltrating lymphocytes. *Front Oncol* (2013) 3:231. doi:10.3389/fonc.2013.00231
89. Bellone M, Calcinotto A, Corti A. Won't you come on in? How to favor lymphocyte infiltration in tumors. *Oncoimmunology* (2012) 1(6):986–8. doi:10.4161/onci.20213

90. Bellone M, Mondino A, Corti A. Vascular targeting, chemotherapy and active immunotherapy: teaming up to attack cancer. *Trends Immunol* (2008) 29(5):235–41. doi:10.1016/j.it.2008.02.003
91. Ravi R, Noonan KA, Pham V, Bedi R, Zhavoronkov A, Ozerov IV, et al. Bifunctional immune checkpoint-targeted antibody-ligand traps that simultaneously disable TGFbeta enhance the efficacy of cancer immunotherapy. *Nat Commun* (2018) 9(1):741. doi:10.1038/s41467-017-02696-6
92. Chen TW, Razak AR, Bedard PL, Siu LL, Hansen AR. A systematic review of immune-related adverse event reporting in clinical trials of immune checkpoint inhibitors. *Ann Oncol* (2015) 26(9):1824–9. doi:10.1093/annonc/mdv182

10

Controlling the Immune Suppressor: Transcription Factors and MicroRNAs Regulating CD73/NT5E

*Theresa Kordaß[1,2], Wolfram Osen[1] and Stefan B. Eichmüller[1]**

[1] GMP & T Cell Therapy Unit, German Cancer Research Center (DKFZ), Heidelberg, Germany, [2] Faculty of Biosciences, University Heidelberg, Heidelberg, Germany

Edited by:
Alexandr Bazhin,
Klinikum der Universität
München, Germany

Reviewed by:
Jörg Wischhusen,
Universität Würzburg, Germany
Ivan Shevchenko,
Ludwig-Maximilians-Universität
München, Germany
Camilla Jandus,
Université de Lausanne,
Switzerland

***Correspondence:**
Stefan B. Eichmüller
s.eichmueller@dkfz.de

The NT5E (CD73) molecule represents an ecto-5′-nucleotidase expressed on the cell surface of various cell types. Hydrolyzing extracellular adenosine monophosphate into adenosine and inorganic phosphate, NT5E performs numerous homeostatic functions in healthy organs and tissues. Importantly, NT5E can act as inhibitory immune checkpoint molecule, since free adenosine generated by NT5E inhibits cellular immune responses, thereby promoting immune escape of tumor cells. MicroRNAs (miRNAs) are small non-coding RNA molecules regulating gene expression on posttranscriptional level through binding to mRNAs, resulting in translational repression or degradation of the targeted mRNA molecule. In tumor cells, miRNA expression patterns are often altered which in turn might affect NT5E surface expression and eventually influence the efficacy of antitumor immune responses. This review describes the diverse roles of NT5E, summarizes current knowledge about transcription factors controlling NT5E expression, and highlights the significance of miRNAs involved in the posttranscriptional regulation of NT5E expression.

Keywords: checkpoint molecule, CD73, NT5E, microRNA, transcription factor, T cell, tumor, A2A receptor

FUNCTIONS OF NT5E IN HEALTHY TISSUE AND TUMORS

The membrane bound NT5E (CD73) is an ecto-5′-nucleotidase (NT5E) hydrolyzing extracellular adenosine monophosphate (AMP) into adenosine and inorganic phosphate (1) (**Figure 1A**). The enzyme consists of a homodimer inserted into the cellular membrane by glycophosphatidylinositol anchors. Besides hydrolyzing AMP to adenosine, NT5E has nucleosidase activity as shown for nicotinamide adenine dinucleotide and nicotinamide mononucleotide (2, 3). NT5E works in concert with ectonucleoside triphosphate diphosphohydrolase-1 (ENTPD1), which is also referred to as CD39, representing another ectonucleotidase acting upstream of NT5E catalyzing the hydrolysis of adenosine triphosphate (ATP) into AMP through two reversible reaction steps, whereas the final NT5E-mediated reaction from AMP to adenosine is largely irreversible (4) (**Figure 1A**). The two C-terminal domains of the NT5E molecule mediate noncovalent homodimer association and harbor the substrate binding sites (2). The molecular structure of NT5E can exhibit open or closed conformation and transition between these two stages occurs during substrate cleavage involving conformational changes enabled by the flexible α-helix connecting the C-terminal domains with the Zn^{2+} binding N-terminal domains (3), the latter being N-glycosylated at four distinct asparagine residues either by mannose saccharide chains or by a mixture of complex glycans and high mannose (2). Besides expression of the full-length molecule NT5EL (NT5E-201, 574 aa), a spliced version lacking exon 7 designated NT5ES (NT5E-203, 525 aa) can be detected in various human tissues and was found intracellularly overexpressed in human hepatocellular carcinoma cell lines (5).

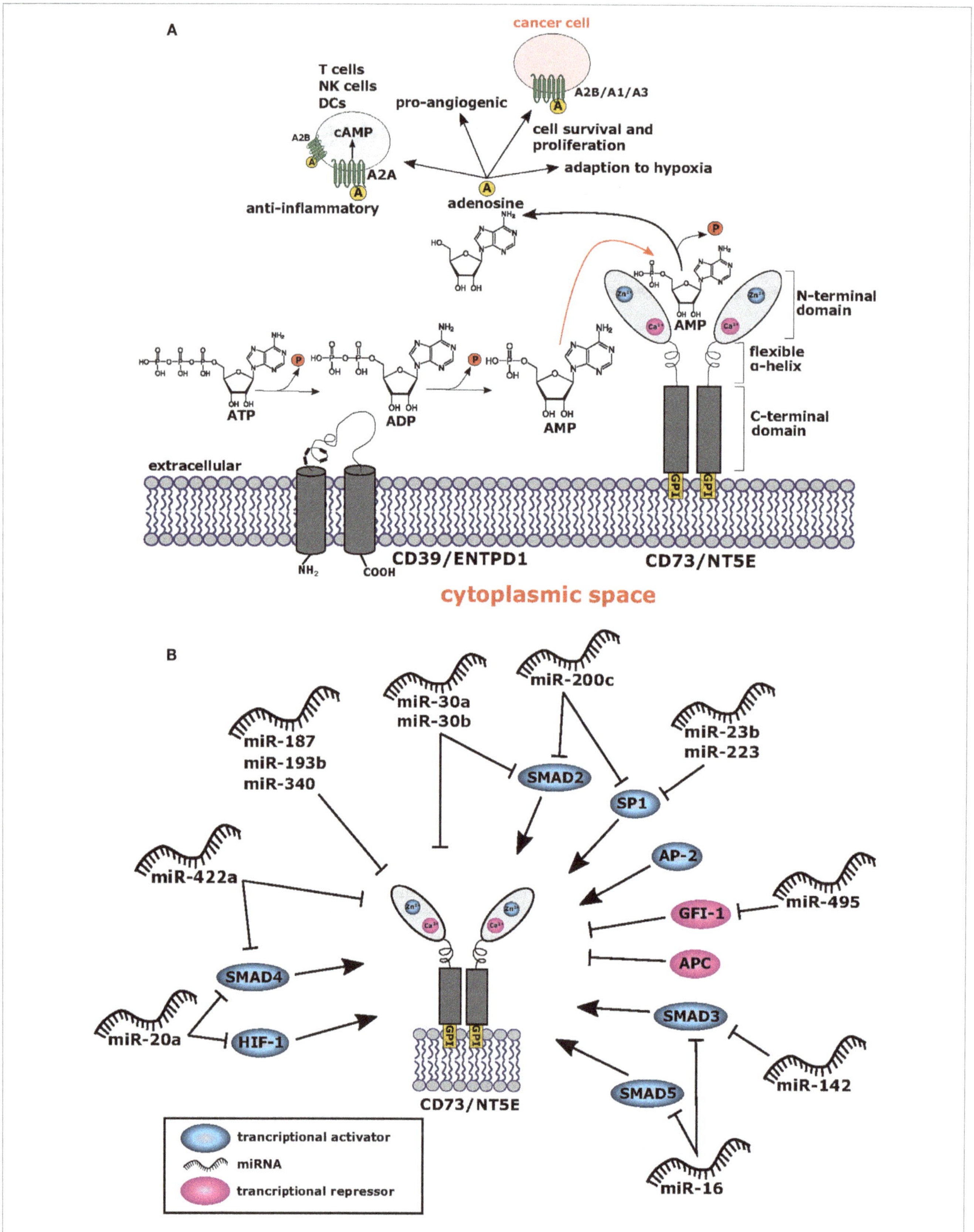

FIGURE 1 | Continued

FIGURE 1 | (A) Structure and function of CD73/NT5E. The membrane bound ecto-5′-nucleotidase NT5E hydrolyzes extracellular adenosine monophosphate (AMP) into adenosine and inorganic phosphate (P). Upstream of NT5E, adenosine triphosphate (ATP) is hydrolyzed *via* two reaction steps into AMP by the enzyme ectonucleoside triphosphate diphosphohydrolase-1 (ENTPD1) (CD39). Adenosine thus produced exerts anti-inflammatory effects by binding to the adenosine A2A receptor (ADORA2A) expressed by T cells, natural killer (NK) cells, and dendritic cells (DCs) resulting in cAMP mediated blocking of their effector functions. To some extent, the A2B receptor (ADORA2B) is also expressed on DCs and macrophages which are suppressed by adenosine. Thus, cancer cells can evade the immune system by upregulating NT5E protein levels. Furthermore, adenosine binds to the A2B receptor expressed by cancer cells leading to tumor cell survival and proliferation. Cancer cells also express the adenosine A1 receptor (ADORA1) and A3 receptor (ADORA3) and binding of adenosine to these receptors leads to tumor cell migration and proliferation *via* signaling through Gαi proteins. Adenosine is also involved in the adaption to hypoxia and shows pro-angiogenic potential. All adenosine receptors are depicted as stylized green transmembrane proteins. Adenosine is also symbolized as yellow circles marked with "A". **(B)** Network of transcription factors and microRNAs (miRNAs) regulating NT5E expression. This network summarizes the current knowledge on regulation of NT5E on transcriptional (TFs) and posttranscriptional level by TFs and miRNAs, respectively. Transcriptional activators are depicted in blue and transcriptional repressors are highlighted in magenta. miRNAs targeting NT5E directly are shown, as well as miRNAs with indirect impact on NT5E expression through targeting of transcriptional regulators.

As depletion of amino acids 404–453 encoded by exon 7 prevents homo dimerization, NT5ES shows impaired substrate binding resulting in abrogated 5′-nucleotidase activity and lack of surface expression. Importantly, overexpression of NT5ES was shown to cause proteasome-mediated degradation of intracellular NT5EL, without affecting expression levels of native NT5EL dimers. Thus, altered splicing patterns commonly observed in many tumors (6–8) might contribute to aberrant NT5E expression levels in cancer cells.

Considering healthy tissue, expression of NT5E is detectable in epithelial cells of the respiratory tract, smooth muscle cells, and cardiac myocytes and other tissues, as can be deduced from the bioGPS mRNA expression data base (9) using the data set of Primary Cell Atlas (10). Under physiological conditions, NT5E has been described as a regulator of epithelial ion transport, thereby preserving mucosal hydration (11). Moreover, NT5E can act as gate keeper on endothelial cells as free adenosine facilitates "resealing" of gaps between vascular endothelial cells left behind by transmigrating neutrophils (12). Furthermore, adenosine generated through NT5E was described to restrict inflammatory immune responses through a negative feedback loop on adenosine receptor expressing neutrophils (13). NT5E has been found expressed on regulatory T cells (T_{reg}) and at even higher levels on anergic $CD4^+$ T cells, thereby preserving self tolerance in healthy individuals and protecting the fetus from maternal immune attack during pregnancy (14, 15).

Interestingly, qualitative differences in NT5E function have been described depending on the NT5E expressing cell type (16, 17). Comparing epithelial cells and lymphocytes, both expressing NT5E, lymphocyte NT5E was found susceptible to phosphatidylinositol phospholipase to greater extent compared to NT5E expressed by epithelial cells (16). In the same study, antibody binding to NT5E triggered shedding from the surface of lymphocytes, but not in the case of epithelial cells. A similar observation was reported by others who proposed NT5E shedding from the surface of B16F10 cells as explanation for absent cell surface staining on murine B16F10 melanoma cells despite detection of intracellular NT5E expression (18). The study by Airas et al. (16) demonstrated also signal transduction activity of NT5E expressed on lymphocytes, whereas NT5E expressing epithelial cells lacked this function. Signal transduction by NT5E appears unexpected since this molecule lacks intracellular signaling domains (**Figure 1A**); however, it has been suggested that NT5E might associate with src protein kinases, thereby facilitating cellular signal transduction as proposed by Wang and colleagues (19, 20). Alternatively, NT5E might also mediate signal transduction directly (19).

In pathophysiological situations, NT5E activity was found relevant for the generation of cardio-protective adenosine in the ischemic myocardium (21) or for adaption to hypoxia (see below). Importantly, NT5E is involved in tumor development. Thus, NT5E has been described to sustain tumor angiogenesis in murine tumor models of breast cancer and prostate cancer (20, 22) as well as in xenograft models of humans breast cancer (23). Likewise, NT5E expression promoted invasion and metastasis of murine and human melanoma cells (24) and of human breast cancer cells (25).

Notably, NT5E plays a significant role as immune-inhibitory checkpoint molecule (26). Thus, infiltration of tumors by NT5E expressing regulatory immune cells such as T_{reg} (27), MDSCs (28), or dendritic cells (DCs) (29) results in accumulation of immunosuppressive adenosine that can activate cAMP signaling in T cells expressing A2A adenosine receptors (ADORA2A). Moreover, adenosine receptors were found to be expressed on DCs, macrophages, MDSCs, and natural killer (NK) cells, implying that adenosine can repress the function of these immune cells (30, 31). Recently, an interesting phenomenon was described showing that T_{reg} undergoing apoptosis within the metabolically abnormal tumor microenvironment release substantial amounts of ATP, that is degraded by the nucleotidases of the faded T_{reg} resulting in accumulating adenosine levels (32). Adenosine can then trigger immune suppressive downstream effects among T cells like inhibition of chemotaxis, proliferation, activation, and effector function (33, 34). In light of its immune suppressive function and due to its expression by various tumor entities, such as melanoma (35–37), triple-negative breast cancer (34, 38), colorectal cancer (CRC) (39), and non-small cell lung cancer (40), NT5E has been considered as target checkpoint molecule for novel tumor immunotherapy approaches (41, 42). Indeed, injection of blocking NT5E-specific ab into tumor bearing mice resulted in reduced outgrowth of NT5E expressing tumors as shown for various tumor entities (43–45). Noteworthy, tumor cells can express adenosine A1 receptor (ADORA1) and ADORA3 receptors coupled to Gαi proteins, fostering tumor cell proliferation and migration (46). Moreover, therapeutic targeting of NT5E using specific inhibitors or blocking antibodies, respectively, has been proposed (22, 34, 38, 47–50) and is presently tested in a phase I clinical trial (NCT02503774).

In addition to its enzymatic function, NT5E can act as a receptor molecule shown to mediate cell–cell adhesion between lymphocytes and endothelial cells (51). Moreover, it was demonstrated that NT5E was can interact with extracellular matrix components (ECM) (34, 52, 53). This interaction occurred independently from enzymatic activity of NT5E, as blocking of ectonucleotidase function by concanavalin A did not affect interaction with ECM components like fibronectin, tenascin C, or collagen 1. In fact, NT5E turned out to mediate cell adhesion and migration *via* interaction with tenascin C (53).

Thus, NT5E appears to support tumor growth at multiple levels, i.e., by suppression of antitumoral immune responses *via* supply of adenosine and through facilitated dissemination of malignant cells from the primary tumor.

TRANSCRIPTIONAL REGULATION OF NT5E EXPRESSION

The promoter region of NT5E contains binding sites for the transcription factors SP1, AP-2, and SMAD proteins as well as cAMP-responsive elements (54, 55) (**Figure 1B**; **Table 1**). Chromatin immunoprecipitation showed that transcription factors SMAD2, SMAD3, SMAD4, SMAD5, and SP1 bind to the rat NT5E promoter, with SMAD5 and SP1 being most efficient (55). As rat and human NT5E transcripts share 89% identity (56), it appears possible that human NT5E expression might be regulated by SMAD transcription factors as well.

Interestingly, hypoxia-inducible factor-1 (HIF-1) can directly bind to the NT5E promoter thereby activating NT5E expression (57), which is in line with the functional role described for NT5E in hypoxia adaptation (79). Thus, hypoxia resulting from uncontrolled tumor cell proliferation (80) might induce HIF mediated upregulation of NT5E expression on tumor cells. Another biochemical cascade often altered in tumors is the β-catenin-dependent Wnt signaling pathway (81). The promoter core sequence of NT5E is flanked upstream by a regulatory region containing consensus motifs for T cell factor 1 (TCF-1), representing a component of Wnt/β-catenin signaling pathway. In fact, expression of β-catenin could drastically enhance expression of NT5E. This upregulation was found to be dependent on the presence of TCF-1. Interestingly, the authors could also show that the antagonist of β-catenin, adenomatous polyposis coli protein, inhibits NT5E expression (59). The activation of NT5E

TABLE 1 | List of transcription factors and miRNAs regulating NT5E.

Target	Regulator	Effect on NT5E	Host cell	Reference
NT5E	SP1	Activation	Human WI-L2	Hansen et al. (54)
			Rat hepatocytes	Fausther et al. (55)
NT5E	TFAP2A	Activation	Human WI-L2	Hansen et al. (54)
NT5E	SMAD2	Activation	Rat hepatocytes	Fausther et al. (55)
NT5E	SMAD3	Activation	Rat hepatocytes	Fausther et al. (55)
NT5E	SMAD4	Activation	Rat hepatocytes	Fausther et al. (55)
NT5E	SMAD5	Activation	Rat hepatocytes	Fausther et al. (55)
NT5E	HIF1A	Activation	Human T84 epithelial cells	Synnestvedt et al. (57)
			Human HepaRG cells	Tak et al. (58)
NT5E	TCF-1/β-catenin	Activation	Human HeLa and Jurkat cells, monkey Cos-7 cells	Spychala and Kitajewski (59)
NT5E	APC	Inhibition	Human SW480 colon cancer cells	Spychala and Kitajewski (59)
NT5E	NFκB/TNFα	Activation	Human HT29 colon cancer cells	Pagnotta et al. (60)
NT5E	PPARγ	Inhibition	Human HT29 colon cancer cells	Pagnotta et al. (60)
NT5E	GFI-1	Inhibition	Murine Th17 cells	Chalmin et al. (61)
NT5E	STAT3	Activation	Murine Th17 cells	Chalmin et al. (61)
NT5E	FOXP3	Activation	Murine T_{reg} cells	Zheng et al. (62)
NT5E	miR-422a	Inhibition	Human SCC61, SQ20B and HaCaT cells	Bonnin et al. (63)
NT5E	miR-30 family	Inhibition	Human colorectal cancer	Xie et al. (64)
			Human gallbladder cancer	Wang et al. (65)
NT5E	miR-340	Inhibition	Human gallbladder cancer	Wang et al. (65)
NT5E	miR-187	Inhibition	Human colon cancer SW480, RKO and SW620	Zhang et al. (66)
NT5E	miR-193b	Inhibition	Human pancreatic cancer	Ikeda et al. (67)
SP1	miR-23b	Inhibition	Human MM and WM tumor cells	Fulciniti et al. (68)
SP1	miR-223	Inhibition	Human gastric cancer MGC-803, SGC-7901 and BGC-823	Hu et al. (69)
SP1	miR-200c	Inhibition	Human gastric cancer MGC-803 and AGS	Tang et al. (70)
SMAD2	miR-200c	Inhibition	Human ATC-derived cells	Braun et al. (71)
SMAD2	miR-30 family	Inhibition	Human ATC-derived cells	Braun et al. (71)
SMAD3	miR-16	Inhibition	Human Osteosarcoma	Jones et al. (72)
SMAD3	miR-142	Inhibition	Human HT29 colon cancer cells	Chanda et al. (73)
			MDA-MB-231 breast cancer cells	Ma et al. (74)
SMAD4	miR-20a	Inhibition	Human HT29 and HCT116 colon cancer cells	Cheng et al. (75)
HIF1A	miR-20a	Inhibition	HeLa cells, primary human macrophages	Poitz et al. (76)
GFI1	miR-495	Activation	Human DAOY and D283 (medulloblastoma) cells	Wang et al. (77)
SMAD4	miR-422a	Inhibition	Human LHCN-M2 muscle cells	Paul et al. (78)

MM, multiple myeloma; WM, Waldenstrom's macroglobulinemia; ATC, anaplastic thyroid carcinoma; miRNAs, microRNAs; HIF-1, hypoxia-inducible factor-1; TCF-1, T cell factor 1; APC, adenomatous polyposis coli; T_{reg}, regulatory T cells.

expression by β-catenin was also confirmed by Pagnotta et al. who furthermore identified NFκB/TNFα as positive transcriptional regulators of NT5E (60). Seeking biomarkers for CRC, the authors applied a translational pathology approach and identified NT5E among others as a prognostic marker. In line with these findings, NT5E levels were found significantly upregulated in tumor specimens compared to normal colonic mucosa samples. Spranger et al. found that active β-catenin signaling was negatively associated with T cell infiltration in human melanoma samples. This was confirmed in authochtonous tumor models with inducible β-catenin expression, where absence of T cells was observed selectively in β-catenin expressing tumors (82). It is tempting to speculate that this immune suppressive effect on T cell infiltration might result from enhanced NT5E expression induced through β-catenin signaling. Of note, besides activating mechanisms on NT5E expression *via* NFκB/TNFα signaling pathways, also negative effects on NT5E expression through of PPARγ have been described (60).

In murine Th17 cells differentiated with IL-6 and TGF-β *in vitro*, IL-6 was found to activate Stat3, while TGF-β suppressed the transcription factor Gfi-1. As shown by the authors Stat3 sustained, whereas Gfi-1 repressed expression of ENTPD1 and NT5E through specific promoter binding, thus demonstrating transcriptional regulation of these exonucleotidases in Th17 cells through IL-6 and TGF-β (61).

A genome-wide analysis to identify forkhead box transcription factor (Foxp3) target genes in mouse led to the identification of Nt5e as one target gene of Foxp3 in mature T_{reg} cells (62). Foxp3 is a specific transcription factor expressed in murine and human T_{reg} cells and in recently activated human T cells (83). Thus, regulation of Nt5e by Foxp3 appears cell type specific and does not necessarily apply the same way to cancer cells. Noteworthy, high expression levels of FOXP3 in ovarian cancer has been identified as a prognostic marker for poor survival of patients (84).

MICRORNAs (miRNAs) REGULATING NT5E EXPRESSION

MicroRNAs are small non-coding RNA molecules that bind to the 3′ untranslated region (3′-UTR) of target mRNAs, thereby blocking translation or inducing degradation of the targeted mRNA molecule, respectively, depending on the degree of complementary among the interacting nucleotide sequences (85). In cancer cells, aberrant miRNA expression patterns resulting in impaired regulation of target mRNA expression is commonly observed. Tumor cell-derived miRNAs have therefore gained relevance as biomarkers and as prognostic factors as described (86–88). Of note, the 3′-UTR of NT5E comprises 1,774 nucleotides (89) (NM_001204813.1), exceeding the average size of a human 3′-UTR (90) approximately threefold. Thus, regulation of NT5E expression by miRNAs appears to be particularly restrictive. To date, only a few miRNAs have been described that directly regulate NT5E expression (**Table 1**). Bonnin and co-workers reported the regulation of NT5E by miR-422a in head and neck squamous cell carcinoma (HNSCC) patients. The authors found a significant negative correlation between expression levels of miR-422a levels and NT5E mRNA. Blocking of endogenous miR-422a by specific antagomiRs resulted in increased NT5E protein levels with enhanced enzymatic activity. Reduced levels of miR-422a correlated with shorter relapse free survival times in HNSCC, potentially due to overexpression of NT5E (63).

Recently, miR-30a was found to target NT5E in CRC (64). In this study, transfection with miR-30a reduced NT5E expression on the mRNA and on protein level and direct interaction of miR-30a with the NT5E 3′-UTR was demonstrated *via* luciferase reporter assays. Similarly, direct regulation of NT5E was described through miR-30a-5p in non-small cell lung cancer (91). Enhanced expression of NT5E was accompanied by reduced miR-30a-5p expression, whereas miR-30a-5p overexpression resulted in downregulated NT5E expression on mRNA and protein levels. At the same time, proliferation, cell migration, and invasion of these cells were significantly reduced. These effects were mimicked by silencing NT5E expression using shRNA directed against NT5E.

Interestingly, the miR-30 family shares the same seed sequence (92). Thus, other miRNAs from this family might also regulate NT5E. Indeed, direct regulation of NT5E by miR-30b was shown by Wang et al. in gall bladder carcinoma (GBC). Including miR-340 in their study, the authors found that overexpression of miR-30b or miR-340 reduced GBC cell proliferation, migration, and invasion. For both miRNAs, direct interaction with the NT5E 3′-UTR could be verified and NT5E overexpression partially reverted these miRNA-mediated effects in GBC cells (65). In CRC, miR-187 levels were found strongly downregulated compared to adjacent normal tissue leading to the establishment of miR-187 expression levels as prognostic marker for CRC patients. In fact, transfection of miR-187 reduced cell proliferation and migration *in vitro* and decelerated tumor growth of CRC lines *in vivo*. In the same study, direct targeting of NT5E by miR-187 was demonstrated (66). Studies focused on miRNAs involved in the MAPK pathway of human pancreatic cancer cell lines revealed miR-193b as a direct binder of the NT5E 3′-UTR. However, in this study, binding specificity using a mutated reporter plasmid was not controlled and effects of miR-193 overexpression on NT5E expression on mRNA and protein level were not analyzed (67).

Considering the extraordinary size of the NT5E 3′-UTR region, the restricted number of validated miRNAs identified so far that directly target NT5E mRNA most likely represent just the tip of the iceberg. Further studies are needed to broaden the spectrum of known miRNAs that directly regulate NT5E surface expression, thereby potentially affecting the tumor cells' vulnerability toward immune attack.

On the other hand, miRNAs can also function *via* indirect circuits, for example, by targeting transcription factors of NT5E, opening an alternative route for miRNA-mediated regulation of NT5E expression. In fact, miR-23b was found to directly suppress expression of transcription factor SP1 in multiple myeloma cells (68), and in gastric cancer, an inhibiting effect of miR-223 on epithelial to mesenchymal transition *via* direct posttranscriptional silencing of SP1 was reported (69). Other authors described miR-200b and miR-200c as direct inhibitors of SP1 transcription within this tumor entity (70). Whether the miRNA-mediated inhibition of SP1 expression resulted also in downstream reduction of NT5E expression levels was not investigated in these studies.

In a study by Braun et al., the authors focused on the identification of miRNAs affecting the invasive potential of anaplastic thyroid carcinoma and found miR-200c and miR-30a–e to target SMAD2 (71), representing another transcriptional activator of NT5E. Similarly, miR-16 might indirectly downregulate NT5E expression, as this miRNA was shown to inhibit expression of the transcription factors SMAD3 and, to lesser extent, SMAD5 in human osteosarcoma lines (72). Furthermore, SMAD3 is also targeted by miR-142-5p as shown in human rotavirus infected cells as well as in human breast and lung cancer cell lines (73, 74).

Further examples of miRNA-targeted transcription factors of NT5E are SMAD4 and HIF1A downregulated by miR-20a-5p (75), and Poitz et al. showed the direct downregulation of HIF1A by miR-20a (76). As mentioned above, miR-422a was shown to directly regulate NT5E, however, SMAD4 has also been described as a direct target of miR-422a (78), suggesting that miR-422a has the capacity to decrease NT5E levels both directly and indirectly. One example for a miRNA that could indirectly lead to an upregulation of NT5E levels is miR-495, which was shown to target one of NT5E's transcriptional repressor GFI1 in medulloblastoma cells (77).

CONCLUSION

NT5E (CD73) has emerged as a novel target for tumor immunotherapy approaches, since functional inhibition of NT5E reversed its immunosuppressive effects resulting in tumor immune attack and eradication of cancer cells by cytotoxic $CD8^+$ T cells and NK cells. Knowledge about NT5E regulation on the transcriptional and posttranscriptional level might provide a deeper understanding how cancer cells acquire aberrant NT5E expression to facilitate immune escape. We suggest a complex regulatory network of activatory and inhibitory transcription factors acting in conjunction with miRNAs to control NT5E expression. Interestingly, certain regulators such as miR-422a exert their effect on NT5E expression both directly as well as indirectly, i.e., through binding to the 3′-UTRs of NT5E mRNA and SMAD4 mRNA, the latter representing a transcriptional activator of NT5E. Even though the 3′-UTR region of NT5E is of extraordinary size, only few miRNAs have been described so far that regulate NT5E expression. Identification of further miRNAs targeting NT5E will help to unravel the complex regulation of NT5E expression in cancer cells.

AUTHOR CONTRIBUTIONS

TK, WO, and SE wrote this paper. TK generated the figures.

REFERENCES

1. Robson SC, Sevigny J, Zimmermann H. The E-NTPDase family of ectonucleotidases: structure function relationships and pathophysiological significance. *Purinergic Signal* (2006) 2(2):409–30. doi:10.1007/s11302-006-9003-5
2. Strater N. Ecto-5'-nucleotidase: structure function relationships. *Purinergic Signal* (2006) 2(2):343–50. doi:10.1007/s11302-006-9000-8
3. Knapp K, Zebisch M, Pippel J, El-Tayeb A, Muller CE, Strater N. Crystal structure of the human ecto-5'-nucleotidase (CD73): insights into the regulation of purinergic signaling. *Structure* (2012) 20(12):2161–73. doi:10.1016/j.str.2012.10.001
4. Antonioli L, Pacher P, Vizi ES, Hasko G. CD39 and CD73 in immunity and inflammation. *Trends Mol Med* (2013) 19(6):355–67. doi:10.1016/j.molmed.2013.03.005
5. Snider NT, Altshuler PJ, Wan S, Welling TH, Cavalcoli J, Omary MB. Alternative splicing of human NT5E in cirrhosis and hepatocellular carcinoma produces a negative regulator of ecto-5'-nucleotidase (CD73). *Mol Biol Cell* (2014) 25(25):4024–33. doi:10.1091/mbc.E14-06-1167
6. Oltean S, Bates DO. Hallmarks of alternative splicing in cancer. *Oncogene* (2014) 33(46):5311–8. doi:10.1038/onc.2013.533
7. Climente-Gonzalez H, Porta-Pardo E, Godzik A, Eyras E. The functional impact of alternative splicing in cancer. *Cell Rep* (2017) 20(9):2215–26. doi:10.1016/j.celrep.2017.08.012
8. Singh B, Eyras E. The role of alternative splicing in cancer. *Transcription* (2017) 8(2):91–8. doi:10.1080/21541264.2016.1268245
9. Wu C, Jin X, Tsueng G, Afrasiabi C, Su AI. BioGPS: building your own mash-up of gene annotations and expression profiles. *Nucleic Acids Res* (2016) 44(D1):D313–6. doi:10.1093/nar/gkv1104
10. Mabbott NA, Baillie JK, Brown H, Freeman TC, Hume DA. An expression atlas of human primary cells: inference of gene function from coexpression networks. *BMC Genomics* (2013) 14:632. doi:10.1186/1471-2164-14-632
11. Strohmeier GR, Lencer WI, Patapoff TW, Thompson LF, Carlson SL, Moe SJ, et al. Surface expression, polarization, and functional significance of CD73 in human intestinal epithelia. *J Clin Invest* (1997) 99(11):2588–601. doi:10.1172/JCI119447
12. Lennon PF, Taylor CT, Stahl GL, Colgan SP. Neutrophil-derived 5'-adenosine monophosphate promotes endothelial barrier function via CD73-mediated conversion to adenosine and endothelial A2B receptor activation. *J Exp Med* (1998) 188(8):1433–43. doi:10.1084/jem.188.8.1433
13. Eltzschig HK, Ibla JC, Furuta GT, Leonard MO, Jacobson KA, Enjyoji K, et al. Coordinated adenine nucleotide phosphohydrolysis and nucleoside signaling in posthypoxic endothelium: role of ectonucleotidases and adenosine A2B receptors. *J Exp Med* (2003) 198(5):783–96. doi:10.1084/jem.20030891
14. Kalekar LA, Schmiel SE, Nandiwada SL, Lam WY, Barsness LO, Zhang N, et al. CD4(+) T cell anergy prevents autoimmunity and generates regulatory T cell precursors. *Nat Immunol* (2016) 17(3):304–14. doi:10.1038/ni.3331
15. Kalekar LA, Mueller DL. Relationship between CD4 regulatory T cells and anergy in vivo. *J Immunol* (2017) 198(7):2527–33. doi:10.4049/jimmunol.1602031
16. Airas L, Niemelä J, Salmi M, Puurunen T, Smith DJ, Jalkanen S. Differential regulation and function of CD73, a glycosyl-phosphatidylinositol-linked 70-kD adhesion molecule, on lymphocytes and endothelial cells. *J Cell Biol* (1997) 136(2):421–31. doi:10.1083/jcb.136.2.421
17. Yegutkin GG, Auvinen K, Rantakari P, Hollmén M, Karikoski M, Grénman R, et al. Ecto-5′-nucleotidase/CD73 enhances endothelial barrier function and sprouting in blood but not lymphatic vasculature. *Eur J Immunol* (2015) 45(2):562–73. doi:10.1002/eji.201444856
18. Koszalka P, Pryszlak A, Golunska M, Kolasa J, Stasilojc G, Skladanowski AC, et al. Inhibition of CD73 stimulates the migration and invasion of B16F10 melanoma cells in vitro, but results in impaired angiogenesis and reduced melanoma growth in vivo. *Oncol Rep* (2014) 31(2):819–27. doi:10.3892/or.2013.2883
19. Zhi X, Wang Y, Yu J, Yu J, Zhang L, Yin L, et al. Potential prognostic biomarker CD73 regulates epidermal growth factor receptor expression in human breast cancer. *IUBMB Life* (2012) 64(11):911–20. doi:10.1002/iub.1086
20. Wang L, Tang S, Wang Y, Xu S, Yu J, Zhi X, et al. Ecto-5′-nucleotidase (CD73) promotes tumor angiogenesis. *Clin Exp Metastasis* (2013) 30(5):671–80. doi:10.1007/s10585-013-9571-z
21. Kitakaze M, Minamino T, Node K, Komamura K, Hori M. Activation of ecto-5'-nucleotidase and cardioprotection by ischemic preconditioning. *Basic Res Cardiol* (1996) 91(1):23–6.

22. Allard B, Turcotte M, Spring K, Pommey S, Royal I, Stagg J. Anti-CD73 therapy impairs tumor angiogenesis. *Int J Cancer* (2014) 134(6):1466–73. doi:10.1002/ijc.28456
23. Zhou X, Zhi X, Zhou P, Chen S, Zhao F, Shao Z, et al. Effects of ecto-5'-nucleotidase on human breast cancer cell growth in vitro and in vivo. *Oncol Rep* (2007) 17(6):1341–6. doi:10.3892/or.17.6.1341
24. Burghoff S, Gong X, Viethen C, Jacoby C, Flogel U, Bongardt S, et al. Growth and metastasis of B16-F10 melanoma cells is not critically dependent on host CD73 expression in mice. *BMC Cancer* (2014) 14:898. doi:10.1186/1471-2407-14-898
25. Wang L, Zhou X, Zhou T, Ma D, Chen S, Zhi X, et al. Ecto-5′-nucleotidase _promotes invasion, migration and adhesion of human breast cancer cells. *J Cancer Res Clin Oncol* (2008) 134(3):365–72. doi:10.1007/s00432-007-0292-z
26. Beavis PA, Stagg J, Darcy PK, Smyth MJ. CD73: a potent suppressor of anti-tumor immune responses. *Trends Immunol* (2012) 33(5):231–7. doi:10.1016/j.it.2012.02.009
27. Alam MS, Kurtz CC, Rowlett RM, Reuter BK, Wiznerowicz E, Das S, et al. CD73 is expressed by human regulatory T helper cells and suppresses proinflammatory cytokine production and *Helicobacter felis*-induced gastritis in mice. *J Infect Dis* (2009) 199(4):494–504. doi:10.1086/596205
28. Ryzhov S, Novitskiy SV, Goldstein AE, Biktasova A, Blackburn MR, Biaggioni I, et al. Adenosinergic regulation of the expansion and immunosuppressive activity of CD11b+Gr1+ cells. *J Immunol* (2011) 187(11):6120–9. doi:10.4049/jimmunol.1101225
29. Berchtold S, Ogilvie ALJ, Bogdan C, Mühl-Zürbes P, Ogilvie A, Schuler G, et al. Human monocyte derived dendritic cells express functional P2X and P2Y receptors as well as ecto-nucleotidases. *FEBS Lett* (1999) 458(3):424–8. doi:10.1016/S0014-5793(99)01197-7
30. Allard B, Beavis PA, Darcy PK, Stagg J. Immunosuppressive activities of adenosine in cancer. *Curr Opin Pharmacol* (2016) 29:7–16. doi:10.1016/j.coph.2016.04.001
31. Young A, Ngiow SF, Barkauskas DS, Sult E, Hay C, Blake SJ, et al. Co-inhibition of CD73 and A2AR adenosine signaling improves anti-tumor Immune responses. *Cancer Cell* (2018) 30(3):391–403. doi:10.1016/j.ccell.2016.06.025
32. Maj T, Wang W, Crespo J, Zhang H, Wang W, Wei S, et al. Oxidative stress controls regulatory T cell apoptosis and suppressor activity and PD-L1-blockade resistance in tumor. *Nat Immunol* (2017) 18:1332. doi:10.1038/ni.3868
33. Sitkovsky MV, Lukashev D, Apasov S, Kojima H, Koshiba M, Caldwell C, et al. Physiological control of immune response and inflammatory tissue damage by hypoxia-inducible factors and adenosine A2A receptors. *Annu Rev Immunol* (2004) 22:657–82. doi:10.1146/annurev.immunol.22.012703.104731
34. Allard B, Turcotte M, Stagg J. Targeting CD73 and downstream adenosine receptor signaling in triple-negative breast cancer. *Expert Opin Ther Targets* (2014) 18(8):863–81. doi:10.1517/14728222.2014.915315
35. Sadej R, Spychala J, Skladanowski AC. Ecto-5'-nucleotidase (eN, CD73) is coexpressed with metastasis promoting antigens in human melanoma cells. *Nucleosides Nucleotides Nucleic Acids* (2006) 25(9–11):1119–23. doi:10.1080/15257770600894188
36. Sadej R, Spychala J, Skladanowski AC. Expression of ecto-5'-nucleotidase (eN, CD73) in cell lines from various stages of human melanoma. *Melanoma Res* (2006) 16(3):213–22. doi:10.1097/01.cmr.0000215030.69823.11
37. Wang H, Lee S, Nigro CL, Lattanzio L, Merlano M, Monteverde M, et al. NT5E (CD73) is epigenetically regulated in malignant melanoma and associated with metastatic site specificity. *Br J Cancer* (2012) 106(8):1446–52. doi:10.1038/bjc.2012.95
38. Buisseret L, Pommey S, Allard B, Garaud S, Bergeron M, Cousineau I, et al. Clinical significance of CD73 in triple-negative breast cancer: multiplex analysis of a phase III clinical trial. *Ann Oncol* (2017) mdx730. doi:10.1093/annonc/mdx730
39. Liu N, Fang XD, Vadis Q. CD73 as a novel prognostic biomarker for human colorectal cancer. *J Surg Oncol* (2012) 106(7):918–9. doi:10.1002/jso.23159
40. Inoue Y, Yoshimura K, Kurabe N, Kahyo T, Kawase A, Tanahashi M, et al. Prognostic impact of CD73 and A2A adenosine receptor expression in non-small-cell lung cancer. *Oncotarget* (2017) 8(5):8738–51. doi:10.18632/oncotarget.14434
41. Allard B, Longhi MS, Robson SC, Stagg J. The ectonucleotidases CD39 and CD73: novel checkpoint inhibitor targets. *Immunol Rev* (2017) 276(1):121–44. doi:10.1111/imr.12528
42. Antonioli L, Novitskiy SV, Sachsenmeier KF, Fornai M, Blandizzi C, Haskó G. Switching off CD73: a way to boost the activity of conventional and targeted antineoplastic therapies. *Drug Discov Today* (2017) 22(11):1686–96. doi:10.1016/j.drudis.2017.06.005
43. Young A, Ngiow SF, Gao Y, Patch A-M, Barkauskas DS, Messaoudene M, et al. A2AR adenosine signaling suppresses natural killer cell maturation in the tumor microenvironment. *Cancer Res* (2018) 78(4):1003–16. doi:10.1158/0008-5472.can-17-2826
44. Stagg J, Divisekera U, McLaughlin N, Sharkey J, Pommey S, Denoyer D, et al. Anti-CD73 antibody therapy inhibits breast tumor growth and metastasis. *Proc Natl Acad Sci U S A* (2010) 107(4):1547–52. doi:10.1073/pnas.0908801107
45. Beavis PA, Divisekera U, Paget C, Chow MT, John LB, Devaud C, et al. Blockade of A2A receptors potently suppresses the metastasis of CD73+ tumors. *Proc Natl Acad Sci U S A* (2013) 110(36):14711–6. doi:10.1073/pnas.1308209110
46. Ohta A. A metabolic immune checkpoint: adenosine in tumor microenvironment. *Front Immunol* (2016) 7(109):1–11. doi:10.3389/fimmu.2016.00109
47. Zhang B. CD73: a novel target for cancer immunotherapy. *Cancer Res* (2010) 70(16):6407–11. doi:10.1158/0008-5472.CAN-10-1544
48. Antonioli L, Yegutkin GG, Pacher P, Blandizzi C, Hasko G. Anti-CD73 in cancer immunotherapy: awakening new opportunities. *Trends Cancer* (2016) 2(2):95–109. doi:10.1016/j.trecan.2016.01.003
49. Geoghegan JC, Diedrich G, Lu X, Rosenthal K, Sachsenmeier KF, Wu H, et al. Inhibition of CD73 AMP hydrolysis by a therapeutic antibody with a dual, non-competitive mechanism of action. *MAbs* (2016) 8(3):454–67. doi:10.1080/19420862.2016.1143182
50. Turcotte M, Allard D, Mittal D, Bareche Y, Buisseret L, Jose V, et al. CD73 promotes resistance to HER2/ErbB2 antibody therapy. *Cancer Res* (2017) 77(20):5652–63. doi:10.1158/0008-5472.CAN-17-0707
51. Airas L, Hellman J, Salmi M, Bono P, Puurunen T, Smith DJ, et al. CD73 is involved in lymphocyte binding to the endothelium: characterization of lymphocyte-vascular adhesion protein 2 identifies it as CD73. *J Exp Med* (1995) 182(5):1603–8. doi:10.1084/jcm.182.5.1603
52. Andrade CM, Lopez PL, Noronha BT, Wink MR, Borojevic R, Margis R, et al. Ecto-5'-nucleotidase/CD73 knockdown increases cell migration and mRNA level of collagen I in a hepatic stellate cell line. *Cell Tissue Res* (2011) 344(2):279–86. doi:10.1007/s00441-011-1140-7
53. Sadej R, Skladanowski AC. Dual, enzymatic and non-enzymatic, function of ecto-5'-nucleotidase (eN, CD73) in migration and invasion of A375 melanoma cells. *Acta Biochim Pol* (2012) 59(4):647–52.
54. Hansen KR, Resta R, Webb CF, Thompson LF. Isolation and characterization of the promoter of the human 5'-nucleotidase (CD73)-encoding gene. *Gene* (1995) 167(1–2):307–12. doi:10.1016/0378-1119(95)00574-9
55. Fausther M, Sheung N, Saiman Y, Bansal MB, Dranoff JA. Activated hepatic stellate cells upregulate transcription of ecto-5'-nucleotidase/CD73 via specific SP1 and SMAD promoter elements. *Am J Physiol Gastrointest Liver Physiol* (2012) 303(8):G904–14. doi:10.1152/ajpgi.00015.2012
56. Zhang Z, Schwartz S, Wagner L, Miller W. A greedy algorithm for aligning DNA sequences. *J ComputBiol* (2000) 7(1–2):203–14. doi:10.1089/10665270050081478
57. Synnestvedt K, Furuta GT, Comerford KM, Louis N, Karhausen J, Eltzschig HK, et al. Ecto-5'-nucleotidase (CD73) regulation by hypoxia-inducible factor-1 mediates permeability changes in intestinal epithelia. *J Clin Invest* (2002) 110(7):993–1002. doi:10.1172/JCI15337
58. Tak E, Jung DH, Kim SH, Park GC, Jun DY, Lee J, et al. Protective role of hypoxia-inducible factor-1alpha-dependent CD39 and CD73 in fulminant acute liver failure. *Toxicol Appl Pharmacol* (2017) 314:72–81. doi:10.1016/j.taap.2016.11.016
59. Spychala J, Kitajewski J. Wnt and beta-catenin signaling target the expression of ecto-5'-nucleotidase and increase extracellular adenosine generation. *Exp Cell Res* (2004) 296(2):99–108. doi:10.1016/j.yexcr.2003.11.001
60. Pagnotta SM, Laudanna C, Pancione M, Sabatino L, Votino C, Remo A, et al. Ensemble of gene signatures identifies novel biomarkers in colorectal cancer activated through PPARgamma and TNFalpha signaling. *PLoS One* (2013) 8(8):e72638. doi:10.1371/journal.pone.0072638
61. Chalmin F, Mignot G, Bruchard M, Chevriaux A, Vegran F, Hichami A, et al. Stat3 and Gfi-1 transcription factors control Th17 cell immunosuppressive activity via the regulation of ectonucleotidase expression. *Immunity* (2012) 36(3):362–73. doi:10.1016/j.immuni.2011.12.019

62. Zheng Y, Josefowicz SZ, Kas A, Chu TT, Gavin MA, Rudensky AY. Genome-wide analysis of Foxp3 target genes in developing and mature regulatory T cells. *Nature* (2007) 445(7130):936–40. doi:10.1038/nature05563
63. Bonnin N, Armandy E, Carras J, Ferrandon S, Battiston-Montagne P, Aubry M, et al. miR-422a promotes loco-regional recurrence by targeting NT5E/CD73 in head and neck squamous cell carcinoma. *Oncotarget* (2016) 7(28):44023–38. doi:10.18632/oncotarget.9829
64. Xie M, Qin H, Luo Q, Huang Q, He X, Yang Z, et al. MicroRNA-30a regulates cell proliferation and tumor growth of colorectal cancer by targeting CD73. *BMC Cancer* (2017) 17(1):305. doi:10.1186/s12885-017-3291-8
65. Wang N, Xiang X, Chen K, Liu P, Zhu A. Targeting of NT5E by miR-30b and miR-340 attenuates proliferation, invasion and migration of gallbladder carcinoma. *Biochimie* (2017) 146:56–67. doi:10.1016/j.biochi.2017.10.027
66. Zhang F, Luo Y, Shao Z, Xu L, Liu X, Niu Y, et al. MicroRNA-187, a downstream effector of TGFbeta pathway, suppresses Smad-mediated epithelial-mesenchymal transition in colorectal cancer. *Cancer Lett* (2016) 373(2):203–13. doi:10.1016/j.canlet.2016.01.037
67. Ikeda Y, Tanji E, Makino N, Kawata S, Furukawa T. MicroRNAs associated with mitogen-activated protein kinase in human pancreatic cancer. *Mol Cancer Res* (2012) 10(2):259–69. doi:10.1158/1541-7786.MCR-11-0035
68. Fulciniti M, Amodio N, Bandi RL, Cagnetta A, Samur MK, Acharya C, et al. miR-23b/SP1/c-myc forms a feed-forward loop supporting multiple myeloma cell growth. *Blood Cancer J* (2016) 6:e380. doi:10.1038/bcj.2015.106
69. Hu J, Shan Z, Hu K, Ren F, Zhang W, Han M, et al. miRNA-223 inhibits epithelial-mesenchymal transition in gastric carcinoma cells via Sp1. *Int J Oncol* (2016) 49(1):325–35. doi:10.3892/ijo.2016.3533
70. Tang H, Deng M, Tang Y, Xie X, Guo J, Kong Y, et al. miR-200b and miR-200c as prognostic factors and mediators of gastric cancer cell progression. *Clin Cancer Res* (2013) 19(20):5602–12. doi:10.1158/1078-0432.CCR-13-1326
71. Braun J, Hoang-Vu C, Dralle H, Huttelmaier S. Downregulation of microRNAs directs the EMT and invasive potential of anaplastic thyroid carcinomas. *Oncogene* (2010) 29(29):4237–44. doi:10.1038/onc.2010.169
72. Jones KB, Salah Z, Del Mare S, Galasso M, Gaudio E, Nuovo GJ, et al. miRNA signatures associate with pathogenesis and progression of osteosarcoma. *Cancer Res* (2012) 72(7):1865–77. doi:10.1158/0008-5472.CAN-11-2663
73. Chanda S, Nandi S, Chawla-Sarkar M. Rotavirus-induced miR-142-5p elicits proviral milieu by targeting non-canonical transforming growth factor beta signalling and apoptosis in cells. *Cell Microbiol* (2016) 18(5):733–47. doi:10.1111/cmi.12544
74. Ma Z, Liu T, Huang W, Liu H, Zhang HM, Li Q, et al. MicroRNA regulatory pathway analysis identifies miR-142-5p as a negative regulator of TGF-beta pathway via targeting SMAD3. *Oncotarget* (2016) 7(44):71504–13. doi:10.18632/oncotarget.12229
75. Cheng D, Zhao S, Tang H, Zhang D, Sun H, Yu F, et al. MicroRNA-20a-5p promotes colorectal cancer invasion and metastasis by downregulating Smad4. *Oncotarget* (2016) 7(29):45199–213. doi:10.18632/oncotarget.9900
76. Poitz DM, Augstein A, Gradehand C, Ende G, Schmeisser A, Strasser RH. Regulation of the Hif-system by micro-RNA 17 and 20a – role during monocyte-to-macrophage differentiation. *Mol Immunol* (2013) 56(4):442–51. doi:10.1016/j.molimm.2013.06.014
77. Wang C, Yun Z, Zhao T, Liu X, Ma X. miR-495 is a predictive biomarker that downregulates GFI1 expression in medulloblastoma. *Cell Physiol Biochem* (2015) 36(4):1430–9. doi:10.1159/000430308
78. Paul R, Lee J, Donaldson AV, Connolly M, Sharif M, Natanek SA, et al. miR-422a suppresses SMAD4 protein expression and promotes resistance to muscle loss. *J Cachexia Sarcopenia Muscle* (2018) 9:119–28. doi:10.1002/jcsm.12236
79. Colgan SP, Eltzschig HK, Eckle T, Thompson LF. Physiological roles for ecto-5'-nucleotidase (CD73). *Purinergic Signal* (2006) 2(2):351–60. doi:10.1007/s11302-005-5302-5
80. Eales KL, Hollinshead KE, Tennant DA. Hypoxia and metabolic adaptation of cancer cells. *Oncogenesis* (2016) 5:e190. doi:10.1038/oncsis.2015.50
81. Zhan T, Rindtorff N, Boutros M. Wnt signaling in cancer. *Oncogene* (2017) 36(11):1461–73. doi:10.1038/onc.2016.304
82. Spranger S, Bao R, Gajewski TF. Melanoma-intrinsic β-catenin signalling prevents anti-tumour immunity. *Nature* (2015) 523:231. doi:10.1038/nature14404
83. Lu L, Barbi J, Pan F. The regulation of immune tolerance by FOXP3. *Nat Rev Immunol* (2017) 17(11):703–17. doi:10.1038/nri.2017.75
84. Wolf D, Wolf AM, Rumpold H, Fiegl H, Zeimet AG, Muller-Holzner E, et al. The expression of the regulatory T cell-specific forkhead box transcription factor FoxP3 is associated with poor prognosis in ovarian cancer. *Clin Cancer Res* (2005) 11(23):8326–31. doi:10.1158/1078-0432.CCR-05-1244
85. Vidigal JA, Ventura A. The biological functions of miRNAs: lessons from in vivo studies. *Trends Cell Biol* (2015) 25(3):137–47. doi:10.1016/j.tcb.2014.11.004
86. Hayes J, Peruzzi PP, Lawler S. MicroRNAs in cancer: biomarkers, functions and therapy. *Trends Mol Med* (2014) 20(8):460–9. doi:10.1016/j.molmed.2014.06.005
87. Hamam R, Ali AM, Alsaleh KA, Kassem M, Alfayez M, Aldahmash A, et al. MicroRNA expression profiling on individual breast cancer patients identifies novel panel of circulating microRNA for early detection. *Sci Rep* (2016) 6:25997. doi:10.1038/srep25997
88. Larrea E, Sole C, Manterola L, Goicoechea I, Armesto M, Arestin M, et al. New concepts in cancer biomarkers: circulating miRNAs in liquid biopsies. *Int J Mol Sci* (2016) 17(5):1–42. doi:10.3390/ijms17050627
89. Dassi E, Re A, Leo S, Tebaldi T, Pasini L, Peroni D, et al. AURA 2: empowering discovery of post-transcriptional networks. *Translation (Austin)* (2014) 2(1):e27738. doi:10.4161/trla.27738
90. Mazumder B, Seshadri V, Fox PL. Translational control by the 3'-UTR: the ends specify the means. *Trends Biochem Sci* (2003) 28(2):91–8. doi:10.1016/S0968-0004(03)00002-1
91. Zhu J, Zeng Y, Li W, Qin H, Lei Z, Shen D, et al. CD73/NT5E is a target of miR-30a-5p and plays an important role in the pathogenesis of non-small cell lung cancer. *Mol Cancer* (2017) 16(1):34. doi:10.1186/s12943-017-0591-1
92. Guess MG, Barthel KK, Harrison BC, Leinwand LA. miR-30 family microRNAs regulate myogenic differentiation and provide negative feedback on the microRNA pathway. *PLoS One* (2015) 10(2):e0118229. doi:10.1371/journal.pone.0118229

11

Successful Anti-CLL1 CAR T-Cell Therapy in Secondary Acute Myeloid Leukemia

Hui Zhang[1*†], *Wen-Ting Gan*[1†], *Wen-Ge Hao*[1], *Peng-Fei Wang*[1], *Zhuo-Yan Li*[1] *and Lung-Ji Chang*[2,3*]

[1] *Department of Pediatric Hematology/Oncology, Guangzhou Women and Children's Medical Center, Guangzhou, China,* [2] *Shenzhen Geno-Immune Medical Institute, Shenzhen, China,* [3] *Department of Molecular Genetics and Microbiology, College of Medicine, University of Florida, Gainesville, FL, United States*

Edited by:
Bin Zhang,
Northwestern University, United States

Reviewed by:
William K. Decker,
Baylor College of Medicine,
United States
Muharrem Muftuoglu,
University of Texas MD Anderson
Cancer Center, United States

***Correspondence:**
Hui Zhang
zhanghuirjh@gwcmc.org
Lung-Ji Chang
lung-ji chang c@szgimi.org

† *These authors have contributed equally to this work*

Secondary acute myeloid leukemia (sAML) is a high-risk AML evolving from heterogenous prior hematological disorders. Compared to de novo AML, sAML has even worse responses to current therapy and thus is associated with lower remission rates, inferior overall survival (OS) and higher relapse rates. Many efforts have been devoted to improving the overall but with limited success, and novel strategy is thus highly needed. Recent research has identified that CLL1 is highly expressed on AML leukemia stem cells and blasts cells but not on normal hematopoietic stem cells. In this case report, we treated a secondary AML patient with anti -CLL1 CAR-T therapy and achieved morphological, immunophenotypic and molecular complete remission for over 10 months. Although only one successful case is presented here, the anti-CLL1 CAR T-cells should be considered as another treatment option for secondary AML in the future.

Keywords: secondary acute myeloid leukemia, myelodysplastic syndrome, myeloproliferative neoplasm, CAR T-cell therapy, CLL1

BACKGROUND

The prognosis of patients with acute myeloid leukemia (AML) has been improving in the last decades through the intensification of combination chemotherapy and hematopoietic stem cell transplantation. However, the 5-year survival rate of patients with AML varies from 33.3–79.5% worldwide, as documented in the recent CONCORD-2 study (1), with a rate of only 40.1% in China.

Secondary AML (sAML) is considered high-risk as it evolves from heterogenous prior hematological disorders such as myelodysplastic syndrome (MDS), myeloproliferative neoplasm (MPN), and other malignancies exposed to cytotoxic agents or radiation therapy (2). Compared to *de novo* AML, sAML has worse response to current therapy, and thus is associated with lower remission rates, inferior overall survival (OS), and higher relapse rates (2). Many efforts have been devoted to improving the OS but with limited success; therefore, a novel strategy is highly needed (3).

Chimeric antigen receptor (CAR) T cells have emerged as a highly effective therapy for relapsed/refractory hematological malignancies (4–6); however, the efficacy of CAR T cells is unclear in AML. Recent research has shown that C-type lectin-like molecule-1 (CLL1) is highly expressed on AML leukemia stem cells (LSCs) and blast cells but not on the normal hematopoietic stem cells (HSCs) (7, 8), suggesting CLL1 as a promising target for novel AML therapy. Intriguingly, several groups have successfully developed CLL1-targeting strategies (9–13). These novel CLL1-directed therapies have shown some efficacy on AML cell lines *ex vivo*, primary human AML cells, and human AML patient-derived xenograft mice and monkey models *in vivo*; however, direct evidence regarding responses in patients with AML has not been reported.

In this case report, we treated a patient with secondary AML using anti-CLL1 CAR-T cells therapy and achieved morphological, immunophenotypic, and molecular complete remission for over a 10-month period. Although only one successful case is presented here, the anti-CLL1 CAR T-cells should be considered as another treatment option for secondary AML in the future.

CASE PRESENTATION

In early July 2018, a 10-year-old girl presented with pancytopenia and an elevated peripheral blood blast percentage while undergoing maintenance treatment for her first B-cell acute lymphoblastic leukemia (ALL) relapse. Bone marrow (BM) aspiration was performed every 2 weeks from July 2018, and blast percentage gradually increased from initial 7.5% to 19.5% within 1 month of observation (**Figure 1**). Furthermore, her medical history showed that she was diagnosed with high-risk B-ALL in October 2012, with a $CD34^{+}CD38^{+}CD10^{+}CD19^{+}CD123^{+}$ immunophenotype. Initially, she was enrolled into the GD-2008-ALL clinical trial (NCT00846703) and then achieved complete remission (CR) after one course of induction therapy, while her minimal residual disease (MRD) evaluated by flow cytometry remained above 0.01% during all treatment phases (**Figure 1**). Unfortunately, she experienced an isolated BM relapse after a 1.5-year cessation of chemotherapy, and her relapse disease showed the same B-ALL immunophenotype as her first diagnosis. Due to the lack of economic support, she was treated with the HKPHOSG-Relapsed-ALL-2007 protocol and experienced persistent fever, pancytopenia, and elevated peripheral blood blast cells during the treatment (**Figure 1**). We then systemically compared samples from her primary diagnosis, along with her first and second instance of relapse. From this comparison, we found that the blast cells from the second relapse sample originated from the myeloid lineage ($CD34^{+}CD38^{+}CD10^{dim}CD19^{dim}CD123^{+}CD33^{+}CLL1^{+}$) and not from the B cell lineage (**Figures 2A–C**). Moreover, we excluded the possibility of MDS-transformed AML because we did not identify a deletion of chromosome 5 or 7, or abnormal localization of immature precursors or marrow fibrosis. Molecular cytogenetic tests indicated the existence of MLL rearrangement, $RUNX1^{R204P}$, and $WT1^{S381fs}$ mutation (**Supplementary Figure 1**, **Supplementary Table 1**). Results were double confirmed by a peer review from the Shenzhen Gene-Immune Medical Institute (GIMI). Based on the 2017 European LeukemiaNet recommendations for AML, she was diagnosed as secondary AML and considered to be in the adverse risk group. Of note, CLL1 was highly expressed on the myeloid blast cells (**Figure 3A**, **Supplementary Figure 2**), which could be a target for CAR T-cell therapy.

Considering the long-term exposure to chemotherapeutic agents and the poor prognosis, her parents decided for her not to receive chemotherapy as a first-line therapy. With the help of GIMI, we developed a chimeric antigen receptor (CAR) containing a CLL1-specific single chain variable fragment, in combination with a fourth-generation CAR lentiviral vector (4SCAR) carrying T cell costimulatory signals for CD28-CD27-CD3z (14). The 4SCAR-CLL1 lentivector transfer efficiency for patient's PBMCs was ~95.06%. The patient received a lymphodepleting chemotherapy (cyclophosphamide 300 mg/m^2/d and fludarabine 30 mg/m^2/d for 4 days) before CAR T-cell transfer to enhance *in vivo* expansion of CAR T-cells, after which she received a single dose (5.8×10^7

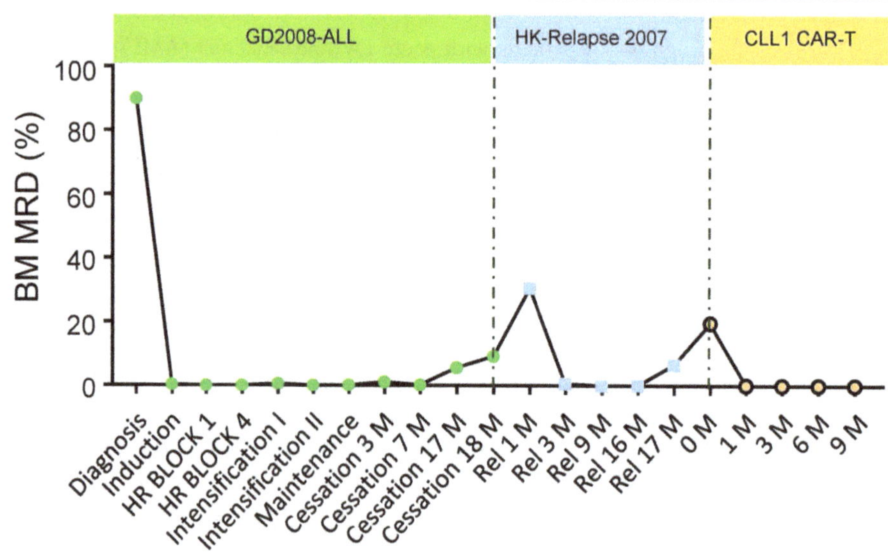

FIGURE 1 | Therapeutic response for the anti-CLL1 CAR-T treatment. Plot of therapeutic response in this sAML during her primary diagnosis, 1st relapse and 2nd relapse including anti-CLL1 CAR-T cells therapy.

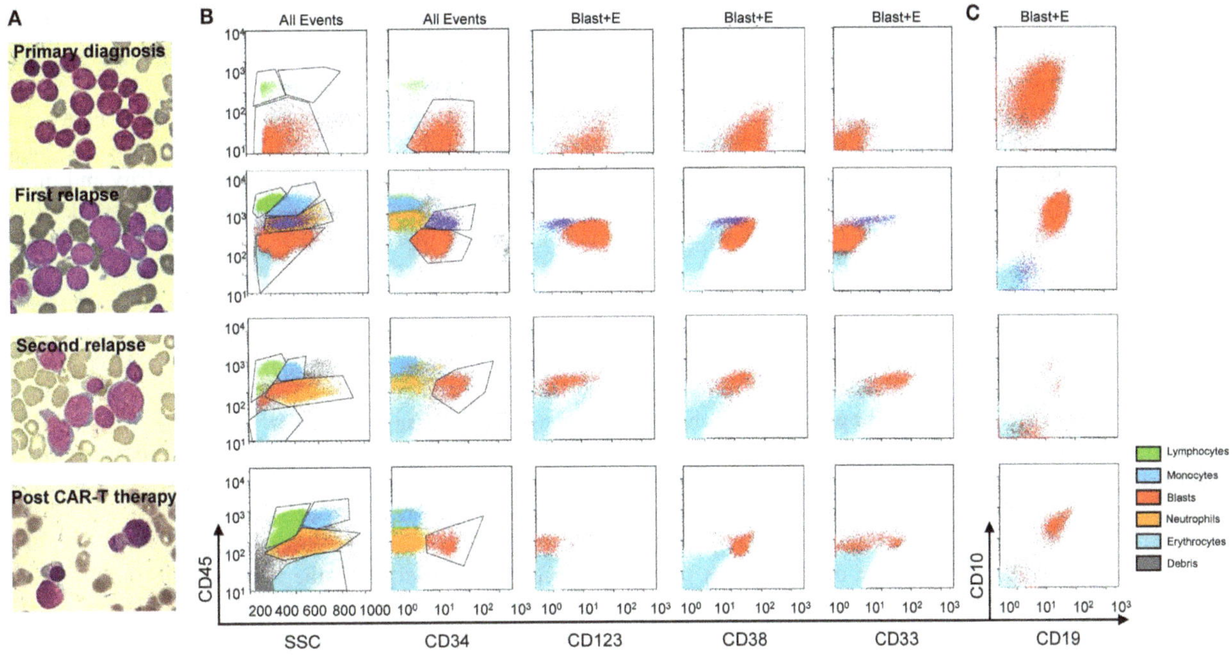

FIGURE 2 | Morphologic and immunophenotypic evolution for this secondary AML case. Morphologic **(A)** (upper, primary diagnosis; upper middle, 1st relapse; lower middle, 2nd relapse; and lower, post anti-CLL1 CAR T-cell therapy) and flow cytometric **(B,C)** features at primary diagnosis (upper panel), 1st relapse (upper middle panel), 2nd relapse (lower middle panel), and post anti-CLL1 CAR T-cell therapy (lower panel) in this secondary AML case; gating: all events (All Events) or blast and erythroid cells (Blast+E). The green, blue, orange, light blue, gray and red dots represent lymphocytes, monocytes, neutrophils, erythrocytes, debris, and blasts population, respectively.

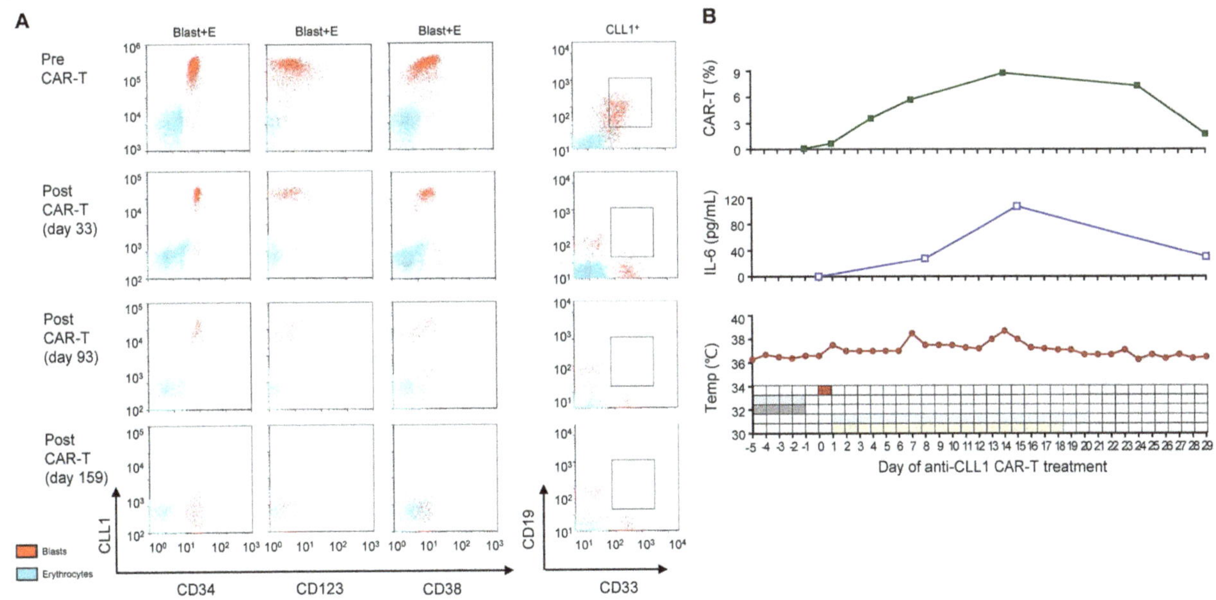

FIGURE 3 | MRD and CRS status during acnti-CLL1 CAR T-cell therapy. **(A)** CLL1 population, intensity, and the blast percentage (gating on CLL$^+$ cells) before (upper panel) and after (lower panel) anti-CLL1 CAR T-cell therapy. The blue and red dots represent erythrocytes and blasts population, respectively. **(B)** Anti-CLL1 CAR T-cells persistence (upper panel), serum IL-6 level (middle panel), and temperature and therapy scheme (low panel) during the first month of anti-CLL1 CAR T- cell therapy in this secondary AML case.

anti-CLL1 CAR-T cells, ~1.9 × 10^6/kg) infusion over 10 min through a peripherally inserted central venous catheter on 11 September 2018. Subsequently, she experienced Grade I-II cytokine release syndrome (CRS) manifested by a temperature ≥38°C; at this time, she developed transient hypotension requiring fluid resuscitation under the CAR T-cell therapy management consensus guidelines (15, 16). Serum IL-6 level reached a peak on day 14 and then gradually decreased, which was consistent with the occurrence of CRS. Following the guidelines, glucocorticoids and tocilizumab intervention were not prescribed (**Figure 3B**). After the completion of CAR T-cell therapy, the patient achieved a morphological CR and was negative for MRD (< 0.1%) on day 29. However, the CLL1$^+$ cells were not completely eliminated until early in the 6 months after CAR T-cell therapy (**Figure 3A**, **Supplementary Table 2**). Upon complete remission, the BM response was monitored monthly during the first 3 months and every 3 months thereafter. Strikingly, the morphologic CR and MRD <0.1% were sustained for ~9 months at the time of this report's submission (**Figures 1–3**, **Supplementary Table 2**). However, we did not check CLL1 expression in peripheral blood samples in this case due to lack of experience. The persistence of anti-CLL1 CAR T-cells in peripheral blood was determined by quantitative real-time PCR, as previously described (17), during treatment and clinical follow-up. An effective expansion was achieved in the first month, which then dropped quickly thereafter; then, a low CAR T-cell level persistence was detected 5 months after CAR T-cell injection (**Figure 3B**). Even with the disappearance of CAR T-cells, a 10 month response (approximately) was achieved using one dose of anti-CLL1 CAR-T monotherapy in this patient, suggesting that anti-CLL1 CAR T-cells should be considered as an alternative strategy for AML or sAML in the future.

DISCUSSION

In this reported case, the main finding was the achievement of a surprisingly long-term complete remission with anti-CLL1 CAR T-cells therapy. Only grade I-II cytokine release syndrome was observed and successfully managed.

Anthracyclines- and cytarabine-based conventional chemotherapy are the main treatments for AML patients; however, both have significant toxicities. In addition, the overall prognosis for patients with this treatment has remained stagnant in the last two decades (18, 19). With the advent of next generation sequencing (NGS), more and more prognostically cytogenetic and molecular markers have been incorporated into AML risk classification and therapy (20–22). For example, tyrosine kinase inhibitors (FLT3-ITD inhibitor), IDH1 inhibitor ivosidenib, IDH2 inhibitor enasidenib, and BCL2 inhibitor venetoclax, monoclonal antibody-based therapy (anti-CD33 therapy); cellular therapy (CAR-T and TCR-engineered T-cell, and NK cell therapies), and novel regimens (decitabine and pracinostat) have been successfully developed (23–25). Although new targeted agents have been extensively introduced into clinical treatment, relapse still remains the most significant issue influencing the survival of patients with AML. Allogeneic hematopoietic stem cell transplantation remains the last hope for these patients, indicating the important role of normal immune reconstitution for successfully treating patients with AML.

In contrast to chemotherapy and new FDA-approved targeting agents, cellular CAR-T cell therapy and cytotoxic T lymphocytes can minimize systemic cytotoxicity and morbidity while generating maximal anti-tumor activity (22). However, in this study, we did observe low anti-CLL1 CAR T-cells expansion during the CAR T-cell therapy. The selection of CD28/CD27 costimulatory signals might be the reason for short-term persistence. CD28 and 4-1-BB are two well-established costimulatory signals for the generation of CAR-T cells. CD28 costimulation can augment T-cell receptor (TCR) signaling and increase TCR sensitivity, which is very helpful in facilitating T-cell responses against weak agonist peptides. Compared to CD28, 4-1-BB costimulation can enhance T-cell expansion and maintenance and rescue T-cells from anergy and exhaustion. The low effective CAR-T cell expansion and the lack of long-term persistence might be the bottleneck in the future clinical application of this therapy.

In conclusion, our prolonged survival observation in this patient with sAML showed that anti-CLL1 CAR-T might be of great potential in AML treatment. Interestingly, Liu F et al. has reported the efficacy of combination CLL1-CD33 CAR-T cells in a 6-year-old girl with sAML transformed from prior faconi anemia and juvenile myelomonocytic leukemia (22). Given that B-cell aplasia is an indicator of CD19 CAR T-cell therapy, frequencies of CLL1 expressing mononuclear cells might be used as an indicator in a similar way, to monitor the efficacy of CAR T-cells. As mentioned above, the persistence of CLL1 expressing mononuclear cells might serve as an indicator of anti-CLL1 CAR-T efficacy and should be included to monitor the anti-CLL1 CAR-T in the future. To our knowledge, this is the second successful case of anti-CLL1 CAR-T application for secondary AML treatment, highlighting its promising potential in the high-risk AML population.

ETHICS STATEMENT

The studies involving human participants were reviewed and approved by GIMI-IRB-16001. Written informed consent to participate in this study was provided by the participants' legal guardian/next of kin. Written informed consent was obtained from the individual(s), and minor(s)' legal guardian/next of kin, for the publication of any potentially identifiable images or data included in this article.

AUTHOR CONTRIBUTIONS

HZ, W-TG, and L-JC performed the research, analyzed the data, and wrote the paper. W-GH and P-FW included the patients and collected clinical data. Z-YL contributed to clinical nursing. All authors critically revised the manuscript and approved the final version.

FUNDING

This work is partially funded by research funds from St. Baldrick's Foundation International Scholar (581580), the Natural Science Foundation of Guangdong Province (2015A030313460), and the Science and Technology Planning Technical Research Project of Shenzhen (JCYJ20170413154349187, JCYJ20170817172416991, JCYJ20170817172541842, and KQTD20140630143254906).

ACKNOWLEDGMENTS

We would like to thank Andy Zhao and Dr. Jun J. Yang for the scientific editing. Also, we would like to thank Editage (www.editage.cn) for English language editing.

SUPPLEMENTARY MATERIAL

Supplementary Figure 1 | MLL-rearrangement detection in this secondary AML patient. Interphase FISH using the LSI MLL dual color, break-apart rearrangement probe set. Interphase nucleus harboring the MLL translocation, 1 fusion signal (yellow), and 2 separate signals (red and green).

Supplementary Figure 2 | The isotype control for flow cytometry. The gray shaded area represented isotype controls for multi-color flow cytometry.

Supplementary Table 1 | Immunophenotypic, cytogenetics and mutation features of this patients.

Supplementary Table 2 | Clinical follow-up during anti-CLL1 CAR-T therapy in this secondary AML case.

REFERENCES

1. Bonaventure A, Harewood R, Stiller CA, Gatta G, Clavel J, Stefan DC, et al. Worldwide comparison of survival from childhood leukaemia for 1995-2009, by subtype, age, and sex (CONCORD-2): a population-based study of individual data for 89 828 children from 198 registries in 53 countries. *Lancet Haematol.* (2017) 4:e202–17. doi: 10.1016/S2352-3026(17)30052-2
2. Granfeldt Østgård LS, Medeiros BC, Sengeløv H, Nørgaard M, Andersen MK, Dufva IH, et al. Epidemiology and clinical significance of secondary and therapy-related acute myeloid leukemia: a national population-based cohort study. *J Clin Oncol.* (2015) 33:3641–9. doi: 10.1200/JCO.2014.60.0890
3. Thol F, Schlenk RF, Heuser M, Ganser A. How I treat refractory and early relapsed acute myeloid leukemia. *Blood.* (2015) 126:319–27. doi: 10.1182/blood-2014-10-551911
4. Vo P, Gooley TA, Rajendran JG, Fisher DR, Orozco JJ, Green DJ, et al. Yttrium-90-labeled anti-CD45 antibody followed by a reduced-intensity hematopoietic cell transplantation for patients with relapsed/refractory leukemia or myelodysplasia. *Haematologica.* (2019). doi: 10.3324/haematol.2019.229492. [Epub ahead of print].
5. Schuster SJ, Bishop MR, Tam CS, Waller EK, Borchmann P, McGuirk JP, et al. Tisagenlecleucel in adult relapsed or refractory diffuse large B-cell lymphoma. *N Engl J Med.* (2019) 380:45–56. doi: 10.1056/NEJMoa1804980
6. Ying Z, Huang XF, Xiang X, Liu X, Kang Y, Song X, et al. A safe and potent anti-CD19 CAR T cell therapy. *Nat Med.* (2019) 25:1–7. doi: 10.1038/s41591-019-0421-7
7. Haubner S, Perna F, Kohnke T, Schmidt C, Berman S, Augsberger C, et al. Coexpression profile of leukemic stem cell markers for combinatorial targeted therapy in AML. *Leukemia.* (2019) 33:64–74. doi: 10.1038/s41375-018-0180-3
8. van Rhenen A, van Dongen GA, Kelder A, Rombouts EJ, Feller N, Moshaver B, et al. The novel AML stem cell associated antigen CLL-1 aids in discrimination between normal and leukemic stem cells. *Blood.* (2007) 110:2659–66. doi: 10.1182/blood-2007-03-083048
9. Jiang YP, Liu BY, Zheng Q, Panuganti S, Chen R, Zhu J, et al. CLT030, a leukemic stem cell-targeting CLL1 antibody-drug conjugate for treatment of acute myeloid leukemia. *Blood Adv.* (2018) 2:1738–49. doi: 10.1182/bloodadvances.2018020107
10. Leong SR, Sukumaran S, Hristopoulos M, Totpal K, Stainton S, Lu E, et al. An anti-CD3/anti-CLL-1 bispecific antibody for the treatment of acute myeloid leukemia. *Blood.* (2017) 129:609–18. doi: 10.1182/blood-2016-08-735365
11. Lin TY, Zhu Y, Li Y, Zhang H, Ma AH, Long Q, et al. Daunorubicin-containing CLL1-targeting nanomicelles have anti-leukemia stem cell activity in acute myeloid leukemia. *Nanomedicine.* (2019) 20:102004. doi: 10.1016/j.nano.2019.04.007
12. Lu H, Zhou Q, Deshmukh V, Phull H, Ma J, Tardif V, et al. Targeting human C-type lectin-like molecule-1 (CLL1) with a bispecific antibody for immunotherapy of acute myeloid leukemia. *Angewandte Chemie.* (2014) 53:9841–5. doi: 10.1002/anie.201405353
13. Wang J, Chen S, Xiao W, Li W, Wang L, Yang S, et al. CAR-T cells targeting CLL-1 as an approach to treat acute myeloid leukemia. *J Hematol Oncol.* (2018) 11:7. doi: 10.1186/s13045-017-0553-5
14. Zhang JP, Zhang R, Tsao ST, Liu YC, Chen X, Lu DP, et al. Sequential allogeneic and autologous CAR-T-cell therapy to treat an immune-compromised leukemic patient. *Blood Adv.* (2018) 2:1691–5. doi: 10.1182/bloodadvances.2018017004
15. Mahadeo KM, Khazal SJ, Abdel-Azim H, Fitzgerald JC, Taraseviciute A, Bollard CM, et al. Management guidelines for paediatric patients receiving chimeric antigen receptor T cell therapy. *Nat Rev Clin Oncol.* (2019) 16:45–63. doi: 10.1038/s41571-018-0075-2
16. Neelapu SS, Tummala S, Kebriaei P, Wierda W, Gutierrez C, Locke FL, et al. Chimeric antigen receptor T-cell therapy - assessment and management of toxicities. *Nat Rev Clin Oncol.* (2018) 15:47–62. doi: 10.1038/nrclinonc.2017.148
17. Wang B, He J, Liu C, Chang LJ. An effective cancer vaccine modality: lentiviral modification of dendritic cells expressing multiple cancer-specific antigens. *Vaccine.* (2006) 24:3477–89. doi: 10.1016/j.vaccine.2006.02.025
18. Döhner H, Estey EH, Amadori S, Appelbaum FR, Büchner T, Burnett AK, et al. Diagnosis and management of acute myeloid leukemia in adults: recommendations from an international expert panel, on behalf of the European LeukemiaNet. *Blood.* (2010) 115:453–74. doi: 10.1182/blood-2009-07-235358
19. Lowenberg B, Pabst T, Vellenga E, van Putten W, Schouten HC, Graux C, et al. Cytarabine dose for acute myeloid leukemia. *N Engl J Med.* (2011) 364:1027–36. doi: 10.1056/NEJMoa1010222
20. Winer ES, Stone RM. Novel therapy in Acute myeloid leukemia (AML): moving toward targeted approaches. *Ther Adv Hematol.* (2019) 10:2040620719860645. doi: 10.1177/2040620719860645
21. Fernandez S, Desplat V, Villacreces A, Guitart AV, Milpied N, Pigneux A, et al. Targeting tyrosine kinases in acute myeloid leukemia: why, who and how? *Int J Mol Sci.* (2019) 20:3429. doi: 10.3390/ijms20143429
22. Lee JB, Chen B, Vasic D, Law AD, Zhang L. Cellular immunotherapy for acute myeloid leukemia: how specific should

it be? *Blood Rev.* (2019) 35:18–31. doi: 10.1016/j.blre.2019.02.001

23. Lichtenegger FS, Krupka C, Haubner S, Kohnke T, Subklewe M. Recent developments in immunotherapy of acute myeloid leukemia. *J Hematol Oncol.* (2017) 10:142. doi: 10.1186/s13045-017-0505-0
24. Benard B, Gentles AJ, Kohnke T, Majeti R, Thomas D. Data mining for mutation-specific targets in acute myeloid leukemia. *Leukemia.* (2019) 33:826–43. doi: 10.1038/s41375-019-0387-y
25. Heuser M, Mina A, Stein EM, Altman JK. How Precision Medicine Is Changing Acute Myeloid Leukemia Therapy. *Am Soc Clin Oncol Educ Book.* (2019) 39:411–20. doi: 10.1200/EDBK_238687

Indoleamine 2,3-Dioxygenase Expression Pattern in the Tumor Microenvironment Predicts Clinical Outcome in Early Stage Cervical Cancer

*A. Marijne Heeren[1,2], Ilse van Dijk[2], Daniella R. A. I. Berry[3], Maryam Khelil[1], Debbie Ferns[1], Jeroen Kole[4], René J. P. Musters[4], Victor L. Thijssen[2], Constantijne H. Mom[5], Gemma G. Kenter[1,5,6], Maaike C. G. Bleeker[3], Tanja D. de Gruijl[2] and Ekaterina S. Jordanova[1]**

[1] Center Gynecological Oncology Amsterdam (CGOA), Department of Obstetrics and Gynecology, VU University Medical Center, Amsterdam, Netherlands, [2] Cancer Center Amsterdam, Departments of Medical Oncology & Radiation Oncology, VU University Medical Center, Amsterdam, Netherlands, [3] Department of Pathology, VU University Medical Center, Amsterdam, Netherlands, [4] Laboratory for Physiology, Institute for Cardiovascular Research, VU University Medical Center, Amsterdam, Netherlands, [5] Center Gynecological Oncology Amsterdam (CGOA), Department of Obstetrics and Gynecology, Academic Medical Center, Amsterdam, Netherlands, [6] Center Gynecological Oncology Amsterdam (CGOA), Department of Gynecology, Netherlands Cancer Institute – Antoni van Leeuwenhoek, Amsterdam, Netherlands

Edited by:
Svetlana Karakhanova, Universität Heidelberg, Germany

Reviewed by:
Graham Robert Leggatt, The University of Queensland, Australia
Antonio Curti, Università degli Studi di Bologna, Italy

***Correspondence:**
Ekaterina S. Jordanova
e.jordanova@vumc.nl

The indoleamine 2,3-dioxygenase (IDO) enzyme can act as an immunoregulator by inhibiting T cell function *via* the degradation of the essential amino acid tryptophan (trp) into kynurenine (kyn) and its derivates. The kyn/trp ratio in serum is a prognostic factor for cervical cancer patients; however, information about the relationship between serum levels and IDO expression in the tumor is lacking. IDO expression was studied in 71 primary and 14 paired metastatic cervical cancer samples by various immunohistochemical (IHC) techniques, including 7-color fluorescent multiparameter IHC, and the link between the concentration of IDO metabolites in serum, clinicopathological characteristics, and the presence of (proliferating) T cells (CD8, Ki67, and FoxP3) was examined. In addition, we compared the relationships between *IDO1* and *IFNG* gene expression and clinical parameters using RNAseq data from 144 cervical tumor samples published by The Cancer Genome Atlas (TCGA). Here, we demonstrate that patchy tumor IDO expression is associated with an increased systemic kyn/trp ratio in cervical cancer ($P = 0.009$), whereas marginal tumor expression at the interface with the stroma is linked to improved disease-free (DFS) ($P = 0.017$) and disease-specific survival ($P = 0.043$). The latter may be related to T cell infiltration and localized IFNγ release inducing IDO expression. Indeed, TCGA analysis of 144 cervical tumor samples revealed a strong and positive correlation between *IDO1* and *IFNG* mRNA expression levels ($P < 0.001$) and a significant association with improved DFS for high *IDO1* and *IFNG* transcript levels ($P = 0.031$). Unexpectedly, IDO+ tumors had higher $CD8^+Ki67^+$ T cell rates ($P = 0.004$). Our data thus indicate that the serum kyn/trp ratio and IDO expression in primary tumor samples are not clear-cut biomarkers for prognosis and stratification of patients with early stage cervical cancer for clinical trials implementing IDO inhibitors. Rather, a marginal IDO expression pattern in the tumor dominantly predicts favorable outcome, which might be related to IFNγ release in the cervical tumor microenvironment.

Keywords: cervical cancer, indoleamine 2,3-dioxygenase, kynurenine, tryptophan, serum, T cells, mRNA, The Cancer Genome Atlas

INTRODUCTION

In cervical cancer, a persistent infection with high-risk human papillomavirus strains (mainly types 16 and -18) is responsible for initiating carcinogenesis (1). Expression of the viral E6 and E7 oncogenes is instrumental in this process, and thereby, cervical cancer is a relatively immunogenic disease, employing various escape mechanisms to avoid the host's immune attack (2).

One of these putative tumor escape mechanisms is the expression of indoleamine 2,3-dioxygenase (IDO), which might be induced by IFNγ secretion by cytotoxic CD8$^+$ T cells in the tumor microenvironment (3, 4). IDO is an intracellular enzyme that is able to catabolize tryptophan along the kynurenine pathway. Tryptophan is an essential amino acid, necessary for protein synthesis and other metabolic cell functions. Contradictory results have been reported about the actual effect of tryptophan depletion (5). Mostly, *in vitro* and *in vivo* mice studies have shown that particularly activated, not resting, T- and natural killer (NK) cells seem to be sensitive to tryptophan-depletion and the presence of kynurenine and its derivates in the microenvironment (6–11). Upon tryptophan depletion, arrest of the cell cycle takes place in the G-phase, which in turn renders T cells more sensitive to apoptosis (6, 12, 13). In addition, it has been shown that IDO-expressing tumors promote differentiation and activation of regulatory T cells (Tregs) (9, 14, 15), which in turn can induce IDO expression in myeloid cells *via* cytotoxic T-lymphocyte-associated protein-4 (CTLA-4)–CD80/86 interactions (16) and recruit myeloid-derived suppressor cells (MDSCs) to the tumor site (17, 18). Whereas the majority of reports point to a detrimental effect of IDO expression and activity on patient outcome in various tumor types (19), others have shown IDO to be associated with favorable outcome (20–26).

In cervical cancer, IDO expression has been observed in primary and metastatic tumor cells and in immune cells, like macrophages, dendritic cells, and NK cells (27–30). In addition, IDO activity, measured by the kynurenine/tryptophan (kyn/trp) ratio, in cervical cancer patients' pretreatment sera has been reported by us and by others to be linked to disease stage and poor prognosis (31, 32). Currently, clinical trials in various tumor types are performed to explore the implementation of IDO inhibitors for cancer therapy (19), but to our knowledge, this does not yet include cervical cancer patients.

Here, for the first time, we searched for a link between IDO expression patterns in the tumor microenvironment and the presence of systemic IDO metabolites in early stage squamous cervical cancer. To this end, we have examined the association between IDO expression patterns in formalin-fixed, paraffin-embedded (FFPE) tumor tissue and the concentrations of IDO metabolites in serum. In addition, we studied the association of IDO expression patterns with clinicopathological features and the presence of proliferating cytotoxic CD8$^+$ T cells and Tregs. Also, we compared the relationships between *IDO1* and *IFNG* gene expression and linked this to survival outcome using RNAseq data from cervical tumor samples published by The Cancer Genome Atlas (TCGA).

Our findings may contribute to the development of predictive biomarkers for clinical trials using IDO inhibitors and to the development of new and more effective immunotherapy strategies for cervical cancer.

MATERIALS AND METHODS

Patient Cohort

Previously, we reported on the measurement of serum levels of IDO metabolites (tryptophan, kynurenine, and 3-hydroxykynurenine) in 251 cervical cancer patients (32). From this cohort, we selected all squamous cell carcinoma patients, diagnosed between 2003 and 2008, with surgery as primary treatment and with sufficient FFPE material available for our study. FFPE tissue blocks with 71 primary tumors (PTs) and 14 paired metastatic lymph nodes were obtained from the archives of the Department of Pathology at the Academic Medical Center (AMC) Amsterdam, The Netherlands. The main clinicopathological features of these patients are summarized in **Table 1**. None of the patients underwent chemotherapy or radiotherapy before surgery. The specimens were anonymously processed and selection of blocks was guided by initial diagnosis and review by the pathologist. Ethical approval was waived according to the regulations in The Netherlands (33).

Immunohistochemistry

Immunohistochemical staining of 71 PTs and 14 metastatic lymph nodes was performed as previously described (34) using Tris/EDTA buffer pH 9.0 for antigen retrieval, mouse-IgG1 anti-IDO antibody (1F8.2, Millipore), and ready to use Poly-HRP-GAM/R/R IgG (ImmunoLogic, The Netherlands). Complexes were visualized using 3,3′-diaminobenzidine tetrahydrochloride (Sigma, USA). Slides were counterstained with hematoxylin.

Multiplex Immunohistochemistry

On a representative subset of patients, quadruple immunofluorescence staining was performed as previously described (35) using Tris/EDTA buffer pH 9.0 for antigen retrieval. Primary antibodies mouse-IgG1 anti-FoxP3 (236A/E7; Abcam, UK), rabbit anti-Ki67 (SP6; ThermoFisher, USA), mouse-IgG2b anti-CD8 (4B11; Novocastra, UK), and secondary antibodies goat anti-mouse IgG1 Alexa Fluor 488, goat anti-Rabbit IgG Alexa Fluor 546, and goat anti-mouse IgG2b Alexa Fluor 647 (all from Thermo Scientific, USA) were used for T cell phenotyping (n = 35). Primary antibodies mouse-IgG1 anti-IDO (1F8.2, Millipore), mouse-IgG2a CD14 (clone 7, Abcam), rabbit anti-HLA-DR (ab137832, Abcam), and secondary antibodies goat anti-mouse IgG1 Alexa Fluor 488, goat anti-mouse IgG2a Alexa Fluor 546, and goat anti-Rabbit IgG Alexa Fluor 647 (all from Thermo Scientific, USA) were used for IDO-positive myeloid cell identification (n = 6). 4′,6-diamidino-2′-phenylindole, dihydrochloride (DAPI; Thermo Scientific, USA) was used as a counterstain, slides were enclosed with mounting medium and coverslips.

Multiplexed immunofluorescence staining was performed on eight patients in order to identify the type of tumor-associated vessels expressing IDO, using the OPAL 7-color fluorescence immunohistochemistry (IHC) Kit (Perkin Elmer, USA). A blocking step for endogenous peroxidase was introduced with

TABLE 1 | Patient distribution according to indoleamine 2,3-dioxygenase (IDO) expression in relation to clinicopathological characteristics.

Clinicopathological characteristics		Total	Tumor cells IDO expression			Tumor cells IDO expression pattern				Tumor-infiltrating immune cells			Stromal immune cells			Tumor-associated vessels		
		n (%)	IDO– *n* (%)	IDO+ *n* (%)	*P*	Patchy *n* (%)	Patchy + margin *n* (%)	Margin *n* (%)	*P*	IDO– *n* (%)	IDO+ *n* (%)	*P*	IDO– *n* (%)	IDO+ *n* (%)	*P*	IDO– *n* (%)	IDO+ *n* (%)	*P*
Number of patients		71 (100)	15 (21)	56 (79)	–	33 (63)	14 (26)	6 (11)	–	33 (54)	28 (46)	–	7 (10)	61 (90)	–	60 (87)	9 (13)	–
Age in years*		44.9	39.0	46.5	***0.010***	45.6	49.4	44.8	*0.499*	43.3	48.1	*0.116*	44.7	45.5	*0.911*	44.8	48.4	*0.276*
FIGO stage#	IBI	55 (77)	10 (14)	45 (63)	*0.260*	25 (47)	11 (21)	6 (11)	*0.535*	23 (38)	24 (39)	*0.222*	4 (6)	50 (74)	*0.147*	48 (70)	6 (9)	*0.396*
	≥IBII	16 (23)	5 (7)	11 (16)		8 (15)	3 (6)	0 (0)		10 (16)	4 (7)		3 (4)	11 (16)		12 (17)	3 (4)	
Tumor size#,a	≤4 cm	59 (84)	10 (14)	49 (70)	***0.034***	28 (54)	13 (25)	6 (12)	*1.000*	27 (45)	23 (38)	*1.000*	6 (9)	51 (76)	*1.000*	51 (75)	7 (10)	*0.611*
	>4 cm	11 (16)	5 (7)	6 (9)		4 (8)	1 (2)	0 (0)		6 (10)	4 (7)		1 (2)	9 (13)		8 (12)	2 (3)	
Parametrium invasion#	No	57 (80)	13 (18)	44 (62)	*0.719*	26 (49)	10 (19)	5 (9)	*0.886*	25 (41)	22 (36)	*0.795*	5 (7)	50 (74)	*0.611*	53 (77)	3 (4)	***0.001***
	Yes	14 (20)	2 (3)	12 (17)		7 (13)	4 (8)	1 (2)		8 (13)	6 (10)		2 (3)	11 (16)		7 (10)	6 (9)	
Vaginal involvement#	No	65 (91)	13 (18)	52 (73)	*0.600*	31 (58)	12 (23)	6 (11)	*0.739*	28 (46)	27 (44)	*0.205*	5 (7)	57 (84)	*0.112*	56 (81)	7 (10)	*0.172*
	Yes	6 (9)	2 (3)	4 (6)		2 (4)	2 (4)	0 (0)		5 (8)	1 (2)		2 (3)	4 (6)		4 (6)	2 (3)	
Lymph node metastases	No	49 (69)	10 (14)	39 (55)	*0.825*	22 (42)	9 (17)	5 (9)	*0.824*	18 (30)	24 (39)	***0.012***	4 (6)	45 (66)	*0.390*	43 (62)	6 (9)	*0.712*
	Yes	22 (31)	5 (7)	17 (24)		11 (21)	5 (9)	1 (2)		15 (25)	4 (6)		3 (4)	16 (24)		17 (25)	3 (4)	

FIGO: International Federation of Gynecology and Obstetrics.

[a]Of one case we do not have information on tumor size.

#P-value measured with Asymptotic Pearson's and Fisher's exact test was used when counts were <5.

**P-value was calculated with Mann–Whitney U test. IDO+, IDO-positive; IDO–, IDO-negative. NB: in three cases, we found it difficult to score IDO+ tumors for their expression pattern (patchy/margin) due to small tumor fields. In some cases (n = 10), we found it difficult to distinguish between IDO-positive immune cells and IDO-positive tumor cells and excluded those cases for scoring expression in infiltrating cells. In some cases (n = 3), we found the staining pattern not convincing due to small stromal fields in the stained tissue section and excluded those cases for scoring stromal IDO+ cells. In some cases (n = 2), we found it difficult to score IDO expression in vessels and excluded those cases.*

P value in bold italic is <0.05.

P value in italic is >0.05

0.3% H_2O_2/methanol for 20 min and an extra fixation step was included for 20 min with 10% neutral buffered formalin (Leica Biosystems, Germany), followed by 2 min in Milli-Q water and 2 min in 0.05% Tween20 in 1× Tris-buffered saline (TBST). The following primary antibodies were used: mouse-IgG1 anti-CD34 (QBEND-10; Cell Sciences), mouse-IgG2a anti-α-smooth muscle (α-sma) actin (1A4; DAKO), mouse-IgG1 anti-CD31 (JC70A; DAKO), mouse-IgG1 anti-IDO (1F8.2, Millipore), mouse-IgG1 anti-podoplanin (D2-40; BIO-RAD), and rabbit anti-galectin-1 (500-P210, PeproTech). Steps were repeated for each primary antibody; microwave treatments were carried out by placing the slides in a plastic tray, after which they were heated in 0.05% ProClin300/Tris-EDTA buffer at pH 9.0 in an 800 W standard microwave at 100% power until boiling point, followed by 15 min at 30% power. Slides were cooled down in ice water, washed in Milli-Q water and in 1× TBST, and were blocked with Normal Antibody Diluent (Immunologic, The Netherlands) for 10 min at room temperature (RT). After that, slides were incubated with primary antibody diluted in Normal Antibody Diluent for 30 min at RT and 30 rounds per minute (rpm) on a shaker. Next, slides were washed 3 × 2 min in 1× TBST at RT and 30 rpm and were subsequently incubated with SuperPicture Polymer Detection Kit—HRP—broad spectrum (Life Technologies, USA) for 20 min at RT and 30 rpm. Afterward, slides were washed 3 × 2 min in 1× TBST and were incubated with Opal fluorochromes (Opal520, Opal570, Opal650, Opal690 Opal540, and Opal620) diluted 1:150 in amplification buffer (all provided by the OPAL 7-color fluorescence IHC Kit) for 10 min at RT and 30 rpm. Slides were then washed 3 × 2 min in TBST. Finally, microwave treatment with AR6 buffer was performed and slides were washed for 2 min in Milli-Q water and for 2 min in TSBT. DAPI working solution (provided by the OPAL 7-color fluorescence IHC Kit) was applied for 5 min at RT and the slides were washed again in Milli-Q water and in 1× TSBT, and then mounted under coverslips with ProLong Diamond antifade mounting medium (Life Technologies, USA).

Imaging and Scoring

The standard IHC stained sections were scored for IDO expression by tumor cells, immune cells, and tumor-associated vessels using an Olympus BX50 bright-field microscope (Olympus, USA) by two investigators (A. Marijne Heeren and Ekaterina S. Jordanova). Primary- and metastatic tumors were designated IDO-negative (<1% of tumor cells expressed IDO) or IDO-positive (≥1% of the tumor cells expressed IDO). Also, tumor cells were divided in different groups: 0, 1–10, 10–50, and >50% positive for IDO, also used by others (27, 30). Furthermore, a distinction was made between patchy (patchy IDO expression throughout the whole tumor field) or marginal (focal staining, on the border between tumor and stroma) expression by tumors. Also, the presence of IDO-expressing tumor-infiltrating immune cells was scored in primary- and metastatic tumor samples either as absent (−) or present (+). Furthermore, IDO expression by stromal immune cells was scored as either present in low numbers (−) or high numbers (+) in stroma of PTs. In the metastatic lymph nodes, scores for IDO-positive immune cells were obtained, high (+) or low (−) numbers, for peritumoral area or in resident lymph node tissue distant from the tumor metastases. Finally, IDO expression by tumor-associated vessels was scored as 0/a few IDO-positive vessels (−) or all vessels positive for IDO (+).

Quadruple immunofluorescence stainings were imaged and analyzed using a digital imaging fluorescence microscope (Axiovert-200M; Zeiss, Germany) and SlideBook 6 Reader [Intelligent Imaging Innovations (3I), USA]. DAPI staining was used to morphologically distinguish tumor fields from stromal and healthy tissue. From each PT, three to five representative areas, including both tumor and stroma, were randomly selected and imaged with a 20× dry objective with 0.3 numerical aperture (NA). CD8-positive, FoxP3-positive, and Ki67-positive cells from digital images were manually enumerated and results were expressed as number of positive cells per square millimeters.

Seven-color multiplex stainings were visualized with Leica TCS SP8 microscope (Leica, Germany), tilescan (3 × 3, 40× oil objective with 1.3 NA) images were generated and viewed using LAS AF Lite software (Leica, Germany). IDO-positive tumor-associated vessels were analyzed for colocalization with the markers CD34, podoplanin, α-sma, galectin-1, and CD31.

TCGA RNAseq Patient Cohort

Level 3 RSEM normalized, log-transformed RNAseq data, profiled using the Illumina HiSeq RNAseq v2, were retrieved from the TCGA data portal (36). Results of the TCGA RNAseq analysis have been described in detail by TCGA Research Network (37). For our analysis, data on 144 cervical SCC patients were used, including downloaded survival data (38), *IDO1* mRNA, and *IFNG* mRNA expression in PT samples.

Statistical Analysis

Statistical analyses were performed using IBM SPSS (IBM, USA) and GraphPad Prism 5 (GraphPad Software, USA) software. Associations between IDO expression patterns in the tumor microenvironment and serum concentrations were performed using the same cutoff "low" (quartiles 1–3) and "high" (quartile 4) as previously been ascribed for survival analysis (32). Fisher's exact test was used to study the association between IDO expression in the tumor microenvironment and serum concentrations of IDO metabolites for (sub)groups with three or more patients. The Mann–Whitney *U* test, Asymptotic Pearson's- or Fisher's exact tests were used for the comparison of IDO expression patterns and clinicopathological characteristics. The log-rank test was performed for survival analyses. Before association, analyses between local IDO protein expression and T cells were carried out, normal distribution was tested using the D'Agostino and Pearson omnibus normality test. Then, based on the observed distribution, Mann–Whitney *U* test or unpaired *t* test were used or the Kruskal–Wallis or one-way ANOVA, with *post hoc* Dunn's Multiple Comparison or Bonferroni's Multiple comparison tests, respectively. Furthermore, correlation analysis between *IDO1* and *IFNG* mRNA levels, retrieved form the TCGA database, was performed by Pearson's correlation. Hierarchical cluster analysis was carried out using Euclidean distance and Ward.D2 clustering methods with the function heatmap.plus in RStudio Version 1.1.423 (RStudio, USA). Survival analysis for *IDO1* mRNA and *IFNG* mRNA were performed using the two acquired clusters (low and high) or using the median as cutoff (low and high).

Comparisons and associations with P-values below 0.05 were considered statistically significantly different.

RESULTS

IDO Expression in PTs

Indoleamine 2,3-dioxygenase protein expression was analyzed by immunohistochemistry. In the PT samples, we observed IDO positivity in tumor cells in a patchy and/or marginal expression pattern. Also, IDO expression was seen in tumor-infiltrating immune cells, stromal immune cells, and tumor-associated vessels. Among patients, various heterogeneous IDO expression patterns were observed (**Figures 1A–F** for representative images and Table S1 in Supplementary Material for IDO IHC scores per patient).

Next, we aimed to further delineate the specific cell subpopulations and vessel types expressing IDO. We hypothesized that most IDO-positive immune cells were monocytic MDSCs or tumor-associated macrophages and tried to identify these cells using multicolor fluorescent immunohistochemistry for IDO, CD14, and HLA-DR in PT section from six cervical cancer patients. IDO-positive tumor- and stroma-infiltrating cells represented a heterogeneous population of immune cells consisting of HLA-DR$^-$CD14$^+$IDO$^+$ MDSC-like cells, HLA-DR$^+$CD14$^+$IDO$^+$ dendritic/macrophage-like cells, HLA-DR$^-$CD14$^-$IDO$^+$-, and HLA-DR$^+$CD14$^-$IDO$^+$ cells (**Figure 2A**). IDO-positive tumor-associated vessels were studied by 7-color multiplex immunohistochemistry using the markers CD31/CD34 (endothelial cell markers), podoplanin (lymphatic endothelial cell marker), α-sma (perivascular cell marker), galectin-1 (activated endothelial cell marker), and IDO. The IDO-positive tumor-associated vessels were predominantly identified as mature blood vessels since most vessels stained positive for α-sma, a marker of pericytes that cover mature vessels (**Figure 2B**). In two patients, IDO expression was also observed in lymphatic (podoplanin-positive) vessels.

IDO Expression in Metastatic Lymph Nodes

In the 14 metastatic lymph node specimens available, we observed IDO positivity in tumor cells, tumor-infiltrating immune cells, immune cells surrounding metastatic tumor cells, and in resident lymph node tissue (**Figures 1G,H**). No IDO-positive vessels were observed. See Table S2 in Supplementary Material for an overview of the IDO IHC scores.

We found no evidence for elevated expression of IDO in the metastatic tumors as compared to the corresponding primary lesions. In one out of 14 metastatic lymph nodes, tumor cells were not detectable in the available tissue sections. In 8 out of 14 metastatic samples, IDO-positive tumor cells were detected. Interestingly, 7 out of 8 metastatic tumors showed a patchy IDO expression pattern. Paired analysis showed that six IDO patchy/patchy + margin expressing PTs retained patchy expression in the metastatic tumor cells, one marginal IDO-expressing PT had a patchy IDO-expressing metastatic tumor, one patchy IDO-expressing PT had a marginal IDO-expressing metastatic tumor, two IDO-negative PTs remained negative for IDO in the metastatic tumor cells and for three IDO-positive (patchy) PTs, corresponding metastatic tumors were negative for IDO (data not shown).

Association Between IDO Expression at the Tumor Site and kyn/trp Ratio in Serum

To determine, in our patient cohort (n = 71), whether IDO-positivity in the PT microenvironment correlates with serum levels of IDO metabolites tryptophan, kynurenine, and 3-hydroxykynurenine, we used previously measured serum levels from a cohort of 251 cervical cancer patients where a high kyn/trp ratio was shown to be detrimental for survival (32). The interquartile concentrations of tryptophan, kynurenine, and 3-hydroxykynurenine and the kyn/trp ratio for the current patient cohort are summarized in **Table 2** and were used for analysis.

We analyzed whether IDO expression in the local tumor microenvironment influenced the levels of IDO metabolites in serum. Notably, we found a significant association between IDO positivity in the PT and a high kyn/trp ratio in serum (P = 0.008, Fisher's exact test) (**Figure 3A**), independent of IDO expression by immune cells (infiltrate and stroma) (**Figure 3B**). Furthermore, patients with both IDO-positive tumors and vessels had significantly more often a high kyn/trp ratio in serum compared to patients with both IDO-negative tumors and vessels (P = 0.001, pairwise Fisher's exact test) and patients with IDO-positive tumors and IDO-negative vessels (P = 0.025, pairwise Fisher's exact test) (**Figure 3C**). Interestingly, we found that the dominance of tumor cell expression on systemic serum levels was independent of the percentage IDO-positive tumor cells (**Figure 3D**), but that the serum kyn/trp ratio was apparently determined by the different IDO expression patterns of the PT. All patients with IDO-negative tumors and marginal IDO-expressing tumors had a low kyn/trp ratio, whereas patients with patchy/patchy + marginal IDO expression had more often a high kyn/trp ratio in serum, which was significantly elevated when compared to patients with IDO-negative tumors (P = 0.009 and P = 0.017 respectively, pairwise Fisher's exact test) (**Figure 3E**).

No associations were found for IDO positivity in the PT microenvironment and the individual IDO metabolites tryptophan, kynurenine, and 3-hydroxykynurenine in serum. Of note, the number of metastatic lymph nodes analyzed was too small for association analysis of IDO expression with serum kyn/trp levels.

IDO Expression in Relation to Clinicopathological Characteristics and Survival

In **Table 1**, the associations between IDO expression patterns and clinicopathological characteristics of the patient cohort are shown.

Interestingly, patients with IDO-positive tumors were older (46.5 vs. 39 years old) (P = 0.010, Mann–Whitney U test) and manifested more often with smaller tumors (≤4 cm) (P = 0.034, Asymptotic Pearson's χ^2-test). However, no difference was observed in survival outcome between patients with IDO-negative and IDO-positive tumors *per se* (**Figures 4A,B**). Remarkably, all patients with marginal, including combined patchy + margin,

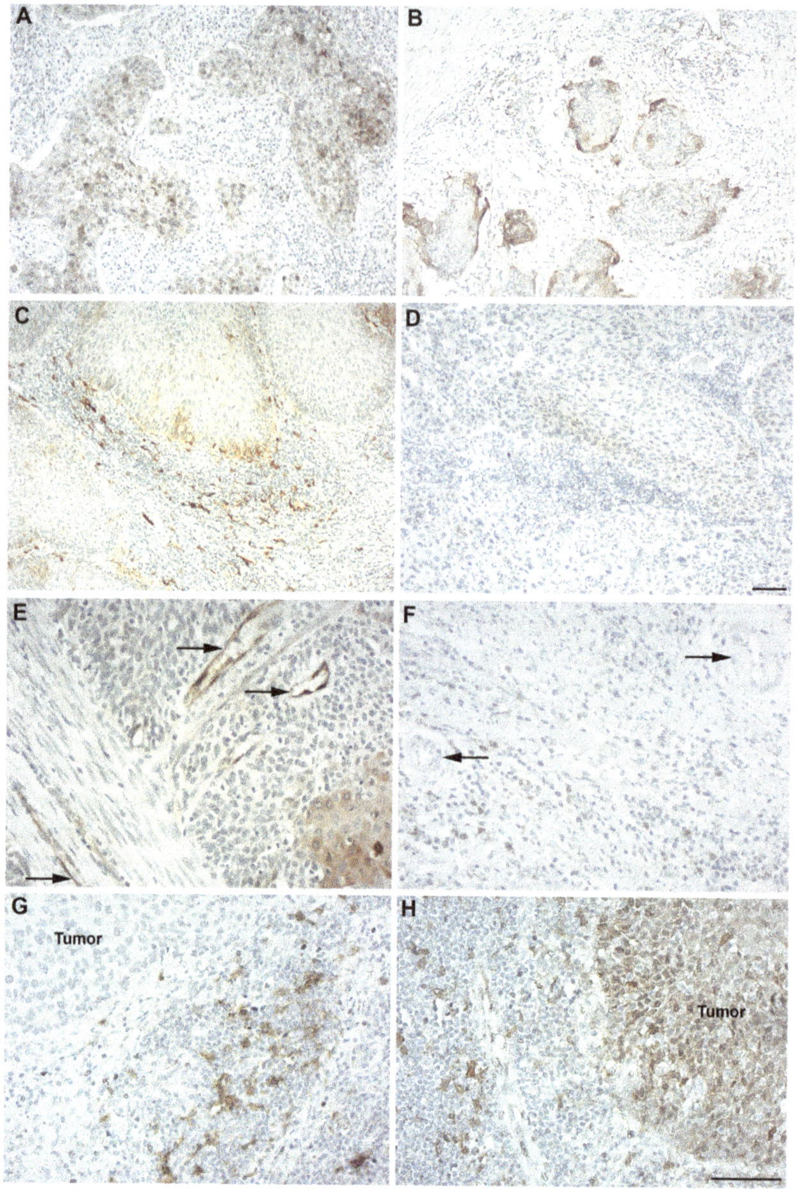

FIGURE 1 | Indoleamine 2,3-dioxygenase (IDO) expression in primary cervical cancer and metastatic lymph nodes. Different patterns for IDO expression (in brown) were detected in primary- and metastatic cervical squamous cell carcinoma. **(A)** Patchy pattern with cytoplasmic IDO expression by primary tumor (PT) cells. **(B)** Marginal IDO expression by PT cells. **(C)** High numbers of IDO-expressing stromal immune cells in a marginal IDO-expressing tumor. **(D)** IDO-negative tumors, with low IDO expression in PT cells and stromal immune cells. **(E)** IDO-positive tumor-associated vessels (indicated by black arrows). **(F)** IDO-negative tumor-associated vessels (indicated by black arrows). **(G)** Metastatic lymph node sample showing metastatic tumor cells negative for IDO and IDO-positive immune cells surrounding the tumor fields. **(H)** Metastatic lymph node sample showing nuclear and cytoplasmic IDO expression by metastatic tumor cells and IDO-positive immune cells. Magnification for **(A–D)** is 100× [scale bar in **(D)** is 100 µm] and for **(E–H)** [scale bar in **(H)** is 100 µm] is 200×.

IDO expression were disease free and still alive after a median follow-up of 60 months. These patients had improved disease-free survival (DFS) ($P = 0.017$, log-rank test) and disease-specific survival (DSS) ($P = 0.043$, log-rank test) as compared to patients with patchy IDO expression only (**Figures 4C,D**).

In addition, patients with IDO-positive tumor-infiltrating immune cells had less often lymph node metastases ($P = 0.012$, Fisher's exact test). Interestingly, patients with IDO-negative tumor-associated vessels had less often parametrium invasion ($P = 0.001$, Fisher's exact test). No further significant correlations were found. IDO expression in tumor-infiltrating immune cells and tumor-associated vessels did not affect survival (data not shown).

IDO Expression in Relation to the Distribution and Localization of T Cells

Next, in order to study the effect of IDO expression on tumor-infiltrating T cell numbers, we quantified cytotoxic

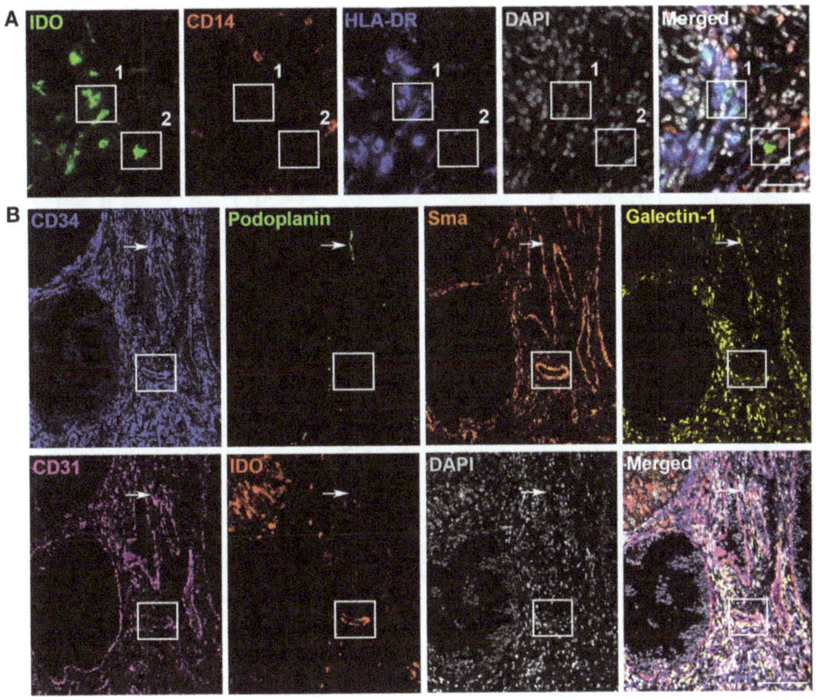

FIGURE 2 | Characterization of indoleamine 2,3-dioxygenase (IDO)-positive immune cells and tumor-associated vessels in primary cervical cancer. Different immune cells expressing IDO were detected in primary cervical cancer. **(A)** Representative immunofluorescence images showing monochromatic IDO (in green), CD14 (in red), HLA-DR (in blue), DAPI (in gray), and the merged panel with IDO, CD14, HLA-DR, and DAPI in the stromal compartment. Box 1 shows $IDO^+CD14^-HLA\text{-}DR^+$ cells and box 2 shows an $IDO^+CD14^-HLA\text{-}DR^-$ cell. Scale bar is 100 µm. **(B)** Representative immunofluorescence tilescan of a IDO-positive tumor showing monochromatic CD34 (in blue), podoplanin (in green), α sma (in glow), galectin-1 (in yellow), CD31 (in pink), IDO (in red), DAPI (in gray), and the merged image. Box indicates an IDO-positive vessel expressing CD34, α-sma, galectin-1, and CD31. Arrow indicates an IDO-negative podoplanin-positive lymphatic vessel. Scale bar is 95 µm.

TABLE 2 | Concentration of indoleamine 2,3-dioxygenase metabolites in serum (n = 71).

	Q1	Q2	Q3	Q4
Tryptophan (µmol/L)	10.86–42.36	42.37–49.73	49.74–55.37	55.38–79.88
Kynurenine (µmol/L)	0.22–1.33	1.34–1.50	1.51–1.64	1.65–2.54
3-Hydroxykynurenine (nmol/L)	3.20–24.89	24.90–32.09	32.10–37.79	37.80–84.90
Kyn/Trp ratio	16.78–25.40	25.41–28.62	28.63–34.91	34.92–52.37

Q, quartile.

$CD8^+$ T cells, $FoxP3^+(CD8^-)$ Tregs, proliferating $CD8^+Ki67^+$ T cells, proliferating $FoxP3^+Ki67^+(CD8^-)$ T cells (proliferative Tregs), and $FoxP3^+CD8^+$ T cells per square millimeters in a representative subset of patients (n = 35) (**Figure 5A**). Nuclear DAPI stain was used to distinguish tumor tissue from stromal tissue. Unexpectedly, we observed higher counts of intratumoral $CD8^+Ki67^+$ T cells in IDO-positive tumors as compared to IDO-negative tumors (P = 0.004, Mann–Whitney U test) (**Figure 5B**). No significant differences were found between IDO-negative- and IDO-positive tumors for any of the other T cell subtypes (**Figure 5C** and data not shown). Also, the IDO expression patterns, marginal, patchy + marginal, or patchy did not affect infiltrating T cell numbers (**Figures 5D,E** and data not shown).

Furthermore, we observed higher rates of intratumoral cytotoxic $CD8^+$ T cells (P = 0.041, Mann–Whitney U test), a higher intratumoral $CD8^+$ T cell/$FoxP3^+$ Treg ratio (P = 0.012, unpaired t test), higher rates of $CD8^+Ki67^+$ T cells both in the stromal (P = 0.004, Mann–Whitney U test) and intratumoral (P < 0.001, Mann–Whitney U test) compartment, in tumors with IDO-positive tumor-infiltrating immune cells (Figures S1A-C in Supplementary Material). Significantly higher rates of intratumoral $CD8^+Ki67^+$ T cells were observed in total IDO-positive PTs (PT+stroma+infiltrate+) vs. partly IDO-positive PTs (PT+stroma+infiltrate−) (Figure S1D in Supplementary Material, both P < 0.01). No further significant associations were found.

IDO1 vs. *IFNG* mRNA Expression

To test whether RNAseq data of PT samples could be used for the validation of IDO protein expression and to study a possible link between IDO and IFNγ (39), we retrieved *IDO1* and *IFNG* gene expression data from 144 cervical SCC patients from TCGA Research Network database (37). Hierarchical clustering revealed two groups: patients with both low *IDO1* and *IFNG* mRNA expression ("Low" group) and patients with both high *IDO1* and *IFNG* mRNA expression ("High" group) (**Figure 6A**). For DSS analysis, no significant associations were found between the two

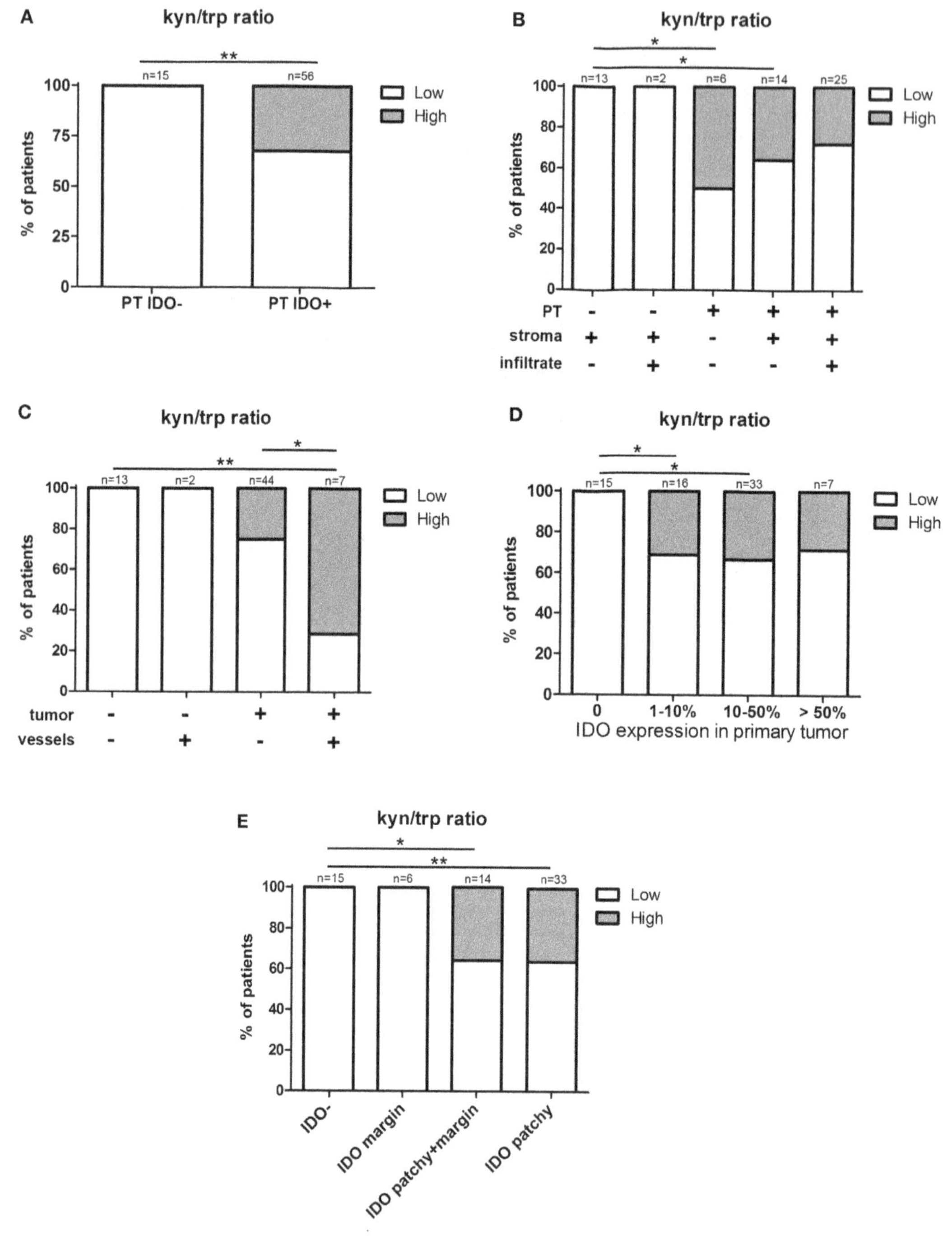

FIGURE 3 | The influence of indoleamine 2,3-dioxygenase (IDO) expression in the local tumor microenvironment on the kyn/trp ratio in serum. Graphs show low (16.78–34.91, white) and high (34.92–52.37, gray) serum kynurenine/tryptophan (kyn/trp) ratio for **(A)** patients with IDO expression (IDO−/IDO+) in primary tumor (PT). Further stratification for expression patterns in **(B)** stroma and infiltrating immune cells (stroma and infiltrate) and **(C)** tumor-associated vessels (vessels). **(D)** Patients with IDO-negative tumors (0%) and patients with IDO-positive tumors divided into groups of 1–10, 10–50, and more than 50% of IDO positivity in tumor cells, and for **(E)** patient groups with different IDO expression patterns including IDO-negative (IDO−), IDO margin, IDO patchy + margin, and patchy IDO expression by PTs. *P* values were calculated excluding subgroups with *n* = 2 or smaller, using (pairwise) Fisher's exact test. **P* = 0.01–0.05 and ***P* = 0.01–0.001.

patient groups (**Figure 6C**). However, DFS analysis showed an improved outcome for patients with "High" *IDO1* and *IFNG* as compared to patients with "Low" *IDO1* and *IFNG* mRNA expression ($P = 0.031$, log-rank test) (**Figure 6B**). Interestingly, *IDO1* and *IFNG* mRNA expression were strongly and significantly correlated ($P < 0.001$, Pearson's correlation) (**Figure 6D**).

Also, when TCGA tumors were divided into two groups based on above- or below-median *IDO1* mRNA (9.92) and *IFNG*

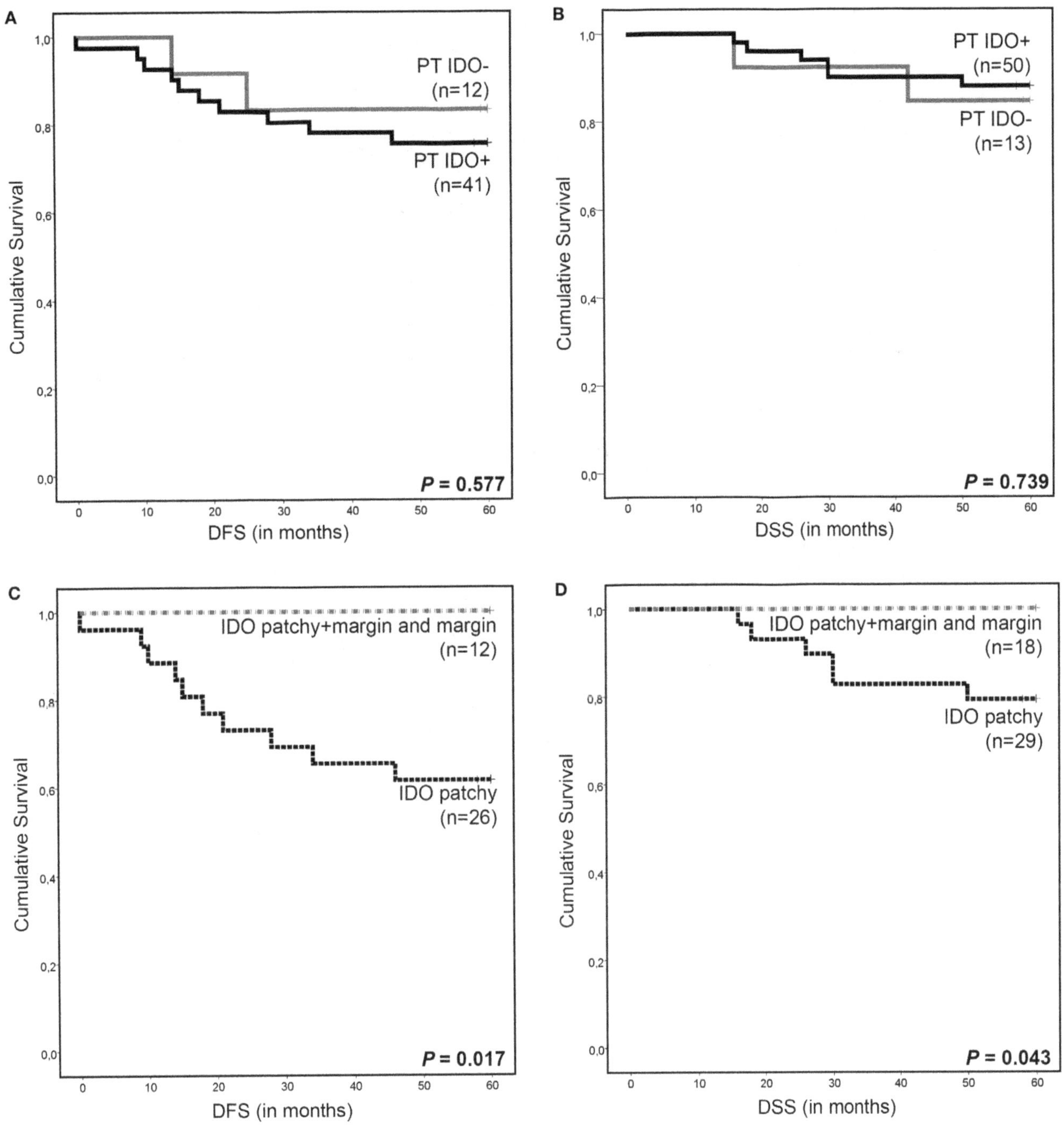

FIGURE 4 | Survival analysis according to indoleamine 2,3-dioxygenase (IDO) expression in cervical cancer. Kaplan–Meier 5-year survival curve shows **(A)** disease-free survival (DFS) and **(B)** disease-specific survival (DSS) for patients with IDO-positive primary tumors (PT IDO+, black line) and IDO-negative (PTs IDO−, gray line). Kaplan–Meier 5-year survival curves show **(C)** DFS and **(D)** DSS for patients with patchy IDO expression (black dotted line), for patients with marginal, including patchy + marginal, IDO expression (gray dotted line) by PT cells. *P* values were calculated between the different groups using the log-rank test. NB: for some patients, DFS and DSS data are missing due to loss of follow-up.

mRNA (3.71) expression levels, *IDO1* mRNA expression was not linked to survival outcome (**Figures 7A,B**), whereas for patients with above median *IFNG* mRNA expression, an improved DFS ($P = 0.008$, log-rank test) and DSS ($P = 0.039$, log-rank test) was observed (**Figures 7C,D**).

DISCUSSION

Expression of the metabolic enzyme IDO is one of the many immune escape mechanisms employed by tumor cells (40). Many clinical trials have investigated, or are currently

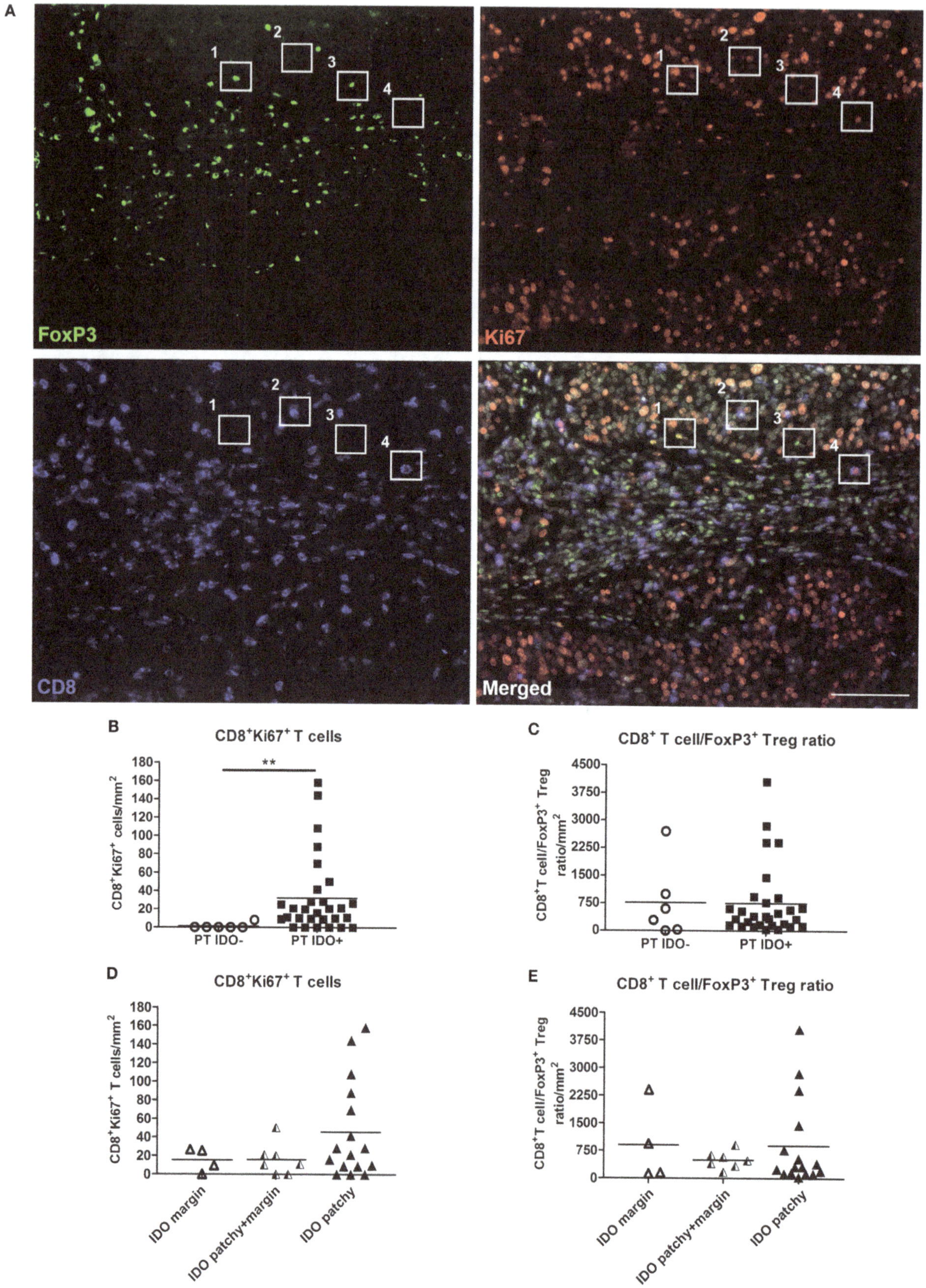

FIGURE 5 | Continued

FIGURE 5 | T cell numbers in relation to indoleamine 2,3-dioxygenase (IDO) expression by primary cervical tumor cells. **(A)** Representative immunofluorescence images showing monochromatic FoxP3 (in green), Ki67 (in red), CD8 (in blue), and the merged panel with FoxP3, Ki67, CD8 and DAPI. In box 1 a proliferating $Ki67^+FoxP3^+$ T cell is depicted, in box 2 a cytotoxic $CD8^+$ T cells is depicted, in box 3 a $FoxP3^+$ Treg is depicted, and in box 4 a proliferating $CD8^+Ki67^+$ T cell is depicted. Scale bar is 100 µm. Scatter plots show intratumoral numbers per square millimeters for **(B)** $CD8^+Ki67^+$ T cells and **(C)** $CD8^+$ T cell/$FoxP3^+$ Treg ratio in IDO-negative ($n = 6$, white dots) and IDO-positive ($n = 29$, black squares) primary tumors (PTs). Scatter plots show intratumoral numbers per square millimeters for **(D)** $CD8^+Ki67^+$ T cells and **(E)** $CD8^+$ T cell/$FoxP3^+$ Treg ratio in PTs with marginal IDO ($n = 4$, white triangles), patchy + marginal IDO ($n = 7$, black/white triangles), and patchy IDO expression ($n = 16$, black triangles). *P* values were calculated using Mann–Whitney *U* test. $^{**}P = 0.004$.

investigating, the effect of IDO inhibitors [i.e., Epacadostat and Indoximod (1-Methyl-D-Tryptophan)], and IDO peptide vaccination in cancer patients (19, 41–44). Currently, patients entering these clinical trials are not stratified for IDO positivity in tumor biopsies and/or systemic kyn/trp levels. Such information could be helpful in order to achieve higher immunotherapy response rates and avoid unnecessary over-treatment. Moreover, it was suggested that IDO activity in serum can be influenced by other factors such as chronic infection, neuropsychiatric diseases, and diet (45–48). Regrettably, extensive studies on the systemic effect of local IDO protein expression are lacking, except for a study in patients with diffuse large B cell lymphoma, which did not find an association between serum kynurenine level and IDO expression in the tumor (49) and a study in prostate cancer wherein a positive correlation between *IDO1* mRNA in PT samples and the kyn/trp ratio in serum was observed (50).

In this study, for the first time, the association between IDO expression in the tumor microenvironment and systemic concentrations of IDO metabolites in cervical cancer patients was comprehensively investigated, using a validated IDO-specific antibody (51). In the current IHC study, we included a subset of patients from the previously reported serum cohort where association between IDO activity and poor survival was observed (32). Interestingly, we did find increased systemic kyn/trp ratio levels in cervical cancer patients with IDO expression by PT cells rather than IDO expression by immune cells. Moreover, the dominance of tumoral IDO expression on kyn/trp serum levels was independent of the percentage of IDO-positive tumor cells, but rather related to patchy IDO expression, with or without marginal IDO expression (at the tumor/stroma interphase), in the PT. Remarkably, this did not directly impact patient survival. This can be explained by the fact that the current cohort consists of patients with early stage of disease (FFPE material is not available for patients with advanced disease), while in the previous serum study, a patient group comprising various disease stages was analyzed. Interestingly, survival analysis showed that patients with marginal IDO expression in the tumor, including combined patchy + marginal expression, manifested with a significantly improved outcome (DFS: $P = 0.017$; DSS: $P = 0.043$). These data are in concordance with another IDO study in cervical cancer by Inaba and colleagues (30). The marginal IDO effect was proposed to be indicative of an effective IFNγ antitumor T cell response inducing, among others, immunomodulatory factors like PD-L1 and IDO expression in tumor cells (39, 52). In line with this hypothesis, we previously reported on an association between marginal PD-L1 expression and improved prognosis in cervical cancer patients (53). In contrast, and in keeping with our PD-L1 data, patchy IDO expression may result from activation of oncogenic signaling pathways leading to intrinsically elevated expression (4, 54). Interestingly, 7 out of 8 metastatic tumors exhibited patchy IDO expression suggesting that this oncogenic signaling is more pronounced in tumors with an aggressive phenotype and poor patient outcome. Possibly, as indicated by the high kyn/trp serum ratio, IDO expression relating to a patchy expression pattern and putative oncogenic signaling occurs at higher levels than the T cell/IFNγ-induced marginal IDO levels. Although, we did not find higher numbers of (proliferating) T cells in tumors with marginal IDO expression, we did confirm a significant correlation between *IDO1* and *IFNG* mRNA expression by analyzing the available TCGA cervical cancer RNA expression data (37). To draw firm conclusions on the role of IFNγ-producing T cells on IDO expression in the complex tumor microenvironment, more in-depth analysis of the location of these cells and corresponding levels of IFNγ relative to IDO-expressing tumor cells should be performed.

Indoleamine 2,3-dioxygenase has been designated as one of the major immune escape mechanisms employed by tumors. In the cervical tumor microenvironment, IDO positivity was observed in tumor cells, immune cells, and in tumor-associated vessels making it a potential therapeutic target. Although the first clinical results on IDO inhibitors show that they are safe and well-tolerated by patients with different tumor types, no major responses have been observed yet (19, 41, 42, 44). IDO inhibitors are not tested yet in cervical cancer. In contrast to other studies that have shown a correlation between IDO expression and lower cytotoxic T cell infiltration rates and higher frequencies of Tregs, as well as an association of IDO levels with poor prognosis in different tumor types, including colorectal cancer (55), endometrial cancer (56, 57), ovarian cancer (58), and breast cancer (59), our findings did not point to a clear-cut association between IDO protein expression and poor patient outcome.

The finding in the current IHC study rather point to IDO expression in tumor cells and in immune cells as a favorable prognostic factor based on association with disease stage (tumor size and lymph node metastases), survival, and infiltration by actively proliferating cytotoxic T cells. In keeping with this notion, we observed a significant correlation between *IDO1* and *IFNG* mRNA expression, with a survival benefit for patients with high levels of *IFNG*, whether or not combined with high levels of *IDO1* expression. A prognostically favorable association for IDO expression has also previously been observed in breast cancer (22, 24), ovarian cancer (60), renal cell cancer (21), vulvar cancer (61), and lung cancer (51). Notably, in literature, there are contradictory results about the actual effect of tryptophan depletion

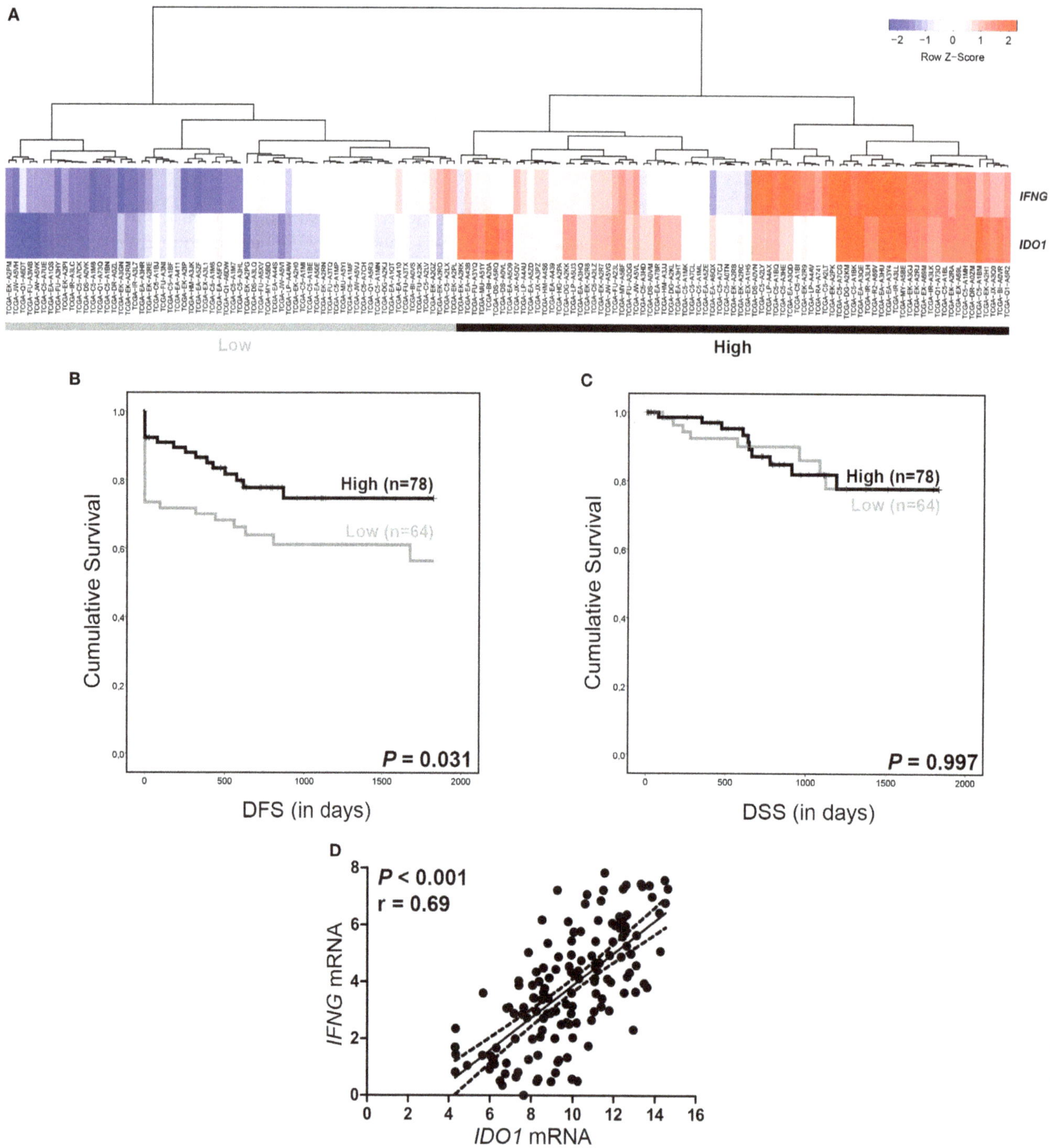

FIGURE 6 | *IDO1* and *IFNG* RNAseq data from The Cancer Genome Atlas. **(A)** Hierarchical clustering of *IDO1* and *IFNG* mRNA (rows) measured on primary tumor samples from 144 cervical SCC patients (columns) reveals a "High" (for both *IDO1* and *IFNG*) and a "Low" (for both *IDO1* and *IFNG*) patient group. Kaplan–Meier 5-year survival curve shows **(B)** disease-free survival (DFS) and **(C)** disease-specific survival (DSS) for patients with both high *IDO1* and *IFNG* (black line) and patients with both low *IDO1* and *IFNG* (gray line), based on hierarchical cluster analysis. **(D)** Graph shows correlation between *IDO1* and *IFNG*. NB: survival data was missing for two patients. *P* values for survival analysis were calculated using the log-rank test. *P* value for correlation analysis was calculated using Pearson's correlation.

on proliferating cells (7, 13, 62), and proof is yet lacking for an immunoregulatory role *in vivo* (5). A recent study using 27 cervical cancer punch biopsies showed a correlation between *IDO1* mRNA levels and a high kyn/trp ratio in primary cervical cancer tissue (63), suggesting the presence of functionally active IDO. However, tryptophan depletion *via* IDO might not be efficient

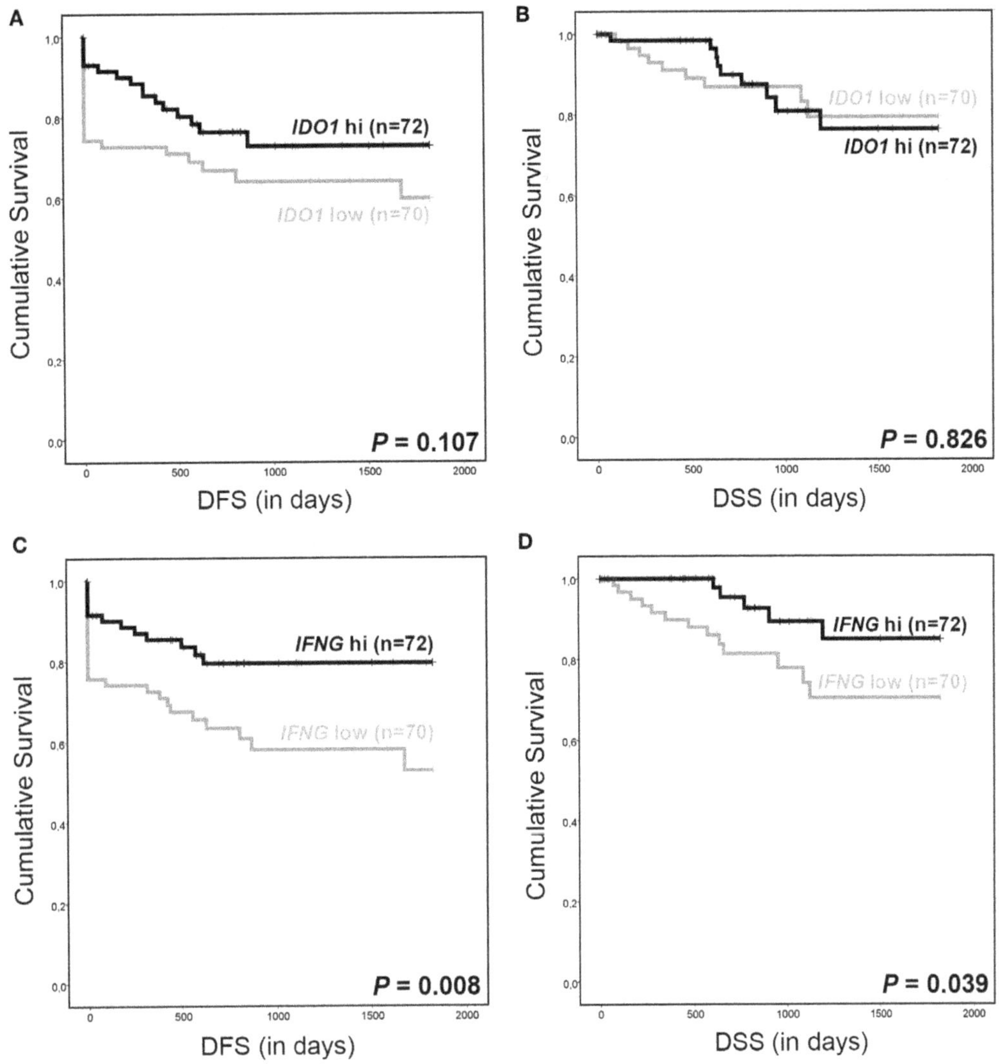

FIGURE 7 | *IDO1* and *IFNG* RNAseq data from The Cancer Genome Atlas. Kaplan–Meier 5-year survival curve shows **(A)** disease-free survival (DFS) and **(B)** disease-specific survival (DSS) for patients with low (gray line, median as cutoff, <9.92) and high (black line, median as cutoff, ≥9.92) *IDO1* mRNA expression. Kaplan–Meier 5-year survival curve shows **(C)** DFS and **(D)** DSS for patients with low (gray line, median as cutoff, <3.71) and high (black line, median as cutoff, ≥3.71) *IFNG* mRNA expression. NB: survival data were missing for two patients. *P* values for survival analysis were calculated using the log-rank test.

enough since tryptophan is able to diffuse rapidly from surrounding tissues into the tumor area (5), or can directly negatively affect the tumor cells themselves (64). This might explain why studies investigating IDO inhibitors in combination with other (immunomodulatory) drugs, like chemotherapy, α-PD-1, and α-CTLA-4, are more promising (43, 65, 66).

This is the first study to apply a multiplex fluorescent immunohistochemistry panel with six different vascular markers for vessel characterization in paraffin-embedded tissue sections. Endothelial IDO expression has previously been reported as an immunoregulatory mechanism in the context of the fetal–maternal interface and of organ transplantation (67–69). In tumors, IDO expression has also been observed in vessels in lymphoma (25, 26), melanoma (70), prostate cancer (50), and renal cell cancer (21). Here, IDO expression was predominantly observed in mature ($CD31^+/CD34^+/\alpha\text{-sma}^+$) tumor-associated blood vessels and in two patients in lymphatic (podoplanin-positive) vessels. IDO-positive vessels were associated with parametrium invasion and higher kyn/trp levels in serum. This is in contrast with another study, which showed IDO to be mainly located in neoangiogenic (CEACAM1-positive) micro-vessels and to correlate with lower rates of tumor cell proliferation (21). However, the number of cases with IDO-positive vessel is small in our study: further analysis on larger cohorts should prove the possible negative effect of IDO-positive vessels on tumor progression.

In conclusion, the effect of IDO in early stage cervical cancer appear to be highly complex. There are several tumor cell expression patterns, many different IDO-positive myeloid cell subtypes as well as varying IDO expression in the vasculature in the tumor microenvironment. Despite this complexity, we have found a dominant effect of patchy IDO expression by PT cells on kyn/trp ratio in serum. Remarkably, marginal IDO expression in tumor fields, independent of the presence of simultaneous patchy IDO expression, was associated with 100% 5-year DSS and DFS. In these patients, the ongoing IFNγ T cell response most likely outweighs any putatively detrimental effect of tryptophan depletion and resulting IDO metabolites. In conclusion, the kyn/trp ratio in serum and *IDO1* mRNA and protein expression *per se* in PTs cannot be used as a clear-cut biomarker for prognosis or to identify early stage cervical cancer patients eligible for clinical trials targeting IDO. Rather, the IDO protein expression patterns in the PT seem vital in this regard.

ETHICS STATEMENT

The specimens were anonymously processed and selection of blocks was guided by initial diagnosis and review by the pathologist. Ethical approval was waived according to the regulations in The Netherlands (http://www.federa.org, 2011).

AUTHOR CONTRIBUTIONS

AH performed the experiments, analyzed the data, and wrote the manuscript. ID performed the experiments and analyzed the data. DB and MK performed the experiments. JK and RM performed technical assistance for microscopy. CM, GK, DF and MB contributed to patient inclusion and the final review of the manuscript. VT contributed to data interpretation and to the final review of the manuscript. EJ and TG conceived and designed the experiments, data interpretation, and final review of the manuscript. All authors read and approved the final manuscript.

ACKNOWLEDGMENTS

We would like to thank Dr. Sanne Samuels for patient inclusion. This work was supported by a research grant from the Dutch Cancer Society (KWF VU 2013-6015).

SUPPLEMENTARY MATERIAL

FIGURE S1 | T cell numbers in relation to IDO expression patterns in primary cervical cancer. Scatter plots show stromal and intratumoral numbers per square millimeters for **(A)** CD8$^+$ T cells, **(B)** CD8$^+$ T cell/Foxp3$^+$ Treg ratio, and **(C)** CD8$^+$Ki67$^+$ T cells in tumors without IDO-positive tumor-infiltrating immune cells (IDO− infiltrate, white dots, $n = 14$) and with IDO-positive tumor-infiltrating immune cells (IDO+ infiltrate, black squares, $n = 17$). Scatter plot shows **(D)** intratumoral numbers of CD8$^+$Ki67$^+$ T cells in different groups of primary tumor expression patterns. *P* values were calculated in **(A–C)** using Mann–Whitney *U* test and unpaired *t* test in case of normal distribution of data. *P* values were calculated excluding subgroups with $n = 2$ or smaller (*) in **(D)** using Kruskal–Wallis test. *$P = 0.01–0.05$, **$P = 0.01–0.001$, and ***$P < 0.001$.

REFERENCES

1. De Sanjose S, Quint WG, Alemany L, Geraets DT, Klaustermeier JE, Lloveras B, et al. Human papillomavirus genotype attribution in invasive cervical cancer: a retrospective cross-sectional worldwide study. *Lancet Oncol* (2010) 11:1048–56. doi:10.1016/S1470-2045(10)70230-8
2. Piersma SJ. Immunosuppressive tumor microenvironment in cervical cancer patients. *Cancer Microenviron* (2011) 4:361–75. doi:10.1007/s12307-011-0066-7
3. Taylor MW, Feng GS. Relationship between interferon-gamma, indoleamine 2,3-dioxygenase, and tryptophan catabolism. *FASEB J* (1991) 5:2516–22. doi:10.1096/fasebj.5.11.1907934
4. Muller AJ, Duhadaway JB, Donover PS, Sutanto-Ward E, Prendergast GC. Inhibition of indoleamine 2,3-dioxygenase, an immunoregulatory target of the cancer suppression gene Bin1, potentiates cancer chemotherapy. *Nat Med* (2005) 11:312–9. doi:10.1038/nm1196
5. Terness P, Chuang JJ, Opelz G. The immunoregulatory role of IDO-producing human dendritic cells revisited. *Trends Immunol* (2006) 27:68–73. doi:10.1016/j.it.2005.12.006
6. Munn DH, Shafizadeh E, Attwood JT, Bondarev I, Pashine A, Mellor AL. Inhibition of T cell proliferation by macrophage tryptophan catabolism. *J Exp Med* (1999) 189:1363–72. doi:10.1084/jem.189.9.1363
7. Frumento G, Rotondo R, Tonetti M, Damonte G, Benatti U, Ferrara GB. Tryptophan-derived catabolites are responsible for inhibition of T and natural killer cell proliferation induced by indoleamine 2,3-dioxygenase. *J Exp Med* (2002) 196:459–68. doi:10.1084/jem.20020121
8. Terness P, Bauer TM, Rose L, Dufter C, Watzlik A, Simon H, et al. Inhibition of allogeneic T cell proliferation by indoleamine 2,3-dioxygenase-expressing dendritic cells: mediation of suppression by tryptophan metabolites. *J Exp Med* (2002) 196:447–57. doi:10.1084/jem.20020052
9. Fallarino F, Grohmann U, You S, Mcgrath BC, Cavener DR, Vacca C, et al. The combined effects of tryptophan starvation and tryptophan catabolites down-regulate T cell receptor zeta-chain and induce a regulatory phenotype in naive T cells. *J Immunol* (2006) 176:6752–61. doi:10.4049/jimmunol.176.11.6752
10. Aldajani WA, Salazar F, Sewell HF, Knox A, Ghaemmaghami AM. Expression and regulation of immune-modulatory enzyme indoleamine 2,3-dioxygenase (IDO) by human airway epithelial cells and its effect on T cell activation. *Oncotarget* (2016) 7:57606–17. doi:10.18632/oncotarget.11586
11. Van De Velde LA, Guo XJ, Barbaric L, Smith AM, Oguin TH III, Thomas PG, et al. Stress kinase GCN2 controls the proliferative fitness and trafficking of cytotoxic T cells independent of environmental amino acid sensing. *Cell Rep* (2016) 17:2247–58. doi:10.1016/j.celrep.2016.10.079
12. Lee GK, Park HJ, Macleod M, Chandler P, Munn DH, Mellor AL. Tryptophan deprivation sensitizes activated T cells to apoptosis prior to cell division. *Immunology* (2002) 107:452–60. doi:10.1046/j.1365-2567.2002.01526.x
13. Munn DH, Sharma MD, Baban B, Harding HP, Zhang Y, Ron D, et al. GCN2 kinase in T cells mediates proliferative arrest and anergy induction in response to indoleamine 2,3-dioxygenase. *Immunity* (2005) 22:633–42. doi:10.1016/j.immuni.2005.03.013
14. Curti A, Pandolfi S, Valzasina B, Aluigi M, Isidori A, Ferri E, et al. Modulation of tryptophan catabolism by human leukemic cells results in the conversion of CD25- into CD25+ T regulatory cells. *Blood* (2007) 109:2871–7.
15. Baban B, Chandler PR, Sharma MD, Pihkala J, Koni PA, Munn DH, et al. IDO activates regulatory T cells and blocks their conversion into Th17-like T cells. *J Immunol* (2009) 183:2475–83. doi:10.4049/jimmunol.0900986
16. Fallarino F, Grohmann U, Hwang KW, Orabona C, Vacca C, Bianchi R, et al. Modulation of tryptophan catabolism by regulatory T cells. *Nat Immunol* (2003) 4:1206–12. doi:10.1038/ni1003
17. Mellor AL, Munn DH. IDO expression by dendritic cells: tolerance and tryptophan catabolism. *Nat Rev Immunol* (2004) 4:762–74. doi:10.1038/nri1457
18. Holmgaard RB, Zamarin D, Li Y, Gasmi B, Munn DH, Allison JP, et al. Tumor-expressed IDO recruits and activates MDSCs in a Treg-dependent manner. *Cell Rep* (2015) 13:412–24. doi:10.1016/j.celrep.2015.08.077

19. Brochez L, Chevolet I, Kruse V. The rationale of indoleamine 2,3-dioxygenase inhibition for cancer therapy. *Eur J Cancer* (2017) 76:167–82. doi:10.1016/j.ejca.2017.01.011
20. Ishio T, Goto S, Tahara K, Tone S, Kawano K, Kitano S. Immunoactivative role of indoleamine 2,3-dioxygenase in human hepatocellular carcinoma. *J Gastroenterol Hepatol* (2004) 19:319–26. doi:10.1111/j.1440-1746.2003.03259.x
21. Riesenberg R, Weiler C, Spring O, Eder M, Buchner A, Popp T, et al. Expression of indoleamine 2,3-dioxygenase in tumor endothelial cells correlates with long-term survival of patients with renal cell carcinoma. *Clin Cancer Res* (2007) 13:6993–7002. doi:10.1158/1078-0432.CCR-07-0942
22. Jacquemier J, Bertucci F, Finetti P, Esterni B, Charafe-Jauffret E, Thibult ML, et al. High expression of indoleamine 2,3-dioxygenase in the tumour is associated with medullary features and favourable outcome in basal-like breast carcinoma. *Int J Cancer* (2012) 130:96–104. doi:10.1002/ijc.25979
23. Yuan F, Liu Y, Fu X, Chen J. Indoleamine-pyrrole 2,3-dioxygenase might be a prognostic biomarker for patients with renal cell carcinoma. *Zhong Nan Da Xue Xue Bao Yi Xue Ban* (2012) 37:649–55. doi:10.3969/j.issn.1672-7347.2012.07.001
24. Soliman H, Rawal B, Fulp J, Lee JH, Lopez A, Bui MM, et al. Analysis of indoleamine 2-3 dioxygenase (IDO1) expression in breast cancer tissue by immunohistochemistry. *Cancer Immunol Immunother* (2013) 62:829–37. doi:10.1007/s00262-013-1393-y
25. Choe JY, Yun JY, Jeon YK, Kim SH, Park G, Huh JR, et al. Indoleamine 2,3-dioxygenase (IDO) is frequently expressed in stromal cells of Hodgkin lymphoma and is associated with adverse clinical features: a retrospective cohort study. *BMC Cancer* (2014) 14:335. doi:10.1186/1471-2407-14-335
26. Nam SJ, Kim S, Paik JH, Kim TM, Heo DS, Kim CW, et al. An increase in indoleamine 2,3-dioxygenase-positive cells in the tumor microenvironment predicts favorable prognosis in patients with diffuse large B-cell lymphoma treated with rituximab, cyclophosphamide, doxorubicin, vincristine, and prednisolone. *Leuk Lymphoma* (2016) 57:1956–60. doi:10.3109/10428194.2015.1117610
27. Uyttenhove C, Pilotte L, Theate I, Stroobant V, Colau D, Parmentier N, et al. Evidence for a tumoral immune resistance mechanism based on tryptophan degradation by indoleamine 2,3-dioxygenase. *Nat Med* (2003) 9:1269–74. doi:10.1038/nm934
28. Nakamura T, Shima T, Saeki A, Hidaka T, Nakashima A, Takikawa O, et al. Expression of indoleamine 2, 3-dioxygenase and the recruitment of Foxp3-expressing regulatory T cells in the development and progression of uterine cervical cancer. *Cancer Sci* (2007) 98:874–81. doi:10.1111/j.1349-7006.2007.00470.x
29. Kobayashi A, Weinberg V, Darragh T, Smith-Mccune K. Evolving immunosuppressive microenvironment during human cervical carcinogenesis. *Mucosal Immunol* (2008) 1:412–20. doi:10.1038/mi.2008.33
30. Inaba T, Ino K, Kajiyama H, Shibata K, Yamamoto E, Kondo S, et al. Indoleamine 2,3-dioxygenase expression predicts impaired survival of invasive cervical cancer patients treated with radical hysterectomy. *Gynecol Oncol* (2010) 117:423–8. doi:10.1016/j.ygyno.2010.02.028
31. Fotopoulou C, Sehouli J, Pschowski R, VON Haehling S, Domanska G, Braicu EI, et al. Systemic changes of tryptophan catabolites via the indoleamine-2,3-dioxygenase pathway in primary cervical cancer. *Anticancer Res* (2011) 31:2629–35.
32. Ferns DM, Kema IP, Buist MR, Nijman HW, Kenter GG, Jordanova ES. Indoleamine-2,3-dioxygenase (IDO) metabolic activity is detrimental for cervical cancer patient survival. *Oncoimmunology* (2015) 4:e981457. doi:10.4161/2162402X.2014.981457
33. Federation of Dutch Medical Scientific Societies. *Federation of Biomedical Scientific Societies. Human Tissue and Medical Research: Code of Conduct for Responsible Use [Internet]*. Rotterdam, The Netherlands (2011). [A4 web-based version, approved October 2015]. Available from: http://Www.Federa.Org
34. Ferns DM, Heeren AM, Samuels S, Bleeker MC, De Gruijl TD, Kenter GG, et al. Classical and non-classical HLA class I aberrations in primary cervical squamous- and adenocarcinomas and paired lymph node metastases. *J Immunother Cancer* (2016) 4:78. doi:10.1186/s40425-016-0184-3
35. Heeren AM, De Boer E, Bleeker MC, Musters RJ, Buist MR, Kenter GG, et al. Nodal metastasis in cervical cancer occurs in clearly delineated fields of immune suppression in the pelvic lymph catchment area. *Oncotarget* (2015) 6:32484–93. doi:10.18632/oncotarget.5398
36. NCI Genomic Data Commons (GDC). *TCGA Data Portal – Project ID: TCGA-CESC*. MD, USA: NCI Center for Cancer Genomics (CCG), National Cancer Institute. Available from: https://Gdc.Cancer.Gov/ (Accessed: March, 2018).
37. Cancer Genome Atlas Research Network, Albert Einstein College Of Medicine, Analytical Biological Services, Barretos Cancer Hospital, Baylor College Of Medicine, Beckman Research Institute of City Of Hope, et al. Integrated genomic and molecular characterization of cervical cancer. *Nature* (2017) 543:378–84. doi:10.1038/nature21386
38. Broad Institute TCGA Genome Data Analysis Center. *Cervical and Endocervical Cancers (CESC)*. Harvard, MA, USA: Broad Institute of MIT. Available from: http://firebrowse.org/ (Accessed: March, 2018).
39. Spranger S, Spaapen RM, Zha Y, Williams J, Meng Y, Ha TT, et al. Up-regulation of PD-L1, IDO, and T(regs) in the melanoma tumor microenvironment is driven by CD8(+) T cells. *Sci Transl Med* (2013) 5:200ra116. doi:10.1126/scitranslmed.3006504
40. Johnson TS, Munn DH. Host indoleamine 2,3-dioxygenase: contribution to systemic acquired tumor tolerance. *Immunol Invest* (2012) 41:765–97. doi:10.3109/08820139.2012.689405
41. Soliman HH, Minton SE, Han HS, Ismail-Khan R, Neuger A, Khambati F, et al. A phase I study of indoximod in patients with advanced malignancies. *Oncotarget* (2016) 7:22928–38. doi:10.18632/oncotarget.8216
42. Beatty GL, O'dwyer PJ, Clark J, Shi JG, Bowman KJ, Scherle PA, et al. First-in-human phase I study of the oral inhibitor of indoleamine 2,3-dioxygenase-1 epacadostat (INCB024360) in patients with advanced solid malignancies. *Clin Cancer Res* (2017) 23:3269–76. doi:10.1158/1078-0432.CCR-16-2272
43. National Library of Medicine. Clinicaltrials.Gov [Internet]. MD, USA: National Institutes of Health. Available from: https://clinicaltrials.gov/ (Accessed: 2018).
44. Kristeleit R, Davidenko I, Shirinkin V, El-Khouly F, Bondarenko I, Goodheart MJ, et al. A randomised, open-label, phase 2 study of the IDO1 inhibitor epacadostat (INCB024360) versus tamoxifen as therapy for biochemically recurrent (CA-125 relapse)-only epithelial ovarian cancer, primary peritoneal carcinoma, or fallopian tube cancer. *Gynecol Oncol* (2017) 146:484–90. doi:10.1016/j.ygyno.2017.07.005
45. Fuchs D, Forsman A, Hagberg L, Larsson M, Norkrans G, Reibnegger G, et al. Immune activation and decreased tryptophan in patients with HIV-1 infection. *J Interferon Res* (1990) 10:599–603. doi:10.1089/jir.1990.10.599
46. Heyes MP, Saito K, Crowley JS, Davis LE, Demitrack MA, Der M, et al. Quinolinic acid and kynurenine pathway metabolism in inflammatory and non-inflammatory neurological disease. *Brain* (1992) 115(Pt 5):1249–73. doi:10.1093/brain/115.5.1249
47. Strasser B, Berger K, Fuchs D. Effects of a caloric restriction weight loss diet on tryptophan metabolism and inflammatory biomarkers in overweight adults. *Eur J Nutr* (2015) 54:101–7. doi:10.1007/s00394-014-0690-3
48. Hestad KA, Engedal K, Whist JE, Farup PG. The relationships among tryptophan, kynurenine, indoleamine 2,3-dioxygenase, depression, and neuropsychological performance. *Front Psychol* (2017) 8:1561. doi:10.3389/fpsyg.2017.01561
49. Ninomiya S, Hara T, Tsurumi H, Goto N, Saito K, Seishima M, et al. Indoleamine 2,3-dioxygenase expression and serum kynurenine concentrations in patients with diffuse large B-cell lymphoma. *Leuk Lymphoma* (2012) 53:1143–5. doi:10.3109/10428194.2011.643472
50. Feder-Mengus C, Wyler S, Hudolin T, Ruszat R, Bubendorf L, Chiarugi A, et al. High expression of indoleamine 2,3-dioxygenase gene in prostate cancer. *Eur J Cancer* (2008) 44:2266–75. doi:10.1016/j.ejca.2008.05.023
51. Schalper KA, Carvajal-Hausdorf D, Mclaughlin J, Altan M, Velcheti V, Gaule P, et al. Differential expression and significance of PD-L1, IDO-1, and B7-H4 in human lung cancer. *Clin Cancer Res* (2017) 23:370–8. doi:10.1158/1078-0432.CCR-16-0150
52. Taube JM, Anders RA, Young GD, Xu H, Sharma R, Mcmiller TL, et al. Colocalization of inflammatory response with B7-h1 expression in human melanocytic lesions supports an adaptive resistance mechanism of immune escape. *Sci Transl Med* (2012) 4:127ra137. doi:10.1126/scitranslmed.3003689
53. Heeren AM, Punt S, Bleeker MC, Gaarenstroom KN, Van Der Velden J, Kenter GG, et al. Prognostic effect of different PD-L1 expression patterns in squamous cell carcinoma and adenocarcinoma of the cervix. *Mod Pathol* (2016) 29:753–63. doi:10.1038/modpathol.2016.64

54. Litzenburger UM, Opitz CA, Sahm F, Rauschenbach KJ, Trump S, Winter M, et al. Constitutive IDO expression in human cancer is sustained by an autocrine signaling loop involving IL-6, STAT3 and the AHR. *Oncotarget* (2014) 5:1038–51. doi:10.18632/oncotarget.1637
55. Brandacher G, Perathoner A, Ladurner R, Schneeberger S, Obrist P, Winkler C, et al. Prognostic value of indoleamine 2,3-dioxygenase expression in colorectal cancer: effect on tumor-infiltrating T cells. *Clin Cancer Res* (2006) 12:1144–51. doi:10.1158/1078-0432.CCR-05-1966
56. Ino K, Yamamoto E, Shibata K, Kajiyama H, Yoshida N, Terauchi M, et al. Inverse correlation between tumoral indoleamine 2,3-dioxygenase expression and tumor-infiltrating lymphocytes in endometrial cancer: its association with disease progression and survival. *Clin Cancer Res* (2008) 14:2310–7. doi:10.1158/1078-0432.CCR-07-4144
57. De Jong RA, Kema IP, Boerma A, Boezen HM, Van Der Want JJ, Gooden MJ, et al. Prognostic role of indoleamine 2,3-dioxygenase in endometrial carcinoma. *Gynecol Oncol* (2012) 126:474–80. doi:10.1016/j.ygyno.2012.05.034
58. Inaba T, Ino K, Kajiyama H, Yamamoto E, Shibata K, Nawa A, et al. Role of the immunosuppressive enzyme indoleamine 2,3-dioxygenase in the progression of ovarian carcinoma. *Gynecol Oncol* (2009) 115:185–92. doi:10.1016/j.ygyno.2009.07.015
59. Yu J, Sun J, Wang SE, Li H, Cao S, Cong Y, et al. Upregulated expression of indoleamine 2, 3-dioxygenase in primary breast cancer correlates with increase of infiltrated regulatory T cells in situ and lymph node metastasis. *Clin Dev Immunol* (2011) 2011:469135. doi:10.1155/2011/469135
60. Mills AM, Peres LC, Meiss A, Ring KL, Modesitt SC, Abbott SE, et al. Targetable immune regulatory molecule expression in high-grade serous ovarian carcinomas in African American Women: a study of PD-L1 and IDO in 112 cases from the African American Cancer Epidemiology Study (AACES). *Int J Gynecol Pathol* (2018). doi:10.1097/PGP.0000000000000494
61. De Jong RA, Toppen NL, Ten Hoor KA, Boezen HM, Kema IP, Hollema H, et al. Status of cellular immunity lacks prognostic significance in vulvar squamous carcinoma. *Gynecol Oncol* (2012) 125:186–93. doi:10.1016/j.ygyno.2011.12.416
62. Sonner JK, Deumelandt K, Ott M, Thome CM, Rauschenbach KJ, Schulz S, et al. The stress kinase GCN2 does not mediate suppression of antitumor T cell responses by tryptophan catabolism in experimental melanomas. *Oncoimmunology* (2016) 5:e1240858. doi:10.1080/2162402X.2016.1240858
63. Hascitha J, Priya R, Jayavelu S, Dhandapani H, Selvaluxmy G, Sunder Singh S, et al. Analysis of kynurenine/tryptophan ratio and expression of IDO1 and 2 mRNA in tumour tissue of cervical cancer patients. *Clin Biochem* (2016) 49:919–24. doi:10.1016/j.clinbiochem.2016.04.008
64. Takikawa O, Kuroiwa T, Yamazaki F, Kido R. Mechanism of interferon-gamma action. Characterization of indoleamine 2,3-dioxygenase in cultured human cells induced by interferon-gamma and evaluation of the enzyme-mediated tryptophan degradation in its anticellular activity. *J Biol Chem* (1988) 263:2041–8.
65. Soliman HH, Jackson E, Neuger T, Dees EC, Harvey RD, Han H, et al. A first in man phase I trial of the oral immunomodulator, indoximod, combined with docetaxel in patients with metastatic solid tumors. *Oncotarget* (2014) 5:8136–46. doi:10.18632/oncotarget.2357
66. Bjoern J, Iversen TZ, Nitschke NJ, Andersen MH, Svane IM. Safety, immune and clinical responses in metastatic melanoma patients vaccinated with a long peptide derived from indoleamine 2,3-dioxygenase in combination with ipilimumab. *Cytotherapy* (2016) 18:1043–55. doi:10.1016/j.jcyt.2016.05.010
67. Daubener W, Schmidt SK, Heseler K, Spekker KH, Mackenzie CR. Antimicrobial and immunoregulatory effector mechanisms in human endothelial cells. Indoleamine 2,3-dioxygenase versus inducible nitric oxide synthase. *Thromb Haemost* (2009) 102:1110–6. doi:10.1160/TH09-04-0250
68. Sedlmayr P, Blaschitz A, Stocker R. The role of placental tryptophan catabolism. *Front Immunol* (2014) 5:230. doi:10.3389/fimmu.2014.00230
69. Schmid PM, Bouazzaoui A, Schmid K, Birner CM, Schach C, Maier LS, et al. Vascular alterations in a murine model of acute graft-versus-host disease are associated with decreased serum levels of adiponectin and an increased activity and vascular expression of indoleamine 2,3-dioxygenase. *Cell Transplant* (2016) 25:2051–62. doi:10.3727/096368916X691646
70. Chevolet I, Speeckaert R, Haspeslagh M, Neyns B, Kruse V, Schreuer M, et al. Peritumoral indoleamine 2,3-dioxygenase expression in melanoma: an early marker of resistance to immune control? *Br J Dermatol* (2014) 171:987–95. doi:10.1111/bjd.13100

13

Immune Checkpoint Inhibition for Pancreatic Ductal Adenocarcinoma: Current Limitations and Future Options

*Derya Kabacaoglu, Katrin J. Ciecielski†, Dietrich A. Ruess† and Hana Algül**

Internal Medicine II, Klinikum rechts der Isar, Technische Universität München, Munich, Germany

Edited by:
Alexandr Bazhin,
Klinikum der Universität München, Germany

Reviewed by:
Carmen Guerra,
Centro Nacional de Investigaciones Oncológicas CNIO—Fundación Cáncer FUCA, Spain
Cara Haymaker,
University of Texas MD Anderson Cancer Center, United States

***Correspondence:**
Hana Algül
hana.alguel@mri.tum.de

†These authors have contributed equally to this work.

Pancreatic ductal adenocarcinoma (PDAC), as the most frequent form of pancreatic malignancy, still is associated with a dismal prognosis. Due to its late detection, most patients are ineligible for surgery, and chemotherapeutic options are limited. Tumor heterogeneity and a characteristic structure with crosstalk between the cancer/malignant cells and an abundant tumor microenvironment (TME) make PDAC a very challenging puzzle to solve. Thus far, targeted therapies have failed to substantially improve the overall survival of PDAC patients. Immune checkpoint inhibition, as an emerging therapeutic option in cancer treatment, shows promising results in different solid tumor types and hematological malignancies. However, PDAC does not respond well to immune checkpoint inhibitors anti-programmed cell death protein 1 (PD-1) or anti-cytotoxic T lymphocyte-associated antigen 4 (CTLA-4) alone or in combination. PDAC with its immune-privileged nature, starting from the early pre-neoplastic state, appears to escape from the antitumor immune response unlike other neoplastic entities. Different mechanisms how cancer cells achieve immune-privileged status have been hypothesized. Among them are decreased antigenicity and impaired immunogenicity *via* both cancer cell-intrinsic mechanisms and an augmented immunosuppressive TME. Here, we seek to shed light on the recent advances in both bench and bedside investigation of immunotherapeutic options for PDAC. Furthermore, we aim to compile recent data about how PDAC adopts immune escape mechanisms, and how these mechanisms might be exploited therapeutically in combination with immune checkpoint inhibitors, such as PD-1 or CTLA-4 antibodies.

Keywords: pancreatic ductal adenocarcinoma, immune checkpoint inhibitors, triple E, antigenicity, immunogenicity, tumor microenvironment

INTRODUCTION

Pancreatic ductal adenocarcinoma (PDAC), as one of the most fatal malignancies in the world, is the fourth leading cause of cancer-related deaths among both men and women in developed countries (1). Its mortality almost equals its incidence: for 2018 alone, 55,440 diagnoses of pancreatic cancer are projected for the United States with 44,330 associated deaths in the same year (2). At the time of diagnosis, only a minority of patients have localized, resectable tumors (10%); while most patients display locally advanced disease (29%) and/or distant metastasis (52%), and the remainder are not even staged (2). The 5-year survival rate of pancreatic cancer is only around 7–8% in the United States, which is likely due to late stage diagnosis (2, 3). The high number of estimated pancreatic cancer-related deaths can be hypothesized to be due to several factors: first, late and unspecific symptoms, as well as a lack of PDAC-specific markers or screening resources result in late diagnosis at an advanced stage. Second, delayed diagnosis leads to low resection rates, since most of the tumor patients present with locally advanced or metastatic disease. And third, PDAC is characterized by a low response to radiotherapy (RT) and chemotherapy, which, at least in part, is due to its dense desmoplastic stroma impairing drug delivery (4–6). Also, targeted therapies including small drug inhibitors of key molecular signaling pathways associated with PDAC progression showed almost none (i.e., MEK and PI3K) or only mild benefits (e.g., EGFR) with a moderate increase in overall survival (7–12). Recent advances in chemotherapeutic options for PDAC appear to provide a survival benefit that will likely not be sufficient to decrease mortality rates (13–15). Hence, in developed countries, PDAC is expected to be the second leading cause of cancer-related deaths by 2030 (1, 16). Impaired efficacy of chemotherapy or targeted therapies in cancer was associated with innate and acquired resistance through genetic and epigenetic instability of cancer cells (17, 18). Immunotherapy offers great potential for the treatment of tumors displaying such resistance. Especially T cells with their ability to generate receptors recognizing the heterogeneous and specific repertoire of tumor-related antigens provide great promise in cancer therapeutics. The adaptive immune response might even form an immunological memory providing long-term tumor control. Studies revealing how T cells function under pathophysiological conditions led to development of immune checkpoint inhibitors, which have been successfully translated into the clinic. Thus far, immune checkpoint inhibition (ICI) has shown promising results for the treatment of solid tumors, including melanomas (19–22), as well as lung (23–27), renal (28, 29), bladder (30–32), and head and neck cancers (33, 34), as well as in hematological malignancies, such as Hodgkin's disease (35, 36) and follicular or diffuse-large B-cell lymphoma (37). Although single-agent treatment with immune checkpoint inhibitors showed great promise with many solid tumors, their effect on PDAC has been quite disappointing (38, 39).

Here, we want to discuss the unique characteristics of PDAC immune evasion and why PDAC is unresponsive toward checkpoint inhibition. First, we will provide details concerning immune checkpoint inhibitors and their mechanism of action. Second, the immune-privileged nature of PDAC will be examined. Then, the antigenic and immunogenic attributes of PDAC and how tumor cell-intrinsic and -extrinsic factors within the tumor microenvironment (TME) regulate immunogenicity will be comprehensively discussed, including options for pharmacological modulation of these mechanisms to increase ICI therapy response in the clinic.

IMMUNE CHECKPOINT INHIBITORS

T cells with their various subsets are involved in the regulation of immune responses in autoimmune diseases, but also against infections and cancer. In TME or in tumor-resident lymph nodes, professional antigen-presenting cells (APCs) such as dendritic cells (DCs) display tumor-specific antigens to naïve T cells through major histocompatibility complexes (MHCs) in a process called priming (40). Antigen presentation through MHC-class II acts on naïve CD4$^+$ T cells, giving rise to Th_1, Th_2, and Foxp3$^+$ regulatory T cell (T_{reg}) subtypes, which are all important for immune response orchestration (41): Th_1 polarization induces cytokines (characterized mainly by IFNγ production) further augmenting MHC expression in APCs (42) and antitumor T cell and macrophage cytotoxic activity (43). Th_2 polarized cells are characterized by IL-4 and IL-13 production, leading to exhaustion of T cells and enhancement of other tumor-promoting responses (44, 45). T_{regs} get activated once the effector T cell activation reaches a threshold. With the release of immunosuppressive cytokines (TGF_β and IL-10) T_{regs} negatively regulate T cell effector function (46). On the other hand, antigen presentation through MHC-class I leads to differentiation of naïve CD8$^+$ T cells into cytotoxic T lymphocytes (CTLs), which are directly able to kill antigen-expressing cancer cells (41). Upon MHC:antigen engagement, activated T cells clonally expand in secondary lymphoid organs, and traffic into the inflammatory sites to execute their functions and release intermediary cytokines and ligands to provoke helper immune cells for further support (40).

T cell-mediated immune response is tightly regulated *via* both the repertoire of immunosuppressive cells in the microenvironment and cell-intrinsic regulation of anergy and exhaustion (47). T cell anergy is the state of T cells in which they are hyporesponsive to triggers of naïve T cell differentiation (47). And T cell exhaustion describes a process by which effector T cells become resistant to persistent reactivation (47). Under physiological conditions, T cell activation upon MHC engagement is balanced *via* co-regulation of both stimulatory and inhibitory signals, referred to as immune checkpoints. The balance between stimulatory and inhibitory signals is crucial to generate self-tolerance and to maintain the ability to fight with non-self. However, tumor cells shift this balance toward their benefit by abrogating co-activatory signals and augmenting co-inhibitory signals ultimately heightening anergy and exhaustion (48).

Cytotoxic T lymphocyte-associated antigen 4 (CTLA-4 or CD152) and programmed cell death protein 1 (PD-1 or CD279) are the most studied co-inhibitory receptors of T cell receptor (TCR) signaling (40). The first antibody against CTLA-4, ipilimumab, was approved in 2011 (19), while pembrolizumab and nivolumab, antibodies that both target PD-1, were approved in 2014 for the treatment of melanoma (20, 21, 38). The clinical success of antibodies targeting CTLA-4 and PD-1 marks a breakthrough as these agents established immunotherapy as a new pillar of cancer treatment strategies next to surgery, chemotherapy, and radiation therapy (49).

After TCR engagement with cognate peptide presented by a MHC molecule, costimulatory receptor CD28 binding with CD80 (B7.1) or CD86 (B7.2) amplifies TCR signaling (50). CTLA-4, on the other hand, has higher affinity for CD80 and CD86, outcompeting CD28 binding (50, 51), and subsequently sequestering CD80 and CD86 from the APC surface (52). Initial TCR activation with CD28 co-activation increases IL-2 release, which induces metabolism, proliferation, and survival in a paracrine manner. However, gradual CTLA-4 accumulation on the T cell membrane replaces the activation signal of CD28, blocking IL-2 accumulation (53). Since B7 proteins are expressed on APCs but not on solid tumor cells, the action of CTLA-4 inhibition is thought to take place in secondary lymphoid organs where early T cell activation occurs. CTLA-4 action on $CD8^+$ CTLs is inhibitory, as shown in several studies (54, 55). Still, the overall inhibitory action of CTLA-4 is thought to mainly show itself through its action on $CD4^+$ $Foxp3^+$ T_{regs}, indirectly modulating $CD8^+$ CTL action (48). T_{regs} produce CTLA-4 constitutively through the action of their subset defining transcription factor Foxp3 (56–58). Deletion of CTLA-4 in T_{regs} reduces their activity, blocking their immune-suppressive action (59, 60). Still, use of CTLA4 antibodies in preclinical mouse models of PDAC did not affect T_{reg} infiltration in tumors while enhancing total $CD4^+$ T cell presence (61). T_{regs} might also mediate effector T cell activation through APCs, impairing their B7 ligand expression, and thereby decreasing the CD28 co-activation signal on effector T cells (52). Overall, CTLA-4 engagement downregulates effector T cell activity, while enhancing T_{reg} immunosuppressive activity (59, 62). Inhibiting CTLA-4 action might enhance immunosurveillance through both its action on effector and T_{regs}.

Programmed cell death protein 1 belongs to the family of CD28 proteins, initiating co-inhibitory signaling upon TCR engagement (63, 64). Ligands of PD-1 receptor PD-L1 (B7-H1 or CD274) and PD-L2 (B7-DC or CD273) belong to the B7 family of proteins (64–67). PD-1 is expressed mostly on late effector phase $CD4^+$ helper T cells and $CD8^+$ cytotoxic T cells in peripheral tissues (63, 68). Especially chronically activated, then exhausted $CD8^+$ cytotoxic T cells show constitutive PD-1 production (69–72). Therefore, PD-1 action is mostly associated with the late phase of immune response, which counterbalances cytotoxic T cell activity. PD-1 is also expressed on T_{regs} and PD-1 blockage leads T_{reg} apoptosis (73). Also, PD-L1 stimulation of naïve T cells can skew differentiation toward the T_{reg} subset (74). Therefore, anti-PD-1 treatment might show an indirect effect on antitumor T cells through its inhibitory actions on T_{regs} (75).

Programmed cell death protein 1 knock out mice show reduced peripheral tolerance and display autoimmunity (76, 77), with a milder phenotype compared with CTLA-4 knock out mice (78, 79). There is a prominent difference between CTLA-4 and PD-1 effects. Anti-CTLA-4 action mostly results in changes in secondary lymphoid organs during the initial phase of naïve T cell activation, while anti-PD-1 treatment targets the effector phase of T cell activation in the periphery where the activated T cells attack the target (40, 48, 80). In addition, CTLA-4 is mobilized to the cell membrane upon TCR engagement in naïve T cells directly from the protein stores, implicating its importance for initial T cell activation (81). By contrast, PD-1 transport requires an initial transcriptional production causing a 6–12 h delay in response upon TCR engagement (48). Considering the differences in mode of action between CTLA-4 and PD-1, PD-1 blockage is thought to be effective in TME (80). Tumor-infiltrating lymphocytes (TILs) in the TME are frequently exhausted due to chronic exposure to the tumor antigens and PD-L1 directly produced by the tumor cells or anti-inflammatory cells of the TME (82). Anti-PD-1 or anti-PD-L1 therapy aims to reduce this exhausted state of TILs in the TME. Of note, PD-1 blockage (e.g., nivolumab) shows milder autoimmunity-related side effects than anti-CTLA-4 treatment (e.g., ipilimumab) in melanoma patients (19, 83). Considering anti-CTLA-4 and PD-1 therapy has implications in different phases of immune response, combination therapy with nivolumab and ipilimumab showed prolonged progression free survival and a higher objective response rate than ipilimumab alone, albeit with concomitant higher toxicity (84).

THE IMMUNE-PRIVILEGED NATURE OF PDAC: IMMUNOSURVEILLANCE AND IMMUNOEDITING

The immunosurveillance hypothesis was proposed by Paul Ehrlich (85) in the early 1900s and later developed further by Thomas and Burnet (86, 87). As a very important concept for cancer immunotherapy, immunosurveillance states that immune cells continually survey somatic cells for any malignant transformation to then destroy them (88). The concept of cancer immunoediting is a byproduct of the immunosurveillance process, in which cancer cells undergo a Darwinian-like selection for their capacity to evade an attack by the immune system (88). The concept of tumor immunoediting proposed by Schreiber and colleagues in 2002 states three different phases of tumor immunoediting: elimination, equilibrium, and escape (i.e., triple E hypothesis) (**Figure 1**) (88, 89). As being more comprehensive than immunosurveillance, immunoediting proposes that not only innate immunity but also adaptive immunity is involved in the elimination process of tumor cells. During the equilibrium phase, tumor cell variants surviving the dynamic but relentless pressure of adaptive and innate immunity undergo a Darwinian-like selection. At the end of the equilibrium phase, many of the tumor cells are dead, whereas new clones generated, likely through genetic instability with better resistance to the immune response, remain. In the escape phase, survivors of the equilibrium phase start to expand in numbers, maintaining an immune-privileged state (89).

Before the wide use of genetically engineered mouse models (GEMMs) of PDAC, human or mouse tumor transplantation into mice had been the main model for preclinical studies of therapeutic response (90). To eliminate simple tissue rejection of tumor xenografts, mostly immune-incompetent mouse models had been utilized. However, these models are unsuitable for studies of the immune response toward tumors. Furthermore, syngeneic murine transplantation models do not provide information regarding the tumorigenesis process. GEMMs for PDAC harboring pancreas-specific expression of mutant Kras recapitulate carcinogenesis of human PDAC, as pre-neoplastic lesions (PanIN) reliably progress to invasive and metastatic cancer (91). In this mouse model, $CD45^+$ leukocytes were shown to accumulate in time as the disease progresses. However, $CD4^+$ T cells observed in PanIN lesions were mostly of the $Foxp3^+$ T_{reg} subtype, accompanied by an abundance of myeloid-derived suppressor cells (MDSCs) and M2 macrophages (92). Strikingly, infiltration by $CD8^+$ antitumor

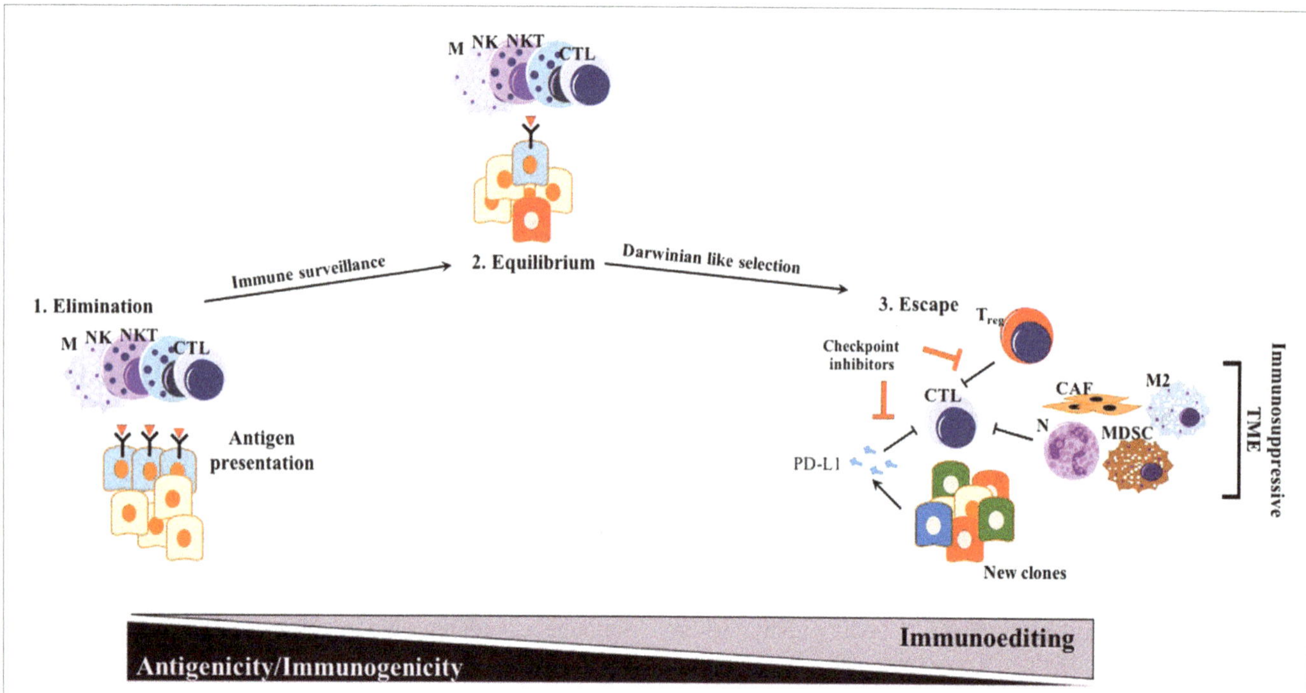

FIGURE 1 | Conventional triple E hypothesis: elimination, equilibrium, and escape. While many solid tumors responding to ICI therapy follow triple E of immunoediting, PDAC is mostly an exception. Generated new clones due to Darwinian-like selection reduce their antigenicity and immunogenicity, escaping from immunosurveillance. Abbreviations: M, macrophages; NK, natural killer; NKT, natural killer T cells; CTLs, cytotoxic T lymphocytes; N, neutrophils; M2, M2 phenotype macrophages; MDSCs, myeloid-derived suppressor cells; T_{reg}, regulatory T cells; CAFs, cancer-associated fibroblasts; ICI, immune checkpoint inhibition.

cytotoxic T cells was very scarce in early PanIN lesions, and only a small portion of advanced tumors actually showed presence of active $CD8^+$ CTLs (92). This spontaneous carcinogenesis model of PDAC highlights the immune-privileged status of PDAC even in the early neoplastic state (92). Unlike for many other solid tumors, the elimination phase of the triple E hypothesis is almost absent or substantially impaired during murine carcinogenesis due to the scarcity of cytotoxic immune cells and the abundant presence of immunosuppressive cells (92). Thus, ablation of T cells did not affect the spontaneous formation of cancer in KPC models (LSL—$Kras^{G12D/+}$; LSL—$Trp53^{R172H/+}$; Pdx—1Cre) (93). However, ectopic expression of a strong neoantigen (e.g., ovalbumin) in cancer cells boosted T cell-mediated immunity, rescuing the elimination phase of the immunoediting sequence. Expression of a single, yet strong, neoantigen thus allowed tumor control *via* CTL infiltration and "Triple E" (immune active) immunoediting. This implies that the scarcity of neoantigens in PDAC is not a result of the elimination step of immunoediting, but rather due to an alternative mechanism more like immune quiescence (**Figure 2**). Because of immune quiescence in tumors with low basal adaptive immune activation, CTLs cannot invade into the TME to initiate conventional immunoediting during carcinogenesis, which is true for the KPC model (93). This model represents human PDAC fairly well, showing an "immune quiescence like" phenotype rather than an "immune active" one (94). Reduced $CD8^+$ CTL and increased $CD4^+$ $Foxp3^+$ T_{reg} infiltration in progressive PDAC has also been validated in human patient samples (95).

In summary, PDAC frequently does not undergo a Darwinian-like selection with respect to the adaptive immune response. Thus, it retains vulnerability toward the natural T cell repertoire. Thus, strategies boosting T cell priming, activation levels, and attraction are promising for the treatment of this cancer (96).

FACTORS DETERMINING THE EFFICACY OF ICI AND FAILURE IN PDAC

Two important factors determine the prospects of immunotherapy of cancer in general, and checkpoint inhibition, in particular, antigenicity and immunogenicity, the latter being modulated by both intrinsic properties of tumor cells and TME (97) (**Figure 3**). Considering the, to date, low efficacy of immunotherapy, and especially checkpoint inhibition in PDAC, a better understanding of the immune escape mechanisms present in PDAC will pave the way for combination factors of checkpoint inhibition for the treatment of this generally intractable disease. A list of selected preclinical mouse model studies focusing on ICI combination therapies in PDAC can be found in **Table 1**.

Antigenicity

Antigenicity refers to the ability of tumor cells to produce and present tumor-specific antigens (TSA) and tumor-associated antigens (TAAs) to the adaptive immune system (97). The bottlenecks of antigenicity include the range of TAA and TSA production, and their ability to be presented to the immune system

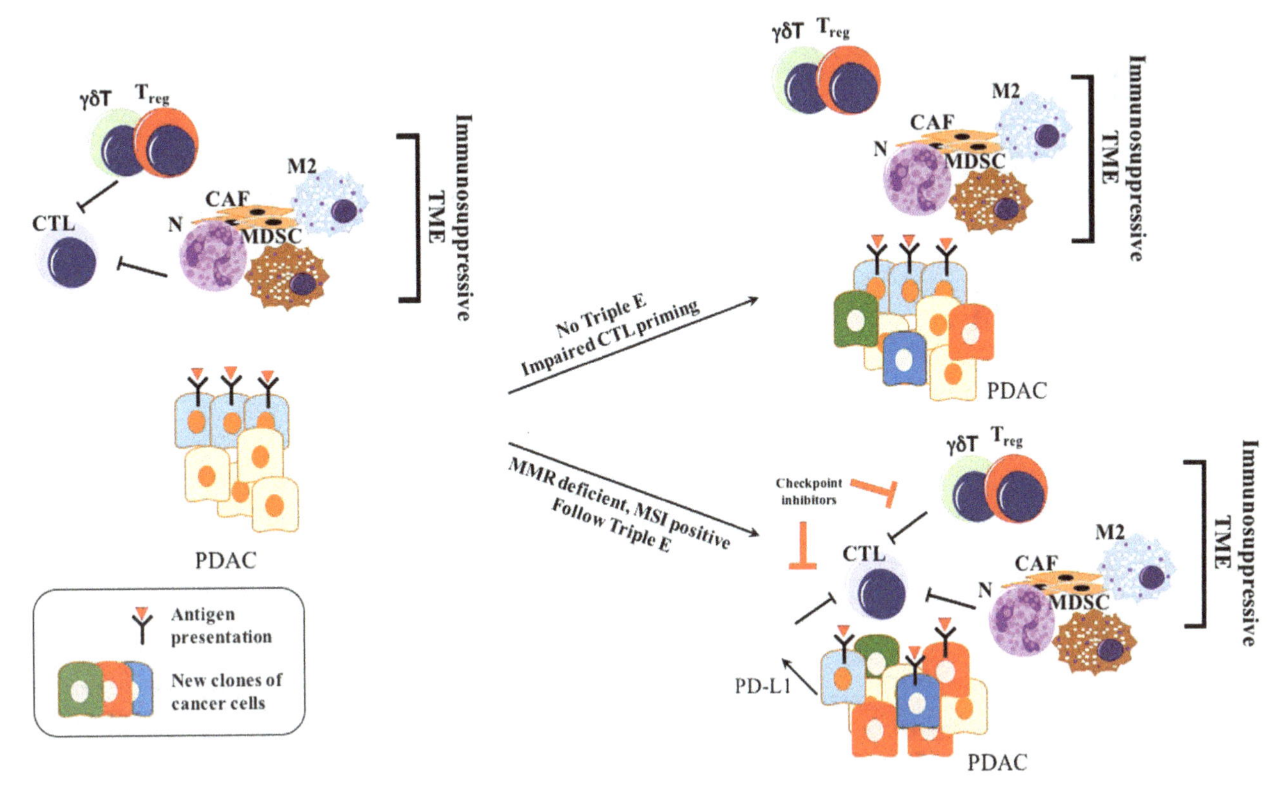

FIGURE 2 | Immunoediting in PDAC: only tumors with genetic instability follow Triple E, while others cannot. Immunosuppressive TME blocks initial CTL priming. Therefore, cancer cells are not forced to undergo Darwinian-like selection. PDAC can still retain its antigenic capacity while impairing immunogenicity making it unresponsive to checkpoint inhibitors. Abbreviations: CTLs, cytotoxic T lymphocytes; N, neutrophils; M2, M2 phenotype macrophages; MDSCs, myeloid-derived suppressor cells; T_{regs}, regulatory T cells; CAFs, cancer-associated fibroblasts; γδT, γδT cells; MMR, mismatch repair; MSI, microsatellite instability; TME, tumor microenvironment.

through MHC complexes (human leukocyte antigen—HLA—in humans) (97, 98). TAAs are overexpressed in cancer cells while their expression is low in normal cells, whereas TSA subtype neoantigens are produced *de novo* upon mutational changes of tumor cells (98). These mutations can favor neoantigen tethering to MHCs, produce a new residue on neoantigens increasing TCR recognition, or generate a proteolytic cleavage site, providing better processing for antigen presentation (99). Since TSAs are expressed only in malignant cells, they provide great specificity for T cell cytotoxicity (98). Epigenetic regulation of TAAs in tumor cells can also represent an important target for T cell action (99). In melanoma patients, even tumors with a low mutational burden, but with a high expression of TAAs, which is likely mediated by epigenetic mechanisms, showed considerable response to immunotherapy (100).

Cancers with high mutation rates such as melanoma, bladder cancer, and lung cancer show better response to check point inhibition compared with other types with a lower mutational burden, for instance, PDAC (101–105). Especially tumors with mismatch repair (MMR) deficiency or with more microsatellite instability (MSI) are shown to respond better to immunotherapy (106). As a matter of fact, impairing MMR through genetic inactivation of mutL homolog 1 gene (MLH1) in PDAC mouse models provoked hypermutation, triggering more neoantigen production. This, in turn, prolonged immunosurveillance with better therapeutic response to immune check point inhibitors (**Figure 2**) (107). Humphris et al. reported that among the 385 resected patient samples only 1% of showed MSI with inactivation of MLH1 and MSH2 (mutS protein homolog 2). This may provide a possible explanation for low response rate to immunotherapy in PDAC (108). Pembrolizumab, a PD-1 antibody, was approved by the Food and Drug Administration in 2017 for solid tumors with MMR defects or MSI, including PDAC (106). Use of DNA damage response (DDR) inhibitors may also enhance the genetic instability of the cancer cells upon exposure to DNA damaging agents, increasing the production of neoantigens. On the other hand, DDR inhibition may show a tumorigenic effect by acting on antitumor immune cells (109). Still, mutational load is not a reliable biomarker for the prediction of response to immunotherapy, considering the patients who were not responding to immunotherapy even if they had a high mutation burden. Likewise, tumors with a low mutational load, such as renal cell carcinomas, responded well to immunotherapy (28, 110).

Recently, Balachandran et al. described a neoantigen quality fitness model identifying long-term survivors of PDAC *via* selecting neoantigens with great resemblance to disease derived peptides (111). On the other hand, a neoantigen quantity model showing more immunosurveillance in response to increasing

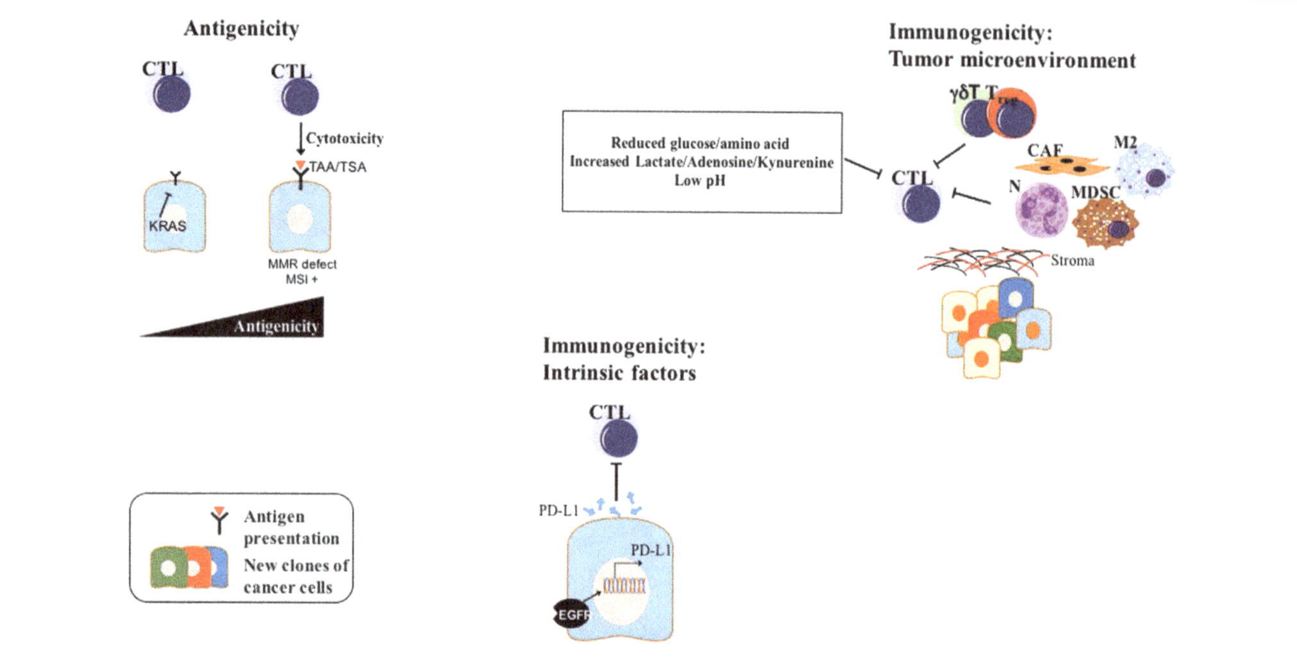

FIGURE 3 | Factors determining ICI efficiency in PDAC: while modulation of antigenicity, intrinsic immunogenicity, and extrinsic immunogenicity *via* TME might be valid for many tumors, drawn examples above are experimentally shown for PDAC. Abbreviations: TAAs, tumor-associated antigens; TSAs, tumor-specific antigens; CTLs, cytotoxic T lymphocytes; N, neutrophils; M2, M2 phenotype macrophages; MDSCs, myeloid-derived suppressor cells; T_{regs}, regulatory T cells; CAFs, cancer-associated fibroblasts; γδT, γδT cells; MMR, mismatch repair; MSI, microsatellite instability; TME, tumor microenvironment; ICI, immune checkpoint inhibition.

neoantigen numbers revealed no long-term survivors by itself. Only tumors showing both, high neoantigen numbers and abundant $CD8^+$ cytotoxic T cell infiltration, were associated with a significant survival benefit for the patients. Supporting the immune quiescence-like phenotype of PDAC, a modest decrease in high-quality neoantigen transcript levels was seen. More strikingly, they identified a loss of high-quality neoantigen expression in metastatic tumors compared with their primary counterparts. In conclusion, identification of hotspot neoantigens and methods to exploit or target them may increase the response to checkpoint inhibition, not only regarding the primary tumor but also regarding metastatic lesions.

Another mode of reduced antigenicity is the loss of antigen presentation, which can reduce immunosurveillance either by blocking priming of naïve T cells, or by making cancer cells invisible to effector T cell function (97, 112). In other cancer types, reduced antigen presentation was achieved by downregulation of MHC class proteins or impaired antigen processing and shuttling (113–116). Oncogenic RAS signaling was shown to reduce antigen presentation in different cancer types, including PDAC (113, 117, 118). Also, HLA-1 and transporter for antigen presentation production was demonstrated to be reduced in human PDAC specimens (113, 117–119). Manipulating cancer cells for enhanced antigen presentation can reinforce the checkpoint inhibition response.

As a matter of fact, Pommier et al. recently showed that disseminated cancer cells (DCCs, metastatic, quiescent single cancer cells) are undergoing a Darwinian-like selection during immune surveillance of metastasis (120). These investigators elegantly showed that only the metastatic cancer cells, negative for MHC-I and CK-19 expression on the surface, could form DCCs, avoiding T cell-mediated killing in pre-immunized mice. ER stress was the barrier for DCCs to maintain a quiescent state, and also to escape from T-cell-mediated immunity. Therefore, to form macrometastasis, in addition to ER stress relieve, a systemic immunity depletion was required. All these results show how important it is for cancer cells (both primary and metastatic tumor cells) to have good quality neoantigens, and a competency to present neoantigens through MHC complexes to immune cells.

The correlation between total neoantigen load and checkpoint inhibition response is absent in PDAC unlike in other, immunogenic tumors, such as melanoma or lung cancer (104, 121–125). This implies that other factors, determined by the immunogenic properties of PDAC, play an important role in the response to immunotherapy of this malignancy.

Immunogenicity

Immunogenicity of cancer refers to its ability to induce an adaptive immune response. Based on comprehensive integrated genomic analysis, PDAC was classified into different subgroups by several studies (126–130). RNA expression analysis identified an immunogenic subtype of PDAC in 25 among 96 PDAC patient specimens. This subtype is associated with an increased immune cell infiltration, and enriched signatures such as $CD4^+$ and $CD8^+$ T cell signaling, antigen presentation, B cell signaling, and most notably CTLA-4 and PD-1 signaling. Signatures enriched in immunogenic subtype might represent predictive biomarkers for immunotherapeutic response in PDAC (130).

TABLE 1 | Selection of studies focusing on immune checkpoint inhibition (ICI) combination therapies in preclinical mouse PDAC model.

Combination approach	Method	Preclinical mouse model	Control group/treatment	Experimental group/treatment	Results	Reference
Oncogenic signaling	MEK inhibition	Subcutaneous transplantation of $KP^{lox/+}C$ mouse cell line	Either MEKi (GSK1120212) or mPD-1-Ab	MEKi and mPD-1-Ab	Reduced tumor growth and possible regression	(140)
Stromal remodeling	FAP^{+} cell depletion	$KP^{R172H}C$ transgenic mouse model with modified *fap* gene driving diphtheria toxin receptor expression in FAP^{+} cell	Only diphtheria toxin (DTx)	DTx with mPD-L1-Ab	Reduced tumor volume	(158)
			Only diphtheria toxin (DTx)	DTx with cytotoxic T lymphocyte-associated antigen 4 (CTLA-4)-Ab	Deceleration of tumor growth	
	CXCR4 inhibition	$KP^{R172H}C$ autochthonous mouse model	CXCR4i (AMD3100) with isotype control	CXCR4i and CTLA-4-Ab	No effect	
			CXCR4i (AMD3100) with isotype control	CXCR4i and mPD-1-Ab	Reduced tumor growth	
	Focal adhesion kinase (FAK) inhibition	Syngeneic and orthotopic tumor transplantation of mouse PDAC cell lines isolated from $KP^{lox/+}C$ mice	Low dose gemcitabine with either FAKi (VS4718) or mPD-1-Ab	Low dose gemcitabine with FAKi and mPD-1-Ab	Reduced tumor burden, improved overall survival	(160)
			Low dose gemcitabine with either FAKi or anti-CTLA4	Low dose gemcitabine with FAKi, and CTLA-4-Ab	No benefit	
			Low dose gemcitabine with FAKi and mPD-1-Ab	Low dose gemcitabine with FAKi and mPD-1-Ab and CTLA-4-Ab	Reduced tumor burden	
		$KP^{lox/lox}C$ autochthonous mouse model	Low dose gemcitabine with mPD-1-Ab and CTLA-4-Ab	Low dose gemcitabine with FAKi and mPD-1-Ab and CTLA-4-Ab	Increased survival, 2/15 mice are long-term survivors	
	Interleukin 6 (IL-6) targeting	Isolated cancer cells from $KP^{R172H}C$ mice and Pan02 cells were subcutaneously transplanted, KPC-luc cells orthotopically transplanted into C57BL/6 mice	Either isotype control or anti-IL-6 or mPD-1-Ab	Anti-IL-6 and mPD-1-Ab in combination	Reduced tumor growth	(169)
		KPC-Brca2 autochthonous mouse model	Isotype control	Anti-IL-6 and mPD-1-Ab in combination	Extended overall survival	
	Hyaluronan depletion	Orthotopic transplanted $KP^{R172H}C$-luc cells or KPC-Brca autochtonous mice	Either *Salmonella*-based sh-IDO (shIDO-ST) delivery or PEGPH20	*Salmonella*-based sh-IDO (shIDO-ST) delivery and PEGPH20	Reduced tumor burden, increased overall survival	(177)
Myeloid compartment	Cluster of differentiation 40 (CD40) agonist	Subcutaneously transplanted $KP^{R172H}C$ cells	Either gemcitabine/nab-paclitaxel or CD40 agonist-Ab	Gemcitabine/nab-paclitaxel and CD40 agonist-Ab	Higher tumor regression, enhanced survival, reduced overall tumor growth rate, maintained T cell memory	(203)
	CXCR2 inhibitors	$KP^{R172H}C$ autochthonous mouse model	mPD-1-Ab treatment with vehicle	mPD-1-Ab treatment with CXCR2 SM (AZ13381758)	Extended survival, 2/14 mice long-term survivors	(212)
	CSF1R inhibitors	Orthotopic transplantation of KC-INK4A/$Arf^{lox/lox}$	Gemcitabine with either vehicle or CTLA-4-Ab or CSF1Ri (PLX3397)	Gemcitabine with CTLA-4-Ab and CSF1Ri	More than 90% reduced tumor progression	(216)
			Either vehicle or CTLA-4-Ab and mPD-1-Ab combination, or CSF1Ri	CTLA-4-Ab, mPD-1-Ab, and CSF1Ri combination	Completely blocked tumor progression, 15% tumor regression	
			Gemcitabine with either vehicle or CTLA-4-Ab and mPD-1-Ab combination, or CSF1R-Ab	Gemcitabine with CTLA-4-Ab, mPD-1-Ab, and CSF1R-Ab combination	Completely blocked tumor progression, 85% tumor regression	
Metabolic regulation	Glucocorticoid treatment	Pre-cachectic $KP^{R172H}C$ autochthonous	Isotype and PBS treatment	CXCR4i (AMD3100) with mPD-L1-Ab	Arrested PDA growth	(254)
			Isotype, PBS, and corticosterone treatment	CXCR4i (AMD3100), mPD-L1-Ab, and corticosterone	PDA is no more arrested, tumor growth in control and experimental groups was same	
Radiotherapy	Radiation with ICI	Subcutaneous transplantation of $KP^{R172H}C$ cell line	Either treatment of CTLA-4-Ab or mPD-1-Ab or radiation, or dual combinations	CTLA-4-Ab, mPD-1-Ab, and radiation triple combination	Extended survival	(269)
	Radiation with CD40 agonist-Ab	Subcutaneous and orthotopic transplantation of $KP^{R172H}C$ cell line	Radiation with CTLA-4-Ab and mPD-1-Ab	Radiation, CTLA-4-Ab, mPD-1-Ab, and CD40 agonist-Ab	Increased abscopal effect, extended survival	(270)

Cytolytic activity is determined by the transcription levels of granzyme A (GZMA) and perforin (PRF1), which are known cytotoxicity markers of $CD8^+$ T cells (131). Interestingly, genetic amplification of MYC and/or deletion of CDKN2A/B were associated with reduced cytolytic activity in TCGA PDAC datasets (125). Mutant Kras-mediated immunosuppression *via* GM-CSF or IL17R production might be another reason for impaired cytolytic activity in PDAC (132–134). Other than oncogenic drivers, stromal composition may have an impact: PDAC with so-called "normal" stroma (127) (i.e., a good version of stroma, characterized by high ACTA2, VIM, and DES pancreatic stellate cell-PSC markers) was associated with a higher cytolytic activity (125). Considering various factors determine cytolytic activity other than neoantigenic capacity, it is important to adapt individualized precision immunotherapy covering different determinants of immunogenicity in PDAC (125, 135). For an ease of understanding, the determinants of immunogenicity can be divided into two: intrinsic and extrinsic factors.

Intrinsic Determinants of Immunogenicity

Antigenic tumors can still evade ICI therapy *via* downregulation of tumor cell-intrinsic immunogenicity (97). In various cancers, stimulation of oncogenic pathways such as PI3K (136, 137), MYC (138), TAZ (139), and JAK-STAT (35) through either excessive ligand production or their mutations induces constitutive PD-L1 production (**Figure 2**). Myeloid cell induction of EGFR and MAPK signaling in PDAC cells enhanced PD-L1 production inhibiting $CD8^+$ T cell infiltration (140). The expression of PD-L1 in various tumors was associated with higher immune cell infiltration and the presence of lymphoid aggregates, and tumors with naturally high levels of PD-L1 in these showed comparably high response rates to anti-PD-1 or anti-PD-L1 (38, 83, 141). Regulation of PD-L1 and other checkpoint inhibitors or oncogenic signaling cascades in cancer cells also constitute an important place for the regulation of tumor immunogenicity (142–144).

Although initial IFNγ production is favorable for CTL activity, chronic exposure may lead to immunoediting in tumor cells. As a result of this, tumors develop genetic or epigenetic modifications in IFNγ signaling components such as IFNγ receptors (IFNGR1 and IFNGR2), JAK-STAT pathway components and IRF1 transcription factors (145, 146). A loss of function mutation on Apelin receptor has recently been identified impairing IFNγ induced JAK-STAT signaling cascade in melanoma (147). Although IFNγ is considered to be antitumorigenic, its induction of PD-L1 transcription in cancer cells might positively correlate to anti-PD-1 or PD-L1 therapy response in established tumors (148). Since IFNγ exposure of cancer cells induces PD-L1 production, mutations in IFNγ signaling components JAK1 and JAK2 would lead to clonal evolution of PD-L1-negative tumor cells, which are not responsive to anti-PD-1 treatment (149). Although no such mutations have been identified in PDAC, personalized medicine can favor the prediction of checkpoint inhibition response through identification of these type of mutations.

Several solid tumors including PDAC showed anti-PD-1 resistance signatures (IPRES) such as enhanced mesenchymal transformation, cell adhesion, extracellular matrix modeling, angiogenesis, hypoxia, and wound healing in TCGA datasets (123). Overall, the differential mutational and transcriptional landscape of tumors does not only determine neoantigen quality and quantity but also regulates several signaling pathways responsible for intrinsic and extrinsic properties of immunogenicity in cancer.

Extrinsic Determinants of Immunogenicity: Modulation of TME

Cytotoxic T lymphocyte infiltration into the TME is essential for ICI therapy (150). Even if the anti-tumor CTL infiltration is seen in many tumor types, PDAC represents an outlier in this manner (92). Starting from the premalignant lesions, its microenvironment restricts the cytotoxic T cell infiltration. The cytotoxic T cell function is limited through the actions of immunosuppressive cells in the TME such as cancer-associated fibroblasts (CAFs), myeloid cells, and inhibitory actions of some T cell subsets, albeit they infiltrate in the TME (97, 151). In support of this, strategies eliminating immunosuppressive populations in the TME enhanced CTL infiltration in various cancers (152, 153). To shift the immunosuppressive environment to a non-immune-privileged status, it is important to be aware of the individual components of the TME and to know how to modulate them.

Stromal Remodeling

The characteristic abundant desmoplastic stroma of PDAC can be both beneficial and harmful in terms of carcinogenesis. Studies showed that transplantation of PDAC cancer cells with pancreatic stellate cells increased tumorigenic potential and metastasis (154). However, depletion of stroma in preclinical mouse models also revealed further accumulation of T_{regs} in the TME showing the dual nature of stromal compartment (155). In a study performed on human PDAC tissues, the fibrotic reaction did not impair TIL infiltration, rather fibrosis associated collagen-I amount positively correlated with effector T cell presence (156). However, previous studies showed the inhibitory actions of αSMA^+ CAFs on $CD8^+$ CTLs in PDAC TME (157, 158). These results indicated the presence of (?) tumor heterogeneity not only in terms of cancer cells but also stromal compartments of PDAC (159).

One study revealed that depletion of CAFs could actually be employed to increase the immunotherapy response of PDAC: fibroblast activation protein (FAP^+) CAFs were shown to induce chemokine (C-X-C motif) ligand 12 (CXCL-12) mediating immunosuppression through limiting effector T cell infiltration (158). Targeted inhibitors of FAP^+ CAFs or CXCL-12 chemokine (C-X-C motif) receptor (CXCR-4) inhibition *via* AMD3100 increased $CD3^+$ T cell accumulation and revealed a synergistic effect with anti-PD-L1 therapy in mouse models (158).

Further studies focusing on focal adhesion kinase (FAK) showed FAK inhibition in cancer cells can remodel stroma, inhibiting immunosuppressive TME cells (160). Combination of FAK inhibitor with gemcitabine and anti-PD-1 increased $CD8^+$ CTL infiltration, reducing tumor burden and prolonging overall survival (160). Even though single agents targeting FAK inhibition in PDAC showed no objective response in clinic (161–163), trials combining iFAK (vs.-4718) with gemcitabine and anti-PD-1 are ongoing (NCT02758587).

The importance of interleukin 6 (IL-6) signaling in PDAC has been shown by several groups revealing its importance on both carcinogenesis and persistency (164–166). CAFs are also responsible for the production of pro-inflammatory cytokines other than myeloid cells such as IL-6 (167). Unfortunately, clinical trials targeting IL-6 alone demonstrated no benefit (168). However, preclinical studies targeting IL-6 in combination with PD-L1 showed decreased αSMA^+ stromal cells and increased $CD3^+$ lymphocyte infiltration in KPC and Panc02 subcutaneous and orthotopic transplantation models and a survival benefit in the KPC-Brca2 autochthonous mouse model (169).

Hyaluronan, an extracellular matrix component, is a linear glycosaminoglycan in PDAC, associated with multiple markers of aggressiveness of cancer for instance increased cell proliferation, invasion, and metastasis (170). High hyaluronan expression correlates with worse prognosis in PDAC patients (171). Several drugs have been developed to deplete stromal hyaluronan, such as PEGPH20. In preclinical models, hyaluronan depletion *via* PEGPH20 remodeled stroma, decreased interstitial fluid pressure, and increased drug delivery by enhancing micro-vessel permeability (172–174). As PEGPH20 increased delivery of chemotherapeutic agents in PDAC preclinical models, the same was seen for monoclonal antibodies (trastuzumab) in breast cancer (175). With the use of transplanted and autochthonous PDAC mouse models, *Salmonella*-based IDO-1 depletion (176) was also enhanced with (by means of gibi mi?) PEGPH20 treatment (177). Vitamin D receptor (VDR) was identified as a PSC master regulator for dynamic regulation of stromal composition. Treatment with VDR ligand reduced inflammation and enhanced gemcitabine delivery and efficacy in a mode of action similar to hyaluronan depletion (178). Based on these results, hyaluronan depletion or VDR activation appear as promising combination partners of checkpoint inhibitor monoclonal antibodies in clinical trials.

Modulation of Immunosuppressive Myeloid Cells

Tumor-associated macrophages (TAMs) differentiate from resident macrophages or mobile inflammatory monocytes (179). TAM polarization can be both beneficial and harmful in terms of carcinogenesis. M1 differentiation of TAMs is known to be antitumorigenic due to their tumoricidal nature *via* releasing pro-inflammatory cytokines. By contrast, the M2 subtype is pro-tumorigenic, since it suppresses immunosurveillance by secreting anti-inflammatory cytokines, e.g., TGF_β and IL-10 or by remodeling tumor stroma (180). Consistent with this, expression of M2-related markers such as CD204 and CD163 negatively correlate with patient survival (181, 182). Derived from immature cells of myeloid origin, MDSCs are known for their neoangiogenic and immune-suppressive activities in TME. MDSCs have been shown to inhibit CTL activity by recruiting T_{reg} subset, modulating amino acid reserves in TME, and pushing T cells toward apoptosis *via* ROS production (183). Also, the presence of immunosuppressive cells such as M2 macrophages, T_{regs}, and MDSCs in PDAC negatively correlates with overall survival (155, 184–188). Both pro- and antitumorigenic properties of neutrophils in cancer are reported, and their inhibitory action on CTL activity is known to be mediated by various mechanisms (189). Considering the complexity of immune cells in TME and their crosstalk with T cell activity, it is challenging but important to modulate these mechanisms to boost ICI response in cancer.

Cluster of differentiation 40 (CD40) is a member of the tumor necrosis factor receptor superfamily and is expressed on APCs including monocyte subsets, DCs, macrophages, and B cells (190). CD40 signaling is important for licensing APCs (to maximize their capacity to present antigens) followed by cross-priming of $CD8^+$ CTL in lymph nodes (191–193). CD40 agonists mediated an enhancement of adaptive antitumor immunity in preclinical mouse models in various cancer types (194–196). By contrast, treatment of KPC mice with CD40 agonist (FGK45) and gemcitabine transiently blocked PDAC development through re-education of tumor-infiltrating macrophages and stromal remodeling, but was not able to invoke an adaptive antitumor immune response (197). On the other hand, subcutaneous transplantation of KPC cancer cells into syngeneic mice revealed that the same treatment strategy induced an adaptive immune response with $CD4^+$ and $CD8^+$ T cell infiltration. Consequently, the authors used another "two tumor" model, in which intact KPC tumors (cancer cells with intact TME) were transplanted into endogenous tumor-bearing KPC mice. Here, gemcitabine with FGK45 treatment induced a $CD4^+$ and $CD8^+$ T cell infiltration into subcutaneous tumor but only $CD4^+$ infiltration into endogenous tumor. The barrier for $CD8^+$ repletion in spontaneous tumors was exceeded through systemic macrophage depletion. Upon deeper analysis, $Ly6C^{low}$ $F4/80^+$ macrophages residing in vicinity of PDAC TME were identified as the responsible physical barrier for CTL infiltration (198). In a similar manner, CTL-mediated antitumor immune responses were not seen in clinical trials with CD40 agonists in various cancers even with the addition of gemcitabine to increase tumor immunogenicity (199–202). CD40 agonist treatment finally acted as a checkpoint co-activator through its action on APCs inducing T cell priming upon gemcitabine/nab-paclitaxel dual treatment (203). In conclusion, PDAC retains its antigenic properties to induce both innate and adaptive immune response. This antigenicity might be increased through the use of chemotherapeutics or targeted therapy. Yet, since PDAC is immunologically cold (i.e., very scarce resident CTL infiltration) to respond to increased antigenicity, mechanisms to enhance CTL infiltration must be elucidated. Combination of gemcitabine with nab-paclitaxel remodels TME to permissive conditions for CTL infiltration, but not with gemcitabine alone (203). Furthermore, once T cell priming barrier is exceeded through CD40 agonist treatment, CTL activity might be more expedited with checkpoint inhibitor usage.

C-X-C motif chemokine receptor 2 (interleukin 8 receptor beta, CXCR-2) is a G-protein-coupled receptor for various CXCL ligands including IL-8. CXCR-2 in a cell type-specific manner can act both as a tumor suppressor where it induces senescence in premalignant lesions of PDAC (204, 205) and as tumor promoting *via* enhancing neutrophil and MDSC recruitment to TME (152, 206–208). Through inhibition of CXCR-2 either genetically or pharmacologically with CXCR-2 pepducin (209, 210) or AZ13381758 (211) inhibitors, Steele et al. showed an enhanced response to anti-PD-1 therapy and decreased metastasis in PDAC (212). The enhanced therapy response is reasoned by reduced infiltration of monocytes and MDSCs, which augments T cell infiltration in TME. Also, they propose that stromal remodeling through T cell recruitment might enhance gemcitabine efficacy in tumors (212, 213).

Colony-stimulating factor 1 receptor (CSF1R) is an important regulator of TAMs' differentiation and sustenance in microenvironment (214, 215). Therefore, inhibition of CSF1R is considered to have potential for cancer therapeutics. Yet, single-agent use targeting CSF1R did not yield clinical benefits in various tumor types (215). In mouse models, treatment of PDAC with CSF1R inhibitors enhanced antitumor immune response; however, this effect was diminished due to the production of checkpoint proteins such as PD-L1 and CTLA-4 (216). Combination of checkpoint inhibitors with CSF1R blockage showed regression of tumors in mouse models (216). CSF1R inhibition was shown to have an effect not only on TAMs but also on CAFs in various subcutaneously transplanted mouse models (217). Recently, CSF1R blockage was shown to enhance the production of granulocyte-specific chemokine expression such as CXCL-1 by CAFs increasing polymorphonuclear MDSC (PMN-MDSC) recruitment as a resistance mechanism (217). PMN-MDSC cells are known for their pro-tumorigenic and anti-immunogenic properties (218). Therefore, combination treatment of CSF1R and CXCR2 inhibitors (see above) targeting, respectively, both TAMs and MDSCs enhanced anti-PD-1 therapy response in transplanted tumor models (217). Considering response enhancement by usage of either CXCR2 or CSF1R inhibitor in combination with immune checkpoint inhibitors, simultaneous use of the three might exploit a broader benefit for therapy response also in PDAC (208, 212).

B Cells

Bruton's tyrosine kinase (BTK) is an enzyme expressed in B cells, macrophages, and mast cells, and targeting BTW in combination with ibrutinib was shown to be effective in chronic lymphocytic leukemia, Mantle cell lymphoma, and Waldenstrom's macroglobulinemia (219–221). Besides targeting BTK, ibrutinib also inhibits interleukin-2-inducible T-cell kinase in T cells, skewing Th differentiation toward Th_1 (222). Because of this effect, dual combination of ibrutinib with anti-PD-L1 inhibitor was shown to have a synergistic effect in a T cell-dependent manner, but not MDSC dependently in studies with mouse transplantation models of lymphoma, breast, and colon cancer (219). In various PDAC preclinical mouse models, ibrutinib demonstrated its antitumorigenic effect *via* depletion of macrophage deposition and fibrosis (220). In another study, on the other hand, ibrutinib enhanced macrophage production of Th_1 differentiation cytokines, while inhibiting Th_2, and augmenting the $CD8^+$ cytotoxic T cell deposition in tumors. The effect on macrophage activity was also dependent on B cells, and B cell-specific BTK signaling, still there was no change in fibrosis (221). Based on these results, checkpoint inhibition in combination with BTK inhibitor ibrutinib might enhance the therapeutic benefit of single use of each in PDAC, accordingly clinical trials are ongoing.

γδT Cells (γδT)

T cells are broadly divided into two subtypes based on the antigen receptor types they express: αβT and γδT (223). While 95% of the $CD3^+$ T cells in blood express αβTCR (includes $CD4^+$ and $CD8^+$ T cells) recognizing MHC class I–II, 5% have γδTCR which does not require MHC engagement for activation: γδT are cytolytic through the release of inflammatory cytokines (224, 225). There are conflicting data about the function of γδT in PDAC, with both pro- and antitumorigenic potential. Isolated γδT were shown to be tumoricidal to PDAC cell lines *in vitro* (226). By contrast, in mouse models, pre-neoplastic lesions with $KRAS^{G12D}$ were shown to recruit IL-17-expressing immune cells including γδT, which accelerated carcinogenesis through IL-17 receptor oncogenic signaling (133). In support of this, genetic and therapeutic depletion of γδT in mouse models prolonged survival. Other than the IL-17-mediated oncogenic effect on PanIN lesions, γδT directed checkpoint receptor inhibitory action (through galectin-9 and PD-L1 expression) on αβT cells, accelerating carcinogenesis. While ablation of $CD4^+$ and $CD8^+$ T cells had no impact on PDAC generation and persistency, this was different upon δTCR knock out: γδT cell deletion increased $CD8^+$ CTL and $CD4^+$ Th_1 tumor infiltration, and skewed $CD4^+$ differentiation toward the Th1 type. More importantly, the immunosuppressive action of γδT cell was not due to an effect on MDSCs or TAMs; instead, it was directly dependent on checkpoint co-inhibitory receptor engagement with antitumor T cells. PD-L1 and Galectin-9 checkpoint inhibition was effective in tumors with γδT cell present, but not in their absence. This implies the importance of personalized medicine, through which the γδT cell presence may be characterized in patients, to predict checkpoint inhibition therapy response (227).

Metabolic Regulation

Enhancing checkpoint inhibition efficiency may also be achieved through regulation of metabolic properties of T cells. For cytotoxic and effector T cell activity, a metabolic switch from a catabolic to anabolic state is important (228–231). While naïve T cells rely mostly on oxidative phosphorylation, activated T cells prefer to switch aerobic glycolysis for faster ATP production (230, 231). In support of this, T cells in anergic state even with TCR engagement and costimulator checkpoint activation can retain their hyporesponsive state in a nutrient poor environment (232). The nutrient poor microenvironment with low glucose and amino acid reservoir is regulated by both cancer cells and the TME (233). Cancer cells, for example, outcompete T cells for glucose uptake having implications for intrinsic immunogenicity regulation (234). Furthermore, glutamine usage by cancer cells also limits its presence in TME, limiting its activator function on T cells (235, 236). ARG-1 (Arginase 1) produced by TAMs and MDSCs degrades arginine (237, 238), while indoleamine 2,3-dioxygenase (IDO-1) produced by cancer cells, TAMs, and MDSCs converts tryptophane to an immunosuppressive metabolite kynurenine reducing T cell activity (239–244). Other than limiting nutrient availability, production of immunosuppressive intermediary metabolic products can also impair T cell activation. Cancer cell production of lactate as a result Warburg effect can impair T cell immunity by both decreasing TME pH and lactate shuttling into T cell (245–247). In addition, adenosine produced by cancer and T_{regs} (248–250), and prostaglandin E2 produced by TAMs and MDSCs are known to inhibit T cell signaling (251). Even though PDAC with its cancer cell and TME components shows similarities in metabolic properties as discussed above, how these metabolic properties effect T cell immunity specifically in PDAC has not been well studied (252). Overall, other than modulation of cytokine–chemokine–receptor axis, nutrient availability and production of immunosuppressive metabolites might also affect the extent of T cell immunity.

The impact of metabolism on checkpoint inhibition efficacy may not be only relevant on a micro environmental but also on a more systemic level. Cachexia is a systemic disorder with an excessive weight loss through the consumption of muscles and adipose tissues (253). Many diseases are associated with cachexia, including cancer in general and PDAC in particular (253). An increase in serum IL-6 levels was shown to impair hepatic ketogenesis inducing cachexia in C26 colon cancer and autochthonous KPC-PDAC mouse models (254–256). Physiologically, the body responded to cachexia with an upregulation of glucocorticoids like (?) corticosterone, which inhibits T cell infiltration into tumors of C26 cells. In support of this, transcriptomics analysis of pre-cachectic and cachectic C26 transplanted mice revealed an impaired immunological phenotype. However, this signature was not seen in the KPC model of PDAC, again implying its innate immunocompromised nature (254). With the use of the CXCR-4 inhibitor AMD3100, this barrier was overcome, increasing T cell infiltration and PD-L1 checkpoint inhibitor efficiency (158, 254). However, with the addition of corticosterone to the AMD3100-PD-L1 combination, the therapeutic effect was diminished (254). These results have multiple implications for PDAC therapeutics: the checkpoint inhibition resistance might be tackled with glucocorticoid synthesis inhibition, though this might first require a prior consideration for CTL infiltration. Second, serum glucocorticoid levels might be important markers for checkpoint inhibition response in PDAC patients. And finally, serum IL-6 depletion might provide further opportunities to increase the checkpoint inhibition efficacy, not only because of its direct effect in the TME but also due to its physiological role in cancer-related cachexia (254).

OTHER COMBINATION STRATEGIES EXPLOITING ANTIGENICITY/ IMMUNOGENICITY OF TUMORS TO ENHANCE CHECKPOINT INHIBITION THERAPY

Approaches including specific inhibitors (small molecules and antibodies) of various signaling pathways are described thus far and listed in **Table 2**. Apparently, combining the classical, untargeted treatment strategies, chemotherapy and RT, with checkpoint inhibition in clinical trials appears reasonable. Other targeted immunotherapeutic options, e.g., oncolytic viruses, vaccines, and chimeric antigen receptor-T cell (CAR-T) therapies aim to treat cancer in a more specific manner with minimal side effects. Selected clinical trials combining immune checkpoint inhibitors with untargeted and other targeted immunotherapeutic options are listed in **Table 3**. Combination therapies can modulate both antigenic and immunogenic landscape of tumors (**Figure 4**). Likely more important than just developing novel combination partners, exact understanding of the mode of action of combination partners, their tolerability and toxicity, a determination of dosing and appropriate sequencing of the combinations are required (257).

Combination of Immune Checkpoint Inhibitors With Untargeted Therapeutic Options

Chemotherapy

The first-line PDAC therapeutics used in clinic are chemotherapeutic agents such as gemcitabine with/without nab-paclitaxel, and FOLFIRINOX (folinic acid, fluorouracil, irinotecan, and oxaliplatin) (258). These agents are known for their ability to induce cytotoxicity due to impaired cell division. The mutagenic effect of chemotherapy (or RT) may enhance neoantigen production and MHC class I antigen presentation on cancer cells, increasing tumor antigenicity (109). Still, even if sub-clones with reactive neoantigenic properties might evolve, they might not be substantial enough to result in a broad clonal response in response to checkpoint inhibition (109). Furthermore, considering that PDAC already retains its antigenic capacity but its immunosuppressive microenvironment is the main barrier to pass as explained above, chemotherapy might exert its effect rather by altering immunogenicity. Immunogenic cell death (ICD) upon chemotherapy releases danger signals and cytokines for the generation of a more immunogenic TME (109). As also seen in the gemcitabine with nab-paclitaxel example above, remodeling of the immunosuppressive TME can bolster up T cell cytotoxicity due to enhanced immunogenicity. Chemotherapy can increase immunogenicity by also its direct action on immunosuppressive cells of TME. For example, fluorouracil and paclitaxel were shown to induce MDSC apoptosis in various tumor models, while low dose gemcitabine was shown to deplete T_{regs} in panc02 orthotopic mouse model (259). Furthermore, it will be important to select chemotherapeutic agents, their dosing and time and sequence of administration with regard to their ability to induce ICD and remodel the microenvironment.

Radiotherapy

Although the use of RT for the treatment of PDAC has been controversially discussed due to rather disappointing results in clinical trials (260), radiation treatment in combination with ICI might be a promising strategy for pancreatic cancer patients. In a phenomenon known as the abscopal response, RT was shown to induce immune responses that mediate regression of metastatic lesions lying outside the field of radiation (261). RT could activate the immune system, increase trafficking of T cells to the tumor, and elicit antitumor immune responses following ICD (262). Several preclinical and clinical studies in different cancer types showed synergistic effects in cohorts treated with RT and immune checkpoint blockade (263–266). Although not many studies have been published thus far, evidence for synergism can also be seen in PDAC and has been related to increased immunogenicity (95, 267, 268). In the PDAC mouse model used by Twyman-Saint

TABLE 2 | Selection of currently ongoing clinical trials evaluating CTLA4 or/and PD1/PD-L1 checkpoint blockade in combination with targeted therapy approaches for pancreatic cancer as indicated.

Combination strategy/ target	Compounds	Entity	Phase	Trial ID
Oncogenic signaling	Cobimetinib (MEK-inh.) + atezolizumab (PD-L1-Ab)	Metastatic PDAC, progressed on chemotherapy	Ib/II	NCT03193190
TME: stroma	Ulocuplumab (CXCR-4-ant.) + nivolumab (PD-1-Ab)	Advanced/metastatic pancreatic cancer (next to SCLC)	I/II	NCT02472977 (terminated 03/2018 due to lack of effic. in short-term ph.)
	BL-8040 (CXCR4-ant.) + pembrolizumab (PD-1-Ab)	(Pretreated) metastatic pancreatic cancer	II	NCT02826486 and NCT02907099
	BL-8040 (CXCR4-ant.) + atezolizumab (PD-L1-Ab)	Metastatic PDAC, progressed on chemotherapy	Ib/II	NCT03193190
	Olaptesed pegol (pegylated oligoribonucleotide, neutralizing CXCL12) ± pembrolizumab (PD-1-Ab)	Metastatic pancreatic cancer (next to CRC)	I/II	NCT03168139
	Defactinib (FAK-inh.) + pembrolizumab (PD-1-Ab)	Advanced pancreatic cancer (next to NSCLC and mesothelioma)	I/II	NCT02758587
	PEGPH20 (pegylated recombinant human hyaluronidase) + atezolizumab (PD-L1-Ab)	Metastatic PDAC, progressed on chemotherapy	I/II	NCT03193190
	PEGPH20 (see above) + avelumab (PD-L1-Ab)	Chemotherapy resistant advanced pancreatic cancer	I	NCT03481920
	Pembrolizumab (PD-1-Ab) ± paricalcitol (vitamin D analog)	Maintenance of pretreated advanced pancreatic cancer in (partial) remission	II	NCT03331562
TME: myeloid	RO7009789 (CD40 ago. Ab) + atezolizumab (PD-L1-Ab)	Locally advanced/metastatic solid tumors	I	NCT02304393
	Cabiralizumab (CSF1R-Ab) + nivolumab (PD-1-Ab)	Advanced solid tumors	I	NCT02526017
	AMG820 (CSF1R-Ab) + pembrolizumab (PD-1-Ab)	Advanced pancreatic cancer (next to CRC and NSCLC)	I/II	NCT02713529
	Pedixartinib (CSF1R-tyrosine kinase inh.) + durvalumab (PD-L1-Ab)	Pretreated advanced/metastatic pancreatic cancer (next to CRC)	I	NCT02777710
	Acalabrutinib (bruton tyrosine kinase inh.) + pembrolizumab (PD-1-Ab)	Metastatic pancreatic cancer	II	NCT02362048
TME: metabolism	Epacadostat (IDO1-inh.) + pembrolizumab (PD-1-Ab)	Previously treated advanced pancreatic cancer (with chromosomal instability/HRRD)	II-withdrawn	NCT03432676

Ab, antibody; inh., inhibitor; ant., antagonist; ago., agonist; CRC, colorectal cancer; HRRD, homologous recombination repair deficiency; IDO1, indoleamine 2,3-dioxygenase 1; NSCLC, non-small cell lung cancer; SCLC, small cell lung cancer; TME, tumor microenvironment; PD-1, programmed cell death protein 1.

Victor et al., any combination of immune checkpoint inhibitor with RT substantially increased overall survival, compared with immune checkpoint blockade with either CTLA-4 antibody or PD-1 antibody alone. The highest response rate and longest overall survival was seen in the triple combination therapy (two checkpoint inhibitors + RT) group (269).

Recently, CD40 agonist treatment was demonstrated to be beneficial upon a RT + ICI regimen in murine pancreatic cancer models (270). While RT alone or in combination with ICI resulted in reduction of irradiated tumor growth, only the triple therapy, RT + αCD40 + ICI (RCP4), affected the growth of both irradiated and unirradiated tumors. These observations were also reflected in the long-term survival. Furthermore, CD4 and CD8 T cells, as well as short-lived myeloid cells were shown to be necessary for optimal response to RCP4 and that RCP4 antitumor immunity. This immunity was dependent on host CD40, Batf3, and IFNγ but not on B cells and canonical innate immune activation pathways. The three therapies all showed non-redundant impact on the antitumor immune response. While RT triggered an early pro-inflammatory stimulus, αCD40 caused systemic myeloid compartment reorganization and ICI increases intratumoral T cell infiltration, thus improving the CD8/T_{reg} cell ratio.

In conclusion, RT can enhance the "visibility" of tumor antigens and make the tumor more immunogenic. While the combination of RT and ICI shows promise in preclinical and clinical trials in various cancer entities, challenges still exist for the safe and efficacious application of the combination. Tumor-type and immune therapy-specific optimization of radiation dose and timing and the identification of potential biomarkers is likely to further enhance the effectiveness (271). Also, the addition of αCD40 agonists appears to be a promising avenue to pursue in clinical PDAC trials.

Combination of Immune Checkpoint Inhibitors With Other Immunotherapeutic Approaches

Oncolytic Viruses

Tumor-targeted oncolytic viruses (TOVs) are viruses that selectively infect, replicate in, and lyse tumor cells, while leaving healthy, normal tissues unharmed. TOVs can have intrinsic tumor-selectivity, making them naturally nonpathogenic to humans and sensitive to antiviral signaling (272) or depend on oncogenic signaling pathways, e.g., constitutively activated RAS (273, 274). Viral tumor specificity can also be genetically

TABLE 3 | Selection of currently ongoing clinical trials evaluating CTLA4 or/and PD1/PD-L1 checkpoint blockade in combination with untargeted and targeted options including other immunotherapeutic approaches for pancreatic cancer as indicated.

Combination strategy/target	Compounds	Entity	Phase	Trial ID
Chemotherapy	Gemcitabine + ipilimumab (CTLA-4-Ab)	Advanced pancreatic cancer	Ib	NCT01473940
	Nab-paclitaxel (±gemcitabine) + nivolumab (PD-1-Ab)	Advanced/metastatic pancreatic adenocarcinoma (next to NSCLC and mBC)	I	NCT02309177
	mFOLFOX6 + pembrolizumab (PD-1-Ab) [+celecoxib (COX-2-inh.) for non-responders]	Advanced gastrointestinal-cancer including pancreatic cancer	I	NCT02268825
Radiotherapy	SBRT 6 Gy × 5 days + durvalumab (PD-L1-Ab), vs. tremelimumab (CTLA-4-Ab) vs. both combined	Unresectable, non-metastatic pancreatic cancer	Ib	NCT02868632
	SBRT 5 Gy × 5 days vs. 8 Gy × 1 day + durvalumab (PD-L1-Ab), vs. tremelimumab (CTLA-4-Ab) vs. both combined	Unresectable pancreatic cancer	I/II	NCT02311361
	Radiotherapy (not defined) + nivolumab (PD-1-Ab) and ipilimumab (CTLA-4-Ab)	Pancreatic cancer, progressed on chemotherapy (next to CRC)	II	NCT03104439
	45–50.4 Gy + PD-1-Ab (not defined)	Unresectable pancreatic cancer	II	NCT03374293
Vaccines	GVAX/Cy ± nivolumab (PD-1-Ab)	Neoadjuvant/adjuvant for resectable pancreatic cancer	I/II	NCT02451982
	GVAX/Cy + CRS-207 ± nivolumab (PD-1-Ab)	Previously treated metastatic pancreatic adenocarcinoma	II	NCT02243371
	CRS-207 (±GVAX/Cy) + nivolumab (PD-1-Ab) and ipilimumab (CTLA-4-Ab)	Previously treated pancreatic cancer	II	NCT03190265
Chemotherapy + vaccine	Capecitabine + CV301 + durvalumab (PD-L1-Ab)	Metastatic pancreatic cancer (next to CRC)	I/II	NCT03376659
Chemotherapy + Vit. D analog	Paricalcitol (vitamin D analog) + pembrolizumab (PD-1-Ab) ± gemcitabine/nab-paclitaxel	Resectable pancreatic cancer, neoadjuvant setting	I	NCT02930902
Chemotherapy + FAK	Defactinib (FAK-inh.) + gemcitabine + pembrolizumab (PD-1-Ab)	Advanced solid tumors	I	NCT02546531
Chemotherapy + CD40	Gemcitabine/nab-paclitaxel + APX005M (CD40-ago.-Ab) ± nivolumab (PD-1-Ab)	Untreated metastatic pancreatic adenocarcinoma	II	NCT03214250
Chemotherapy + CSF1R	Cabiralizumab (CSF1R-Ab) + nivolumab (PD-1-Ab) ± different chemotherapeutic regimens	Pretreated, progressed metastatic pancreatic adenocarcinoma	II	NCT03336216
Radiotherapy + vaccine	SBRT 6.6 Gy × 5 days + GVAX/Cy + nivolumab (PD-1-Ab)	Borderline resectable pancreatic cancer, no previous therapy	II	NCT03161379
Radiotherapy + vaccine	SBRT 6.6 Gy × 5 days + GVAX/Cy + pembrolizumab (PD-1-Ab)	Locally advanced pancreatic cancer	II	NCT02648282
CSF1R + vaccine	IMC-CS4 (CSF1R-Ab) + GVAX/Cy + pembrolizumab (PD-1-Ab)	Borderline resectable pancreatic adenocarcinoma	I	NCT03153410
IDO1 + vaccine	Epacadostat (IDO1-inh.) + CRS-207 (±GVAX/Cy) + pembrolizumab (PD-1-Ab)	Metastatic pancreatic cancer progressed on prior chemotherapy	II	NCT03006302
ACT	Autologous TIL, ipilimumab (CTLA-4-Ab), nivolumab (PD-1-Ab), proleukin, Cy., fludara	Cancer patients across all diagnoses	I/II	NCT03296137

Ab, antibody; inh., inhibitor; ago., agonist; CRC, colorectal cancer; CRS-207, Listeria-based mesothelin vaccine; CV301, CEA/MUC1 prime-boost vaccine based on modified vaccinia Ankara-Bavarian Nordic (MVA-BN), a recombinant fowlpox viral vector (foe the boost) and TRICOM, which is comprised of three costimulatory molecules B7-1, ICAM-1, and LFA-3; Cy, cyclophosphamide; GVAX, irradiated pancreatic cancer cells, genetically modified to express GM-CSF; IDO1, indoleamine 2,3-dioxygenase 1; mBC, metastatic breast cancer; NSCLC, non-small cell lung cancer; SBRT, stereotactic body radiation therapy; ACT, adoptive cell therapy; TIL, tumor-infiltrating lymphocyte; CTLA-4, cytotoxic T lymphocyte-associated antigen 4; PD-1, programmed cell death protein 1.

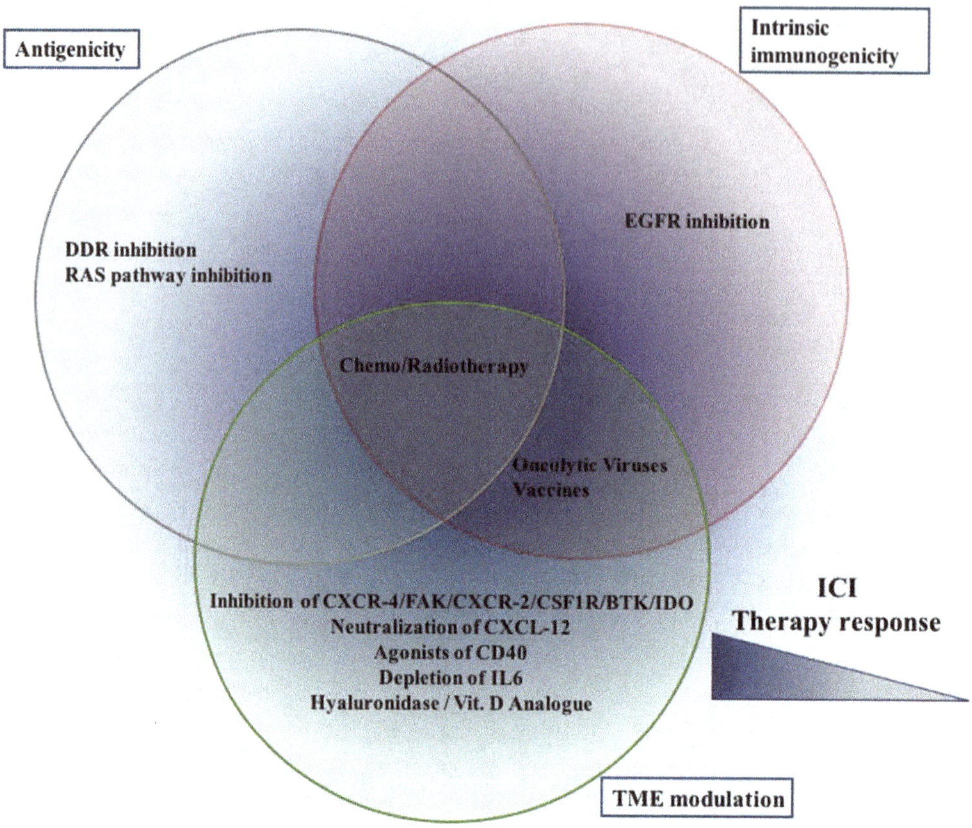

FIGURE 4 | Combination therapeutic options to increase ICI efficiency: while given therapeutic options are placed in the corresponding cluster, only published data thus far are taken into consideration. This still does not eliminate their potential to affect other aspects. While treatments focusing on a single aspect (either one of antigenicity/intrinsic immunogenicity/TME modulation) might be effective, the best synergism will probably be achieved through combinations focusing on all aspects. Abbreviations: ICI, immune checkpoint inhibition, DDR, DNA damage response.

engineered by deleting genes required for replication in normal tissues (273) or by placing viral replication under the control of a tumor-specific promoter (274–276), TOVs can also be designed to express tumor-specific cell surface receptors (277, 278). TOVs can thus be engineered to increase safety, efficacy, and tissue tropism.

The advantages of TOVs are their specificity, modest toxicity, low probability for resistance, and most importantly, their induction of an inflammatory cascade and engagement of the adaptive immune system (273). In contrast to any other drug, the therapeutic dose of TOVs increases over time, as the virus replicates and spreads to neighboring cells (273). Although TOVs directly lyse infected malignant cells, causing acute tumor debulking, it is the ability of the virus to spread from cell to cell and potentiate an inflammatory response through ICD that make oncolytic viruses such promising new therapies (279–281). However, oncolytic virus therapy faces challenges in solid tumors and especially PDAC. These challenges, i.e., overcoming the TME, avoiding neutralization by the host immune system, and acquired resistance in tumor cells culminate in the main problem, i.e., the systemic delivery of TOVs for the targeting of metastatic cancer cells (282). Thus, it is not surprising that thus far, no studies investigating ICI and oncolytic viral therapy in pancreatic cancer have been published. However, Mahalingam et al. (283) conducted a phase II study of pelareorep, a proprietary replication-competent isolate of reovirus type 3 dearing in combination with gemcitabine in advanced PDAC and observed the upregulation of PD-L1 in following treatment. They suggested to investigate the combination of oncolytic virus therapy with anti-PD-L1 inhibitors in PDAC.

Congruent with this finding, recent research in other cancer entities revealed that antiviral immunological events induced by the administration of oncolytic viruses can turn tumors "hot" (284, 285) and establish a TME that is conducive for enhancing the efficacy of checkpoint inhibitors (286–288). Using intravenous infusion of oncolytic human orthoreovirus, Samson et al. (288) found that TOV treatment increases cytotoxic T cell tumor infiltration, upregulates IFN-regulated gene expression, and the PD-1/PD-L1 axis in tumors, *via* an IFN-mediated mechanism. And finally, addition of PD-1 blockade to reovirus treatment enhanced systemic therapy in a preclinical glioma model. In their simultaneously published triple-negative breast cancer

(TNBC) study, Bourgeois-Daigneault et al. (286) reported that TOV therapy sensitizes otherwise refractory TNBC to immune checkpoint blockade, preventing relapse in most of the treated animals.

In conclusion, once the problem of systemic delivery is solved, oncolytic viruses are not only valuable therapies in terms of tumor debulking but are also useful in a "prime and boost" approach in combination with ICIs.

Vaccines

Another promising approach to enhance the immunogenicity of pancreatic cancer cells and boost the antitumor T cell response is the use of cancer vaccines. Vaccines have been designed to generate a humoral/cellular immune response with the aim of stimulating the host immune system to recognize and eliminate tumor cells with specific effector and memory T cells. There are two major categories of tumor vaccines: whole cell vaccines and antigen-specific vaccines (289). A brief review on the different vaccines currently investigated for pancreatic cancer can be found in the publication by Skelton et al. (290). Although early studies using single-agent tumor vaccines against PDAC showed improved immune profiles, they were largely unable to produce a positive clinical response (291). This can be explained by the upregulation of immunosuppressive signaling, as well as other immune modulating mechanisms, which negate the positive effects of the vaccine (267, 292).

The induction of T cell infiltration and PD-L1 expression in the TME by vaccine treatment was hypothesized to prime PDACs for anti-PD-1/PD-L1 therapies. Indeed, the whole cell vaccine GVAX, consisting of two allogeneic irradiated PDAC cell lines engineered to secrete GM-CSF, converted a non-immunogenic or "cold" neoplasm into an immunogenic or "hot" neoplasm by inducing infiltration of T cells and development of tertiary lymphoid structures (267, 285). In a subsequent phase Ib study, Le et al. (293) were able to show that the combination of GVAX with ipilimumab induced objective responses in patients with metastatic PDAC that were not observed with either single therapy alone.

Preclinical data suggested beneficial effects when two vaccination treatments were co-implemented, e.g., GVAX and CRS-207, a live-attenuated *Listeria monocytogenes* vaccine expressing the TAA mesothelin, in a sequential combination—a so-called prime/boost approach. The first vaccine was given to initiate or "prime" the immune system, and this immune response was then "boosted" following re-administration of antigen resulting in the induction of a synergistic enhancement of T cell induction and antitumor effect (289). Based on the preclinical data, a phase II trial (NCT01417000) was conducted resulting in the conclusion that heterologous prime/boost with Cy/GVAX and CRS-207 extended the survival of patients with pancreatic cancer, with minimal toxicity (294). Unfortunately, a subsequent phase IIb trial of CRS-207 and GVAX (NCT02004262) did not show a significant difference in overall survival between the groups treated with either CRS-207/GVAX or CRS207 alone and the group treated with chemotherapy, i.e., physicians' choice of therapies including: gemcitabine, capecitabine, fluorouracil, leucovorin, irinotecan, and erlotinib.

Although the last mentioned study was quite a set-back, the strategy of combining different immunotherapy options with each other still holds a merit, especially for "prime and boost" approach.

Chimeric Antigen Receptor (CAR)—T Cell Therapy

Chimeric antigen receptors are fusion proteins that can be comprised of three major domains. These are the antigen-specific ectodomain, commonly derived from a single-chain variable antibody-fragment (scFv); a transmembrane domain fused to a spacer that links to the ectodomain; and an endodomain consisting of different cytoplasmic proteins responsible for T cell activation (295). Unlike endogenous TCRs, CARs recognize their target antigen in an MHC (or HLA)-independent manner, due to their engineered antibody fragment. Upon antigen recognition, CAR-T cells are activated, leading to cytokine secretion, T cell proliferation, and antigen-specific cytotoxicity (296). The production of CAR-T cells for adoptive T cell transfer requires the isolation, stimulation, expansion, transduction, i.e., viral vector-mediated insertion of specific CAR genes, and ultimately reinfusion of autologous or allogeneic T cells (297–299).

Although impressive clinical activities of CAR-T cells in hematological malignancies were reported, CAR T-cell trials in solid tumors have yet to yield the same level of success (300, 301). The most prominent obstacles standing in the way of successful CAR-T cell therapy are (1) lack of ideal TSAs, (2) inefficient trafficking of CAR-T cells to tumor sites, (3) the immune-suppressive TME, and (4) the risk of developing on-target/off-tumor toxicities, i.e., the attack of normal cells expressing the targeted tumor antigen (296).

While the investigation of CAR-T cells in pancreatic cancer is still in early stages, it is fair to say that the first above mentioned obstacle does not apply. PDAC exhibits a number of TSAs and, conceptually, is a promising candidate tumor for investigating CAR T-cell therapy. Thus far, there have been preclinical studies on various pancreatic cancer cell surface antigens, namely, MSLN, CEA, MUC1, PSCA, CD24, HER2, and natural killer receptors (302).

The main obstacles in pancreatic cancer are most likely the strong immunosuppressive TME, already discussed in this review, and improper homing and inefficient infiltration of CAR T-cells to the tumor bed. Especially challenging is the high number of infiltrating T_{regs} and MDSCs, which can deactivate CAR-T cells through cytokines inhibitory cytokines such as TGF_{β} and IL-10, and the upregulation of inhibitory receptors, e.g., PD-1 on adoptively transferred CAR-T cells after homing to the tumor (95, 302–304). T cell hypofunction was reversed when the cells were isolated from the tumor, or after treatment with a blocking PD-1 antibody (304–306), and there are promising preclinical studies on CAR-T cells engineered to secrete PD-1 checkpoint inhibitors (307, 308) or PD-1 dominant negative receptor (304).

These results provide rationale for combination therapies, with CAR-T cells and checkpoint blockade, as a new strategy to overcome the tumor escape and to further strengthen CAR-T cells, especially in patients with PDAC shown to express high levels of PD-L1.

Adoptive Cell Therapy (ACT) With Endogenous TILs

Adoptive cell therapy using endogenous TILs taken from surgically resected tumors, expanded *in vitro*, and re-infused back into the patient, is a promising approach for otherwise untreatable cancer types (309). In metastatic melanoma patients, for example, TIL-ACT was associated with a 20% complete response lasting beyond 3 years (310). Gastrointestinal tumor patients with $CD3^+$ T cell infiltration showed a higher rate of progression-free survival (311), and pancreatic adenocarcinomas containing both $CD4^+$ and $CD8^+$ T cells correlated with an improved prognosis and significantly greater 5-year survival (181, 312, 313). This evidence of a host T cell immune response in patients with pancreatic adenocarcinoma drove both Hall et al. (309) and Poschke et al. (314) to expand and analyze the T cell repertoire in resected primary PDAC specimen. Contrary to the common description of PDAC as an immunologically "cold" tumor, they found that most resectable PDA tumors actually contained significant numbers of T-cells and, along with that, tertiary lymphoid structures in which clonal T-cell expansion takes place and were able to expand them *in vitro* using high levels of IL-2 (309, 314). The majority of these TILs were $CD4^+$ T cells and were highly activated and resembled those extracted from melanoma samples. Media supplemented with anti-4-1BB significantly increased the TIL yield per fragment and shifted the T cell population to predominantly $CD8^+$ cells compared with control cultures. The population of 4-1BB positive $CD8^+$ lymphocytes represented the population of tumor-resident TILs specific for expressed tumor antigens on the surface of pancreatic adenocarcinoma cells (309, 314).

Thus far, there has been no studies investigating the combination of TIL ACT and ICI in pancreatic cancer. However, pretreating PDAC patients with immune checkpoint inhibitors and thus enriching the population of tumor-specific lymphocytes prior to surgical resection might be a worthwhile strategy. This way the yield of tumor reactive cells could be increased, the expansion time and the time between surgery and infusion shortened, and thus the risk of recurrent growth during the expansion period decreased.

This is exactly the approach taken by Mullinax et al. when analyzing the combination of TIL ACT and Ipilimumab in a clinical pilot study (NCT01701674) for metastatic melanoma, and in clinical trials for metastatic ovarian cancer (NCT03287674). The pretreatment with Ipilimumab followed by ACT in metastatic melanoma patients was reported as feasible, well tolerated, and associated with a low rate of attrition due to progression during cell expansion (315). The investigators are currently recruiting patients for a similar trial in metastatic melanoma, now including 4-1BB (NCT02652455), and another study with a similar design is currently recruiting patients with locally advanced or metastatic cancers of various types (NCT03296137).

Considering the positive results in metastatic melanoma, as well as the similarity in the population of extractable T cells from melanoma and PDAC, the investigation of ICI + TIL ACT in PDAC is recommendable.

CONCLUDING REMARKS

The revolution of immunotherapy is changing our perspective in cancer therapeutics. For some solid tumors, immunotherapy has already entered into clinical practice. While PDAC is unresponsive and refractory to many of the conventional therapies, immunotherapy holds a promise for future improvement. However, single-agent ICI has largely failed. Based on the findings thus far, the decisive drawback for ICI efficiency in PDAC is the initial T cell priming. Only less than 1% of human PDAC samples are projected to show aberrant genomic instability, enabling T cell priming despite the immunosuppressive microenvironment. However, this does not mean the other 99% are not antigenic, rather its antigenic strength likely cannot beat reduced immunogenicity. Each patient, each tumor, and each cancer cell are distinct. T cells might provide the best repertoire for the recognition of each single difference, yet to overcome immunogenic obstacles, combination strategies are required. Development of the best combinations comes along with better characterization of the patient samples. Characterization of these samples might help us to better classify the individual distinctions that patients, tumors, and cancer cells have, and to find the best combination partners with checkpoint inhibition. Even though complete regression of the primary tumor might not be achieved, reduction and control of metastasis can still provide a considerable prognostic value in PDAC patients. While we know that metastatic lesions evade the expression of high quality neoantigens of their cognate primary tumor and antigen presenting machinery, they might still retain their unique antigenic and immunogenic master regulators to be targeted. Most importantly, T cell memory provides the best tool to minimize disease recurrence, therefore strategies exploiting T cell memory may provide long-term disease control. Before achieving T cell memory, to make PDAC responsive to first time checkpoint inhibition, we have to elucidate and exploit the mechanisms discussed above: (1) increasing initial T cell priming, (2) exceeding immunosuppressive TME, and (3) inhibiting compensatory mechanisms of T cell anergy and exhaustion.

AUTHOR CONTRIBUTIONS

DK wrote the manuscript, prepared the figures and tables. KC wrote and edited the manuscript. DR provided the tables and edited the manuscript. HA edited and supervised the manuscript.

ACKNOWLEDGMENTS

We thank to Munich International Max Planck Research Schools-Life Sciences Program (IMPRS-LS) for their financial support of DK. We thank to Dr. Med. Vet. Joerg Steiner and M. A. Zeynep Yueksel for their help during the revision of the manuscript.

REFERENCES

1. Rahib L, Smith BD, Aizenberg R, Rosenzweig AB, Fleshman JM, Matrisian LM. Projecting cancer incidence and deaths to 2030: the unexpected burden of thyroid, liver, and pancreas cancers in the United States. *Cancer Res* (2014) 74:2913–21. doi:10.1158/0008-5472.CAN-14-0155
2. Siegel RL, Miller KD, Jemal A. Cancer statistics, 2018. *CA Cancer J Clin* (2018) 68:7–30. doi:10.3322/caac.21442
3. Siegel RL, Miller KD, Jemal A. Cancer statistics, 2017. *CA Cancer J Clin* (2017) 67:7–30. doi:10.3322/caac.21387
4. Kleeff J, Korc M, Apte M, La Vecchia C, Johnson CD, Biankin AV, et al. Pancreatic cancer. *Nat Rev Dis Prim* (2016) 2:1–22. doi:10.1038/nrdp.2016.22
5. Neesse A, Algül H, Tuveson DA, Gress TM. Stromal biology and therapy in pancreatic cancer: a changing paradigm. *Gut* (2015) 64:1476–84. doi:10.1136/gutjnl-2015-309304
6. Hidalgo M. Pancreatic cancer. *N Engl J Med* (2010) 362:1605–17. doi:10.1056/NEJMra0901557
7. Ko AH, Bekaii-Saab T, Van Ziffle J, Mirzoeva OM, Joseph NM, Talasaz AA, et al. A multicenter, open-label phase II clinical trial of combined MEK plus EGFR inhibition for chemotherapy-refractory advanced pancreatic adenocarcinoma. *Clin Cancer Res* (2016) 22:61–8. doi:10.1158/1078-0432.CCR-15-0979
8. Bedard PL, Tabernero J, Janku F, Wainberg ZA, Paz-Ares L, Vansteenkiste J, et al. A Phase Ib dose-escalation study of the oral pan-PI3K inhibitor buparlisib (BKM120) in combination with the oral MEK1/2 inhibitor trametinib (GSK1120212) in patients with selected advanced solid tumors. *Clin Cancer Res* (2015) 21:730–8. doi:10.1158/1078-0432.CCR-14-1814
9. Tolcher AW, Bendell JC, Papadopoulos KP, Burris HA, Patnaik A, Jones SF, et al. A phase IB trial of the oral MEK inhibitor trametinib (GSK1120212) in combination with everolimus in patients with advanced solid tumors. *Ann Oncol* (2015) 26:58–64. doi:10.1093/annonc/mdu482
10. Wolpin BM, Hezel AF, Abrams T, Blaszkowsky LS, Meyerhardt JA, Chan JA, et al. Oral mTOR inhibitor everolimus in patients with gemcitabine-refractory metastatic pancreatic cancer. *J Clin Oncol* (2009) 27:193–8. doi:10.1200/JCO.2008.18.9514
11. Infante JR, Somer BG, Park JO, Li C-P, Scheulen ME, Kasubhai SM, et al. A randomised, double-blind, placebo-controlled trial of trametinib, an oral MEK inhibitor, in combination with gemcitabine for patients with untreated metastatic adenocarcinoma of the pancreas. *Eur J Cancer* (2014) 50:2072–81. doi:10.1016/j.ejca.2014.04.024
12. Bodoky G, Timcheva C, Spigel DR, La Stella PJ, Ciuleanu TE, Pover G, et al. A phase II open-label randomized study to assess the efficacy and safety of selumetinib (AZD6244 [ARRY-142886]) versus capecitabine in patients with advanced or metastatic pancreatic cancer who have failed first-line gemcitabine therapy. *Invest New Drugs* (2012) 30:1216–23. doi:10.1007/s10637-011-9687-4
13. Conroy T, Desseigne F, Ychou M, Bouché O, Guimbaud R, Bécouarn Y, et al. FOLFIRINOX versus gemcitabine for metastatic pancreatic cancer. *N Engl J Med* (2011) 364:1817–25. doi:10.1056/NEJMoa1011923
14. Von Hoff DD, Ervin T, Arena FP, Chiorean EG, Infante J, Moore M, et al. Increased survival in pancreatic cancer with nab-paclitaxel plus gemcitabine. *N Engl J Med* (2013) 369:1691–703. doi:10.1056/NEJMoa1304369
15. Goldstein D, El-Maraghi RH, Hammel P, Heinemann V, Kunzmann V, Sastre J, et al. Nab-paclitaxel plus gemcitabine for metastatic pancreatic cancer: long-term survival from a phase III trial. *J Natl Cancer Inst* (2015) 107. doi:10.1093/jnci/dju413
16. Ferlay J, Soerjomataram I, Dikshit R, Eser S, Mathers C, Rebelo M, et al. Cancer incidence and mortality worldwide: sources, methods and major patterns in GLOBOCAN 2012. *Int J Cancer* (2015) 136:E359–86. doi:10.1002/ijc.29210
17. Housman G, Byler S, Heerboth S, Lapinska K, Longacre M, Snyder N, et al. Drug resistance in cancer: an overview. *Cancers* (2014) 6:1769–92. doi:10.3390/cancers6031769
18. Groenendijk FH, Bernards R. Drug resistance to targeted therapies: Déjà vu all over again. *Mol Oncol* (2014) 8:1067–83. doi:10.1016/j.molonc.2014.05.004
19. Hodi FS, O'Day SJ, McDermott DF, Weber RW, Sosman JA, Haanen JB, et al. Improved survival with ipilimumab in patients with metastatic melanoma. *N Engl J Med* (2010) 363:711–23. doi:10.1056/NEJMoa1003466
20. Ribas A, Puzanov I, Dummer R, Schadendorf D, Hamid O, Robert C, et al. Pembrolizumab versus investigator-choice chemotherapy for ipilimumab-refractory melanoma (KEYNOTE-002): a randomised, controlled, phase 2 trial. *Lancet Oncol* (2015) 16:908–18. doi:10.1016/S1470-2045(15)00083-2
21. Robert C, Schachter J, Long GV, Arance A, Grob JJ, Mortier L, et al. Pembrolizumab versus ipilimumab in advanced melanoma. *N Engl J Med* (2015) 372:2521–32. doi:10.1056/NEJMoa1503093
22. Weber JS, D'Angelo SP, Minor D, Hodi FS, Gutzmer R, Neyns B, et al. Nivolumab versus chemotherapy in patients with advanced melanoma who progressed after anti-CTLA-4 treatment (CheckMate 037): a randomised, controlled, open-label, phase 3 trial. *Lancet Oncol* (2015) 16:375–84. doi:10.1016/S1470-2045(15)70076-8
23. Rizvi NA, Mazières J, Planchard D, Stinchcombe TE, Dy GK, Antonia SJ, et al. Activity and safety of nivolumab, an anti-PD-1 immune checkpoint inhibitor, for patients with advanced, refractory squamous non-small-cell lung cancer (CheckMate 063): a phase 2, single-arm trial. *Lancet Oncol* (2015) 16:257–65. doi:10.1016/S1470-2045(15)70054-9
24. Garon EB, Rizvi NA, Hui R, Leighl N, Balmanoukian AS, Eder JP, et al. Pembrolizumab for the treatment of non-small-cell lung cancer. *N Engl J Med* (2015) 372:2018–28. doi:10.1056/NEJMoa1501824
25. Reck M, Rodríguez-Abreu D, Robinson AG, Hui R, Csőszi T, Fülöp A, et al. Pembrolizumab versus chemotherapy for PD-L1-positive non-small-cell lung cancer. *N Engl J Med* (2016) 375:1823–33. doi:10.1056/NEJMoa1606774
26. Borghaei H, Paz-Ares L, Horn L, Spigel DR, Steins M, Ready NE, et al. Nivolumab versus docetaxel in advanced nonsquamous non-small-cell lung cancer. *N Engl J Med* (2015) 373:1627–39. doi:10.1056/NEJMoa1507643
27. Taylor M, Antonia S, Bendell J, Calvo E, Jager D, Braud F, et al. Phase I/II study of nivolumab with or without ipilimumab for treatment of recurrent small cell lung cancer (SCLC): CA209-032. *J Immunother Cancer* (2015) 3:P376. doi:10.1186/2051-1426-3-S2-P376
28. Motzer RJ, Rini BI, McDermott DF, Redman BG, Kuzel TM, Harrison MR, et al. Nivolumab for metastatic renal cell carcinoma: results of a randomized phase II trial. *J Clin Oncol* (2015) 33:1430–7. doi:10.1200/JCO.2014.59.0703
29. Weinstock M, McDermott D. Targeting PD-1/PD-L1 in the treatment of metastatic renal cell carcinoma. *Ther Adv Urol* (2015) 7:365–77. doi:10.1177/1756287215597647
30. Powles T, Eder JP, Fine GD, Braiteh FS, Loriot Y, Cruz C, et al. MPDL3280A (anti-PD-L1) treatment leads to clinical activity in metastatic bladder cancer. *Nature* (2014) 515:558–62. doi:10.1038/nature13904
31. Powles T, O'Donnell PH, Massard C, Arkenau H-T, Friedlander TW, Hoimes CJ, et al. Efficacy and safety of durvalumab in locally advanced or metastatic urothelial carcinoma. *JAMA Oncol* (2017) 3:e172411. doi:10.1001/jamaoncol.2017.2411
32. Massard C, Gordon MS, Sharma S, Rafii S, Wainberg ZA, Luke J, et al. Safety and efficacy of durvalumab (MEDI4736), an anti-programmed cell death ligand-1 immune checkpoint inhibitor, in patients with advanced urothelial bladder cancer. *J Clin Oncol* (2016) 34:3119–25. doi:10.1200/JCO.2016.67.9761
33. Seiwert TY, Haddad RI, Gupta S, Mehra R, Tahara M, Berger R, et al. Antitumor activity and safety of pembrolizumab in patients (pts) with advanced squamous cell carcinoma of the head and neck (SCCHN): preliminary results from KEYNOTE-012 expansion cohort. *J Clin Oncol* (2015) 33:LBA6008. doi:10.1200/jco.2015.33.18_suppl.lba6008
34. Seiwert TY, Burtness B, Mehra R, Weiss J, Berger R, Eder JP, et al. Safety and clinical activity of pembrolizumab for treatment of recurrent or metastatic squamous cell carcinoma of the head and neck (KEYNOTE-012): an open-label, multicentre, phase 1b trial. *Lancet Oncol* (2016) 17:956–65. doi:10.1016/S1470-2045(16)30066-3
35. Ansell SM, Lesokhin AM, Borrello I, Halwani A, Scott EC, Gutierrez M, et al. PD-1 blockade with nivolumab in relapsed or refractory Hodgkin's lymphoma. *N Engl J Med* (2015) 372:311–9. doi:10.1056/NEJMoa1411087
36. Armand P, Shipp MA, Ribrag V, Michot JM, Zinzani PL, Kuruvilla J, et al. Programmed death-1 blockade with pembrolizumab in patients with classical Hodgkin lymphoma after brentuximab vedotin failure. *J Clin Oncol* (2016) 34:3733–9. doi:10.1200/JCO.2016.67.3467
37. Lesokhin AM, Ansell SM, Armand P, Scott EC, Halwani A, Gutierrez M, et al. Nivolumab in patients with relapsed or refractory hematologic malignancy:

preliminary results of a phase Ib study. *J Clin Oncol* (2016) 34:2698–704. doi:10.1200/JCO.2015.65.9789
38. Brahmer JR, Tykodi SS, Chow LQM, Hwu W-J, Topalian SL, Hwu P, et al. Safety and activity of anti-PD-L1 antibody in patients with advanced cancer. *N Engl J Med* (2012) 366:2455–65. doi:10.1056/NEJMoa1200694
39. Royal RE, Levy C, Turner K, Mathur A, Hughes M, Kammula US, et al. Phase 2 trial of single agent ipilimumab (anti-CTLA-4) for locally advanced or metastatic pancreatic adenocarcinoma. *J Immunother* (2010) 33:828–33. doi:10.1097/CJI.0b013e3181eec14c
40. Pardoll DM. The blockade of immune checkpoints in cancer immunotherapy. *Nat Rev Cancer* (2012) 12:252–64. doi:10.1038/nrc3239
41. Gao GF, Rao Z, Bell JI. Molecular coordination of αβ T-cell receptors and coreceptors CD8 and CD4 in their recognition of peptide-MHC ligands. *Trends Immunol* (2002) 23:408–13. doi:10.1016/S1471-4906(02) 02282-2
42. Steimle V, Siegrist C, Mottet A, Lisowska-Grospierre B, Mach B. Regulation of MHC class II expression by interferon-gamma mediated by the transactivator gene CIITA. *Science* (1994) 265:106–9. doi:10.1126/science.8016643
43. Stout RD, Bottomly K. Antigen-specific activation of effector macrophages by IFN-gamma producing (TH1) T cell clones. Failure of IL-4-producing (TH2) T cell clones to activate effector function in macrophages. *J Immunol* (1989) 142:760–5.
44. Dobrzanski MJ. Expanding roles for CD4 T cells and their subpopulations in tumor immunity and therapy. *Front Oncol* (2013) 3:63. doi:10.3389/fonc.2013.00063
45. DeNardo DG, Barreto JB, Andreu P, Vasquez L, Tawfik D, Kolhatkar N, et al. CD4+T cells regulate pulmonary metastasis of mammary carcinomas by enhancing protumor properties of macrophages. *Cancer Cell* (2009) 16:91–102. doi:10.1016/j.ccr.2009.06.018
46. Tanaka A, Sakaguchi S. Regulatory T cells in cancer immunotherapy. *Cell Res* (2017) 27:109–18. doi:10.1038/cr.2016.151
47. Crespo J, Sun H, Welling TH, Tian Z, Zou W. T cell anergy, exhaustion, senescence, and stemness in the tumor microenvironment. *Curr Opin Immunol* (2013) 25:214–21. doi:10.1016/j.coi.2012.12.003
48. Topalian SL, Drake CG, Pardoll DM. Immune checkpoint blockade: a common denominator approach to cancer therapy. *Cancer Cell* (2015) 27:451–61. doi:10.1016/j.ccell.2015.03.001
49. Iwai Y, Hamanishi J, Chamoto K, Honjo T. Cancer immunotherapies targeting the PD-1 signaling pathway. *J Biomed Sci* (2017) 24:26. doi:10.1186/s12929-017-0329-9
50. Schwartz RH. Costimulation of T lymphocytes: the role of CD28, CTLA-4, and B7/BB1 in interleukin-2 production and immunotherapy. *Cell* (1992) 71:1065–8. doi:10.1016/S0092-8674(05)80055-8
51. Linsley PS, Greene JL, Brady W, Bajorath J, Ledbetter JA, Peach R. Human B7-1 (CD80) and B7-2 (CD86) bind with similar avidities but distinct kinetics to CD28 and CTLA-4 receptors. *Immunity* (1994) 1:793–801. doi:10.1016/S1074-7613(94)80021-9
52. Qureshi OS, Zheng Y, Nakamura K, Attridge K, Manzotti C, Schmidt EM, et al. Trans-endocytosis of CD80 and CD86: a molecular basis for the cell-extrinsic function of CTLA-4. *Science* (2011) 332:600–3. doi:10.1126/science.1202947
53. Krummel MF, Allison JP. CTLA-4 engagement inhibits IL-2 accumulation and cell cycle progression upon activation of resting T cells. *J Exp Med* (1996) 183:2533–40. doi:10.1084/jem.183.6.2533
54. Fallarino F, Fields PE, Gajewski TF. B7-1 engagement of cytotoxic T lymphocyte antigen 4 inhibits T cell activation in the absence of CD28. *J Exp Med* (1998) 188:205–10. doi:10.1084/jem.188.1.205
55. Chambers CA, Sullivan TJ, Truong T, Allison JP. Secondary but not primary T cell responses are enhanced in CTLA-4-deficient CD8+ T cells. *Eur J Immunol* (1998) 28:3137–43. doi:10.1002/(SICI)1521-4141(199810)28:10<3137::AID-IMMU3137>3.0.CO;2-X
56. Takahashi T, Tagami T, Yamazaki S, Uede T, Shimizu J, Sakaguchi N, et al. Immunologic self-tolerance maintained by $Cd25^+$ $Cd4^+$ regulatory T cells constitutively expressing cytotoxic T lymphocyte-associated antigen 4. *J Exp Med* (2000) 192:303–10. doi:10.1084/jem.192.2.303
57. Hori S, Nomura T, Sakaguchi S. Control of regulatory T cell development by the transcription factor Foxp3. *Science* (2003) 299:1057–61. doi:10.1126/science.1079490
58. Fontenot JD, Gavin MA, Rudensky AY. Foxp3 programs the development and function of CD4+CD25+ regulatory T cells. *Nat Immunol* (2003) 4:330–6. doi:10.1038/ni904
59. Wing K, Onishi Y, Prieto-Martin P, Yamaguchi T, Miyara M, Fehervari Z, et al. CTLA-4 control over Foxp3+ regulatory T cell function. *Science* (2008) 322:271–5. doi:10.1126/science.1160062
60. Klocke K, Holmdahl R, Wing K. CTLA-4 expressed by FOXP3+ regulatory T cells prevents inflammatory tissue attack and not T-cell priming in arthritis. *Immunology* (2017) 152:125–37. doi:10.1111/imm.12754
61. Bengsch F, Knoblock DM, Liu A, McAllister F, Beatty GL. CTLA-4/CD80 pathway regulates T cell infiltration into pancreatic cancer. *Cancer Immunol Immunother* (2017) 66:1609–17. doi:10.1007/s00262-017-2053-4
62. Peggs KS, Quezada SA, Chambers CA, Korman AJ, Allison JP. Blockade of CTLA-4 on both effector and regulatory T cell compartments contributes to the antitumor activity of anti–CTLA-4 antibodies. *J Exp Med* (2009) 206:1717–25. doi:10.1084/jem.20082492
63. Ishida Y, Agata Y, Shibahara K, Honjo T. Induced expression of PD-1, a novel member of the immunoglobulin gene superfamily, upon programmed cell death. *EMBO J* (1992) 11:3887–95.
64. Freeman GJ, Long AJ, Iwai Y, Bourque K, Chernova T, Nishimura H, et al. Engagement of the Pd-1 immunoinhibitory receptor by a novel B7 family member leads to negative regulation of lymphocyte activation. *J Exp Med* (2000) 192:1027–34. doi:10.1084/jem.192.7.1027
65. Dong H, Zhu G, Tamada K, Chen L. B7-H1, a third member of the B7 family, co-stimulates T-cell proliferation and interleukin-10 secretion. *Nat Med* (1999) 5:1365–9. doi:10.1038/70932
66. Latchman Y, Wood CR, Chernova T, Chaudhary D, Borde M, Chernova I, et al. PD-L2 is a second ligand for PD-1 and inhibits T cell activation. *Nat Immunol* (2001) 2:261–8. doi:10.1038/85330
67. Tseng SY, Otsuji M, Gorski K, Huang X, Slansky JE, Pai SI, et al. B7-DC, a new dendritic cell molecule with potent costimulatory properties for T cells. *J Exp Med* (2001) 193:839–46. doi:10.1084/jem.193.7.839
68. Agata Y, Kawasaki A, Nishimura H, Ishida Y, Tsubata T, Yagita H, et al. Expression of the PD-1 antigen on the surface of stimulated mouse T and B lymphocytes. *Int Immunol* (1996) 8:765–72. doi:10.1093/intimm/8.5.765
69. Youngblood B, Oestreich KJ, Ha SJ, Duraiswamy J, Akondy RS, West EE, et al. Chronic virus infection enforces demethylation of the locus that encodes PD-1 in antigen-specific CD8+ T cells. *Immunity* (2011) 35:400–12. doi:10.1016/j.immuni.2011.06.015
70. Iwai Y, Terawaki S, Ikegawa M, Okazaki T, Honjo T. PD-1 inhibits antiviral immunity at the effector phase in the liver. *J Exp Med* (2003) 198:39–50. doi:10.1084/jem.20022235
71. Barber DL, Wherry EJ, Masopust D, Zhu B, Allison JP, Sharpe AH, et al. Restoring function in exhausted CD8 T cells during chronic viral infection. *Nature* (2006) 439:682–7. doi:10.1038/nature04444
72. Staron MM, Gray SM, Marshall HD, Parish IA, Chen JH, Perry CJ, et al. The transcription factor FoxO1 sustains expression of the inhibitory receptor PD-1 and survival of antiviral CD8+ T cells during chronic infection. *Immunity* (2014) 41:802–14. doi:10.1016/j.immuni.2014.10.013
73. Asano T, Meguri Y, Yoshioka T, Kishi Y, Iwamoto M, Nakamura M, et al. PD-1 modulates regulatory T-cell homeostasis during low-dose interleukin-2 therapy. *Blood* (2017) 129:2186–97. doi:10.1182/blood-2016-09-741629
74. Wang L, Pino-Lagos K, De Vries VC, Guleria I, Sayegh MH, Noelle RJ. Programmed death 1 ligand signaling regulates the generation of adaptive Foxp3+ CD4+ regulatory T cells. *Proc Natl Acad Sci U S A* (2008) 105:9331–6. doi:10.1073/pnas.0710441105
75. Wang C, Thudium KB, Han M, Wang X-T, Huang H, Feingersh D, et al. In vitro characterization of the anti-PD-1 antibody nivolumab, BMS-936558, and in vivo toxicology in non-human primates. *Cancer Immunol Res* (2014) 2:846–56. doi:10.1158/2326-6066.CIR-14-0040
76. Nishimura H, Nose M, Hiai H, Minato N, Honjo T. Development of lupus-like autoimmune diseases by disruption of the PD-1 gene encoding an ITIM motif-carrying immunoreceptor. *Immunity* (1999) 11:141–51. doi:10.1016/S1074-7613(00)80089-8
77. Nishimura H, Okazaki T, Tanaka Y, Nakatani K, Hara M, Matsumori A, et al. Autoimmune dilated cardiomyopathy in PD-1 receptor-deficient mice. *Science* (2001) 291:319–22. doi:10.1126/science.291.5502.319
78. Tivol EA, Borriello F, Schweitzer AN, Lynch WP, Bluestone JA, Sharpe AH. Loss of CTLA-4 leads to massive lymphoproliferation and fatal multiorgan

tissue destruction, revealing a critical negative regulatory role of CTLA-4. *Immunity* (1995) 3:541–7. doi:10.1016/1074-7613(95)90125-6

79. Waterhouse P, Penninger JM, Timms E, Wakeham A, Shahinian A, Lee KP, et al. Lymphoproliferative disorders with early lethality in mice deficient in Ctla-4. *Science* (1995) 270:985–8. doi:10.1126/science.270.5238.985
80. Keir ME, Butte MJ, Freeman GJ, Sharpe AH. PD-1 and its ligands in tolerance and immunity. *Annu Rev Immunol* (2008) 26:677–704. doi:10.1146/annurev.immunol.26.021607.090331
81. Linsley PS, Bradshaw J, Greene JA, Peach R, Bennett KL, Mittler RS. Intracellular trafficking of CTLA-4 and focal localization towards sites of TCR engagement. *Immunity* (1996) 4:535–43. doi:10.1016/S1074-7613(00)80480-X
82. Davoodzadeh Gholami M, Kardar GA, Saeedi Y, Heydari S, Garssen J, Falak R. Exhaustion of T lymphocytes in the tumor microenvironment: significance and effective mechanisms. *Cell Immunol* (2017) 322:1–14. doi:10.1016/j.cellimm.2017.10.002
83. Topalian SL, Hodi FS, Brahmer JR, Gettinger SN, Smith DC, McDermott DF, et al. Safety, activity, and immune correlates of anti-PD-1 antibody in cancer. *N Engl J Med* (2012) 366:2443–54. doi:10.1056/NEJMoa1200690
84. Larkin J, Chiarion-Sileni V, Gonzalez R, Grob JJ, Cowey CL, Lao CD, et al. Combined nivolumab and ipilimumab or monotherapy in untreated melanoma. *N Engl J Med* (2015) 373:23–34. doi:10.1056/NEJMoa1504030
85. Ehrlich P. Vol. II. Immunology and cancer research. In: Himmelweit F, Marquardt M, Dale H, editors. *Collected Papers of Paul Ehrlich: In Four Volumes Including a Complete Bibliography*. London: Pergamon Press (1960).
86. Burnet FM. Immunological surveillance in neoplasia. *Immunol Rev* (1971) 7:3–25. doi:10.1111/j.1600-065X.1971.tb00461.x
87. Thomas L. On immunosurveillance in human cancer. *Yale J Biol Med* (1982) 55:329–33.
88. Dunn GP, Bruce AT, Ikeda H, Old LJ, Schreiber RD. Cancer immunoediting: from immunosurveillance to tumor escape. *Nat Immunol* (2002) 3:991–8. doi:10.1038/ni1102-991
89. Dunn GP, Old LJ, Schreiber RD. The three Es of cancer immunoediting. *Annu Rev Immunol* (2004) 22:329–60. doi:10.1146/annurev.immunol.22.012703.104803
90. Gopinathan A, Morton JP, Jodrell DI, Sansom OJ. GEMMs as preclinical models for testing pancreatic cancer therapies. *Dis Model Mech* (2015) 8:1185–200. doi:10.1242/dmm.021055
91. Hingorani SR, Petricoin EF, Maitra A, Rajapakse V, King C, Jacobetz MA, et al. Preinvasive and invasive ductal pancreatic cancer and its early detection in the mouse. *Cancer Cell* (2003) 4:437–50. doi:10.1016/S1535-6108(03)00309-X
92. Clark CE, Hingorani SR, Mick R, Combs C, Tuveson DA, Vonderheide RH. Dynamics of the immune reaction to pancreatic cancer from inception to invasion. *Cancer Res* (2007) 67:9518–27. doi:10.1158/0008-5472.CAN-07-0175
93. Evans RA, Diamond MS, Rech AJ, Chao T, Richardson MW, Lin JH, et al. Lack of immunoediting in murine pancreatic cancer reversed with neoantigen. *JCI Insight* (2016) 1. doi:10.1172/jci.insight.88328
94. Foley K, Kim V, Jaffee E, Zheng L. Current progress in immunotherapy for pancreatic cancer. *Cancer Lett* (2016) 381:244–51. doi:10.1016/j.canlet.2015.12.020
95. Hiraoka N, Onozato K, Kosuge T, Hirohashi S. Prevalence of FOXP3+ regulatory T cells increases during the progression of pancreatic ductal adenocarcinoma and its premalignant lesions. *Clin Cancer Res* (2006) 12:5423–34. doi:10.1158/1078-0432.CCR-06-0369
96. Vonderheide RH. The immune revolution: a case for priming, not checkpoint. *Cancer Cell* (2018) 33:563–9. doi:10.1016/j.ccell.2018.03.008
97. Beatty GL, Gladney WL. Immune escape mechanisms as a guide for cancer immunotherapy. *Clin Cancer Res* (2015) 21:687–92. doi:10.1158/1078-0432.CCR-14-1860
98. Yarchoan M, Johnson BA, Lutz ER, Laheru DA, Jaffee EM. Targeting neoantigens to augment antitumour immunity. *Nat Rev Cancer* (2017) 17:209–22. doi:10.1038/nrc.2016.154
99. Topalian SL, Taube JM, Anders RA, Pardoll DM. Mechanism-driven biomarkers to guide immune checkpoint blockade in cancer therapy. *Nat Rev Cancer* (2016) 16:275–87. doi:10.1038/nrc.2016.36
100. Coulie PG, Van Den Eynde BJ, Van Der Bruggen P, Boon T. Tumour antigens recognized by T lymphocytes: at the core of cancer immunotherapy. *Nat Rev Cancer* (2014) 14:135–46. doi:10.1038/nrc3670
101. Campbell BB, Light N, Fabrizio D, Zatzman M, Fuligni F, de Borja R, et al. Comprehensive analysis of hypermutation in human cancer. *Cell* (2017) 171:1042.e–56.e. doi:10.1016/j.cell.2017.09.048
102. Vogelstein B, Papadopoulos N, Velculescu VE, Zhou S, Diaz LA, Kinzler KW. Cancer genome landscapes. *Science* (2013) 339:1546–58. doi:10.1126/science.1235122
103. Goodman AM, Kato S, Bazhenova L, Patel SP, Frampton GM, Miller V, et al. Tumor mutational burden as an independent predictor of response to immunotherapy in diverse cancers. *Mol Cancer Ther* (2017) 16(11):2598–608. doi:10.1158/1535-7163.MCT-17-0386
104. Rizvi NA, Hellmann MD, Snyder A, Kvistborg P, Makarov V, Havel JJ, et al. Mutational landscape determines sensitivity to PD-1 blockade in non-small cell lung cancer. *Science* (2015) 348:124–8. doi:10.1126/science.aaa1348
105. Yarchoan M, Hopkins A, Jaffee EM. Tumor mutational burden and response rate to PD-1 inhibition. *N Engl J Med* (2017) 377:2500–1. doi:10.1056/NEJMc1713444
106. Le DT, Durham JN, Smith KN, Wang H, Bartlett BR, Aulakh LK, et al. Mismatch repair deficiency predicts response of solid tumors to PD-1 blockade. *Science* (2017) 357:409–13. doi:10.1126/science.aan6733
107. Germano G, Lamba S, Rospo G, Barault L, Magri A, Maione F, et al. Inactivation of DNA repair triggers neoantigen generation and impairs tumour growth. *Nature* (2017) 552:1–5. doi:10.1038/nature24673
108. Humphris JL, Patch AM, Nones K, Bailey PJ, Johns AL, McKay S, et al. Hypermutation in pancreatic cancer. *Gastroenterology* (2017) 152:68.e–74.e. doi:10.1053/j.gastro.2016.09.060
109. Brown JS, Sundar R, Lopez J. Combining DNA damaging therapeutics with immunotherapy: more haste, less speed. *Br J Cancer* (2018) 118:312–24. doi:10.1038/bjc.2017.376
110. Lawrence MS, Stojanov P, Polak P, Kryukov GV, Cibulskis K, Sivachenko A, et al. Mutational heterogeneity in cancer and the search for new cancer-associated genes. *Nature* (2013) 499:214–8. doi:10.1038/nature12213
111. Balachandran VP, Luksza M, Zhao JN, Makarov V, Moral JA, Remark R, et al. Identification of unique neoantigen qualities in long-term survivors of pancreatic cancer. *Nature* (2017) 551:S12–6. doi:10.1038/nature24462
112. de Charette M, Marabelle A, Houot R. Turning tumour cells into antigen presenting cells: the next step to improve cancer immunotherapy? *Eur J Cancer* (2016) 68:134–47. doi:10.1016/j.ejca.2016.09.010
113. Delp K, Momburg F, Hilmes C, Huber C, Seliger B. Functional deficiencies of components of the MHC class I antigen pathway in human tumors of epithelial origin. *Bone Marrow Transplant* (2000) 25:S88–95. doi:10.1038/sj.bmt.1702363
114. Herrmann F, Lehr HA, Drexler I, Sutter G, Hengstler J, Wollscheid U, et al. HER-2/neu-mediated regulation of components of the MHC class I antigen-processing pathway. *Cancer Res* (2004) 64:215–20. doi:10.1158/0008-5472.CAN-2522-2
115. Paulson KG, Tegeder A, Willmes C, Iyer JG, Afanasiev OK, Schrama D, et al. Downregulation of MHC-I expression is prevalent but reversible in Merkel cell carcinoma. *Cancer Immunol Res* (2014) 2:1071–9. doi:10.1158/2326-6066.CIR-14-0005
116. Leone P, Shin EC, Perosa F, Vacca A, Dammacco F, Racanelli V. MHC class I antigen processing and presenting machinery: organization, function, and defects in tumor cells. *J Natl Cancer Inst* (2013) 105:1172–87. doi:10.1093/jnci/djt184
117. Lohmann S, Wollscheid U, Huber C, Seliger B. Multiple levels of MHC class I down-regulation by ras oncogenes. *Scand J Immunol* (1996) 43:537–44. doi:10.1046/j.1365-3083.1996.d01-73.x
118. Seliger B, Harders C, Wollscheid U, Staege MS, Reske-Kunz AB, Huber C. Suppression of MHC class I antigens in oncogenic transformants: association with decreased recognition by cytotoxic T lymphocytes. *Exp Hematol* (1996) 24:1275–9.
119. Mimura K, Shiraishi K, Mueller A, Izawa S, Kua L-F, So J, et al. The MAPK pathway is a predominant regulator of HLA-A expression in esophageal and gastric cancer. *J Immunol* (2013) 191:6261–72. doi:10.4049/jimmunol.1301597
120. Pommier A, Anaparthy N, Memos N, Kelley ZL, Gouronnec A, Yan R, et al. Unresolved endoplasmic reticulum stress engenders immune-resistant, latent pancreatic cancer metastases. *Science* (2018) 360:eaao4908. doi:10.1126/science.aao4908

121. Snyder A, Makarov V, Merghoub T, Yuan J, Zaretsky JM, Desrichard A, et al. Genetic basis for clinical response to CTLA-4 blockade in melanoma. *N Engl J Med* (2014) 371:2189–99. doi:10.1056/NEJMoa1406498
122. Van Allen EM, Miao D, Schilling B, Shukla SA, Blank C, Zimmer L, et al. Genomic correlates of response to CTLA-4 blockade in metastatic melanoma. *Science* (2015) 350:207–11. doi:10.1126/science.aad0095
123. Hugo W, Zaretsky JM, Sun L, Song C, Moreno BH, Hu-Lieskovan S, et al. Genomic and transcriptomic features of response to anti-PD-1 therapy in metastatic melanoma. *Cell* (2016) 165:35–44. doi:10.1016/j.cell.2016.02.065
124. Bailey P, Chang DK, Forget MA, Lucas FAS, Alvarez HA, Haymaker C, et al. Exploiting the neoantigen landscape for immunotherapy of pancreatic ductal adenocarcinoma. *Sci Rep* (2016) 6:1–8. doi:10.1038/srep35848
125. Balli D, Rech AJ, Stanger BZ, Vonderheide RH. Immune cytolytic activity stratifies molecular subsets of human pancreatic cancer. *Clin Cancer Res* (2017) 23:3129–38. doi:10.1158/1078-0432.CCR-16-2128
126. Collisson EA, Sadanandam A, Olson P, Gibb WJ, Truitt M, Gu S, et al. Subtypes of pancreatic ductal adenocarcinoma and their differing responses to therapy. *Nat Med* (2011) 17:500–3. doi:10.1038/nm.2344
127. Moffitt RA, Marayati R, Flate EL, Volmar KE, Loeza SGH, Hoadley KA, et al. Virtual microdissection identifies distinct tumor- and stroma-specific subtypes of pancreatic ductal adenocarcinoma. *Nat Genet* (2015) 47:1168–78. doi:10.1038/ng.3398
128. Biankin AV, Waddell N, Kassahn KS, Gingras MC, Muthuswamy LB, Johns AL, et al. Pancreatic cancer genomes reveal aberrations in axon guidance pathway genes. *Nature* (2012) 491:399–405. doi:10.1038/nature11547
129. Waddell N, Pajic M, Patch AM, Chang DK, Kassahn KS, Bailey P, et al. Whole genomes redefine the mutational landscape of pancreatic cancer. *Nature* (2015) 518:495–501. doi:10.1038/nature14169
130. Bailey P, Chang DK, Nones K, Johns AL, Patch AM, Gingras MC, et al. Genomic analyses identify molecular subtypes of pancreatic cancer. *Nature* (2016) 531:47–52. doi:10.1038/nature16965
131. Rooney MS, Shukla SA, Wu CJ, Getz G, Hacohen N. Molecular and genetic properties of tumors associated with local immune cytolytic activity. *Cell* (2015) 160:48–61. doi:10.1016/j.cell.2014.12.033
132. Pylayeva-Gupta Y, Lee KE, Hajdu CH, Miller G, Bar-Sagi D. Oncogenic Kras-induced GM-CSF production promotes the development of pancreatic neoplasia. *Cancer Cell* (2012) 21:836–47. doi:10.1016/j.ccr.2012.04.024
133. McAllister F, Bailey JM, Alsina J, Nirschl CJ, Sharma R, Fan H, et al. Oncogenic kras activates a hematopoietic-to-epithelial IL-17 signaling axis in preinvasive pancreatic neoplasia. *Cancer Cell* (2014) 25:621–37. doi:10.1016/j.ccr.2014.03.014
134. Vonderheide RH. Tumor-promoting inflammatory networks in pancreatic neoplasia: another reason to loathe kras. *Cancer Cell* (2014) 25:553–4. doi:10.1016/j.ccr.2014.04.020
135. Zhang J, Wolfgang C, Zheng L. Precision immuno-oncology: prospects of individualized immunotherapy for pancreatic cancer. *Cancers (Basel)* (2018) 10:39. doi:10.3390/cancers10020039
136. Lastwika KJ, Wilson W, Li QK, Norris J, Xu H, Ghazarian SR, et al. Control of PD-L1 expression by oncogenic activation of the AKT-mTOR pathway in non-small cell lung cancer. *Cancer Res* (2016) 76:227–38. doi:10.1158/0008-5472.CAN-14-3362
137. Parsa AT, Waldron JS, Panner A, Crane CA, Parney IF, Barry JJ, et al. Loss of tumor suppressor PTEN function increases B7-H1 expression and immunoresistance in glioma. *Nat Med* (2007) 13:84–8. doi:10.1038/nm1517
138. Casey SC, Tong L, Li Y, Do R, Walz S, Fitzgerald KN, et al. MYC regulates the antitumor immune response through CD47 and PD-L1. *Science* (2016) 352:227–31. doi:10.1126/science.aac9935
139. Feng J, Yang H, Zhang Y, Wei H, Zhu Z, Zhu B, et al. Tumor cell-derived lactate induces TAZ-dependent upregulation of PD-L1 through GPR81 in human lung cancer cells. *Oncogene* (2017) 36:5829–39. doi:10.1038/onc.2017.188
140. Zhang Y, Velez-Delgado A, Mathew E, Li D, Mendez FM, Flannagan K, et al. Myeloid cells are required for PD-1/PD-L1 checkpoint activation and the establishment of an immunosuppressive environment in pancreatic cancer. *Gut* (2017) 66:124–36. doi:10.1136/gutjnl-2016-312078
141. Hamid O, Robert C, Daud A, Hodi FS, Hwu W-J, Kefford R, et al. Safety and tumor responses with lambrolizumab (anti-PD-1) in melanoma. *N Engl J Med* (2013) 369:134–44. doi:10.1056/NEJMoa1305133
142. Khandelwal N, Breinig M, Speck T, Michels T, Kreutzer C, Sorrentino A, et al. A high-throughput RNAi screen for detection of immune-checkpoint molecules that mediate tumor resistance to cytotoxic T lymphocytes. *EMBO Mol Med* (2015) 7:450–63. doi:10.15252/emmm.201404414
143. Lim SO, Li CW, Xia W, Cha JH, Chan LC, Wu Y, et al. Deubiquitination and stabilization of PD-L1 by CSN5. *Cancer Cell* (2016) 30:925–39. doi:10.1016/j.ccell.2016.10.010
144. Lu C, Paschall AV, Shi H, Savage N, Waller JL, Sabbatini ME, et al. The MLL1-H3K4me3 axis-mediated PD-L1 expression and pancreatic cancer immune evasion. *J Natl Cancer Inst* (2017) 109. doi:10.1093/jnci/djw283
145. Dunn GP, Bruce AT, Sheehan KCF, Shankaran V, Uppaluri R, Bui JD, et al. A critical function for type I interferons in cancer immunoediting. *Nat Immunol* (2005) 6:722–9. doi:10.1038/ni1213
146. Gao J, Shi LZ, Zhao H, Chen J, Xiong L, He Q, et al. Loss of IFN-γ pathway genes in tumor cells as a mechanism of resistance to anti-CTLA-4 therapy. *Cell* (2016) 167:397.e–404.e. doi:10.1016/j.cell.2016.08.069
147. Patel SJ, Sanjana NE, Kishton RJ, Eidizadeh A, Vodnala SK, Cam M, et al. Identification of essential genes for cancer immunotherapy. *Nature* (2017) 548:537–42. doi:10.1038/nature23477
148. Mandai M, Hamanishi J, Abiko K, Matsumura N, Baba T, Konishi I. Dual faces of ifnγ in cancer progression: a role of pd-l1 induction in the determination of pro and antitumor immunity. *Clin Cancer Res* (2016) 22:2329–34. doi:10.1158/1078-0432.CCR-16-0224
149. Shin DS, Zaretsky JM, Escuin-Ordinas H, Garcia-Diaz A, Hu-Lieskovan S, Kalbasi A, et al. Primary resistance to PD-1 blockade mediated by JAK1/2 mutations. *Cancer Discov* (2017) 7:188–201. doi:10.1158/2159-8290.CD-16-1223
150. Cogdill AP, Andrews MC, Wargo JA. Hallmarks of response to immune checkpoint blockade. *Br J Cancer* (2017) 117:1–7. doi:10.1038/bjc.2017.136
151. Mellor AL, Munn DH. Creating immune privilege: active local suppression that benefits friends, but protects foes. *Nat Rev Immunol* (2008) 8:74–80. doi:10.1038/nri2264
152. Highfill SL, Cui Y, Giles AJ, Smith JP, Zhang H, Morse E, et al. Disruption of CXCR2-mediated MDSC tumor trafficking enhances anti-PD1 efficacy. *Sci Transl Med* (2014) 6:237ra67. doi:10.1126/scitranslmed.3007974
153. Lesokhin AM, Hohl TM, Kitano S, Cortez C, Hirschhorn-Cymerman D, Avogadri F, et al. Monocytic CCR2+ myeloid-derived suppressor cells promote immune escape by limiting activated CD8 T-cell infiltration into the tumor microenvironment. *Cancer Res* (2012) 72:876–86. doi:10.1158/0008-5472.CAN-11-1792
154. Hwang RF, Moore T, Arumugam T, Ramachandran V, Amos KD, Rivera A, et al. Cancer-associated stromal fibroblasts promote pancreatic tumor progression. *Cancer Res* (2008) 68:918–26. doi:10.1158/0008-5472.CAN-07-5714
155. Özdemir BC, Pentcheva-Hoang T, Carstens JL, Zheng X, Wu CC, Simpson TR, et al. Depletion of carcinoma-associated fibroblasts and fibrosis induces immunosuppression and accelerates pancreas cancer with reduced survival. *Cancer Cell* (2014) 25:719–34. doi:10.1016/j.ccr.2014.04.005
156. Carstens JL, De Sampaio PC, Yang D, Barua S, Wang H, Rao A, et al. Spatial computation of intratumoral T cells correlates with survival of patients with pancreatic cancer. *Nat Commun* (2017) 8:15095. doi:10.1038/ncomms15095
157. Ene-Obong A, Clear AJ, Watt J, Wang J, Fatah R, Riches JC, et al. Activated pancreatic stellate cells sequester CD8+ T cells to reduce their infiltration of the juxtatumoral compartment of pancreatic ductal adenocarcinoma. *Gastroenterology* (2013) 145:1121–32. doi:10.1053/j.gastro.2013.07.025
158. Feig C, Jones JO, Kraman M, Wells RJB, Deonarine A, Chan DS, et al. Targeting CXCL12 from FAP-expressing carcinoma-associated fibroblasts synergizes with anti-PD-L1 immunotherapy in pancreatic cancer. *Proc Natl Acad Sci U S A* (2013) 110:20212–7. doi:10.1073/pnas.1320318110
159. Johnson BA, Yarchoan M, Lee V, Laheru DA, Jaffee EM. Strategies for increasing pancreatic tumor immunogenicity. *Clin Cancer Res* (2017) 23:1656–69. doi:10.1158/1078-0432.CCR-16-2318
160. Jiang H, Hegde S, Knolhoff BL, Zhu Y, Herndon JM, Meyer MA, et al. Targeting focal adhesion kinase renders pancreatic cancers responsive to checkpoint immunotherapy. *Nat Med* (2016) 22:851–60. doi:10.1038/nm.4123
161. Infante JR, Camidge DR, Mileshkin LR, Chen EX, Hicks RJ, Rischin D, et al. Safety, pharmacokinetic, and pharmacodynamic phase I dose-escalation trial of PF-00562271, an inhibitor of focal adhesion kinase, in advanced solid tumors. *J Clin Oncol* (2012) 30:1527–33. doi:10.1200/JCO.2011.38.9346

162. Jones SF, Siu LL, Bendell JC, Cleary JM, Razak ARA, Infante JR, et al. A phase i study of VS-6063, a second-generation focal adhesion kinase inhibitor, in patients with advanced solid tumors. *Invest New Drugs* (2015) 33:1100–7. doi:10.1007/s10637-015-0282-y
163. Soria JC, Gan HK, Blagden SP, Plummer R, Arkenau HT, Ranson M, et al. A phase I, pharmacokinetic and pharmacodynamic study of GSK2256098, a focal adhesion kinase inhibitor, in patients with advanced solid tumors. *Ann Oncol* (2016) 27:2268–74. doi:10.1093/annonc/mdw427
164. Lesina M, Kurkowski MU, Ludes K, Rose-John S, Treiber M, Klöppel G, et al. Stat3/Socs3 activation by IL-6 transsignaling promotes progression of pancreatic intraepithelial neoplasia and development of pancreatic cancer. *Cancer Cell* (2011) 19:456–69. doi:10.1016/j.ccr.2011.03.009
165. Fukuda A, Wang SC, Morris JP, Folias AE, Liou A, Kim GE, et al. Stat3 and MMP7 contribute to pancreatic ductal adenocarcinoma initiation and progression. *Cancer Cell* (2011) 19:441–55. doi:10.1016/j.ccr.2011.03.002
166. Kang R, Loux T, Tang D, Schapiro NE, Vernon P, Livesey KM, et al. The expression of the receptor for advanced glycation endproducts (RAGE) is permissive for early pancreatic neoplasia. *Proc Natl Acad Sci U S A* (2012) 109:7031–6. doi:10.1073/pnas.1113865109
167. Zhang Y, Yan W, Collins MA, Bednar F, Rakshit S, Zetter BR, et al. Interleukin-6 is required for pancreatic cancer progression by promoting MAPK signaling activation and oxidative stress resistance. *Cancer Res* (2013) 73:6359–74. doi:10.1158/0008-5472.CAN-13-1558-T
168. Angevin E, Tabernero J, Elez E, Cohen SJ, Bahleda R, van Laethem J-L, et al. A phase I/II, multiple-dose, dose-escalation study of siltuximab, an anti-interleukin-6 monoclonal antibody, in patients with advanced solid tumors. *Clin Cancer Res* (2014) 20:2192–204. doi:10.1158/1078-0432.CCR-13-2200
169. Mace TA, Shakya R, Pitarresi JR, Swanson B, McQuinn CW, Loftus S, et al. IL-6 and PD-L1 antibody blockade combination therapy reduces tumour progression in murine models of pancreatic cancer. *Gut* (2018) 67:320–32. doi:10.1136/gutjnl-2016-311585
170. Sato N, Kohi S, Hirata K, Goggins M. Role of hyaluronan in pancreatic cancer biology and therapy: once again in the spotlight. *Cancer Sci* (2016) 107:569–75. doi:10.1111/cas.12913
171. Cheng XB, Sato N, Kohi S, Yamaguchi K. Prognostic impact of hyaluronan and its regulators in pancreatic ductal adenocarcinoma. *PLoS One* (2013) 8:e80765. doi:10.1371/journal.pone.0080765
172. Jacobetz MA, Chan DS, Neesse A, Bapiro TE, Cook N, Frese KK, et al. Hyaluronan impairs vascular function and drug delivery in a mouse model of pancreatic cancer. *Gut* (2013) 62:112–20. doi:10.1136/gutjnl-2012-302529
173. Provenzano PP, Cuevas C, Chang AE, Goel VK, Von Hoff DD, Hingorani SR. Enzymatic targeting of the stroma ablates physical barriers to treatment of pancreatic ductal adenocarcinoma. *Cancer Cell* (2012) 21:418–29. doi:10.1016/j.ccr.2012.01.007
174. Thompson CB, Shepard HM, O'Connor PM, Kadhim S, Jiang P, Osgood RJ, et al. Enzymatic depletion of tumor hyaluronan induces antitumor responses in preclinical animal models. *Mol Cancer Ther* (2010) 9:3052–64. doi:10.1158/1535-7163.MCT-10-0470
175. Singha NC, Nekoroski T, Zhao C, Symons R, Jiang P, Frost GI, et al. Tumor-associated hyaluronan limits efficacy of monoclonal antibody therapy. *Mol Cancer Ther* (2015) 14:523–32. doi:10.1158/1535-7163.MCT-14-0580
176. Blache CA, Manuel ER, Kaltcheva TI, Wong AN, Ellenhorn JDI, Blazar BR, et al. Systemic delivery of *Salmonella typhimurium* transformed with IDO shRNA enhances intratumoral vector colonization and suppresses tumor growth. *Cancer Res* (2012) 72:6447–56. doi:10.1158/0008-5472.CAN-12-0193
177. Manuel ER, Chen J, D'Apuzzo M, Lampa MG, Kaltcheva TI, Thompson CB, et al. *Salmonella*-based therapy targeting indoleamine 2,3-dioxygenase coupled with enzymatic depletion of tumor hyaluronan induces complete regression of aggressive pancreatic tumors. *Cancer Immunol Res* (2015) 3:1096–107. doi:10.1158/2326-6066.CIR-14-0214
178. Sherman MH, Yu RT, Engle DD, Ding N, Atkins AR, Tiriac H, et al. Vitamin D receptor-mediated stromal reprogramming suppresses pancreatitis and enhances pancreatic cancer therapy. *Cell* (2014) 159:80–93. doi:10.1016/j.cell.2014.08.007
179. Kumar V, Patel S, Tcyganov E, Gabrilovich DI. The nature of myeloid-derived suppressor cells in the tumor microenvironment. *Trends Immunol* (2016) 37:208–20. doi:10.1016/j.it.2016.01.004
180. Sica A, Larghi P, Mancino A, Rubino L, Porta C, Totaro MG, et al. Macrophage polarization in tumour progression. *Semin Cancer Biol* (2008) 18:349–55. doi:10.1016/j.semcancer.2008.03.004
181. Ino Y, Yamazaki-Itoh R, Shimada K, Iwasaki M, Kosuge T, Kanai Y, et al. Immune cell infiltration as an indicator of the immune microenvironment of pancreatic cancer. *Br J Cancer* (2013) 108:914–23. doi:10.1038/bjc.2013.32
182. Protti MP, De Monte L. Immune infiltrates as predictive markers of survival in pancreatic cancer patients. *Front Physiol* (2013) 4:210. doi:10.3389/fphys.2013.00210
183. Monu NR, Frey AB. Myeloid-derived suppressor cells and anti-tumor T cells: a complex relationship. *Immunol Invest* (2012) 41:595–613. doi:10.3109/08820139.2012.673191
184. Shibuya KC, Goel VK, Xiong W, Sham JG, Pollack SM, Leahy AM, et al. Pancreatic ductal adenocarcinoma contains an effector and regulatory immune cell infiltrate that is altered by multimodal neoadjuvant treatment. *PLoS One* (2014) 9:e96565. doi:10.1371/journal.pone.0096565
185. Tassi E, Gavazzi F, Albarello L, Senyukov V, Longhi R, Dellabona P, et al. Carcinoembryonic antigen-specific but not antiviral CD4+ T cell immunity is impaired in pancreatic carcinoma patients. *J Immunol* (2008) 181:6595–603. doi:10.4049/jimmunol.181.9.6595
186. De Monte L, Reni M, Tassi E, Clavenna D, Papa I, Recalde H, et al. Intratumor T helper type 2 cell infiltrate correlates with cancer-associated fibroblast thymic stromal lymphopoietin production and reduced survival in pancreatic cancer. *J Exp Med* (2011) 208:469–78. doi:10.1084/jem.20101876
187. Soares KC, Rucki AA, Kim V, Foley K, Solt S, Wolfgang CL, et al. TGF-β blockade depletes T regulatory cells from metastatic pancreatic tumors in a vaccine dependent manner. *Oncotarget* (2015) 6:43005–15. doi:10.18632/oncotarget.5656
188. Soares KC, Rucki AA, Wu AA, Olino K, Xiao Q, Chai Y, et al. PD-1/PD-L1 blockade together with vaccine therapy facilitates effector T-cell infiltration into pancreatic tumors. *J Immunother* (2015) 38:1–11. doi:10.1097/CJI.0000000000000062
189. Leliefeld PHC, Koenderman L, Pillay J. How neutrophils shape adaptive immune responses. *Front Immunol* (2015) 6:471. doi:10.3389/fimmu.2015.00471
190. Quezada SA, Jarvinen LZ, Lind EF, Noelle RJ. CD40/CD154 interactions at the interface of tolerance and immunity. *Annu Rev Immunol* (2004) 22:307–28. doi:10.1146/annurev.immunol.22.012703.104533
191. Schoenberger SP, Toes REM, Van der Voort EIH, Offringa R, Melief CJM. T-cell help for cytotoxic T-lymphocytes is mediated by CD40-CD40L interactions. *Nature* (1998) 393:480–3. doi:10.1038/31002
192. Bennett SRM, Carbone FR, Karamalis F, Flavell RA, Miller JFAP, Heath WR. Help for cytotoxic-T-cell responses is mediated by CD40 signalling. *Nature* (1998) 393:478–80. doi:10.1038/30996
193. Ridge JP, Di Rosa F, Matzinger P. A conditioned dendritic cell can be a temporal bridge between a CD4+ T-helper and a T-killer cell. *Nature* (1998) 393:474–8. doi:10.1038/30989
194. French RR, Chan HTC, Tutt AL, Glennie MJ. CD40 antibody evokes a cytotoxic T-cell response that eradicates lymphoma and bypasses T-cell help. *Nat Med* (1999) 5:548–53. doi:10.1038/8426
195. Diehl L, Den Boer AT, Schoenberger SP, Van Der Voort EIH, Schumacher TNM, Melief CJM, et al. CD40 activation in vivo overcomes peptide-induced peripheral cytotoxic T-lymphocyte tolerance and augments anti-tumor vaccine efficacy. *Nat Med* (1999) 5:774–9. doi:10.1038/10495
196. Sotomayor EM, Borrello I, Tubb E, Rattis FM, Bien H, Lu Z, et al. Conversion of tumor-specific CD4+ T-cell tolerance to T-cell priming through in vivo ligation of cd40. *Nat Med* (1999) 5:780–7. doi:10.1038/10503
197. Beatty GL, Chiorean EG, Fishman MP, Saboury B, Teitelbaum UR, Sun W, et al. CD40 agonists alter tumor stroma and show efficacy against pancreatic carcinoma in mice and humans. *Science* (2011) 331:1612–6. doi:10.1126/science.1198443
198. Beatty GL, Winograd R, Evans RA, Long KB, Luque SL, Lee JW, et al. Exclusion of T cells from pancreatic carcinomas in mice is regulated by $Ly6C^{low}$ $F4/80^{+}$ extratumoral macrophages. *Gastroenterology* (2015) 149:201–10. doi:10.1053/j.gastro.2015.04.010
199. Vonderheide RH, Burg JM, Mick R, Trosko JA, Li D, Shaik MN, et al. Phase I study of the CD40 agonist antibody CP-870,893 combined with carboplatin and paclitaxel in patients with advanced solid tumors. *Oncoimmunology* (2013) 2:e23033. doi:10.4161/onci.23033

200. Vonderheide RH, Flaherty KT, Khalil M, Stumacher MS, Bajor DL, Hutnick NA, et al. Clinical activity and immune modulation in cancer patients treated with CP-870,893, a novel CD40 agonist monoclonal antibody. *J Clin Oncol* (2007) 25:876–83. doi:10.1200/JCO.2006.08.3311
201. Nowak AK, Cook AM, McDonnell AM, Millward MJ, Creaney J, Francis RJ, et al. A phase 1b clinical trial of the CD40-activating antibody CP-870,893 in combination with cisplatin and pemetrexed in malignant pleural mesothelioma. *Ann Oncol* (2015) 26:2483–90. doi:10.1093/annonc/mdv387
202. Beatty GL, Torigian DA, Chiorean EG, Saboury B, Brothers A, Alavi A, et al. A phase I study of an agonist CD40 monoclonal antibody (CP-870,893) in combination with gemcitabine in patients with advanced pancreatic ductal adenocarcinoma. *Clin Cancer Res* (2013) 19:6286–95. doi:10.1158/1078-0432.CCR-13-1320
203. Byrne KT, Vonderheide RH. CD40 stimulation obviates innate sensors and drives T cell immunity in cancer. *Cell Rep* (2016) 15:2719–32. doi:10.1016/j.celrep.2016.05.058
204. Acosta JC, O'Loghlen A, Banito A, Guijarro MV, Augert A, Raguz S, et al. Chemokine signaling via the CXCR2 receptor reinforces senescence. *Cell* (2008) 133:1006–18. doi:10.1016/j.cell.2008.03.038
205. Lesina M, Wörmann SM, Morton J, Diakopoulos KN, Korneeva O, Wimmer M, et al. RelA regulates CXCL1/CXCR2-dependent oncogene-induced senescence in murine Kras-driven pancreatic carcinogenesis. *J Clin Invest* (2016) 126:2919–32. doi:10.1172/JCI86477
206. Cacalano G, Lee J, Kikly K, Ryan AM, Pitts-Meek S, Hultgren B, et al. Neutrophil and B cell expansion in mice that lack the murine IL-8 receptor homolog. *Science* (1994) 265:682–4. doi:10.1126/science.8036519
207. Eash KJ, Greenbaum AM, Gopalan PK, Link DC. CXCR2 and CXCR4 antagonistically regulate neutrophil trafficking from murine bone marrow. *J Clin Invest* (2010) 120:2423–31. doi:10.1172/JCI41649
208. Chao T, Furth EE, Vonderheide RH. CXCR2-dependent accumulation of tumor-associated neutrophils regulates T-cell immunity in pancreatic ductal adenocarcinoma. *Cancer Immunol Res* (2016) 4:968–82. doi:10.1158/2326-6066.CIR-16-0188
209. Kaneider NC, Agarwal A, Leger AJ, Kuliopulos A. Reversing systemic inflammatory response syndrome with chemokine receptor pepducins. *Nat Med* (2005) 11:661–5. doi:10.1038/nm1245
210. Jamieson T, Clarke M, Steele CW, Samuel MS, Neumann J, Jung A, et al. Inhibition of CXCR2 profoundly suppresses inflammation-driven and spontaneous tumorigenesis. *J Clin Invest* (2012) 122:3127–44. doi:10.1172/JCI61067
211. Nicholls DJ, Wiley K, Dainty I, MacIntosh F, Phillips C, Gaw A, et al. Pharmacological characterization of AZD5069, a slowly reversible CXC chemokine receptor 2 antagonist. *J Pharmacol Exp Ther* (2015) 353:340–50. doi:10.1124/jpet.114.221358
212. Steele CW, Karim SA, Leach JDG, Bailey P, Upstill-Goddard R, Rishi L, et al. CXCR2 inhibition profoundly suppresses metastases and augments immunotherapy in pancreatic ductal adenocarcinoma. *Cancer Cell* (2016) 29:832–45. doi:10.1016/j.ccell.2016.04.014
213. Stromnes IM, Schmitt TM, Hulbert A, Brockenbrough JS, Nguyen HN, Cuevas C, et al. T cells engineered against a native antigen can surmount immunologic and physical barriers to treat pancreatic ductal adenocarcinoma. *Cancer Cell* (2015) 28:638–52. doi:10.1016/j.ccell.2015.09.022
214. Lin EY, Nguyen AV, Russell RG, Pollard JW. Colony-stimulating factor 1 promotes progression of mammary tumors to malignancy. *J Exp Med* (2001) 193:727–40. doi:10.1084/jem.193.6.727
215. Cannarile MA, Weisser M, Jacob W, Jegg A-M, Ries CH, Rüttinger D. Colony-stimulating factor 1 receptor (CSF1R) inhibitors in cancer therapy. *J Immunother Cancer* (2017) 5:53. doi:10.1186/s40425-017-0257-y
216. Zhu Y, Knolhoff BL, Meyer MA, Nywening TM, West BL, Luo J, et al. CSF1/CSF1R blockade reprograms tumor-infiltrating macrophages and improves response to T-cell checkpoint immunotherapy in pancreatic cancer models. *Cancer Res* (2014) 74:5057–69. doi:10.1158/0008-5472.CAN-13-3723
217. Kumar V, Donthireddy L, Marvel D, Condamine T, Wang F, Lavilla-Alonso S, et al. Cancer-associated fibroblasts neutralize the anti-tumor effect of CSF1 receptor blockade by inducing PMN-MDSC infiltration of tumors. *Cancer Cell* (2017) 32:654–68.e5. doi:10.1016/j.ccell.2017.10.005
218. Zhou J, Nefedova Y, Lei A, Gabrilovich D. Neutrophils and PMN-MDSC: their biological role and interaction with stromal cells. *Semin Immunol* (2018) 35:19–28. doi:10.1016/j.smim.2017.12.004
219. Sagiv-Barfi I, Kohrt HEK, Czerwinski DK, Ng PP, Chang BY, Levy R. Therapeutic antitumor immunity by checkpoint blockade is enhanced by ibrutinib, an inhibitor of both BTK and ITK. *Proc Natl Acad Sci U S A* (2015) 112:E966–72. doi:10.1073/pnas.1500712112
220. Masso-Valles D, Jauset T, Serrano E, Sodir NM, Pedersen K, Affara NI, et al. Ibrutinib exerts potent antifibrotic and antitumor activities in mouse models of pancreatic adenocarcinoma. *Cancer Res* (2015) 75:1675–81. doi:10.1158/0008-5472.CAN-14-2852
221. Gunderson AJ, Kaneda MM, Tsujikawa T, Nguyen AV, Affara NI, Ruffell B, et al. Bruton tyrosine kinase-dependent immune cell cross-talk drives pancreas cancer. *Cancer Discov* (2016) 6:270–85. doi:10.1158/2159-8290.CD-15-0827
222. Dubovsky JA, Beckwith KA, Natarajan G, Woyach JA, Jaglowski S, Zhong Y, et al. Ibrutinib is an irreversible molecular inhibitor of ITK driving a Th1-selective pressure in T lymphocytes. *Blood* (2013) 122:2539–49. doi:10.1182/blood-2013-06-507947
223. Zou C, Zhao P, Xiao Z, Han X, Fu F, Fu L. γδ T cells in cancer immunotherapy. *Oncotarget* (2017) 8(5):8900–9. doi:10.18632/oncotarget.13051
224. Tanaka Y, Morita CT, Tanaka Y, Nieves E, Brenner MB, Bloom BR. Natural and synthetic non-peptide antigens recognized by human γδ T cells. *Nature* (1995) 375:155–8. doi:10.1038/375155a0
225. Lawand M, Déchanet-Merville J, Dieu-Nosjean MC. Key features of gamma-delta T-cell subsets in human diseases and their immunotherapeutic implications. *Front Immunol* (2017) 8:761. doi:10.3389/fimmu.2017.00761
226. Oberg HH, Peipp M, Kellner C, Sebens S, Krause S, Petrick D, et al. Novel bispecific antibodies increase GD T-cell cytotoxicity against pancreatic cancer cells. *Cancer Res* (2014) 74:1349–60. doi:10.1158/0008-5472.CAN-13-0675
227. Daley D, Zambirinis CP, Seifert L, Akkad N, Mohan N, Werba G, et al. γδ T cells support pancreatic oncogenesis by restraining αβ T cell activation. *Cell* (2016) 166:1485.e–99.e. doi:10.1016/j.cell.2016.07.046
228. Michalek RD, Gerriets VA, Jacobs SR, Macintyre AN, MacIver NJ, Mason EF, et al. Cutting edge: distinct glycolytic and lipid oxidative metabolic programs are essential for effector and regulatory CD4+ T cell subsets. *J Immunol* (2011) 186:3299–303. doi:10.4049/jimmunol.1003613
229. van der Windt GJW, Pearce EL. Metabolic switching and fuel choice during T-cell differentiation and memory development. *Immunol Rev* (2012) 249:27–42. doi:10.1111/j.1600-065X.2012.01150.x
230. Wang R, Dillon CP, Shi LZ, Milasta S, Carter R, Finkelstein D, et al. The transcription factor myc controls metabolic reprogramming upon T lymphocyte activation. *Immunity* (2011) 35:871–82. doi:10.1016/j.immuni.2011.09.021
231. Chang C-H, Curtis JD, Maggi LB, Faubert B, Villarino AV, O'Sullivan D, et al. Posttranscriptional control of T cell effector function by aerobic glycolysis. *Cell* (2013) 153:1239–51. doi:10.1016/j.cell.2013.05.016
232. Zheng Y, Delgoffe GM, Meyer CF, Chan W, Powell JD. Anergic T cells are metabolically anergic. *J Immunol* (2009) 183:6095–101. doi:10.4049/jimmunol.0803510
233. Renner K, Singer K, Koehl GE, Geissler EK, Peter K, Siska PJ, et al. Metabolic hallmarks of tumor and immune cells in the tumor microenvironment. *Front Immunol* (2017) 8:248. doi:10.3389/fimmu.2017.00248
234. Chang CH, Qiu J, O'Sullivan D, Buck MD, Noguchi T, Curtis JD, et al. Metabolic competition in the tumor microenvironment is a driver of cancer progression. *Cell* (2015) 162:1229–41. doi:10.1016/j.cell.2015.08.016
235. Carr EL, Kelman A, Wu GS, Gopaul R, Senkevitch E, Aghvanyan A, et al. Glutamine uptake and metabolism are coordinately regulated by ERK/MAPK during T lymphocyte activation. *J Immunol* (2010) 185:1037–44. doi:10.4049/jimmunol.0903586
236. Speiser DE, Ho P-C, Verdeil G. Regulatory circuits of T cell function in cancer. *Nat Rev Immunol* (2016) 16:599–611. doi:10.1038/nri.2016.80
237. Rodriguez PC, Hernandez CP, Quiceno D, Dubinett SM, Zabaleta J, Ochoa JB, et al. Arginase I in myeloid suppressor cells is induced by COX-2 in lung carcinoma. *J Exp Med* (2005) 202:931–9. doi:10.1084/jem.20050715
238. Rodriguez PC, Ernstoff MS, Hernandez C, Atkins M, Zabaleta J, Sierra R, et al. Arginase I-producing myeloid-derived suppressor cells in renal cell carcinoma are a subpopulation of activated granulocytes. *Cancer Res* (2009) 69:1553–60. doi:10.1158/0008-5472.CAN-08-1921
239. Löb S, Königsrainer A, Zieker D, Brücher BLDM, Rammensee HG, Opelz G, et al. IDO1 and IDO2 are expressed in human tumors: levo- but not dextro-1-methyl tryptophan inhibits tryptophan catabolism. *Cancer Immunol Immunother* (2009) 58:153–7. doi:10.1007/s00262-008-0513-6

240. Braun D, Longman RS, Albert ML. A two-step induction of indoleamine 2,3 dioxygenase (IDO) activity during dendritic-cell maturation. *Blood* (2005) 106:2375–81. doi:10.1182/blood-2005-03-0979
241. Uyttenhove C, Pilotte L, Théate I, Stroobant V, Colau D, Parmentier N, et al. Evidence for a tumoral immune resistance mechanism based on tryptophan degradation by indoleamine 2,3-dioxygenase. *Nat Med* (2003) 9:1269–74. doi:10.1038/nm934
242. Munn DH, Shafizadeh E, Attwood JT, Bondarev I, Pashine A, Mellor AL. Inhibition of t cell proliferation by macrophage tryptophan catabolism. *J Exp Med* (1999) 189:1363–72. doi:10.1084/jem.189.9.1363
243. Fallarino F, Grohmann U, Vacca C, Bianchi R, Orabona C, Spreca A, et al. T cell apoptosis by tryptophan catabolism. *Cell Death Differ* (2002) 9:1069–77. doi:10.1038/sj.cdd.4401073
244. Platten M, Wick W, Van Den Eynde BJ. Tryptophan catabolism in cancer: beyond IDO and tryptophan depletion. *Cancer Res* (2012) 72:5435–40. doi:10.1158/0008-5472.CAN-12-0569
245. Fischer K, Hoffmann P, Voelkl S, Meidenbauer N, Ammer J, Edinger M, et al. Inhibitory effect of tumor cell-derived lactic acid on human T cells. *Blood* (2007) 109:3812–9. doi:10.1182/blood-2006-07-035972
246. Mendler AN, Hu B, Prinz PU, Kreutz M, Gottfried E, Noessner E. Tumor lactic acidosis suppresses CTL function by inhibition of p38 and JNK/c-Jun activation. *Int J Cancer* (2012) 131:633–40. doi:10.1002/ijc.26410
247. Calcinotto A, Filipazzi P, Grioni M, Iero M, De Milito A, Ricupito A, et al. Modulation of microenvironment acidity reverses anergy in human and murine tumor-infiltrating T lymphocytes. *Cancer Res* (2012) 72:2746–56. doi:10.1158/0008-5472.CAN-11-1272
248. Huang S, Apasov S, Koshiba M, Sitkovsky M. Role of A2a extracellular adenosine receptor-mediated signaling in adenosine-mediated inhibition of T-cell activation and expansion. *Blood* (1997) 90:1600–10.
249. Ohta A, Sitkovsky M. Extracellular adenosine-mediated modulation of regulatory T cells. *Front Immunol* (2014) 5. doi:10.3389/fimmu.2014.00304
250. Ohta A. A metabolic immune checkpoint: adenosine in tumor microenvironment. *Front Immunol* (2016) 7:1–11. doi:10.3389/fimmu.2016.00109
251. Sreeramkumar V, Fresno M, Cuesta N. Prostaglandin E2 and T cells: friends or foes? *Immunol Cell Biol* (2012) 90:579–86. doi:10.1038/icb.2011.75
252. Halbrook CJ, Lyssiotis CA. Employing metabolism to improve the diagnosis and treatment of pancreatic cancer. *Cancer Cell* (2017) 31:5–19. doi:10.1016/j.ccell.2016.12.006
253. Mueller TC, Burmeister MA, Bachmann J, Martignoni ME. Cachexia and pancreatic cancer: are there treatment options? *World J Gastroenterol* (2014) 20:9361–73. doi:10.3748/wjg.v20.i28.9361
254. Flint TR, Janowitz T, Connell CM, Roberts EW, Denton AE, Coll AP, et al. Tumor-induced IL-6 reprograms host metabolism to suppress anti-tumor immunity. *Cell Metab* (2016) 24:672–84. doi:10.1016/j.cmet.2016.10.010
255. Bonetto A, Aydogdu T, Kunzevitzky N, Guttridge DC, Khuri S, Koniaris LG, et al. STAT3 activation in skeletal muscle links muscle wasting and the acute phase response in cancer cachexia. *PLoS One* (2011) 6:e22538. doi:10.1371/journal.pone.0022538
256. Bonetto A, Aydogdu T, Jin X, Zhang Z, Zhan R, Puzis L, et al. JAK/STAT3 pathway inhibition blocks skeletal muscle wasting downstream of IL-6 and in experimental cancer cachexia. *Am J Physiol Endocrinol Metab* (2012) 303:E410–21. doi:10.1152/ajpendo.00039.2012
257. Gotwals P, Cameron S, Cipolletta D, Cremasco V, Crystal A, Hewes B, et al. Prospects for combining targeted and conventional cancer therapy with immunotherapy. *Nat Rev Cancer* (2017) 17:286–301. doi:10.1038/nrc.2017.17
258. Ruess DA, Görgülü K, Wörmann SM, Algül H. Pharmacotherapeutic management of pancreatic ductal adenocarcinoma: current and emerging concepts. *Drugs Aging* (2017) 34:331–57. doi:10.1007/s40266-017-0453-y
259. Zheng Y, Dou Y, Duan L, Cong C, Gao A, Lai Q, et al. Using chemo-drugs or irradiation to break immune tolerance and facilitate immunotherapy in solid cancer. *Cell Immunol* (2015) 294:54–9. doi:10.1016/j.cellimm.2015.02.003
260. Kim SK, Wu CC, Horowitz DP. Stereotactic body radiotherapy for the pancreas: a critical review for the medical oncologist. *J Gastrointest Oncol* (2016) 7:479–86. doi:10.21037/jgo.2015.10.01
261. Kalina JL, Neilson DS, Comber AP, Rauw JM, Alexander AS, Vergidis J, et al. Immune modulation by androgen deprivation and radiation therapy: implications for prostate cancer immunotherapy. *Cancers* (2017) 9:13. doi:10.3390/cancers9020013
262. Burnette B, Weichselbaum RR. Radiation as an immune modulator. *Semin Radiat Oncol* (2013) 23:273–80. doi:10.1016/j.semradonc.2013.05.009
263. Postow MA, Callahan MK, Barker CA, Yamada Y, Yuan J, Kitano S, et al. Immunologic correlates of the abscopal effect in a patient with melanoma. *N Engl J Med* (2012) 366:925–31. doi:10.1056/NEJMoa1112824
264. Formenti SC, Demaria S. Combining radiotherapy and cancer immunotherapy: a paradigm shift. *J Natl Cancer Inst* (2013) 105:256–65. doi:10.1093/jnci/djs629
265. Golden EB, Demaria S, Schiff PB, Chachoua A, Formenti SC. An abscopal response to radiation and ipilimumab in a patient with metastatic non-small cell lung cancer. *Cancer Immunol Res* (2013) 1:365–72. doi:10.1158/2326-6066.CIR-13-0115
266. Deng L, Liang H, Burnette B, Beckett M, Darga T, Weichselbaum RR, et al. Irradiation and anti-PD-L1 treatment synergistically promote antitumor immunity in mice. *J Clin Invest* (2014) 124:687–95. doi:10.1172/JCI67313
267. Lutz ER, Wu AA, Bigelow E, Sharma R, Mo G, Soares K, et al. Immunotherapy converts nonimmunogenic pancreatic tumors into immunogenic foci of immune regulation. *Cancer Immunol Res* (2014) 2:616–31. doi:10.1158/2326-6066.CIR-14-0027
268. Azad A, Yin Lim S, D'Costa Z, Jones K, Diana A, Sansom OJ, et al. PD-L1 blockade enhances response of pancreatic ductal adenocarcinoma to radiotherapy. *EMBO Mol Med* (2017) 9:167–80. doi:10.15252/emmm.201606674
269. Twyman-Saint Victor C, Rech AJ, Maity A, Rengan R, Pauken KE, Stelekati E, et al. Radiation and dual checkpoint blockade activate non-redundant immune mechanisms in cancer. *Nature* (2015) 520:373–7. doi:10.1038/nature14292
270. Rech AJ, Dada H, Kotzin JJ, Henao-Mejia J, Minn AJ, Twyman-Saint Victor C, et al. Radiotherapy and CD40 activation separately augment immunity to checkpoint blockade in cancer. *Cancer Res* (2018) 78:4282–91. doi:10.1158/0008-5472.CAN-17-3821
271. Wang Y, Deng W, Li N, Neri S, Sharma A, Jiang W, et al. Combining immunotherapy and radiotherapy for cancer treatment: current challenges and future directions. *Front Pharmacol* (2018) 9:185. doi:10.3389/fphar.2018.00185
272. Naik S, Russell SJ. Engineering oncolytic viruses to exploit tumor specific defects in innate immune signaling pathways. *Expert Opin Biol Ther* (2009) 9:1163–76. doi:10.1517/14712590903170653
273. Chiocca EA, Rabkin SD. Oncolytic viruses and their application to cancer immunotherapy. *Cancer Immunol Res* (2014) 2:295–300. doi:10.1158/2326-6066.CIR-14-0015
274. Wong HH, Lemoine NR, Wang Y. Oncolytic viruses for cancer therapy: overcoming the obstacles. *Viruses* (2010) 2:78–106. doi:10.3390/v2010078
275. Pan W, Bodempudi V, Esfandyari T, Farassati F. Utilizing Ras signaling pathway to direct selective replication of herpes simplex virus-1. *PLoS One* (2009) 4:e6514. doi:10.1371/journal.pone.0006514
276. Doloff JC, Waxman DJ, Jounaidi Y. Human telomerase reverse transcriptase promoter-driven oncolytic adenovirus with E1B-19 kDa and E1B-55 kDa gene deletions. *Hum Gene Ther* (2008) 19:1383–99. doi:10.1089/hum.2008.056
277. Nishimoto T, Yoshida K, Miura Y, Kobayashi A, Hara H, Ohnami S, et al. Oncolytic virus therapy for pancreatic cancer using the adenovirus library displaying random peptides on the fiber knob. *Gene Ther* (2009) 16:669–80. doi:10.1038/gt.2009.1
278. Conner J, Braidwood L, Brown SM. A strategy for systemic delivery of the oncolytic herpes virus HSV1716: redirected tropism by antibody-binding sites incorporated on the virion surface as a glycoprotein D fusion protein. *Gene Ther* (2008) 15:1579–92. doi:10.1038/gt.2008.121
279. Lichty BD, Breitbach CJ, Stojdl DF, Bell JC. Going viral with cancer immunotherapy. *Nat Rev Cancer* (2014) 14:559–67. doi:10.1038/nrc3770
280. Sobol PT, Boudreau JE, Stephenson K, Wan Y, Lichty BD, Mossman KL. Adaptive antiviral immunity is a determinant of the therapeutic success of oncolytic virotherapy. *Mol Ther* (2011) 19:335–44. doi:10.1038/mt.2010.264
281. Janeway CA, Medzhitov R. Innate immune recognition. *Annu Rev Immunol* (2002) 20:197–216. doi:10.1146/annurev.immunol.20.083001.084359
282. Rahal A, Musher B. Oncolytic viral therapy for pancreatic cancer. *J Surg Oncol* (2017) 116:94–103. doi:10.1002/jso.24626
283. Mahalingam D, Goel S, Aparo S, Patel Arora S, Noronha N, Tran H, et al. A phase II study of pelareorep (REOLYSIN®) in combination with gemcitabine for patients with advanced pancreatic adenocarcinoma. *Cancers* (2018) 10:160. doi:10.3390/cancers10060160

284. Gujar S, Pol JG, Kim Y, Lee PW, Kroemer G. Antitumor benefits of antiviral immunity: an underappreciated aspect of oncolytic virotherapies. *Trends Immunol* (2018) 39(3):209–21. doi:10.1016/j.it.2017.11.006
285. Lutz ER, Kinkead H, Jaffee EM, Zheng L. Priming the pancreatic cancer tumor microenvironment for checkpoint-inhibitor immunotherapy. *Oncoimmunology* (2014) 3:e962401. doi:10.4161/21624011.2014.962401
286. Bourgeois-Daigneault M-C, Roy D, Aitken A, El Sayes N, Martin N, Varrette O, et al. Neo-adjuvant oncolytic virotherapy prior to surgery sensitizes triple-negative breast cancer to immune checkpoint therapy. *Sci Transl Med* (2018) 10:1–12. doi:10.1126/scitranslmed.aao1641
287. Lee P, Gujar S. Potentiating prostate cancer immunotherapy with oncolytic viruses. *Nat Rev Urol* (2018) 15:235–50. doi:10.1038/nrurol.2018.10
288. Samson A, Scott KJ, Taggart D, West EJ, Wilson E, Nuovo GJ, et al. Intravenous delivery of oncolytic reovirus to brain tumor patients immunologically primes for subsequent checkpoint blockade. *Sci Transl Med* (2018) 10. doi:10.1126/scitranslmed.aam7577
289. Blair AB, Zheng L. Rational combinations of immunotherapy for pancreatic ductal adenocarcinoma. *Chin Clin Oncol* (2017) 6:31–31. doi:10.21037/cco.2017.06.04
290. Skelton RA, Javed A, Zheng L, He J. Overcoming the resistance of pancreatic cancer to immune checkpoint inhibitors. *J Surg Oncol* (2017) 116:55–62. doi:10.1002/jso.24642
291. Jaffee EM, Hruban RH, Canto M, Kern SE. Focus on pancreas cancer. *Cancer Cell* (2002) 2:25–8. doi:10.1016/S1535-6108(02)00093-4
292. Melero I, Gaudernack G, Gerritsen W, Huber C, Parmiani G, Scholl S, et al. Therapeutic vaccines for cancer: an overview of clinical trials. *Nat Rev Clin Oncol* (2014) 11:509–24. doi:10.1038/nrclinonc.2014.111
293. Le DT, Lutz E, Uram JN, Sugar EA, Onners B, Solt S, et al. Evaluation of ipilimumab in combination with allogeneic pancreatic tumor cells transfected with a GM-CSF gene in previously treated pancreatic cancer. *J Immunother* (2013) 36:382–9. doi:10.1097/CJI.0b013e31829fb7a2
294. Le DT, Wang-Gillam A, Picozzi V, Greten TF, Crocenzi T, Springett G, et al. Safety and survival with GVAX pancreas prime and *Listeria monocytogenes*-expressing mesothelin (CRS-207) boost vaccines for metastatic pancreatic cancer. *J Clin Oncol* (2015) 33:1325–33. doi:10.1200/JCO.2014.57.4244
295. Abate-Daga D, Davila ML. CAR models: next-generation CAR modifications for enhanced T-cell function. *Mol Ther Oncolytics* (2016) 3:16014. doi:10.1038/mto.2016.14
296. Marin-Acevedo JA, Soyano AE, Dholaria B, Knutson KL, Lou Y. Cancer immunotherapy beyond immune checkpoint inhibitors. *J Hematol Oncol* (2018) 11:8. doi:10.1186/s13045-017-0552-6
297. Zhang C, Liu J, Zhong JF, Zhang X. Engineering CAR-T cells. *Biomark Res* (2017) 5:22. doi:10.1186/s40364-017-0102-y
298. Dotti G, Gottschalk S, Savoldo B, Brenner MK. Design and development of therapies using chimeric antigen receptor-expressing T cells. *Immunol Rev* (2014) 257:107–26. doi:10.1111/imr.12131
299. Kenderian SS, Ruella M, Gill S, Kalos M. Chimeric antigen receptor T-cell therapy to target hematologic malignancies. *Cancer Res* (2014) 74:6383–9. doi:10.1158/0008-5472.CAN-14-1530
300. Brown CE, Adusumilli PS. Next frontiers in CAR T-cell therapy. *Mol Ther oncolytics* (2016) 3:16028. doi:10.1038/mto.2016.28
301. Yu S, Li A, Liu Q, Li T, Yuan X, Han X, et al. Chimeric antigen receptor T cells: a novel therapy for solid tumors. *J Hematol Oncol* (2017) 10:78. doi:10.1186/s13045-017-0444-9
302. DeSelm CJ, Tano ZE, Varghese AM, Adusumilli PS. CAR T-cell therapy for pancreatic cancer. *J Surg Oncol* (2017) 116:63–74. doi:10.1002/jso.24627
303. Bauer C, Kühnemuth B, Duewell P, Ormanns S, Gress T, Schnurr M. Prevailing over T cell exhaustion: new developments in the immunotherapy of pancreatic cancer. *Cancer Lett* (2016) 381:259–68. doi:10.1016/j.canlet.2016.02.057
304. Cherkassky L, Morello A, Villena-Vargas J, Feng Y, Dimitrov DS, Jones DR, et al. Human CAR T cells with cell-intrinsic PD-1 checkpoint blockade resist tumor-mediated inhibition. *J Clin Invest* (2016) 126:3130–44. doi:10.1172/JCI83092
305. Moon EK, Wang L-CS, Dolfi DV, Wilson CB, Ranganathan R, Sun J, et al. Multifactorial T cell hypofunction that is reversible can limit the efficacy of chimeric antibody receptor-transduced human T cells in solid tumors. *Clin Cancer Res* (2014) 20:4262–73. doi:10.1158/1078-0432.CCR-13-2627
306. John LB, Devaud C, Duong CPM, Yong CS, Beavis PA, Haynes NM, et al. Anti-PD-1 antibody therapy potently enhances the eradication of established tumors by gene-modified T cells. *Clin Cancer Res* (2013) 19:5636–46. doi:10.1158/1078-0432.CCR-13-0458
307. Suarez ER, Chang D-K, Sun J, Sui J, Freeman GJ, Signoretti S, et al. Chimeric antigen receptor T cells secreting anti-PD-L1 antibodies more effectively regress renal cell carcinoma in a humanized mouse model. *Oncotarget* (2016) 7:34341–55. doi:10.18632/oncotarget.9114
308. Li S, Siriwon N, Zhang X, Yang S, Jin T, He F, et al. Enhanced cancer immunotherapy by chimeric antigen receptor-modified T cells engineered to secrete checkpoint inhibitors. *Clin Cancer Res* (2017) 23:6982–92. doi:10.1158/1078-0432.CCR-17-0867
309. Hall ML, Liu H, Malafa M, Centeno B, Hodul PJ, Pimiento J, et al. Expansion of tumor-infiltrating lymphocytes (TIL) from human pancreatic tumors. *J Immunother Cancer* (2016) 4:61. doi:10.1186/s40425-016-0164-7
310. Rosenberg SA, Yang JC, Sherry RM, Kammula US, Hughes MS, Phan GQ, et al. Durable complete responses in heavily pretreated patients with metastatic melanoma using T-cell transfer immunotherapy. *Clin Cancer Res* (2011) 17:4550–7. doi:10.1158/1078-0432.CCR-11-0116
311. Rusakiewicz S, Semeraro M, Sarabi M, Desbois M, Locher C, Mendez R, et al. Immune infiltrates are prognostic factors in localized gastrointestinal stromal tumors. *Cancer Res* (2013) 73:3499–510. doi:10.1158/0008-5472.CAN-13-0371
312. Fukunaga A, Miyamoto M, Cho Y, Murakami S, Kawarada Y, Oshikiri T, et al. CD8+ tumor-infiltrating lymphocytes together with CD4+ tumor-infiltrating lymphocytes and dendritic cells improve the prognosis of patients with pancreatic adenocarcinoma. *Pancreas* (2004) 28:e26–31. doi:10.1097/00006676-200401000-00023
313. Sideras K, Braat H, Kwekkeboom J, van Eijck CH, Peppelenbosch MP, Sleijfer S, et al. Role of the immune system in pancreatic cancer progression and immune modulating treatment strategies. *Cancer Treat Rev* (2014) 40:513–22. doi:10.1016/j.ctrv.2013.11.005
314. Poschke I, Faryna M, Bergmann F, Flossdorf M, Lauenstein C, Hermes J, et al. Identification of a tumor-reactive T-cell repertoire in the immune infiltrate of patients with resectable pancreatic ductal adenocarcinoma. *Oncoimmunology* (2016) 5:e1240859. doi:10.1080/2162402X.2016.1240859
315. Mullinax JE, Hall M, Prabhakaran S, Weber J, Khushalani N, Eroglu Z, et al. Combination of ipilimumab and adoptive cell therapy with tumor-infiltrating lymphocytes for patients with metastatic melanoma. *Front Oncol* (2018) 8:44. doi:10.3389/fonc.2018.00044

14

Circulating T Cell Subpopulations Correlate with Immune Responses at the Tumor Site and Clinical Response to PD1 Inhibition in Non-Small Cell Lung Cancer

Nataly Manjarrez-Orduño[1], Laurence C. Menard[1], Selena Kansal[1], Paul Fischer[1], Bijal Kakrecha[1], Can Jiang[1], Mark Cunningham[1], Danielle Greenawalt[1], Vishal Patel[1], Minghui Yang[1], Ryan Golhar[1], Julie A. Carman[1], Sergey Lezhnin[2], Hongyue Dai[2], Paul S. Kayne[1], Suzanne J. Suchard[1], Steven H. Bernstein[1†] and Steven G. Nadler[1]*

[1] *Bristol-Myers Squibb, Princeton, NJ, United States,* [2] *M2GEN, Tampa, FL, United States*

Edited by:
Amedeo Amedei,
Università degli Studi di Firenze, Italy

Reviewed by:
Haidong Dong,
Mayo Clinic College of Medicine & Science, United States
Rodabe N. Amaria,
University of Texas MD Anderson Cancer Center, United States
Kawaljit Kaur,
University of California, Los Angeles, United States

***Correspondence:**
Nataly Manjarrez-Orduño
nataly.manjarrezorduno@bms.com

†Present address:
Steven H. Bernstein,
Turnstone Biologics, Ottawa, ON, United States

Agents targeting the PD1–PDL1 axis have transformed cancer therapy. Factors that influence clinical response to PD1–PDL1 inhibitors include tumor mutational burden, immune infiltration of the tumor, and local PDL1 expression. To identify peripheral correlates of the anti-tumor immune response in the absence of checkpoint blockade, we performed a retrospective study of circulating T cell subpopulations and matched tumor gene expression in melanoma and non-small cell lung cancer (NSCLC) patients. Notably, both melanoma and NSCLC patients whose tumors exhibited increased inflammatory gene transcripts presented high $CD4^+$ and $CD8^+$ central memory T cell (CM) to effector T cell (Eff) ratios in blood. Consequently, we evaluated CM/Eff T cell ratios in a second cohort of NSCLC. The data showed that high CM/Eff T cell ratios correlated with increased tumor PDL1 expression. Furthermore, of the 22 patients within this NSCLC cohort who received nivolumab, those with high CM/Eff T cell ratios, had longer progression-free survival (PFS) (median survival: 91 vs. 215 days). These findings show that by providing a window into the state of the immune system, peripheral T cell subpopulations inform about the state of the anti-tumor immune response and identify potential blood biomarkers of clinical response to checkpoint inhibitors in melanoma and NSCLC.

Keywords: T cells subpopulations, melanoma, lung cancer, checkpoint blockade, PD1 and PDL1

INTRODUCTION

Since their initial approval for the treatment of melanoma in 2014, anti-PD1 agents have transformed cancer therapy, more than doubling median overall survival rates for melanoma (1) and non-small cell lung cancer (NSCLC) (2). It is clear that not every patient or cancer type benefits from an anti-PD1 agent. As the PD1/PDL1 regulatory pathway inhibits the effector activity of T cells, the efficacy of an anti-PD1 agent depends not only on the presence of a counter-ligand to inhibit but also more importantly, on the availability of tumor-specific T cells whose activity can be unleashed by the therapeutic agent (3).

The quest to identify cancer patients who will benefit from therapy includes several companion and complementary diagnostic assays performed on tumor biopsies. These assays aim to identify PDL1 expression in the tumor and tumor microenvironment (4), and tumor mutation burden

(TMB) as a surrogate measure of neoantigen availability (5). In recent findings, the presence of an active immune infiltrate, evaluated through the expression of transcripts associated with $CD8^+$ T cell function, correlates highly with a positive clinical outcome toward anti-PD1 agents (6).

The determination of a patient's probability of response to anti-PD1/PDL1 agents is critical to inform a course of treatment and requires the identification of readily assessable biomarkers. While tissue biopsies provide a window into the immune response unfolding within the tumor microenvironment, tumor heterogeneity and the presence of multiple tumor sites can lead to mischaracterization of the magnitude of the anti-tumor immune response (7). In addition, the extent of this response depends on the state of the host's immune system. Factors such as genetic background, age, gender, and therapies such as chemotherapy and radiotherapy affect the immune system (8). This heterogeneity creates a need to improve the evaluation of the status of the immune system in cancer patients and its associated clinical outcomes. The dynamic nature of tumor evolution in response to therapy means that long-lasting clinical responses require an immune system fit to adapt to this changing environment (9).

An effective immune response toward a tumor requires neoantigen availability (5) and presentation to T cells, and subsequently the entry of antigen-exposed, activated T cells to the tumor. The tumor, in turn, can downregulate the immune response by expressing PDL1, which activates a regulatory mechanism in the T cell through its interaction with PD1 (3).

To determine if blood T cell subpopulations reflect the immune response against the tumor, we performed a cross-sectional, retrospective analysis of peripheral T cells and matched tumor gene expression in melanoma and NSCLC samples collected before checkpoint inhibitors became part of the standard of care. We observed a correlation between the degree of expression of inflammatory transcripts in the tumor and the percentages of circulating central memory (CM) and effector (Eff) $CD4^+$ and $CD8^+$ T cells, expressed as independent $CD4^+$ and $CD8^+$ CM/Eff T cell ratios. High CM/Eff T cell ratios correlate with inflamed tumors. Given that tumor inflammation correlates with good clinical response to checkpoint inhibitors, we tested whether high CM/Eff T cell ratios correlate with clinical outcome in a cohort of nivolumab-treated NSCLC patients. In this cohort, those patients with high CM/Eff T cell ratios experienced more prolonged progression-free survival (PFS). Given that melanoma and NSCLC patients with inflamed tumors, as well as NSCLC patients with longer PFS have high CM/Eff T cell ratios, we propose that measurement of these ratios in an easily accessible peripheral blood sample is a convenient biomarker of the state of the T cell arm of the immune system. These findings represent progress in the characterization of peripheral immunity, immune state, and its relationship to the inflammatory status of the tumor.

MATERIALS AND METHODS

Tissues and PBMC

Banked PBMC and matched flash frozen tumor samples from melanoma and NSCLC patients were obtained in collaboration with M2GEN and Moffitt Cancer Center (Tampa, FL, USA) and consented through their Total Cancer Care protocol. Control PBMC were obtained from the Bristol-Myers Squibb employee volunteer blood donation program (**Table 1**).

For the second NSCLC cohort, we obtained blood samples from 57 patients with NSCLC from a commercial vendor (MT group, CA, USA). A subset of these samples ($n = 22$) are from patients before receiving nivolumab as part of their clinical care. A second blood sample and clinical evaluation was obtained between 8 and 12 weeks after the start of the treatment. Control blood samples were obtained from the BMS employee volunteer blood program and processed simultaneously.

Flow Cytometry

PBMC were stained for viability with Near Infrared dye (Molecular Probes), blocked and incubated in an antibody mix containing anti-CD127-AF488 (Clone A0195D5), anti-PD1-PE (Clone EH12), anti-CD8-APC-R700 (RPA-T8), anti-CD28-BV650 (CD28.2), anti-CCR7-BV421 (GO43H7), anti-CD25-PECy7 (M-A251), anti-PD-1-PE (EH12), anti-CD45RA-BUV395 (HI100) anti-CD4-BUV495 (SK3), and anti-CD3 BUV737 (SK7).

Whole blood samples were collected and shipped overnight. Whole blood was then stained for viability with Near Infrared dye (Molecular Probes) followed by wash and surface staining with an antibody mix containing: anti-CD45-BV480 (Clone HI30), anti-CD4-AF700 (SK3), anti-CD8-BUV395 (RPA-T8), anti-CD3-BUV496 (UCHT1), anti-CCR7-BV711 (GO43H7), anti-PD-1-APC (MIH4), and anti-CD45RO-BV421 (UCHL1). All samples were read on a BD Fortessa instrument and analyzed with FlowJo. Spanning Tree Progression of Density Normalized Events (SPADE) analysis (10) were implemented on Cytobank (www.cytobank.org). Independent clustering of either $CD4^+$ or $CD8^+$ T cells used CD45RA, CCR7, and CD28. Both the circles and color scale denote the number of cells in the cluster.

Gene Expression and Inflammatory Signature

Total RNA was isolated from frozen tumor using AllPrep DNA/RNA/miRNA kit (Qiagen, Valencia, CA, USA) following manufacturer's recommended protocols. After assessing RNA quality, sequencing libraries were made using the TruSeq Stranded mRNA HT kit (Illumina, San Diego, CA, USA). Libraries were run on an illumina HiSeq 2500 at EA Genomics Services. Paired end FASTQ files were stored in AWS S3, and all analysis took place on AWS EC2 c3.8× large instances created by StarCluster (11).

TABLE 1 | Patient characteristics and demographics.

Cohort	Patients (*n*)	Mean age (SD), years	Male, *n*	Stage II, *n* (%)	Stage III, *n* (%)	Stage IV, *n* (%)
Control	27	54.9 (8.5)	12			
Melanoma	43	63.7 (15.0)	31	1 (2.3)	17 (39.5)	25 (58.1)
Nonsquamous NSCLC	40	65.7 (11.8)	15	16 (4.00)	12 (30.0)	12 (30.0)

Gene and isoform expression were calculated using RSEM (12) v1.1.13 and the UCSC hg19 genome annotation. An additional step of calculating gene and isoform quantile normalized read counts was performed using a custom Perl script. Inflammation gene expression scores were calculated based on the gene signature described in Spranger et al. (6) by calculating the mean of the log2, centered normalized data. Genes included in the signature include *CD8A*, *CCL2*, *CCL3*, *CCL4*, *CXCL9*, *CXCL10*, *ICOS*, *GZMK*, *IRF1*, *HLA-DMA*, *HLA-DMB*, *HLA-DOA*, and *HLA-DOB*. The scores where then split based on quantiles of the normal distribution as inflamed, intermediate, and non-inflamed.

Statistics and Visualizations

Comparisons of T cell subpopulations were performed using Student's *t*-test. For non-normal distributions, data were log-transformed before *t*-test. All reported *p*-values were corrected for multiple comparisons (**Figures 1A** and **3A**).

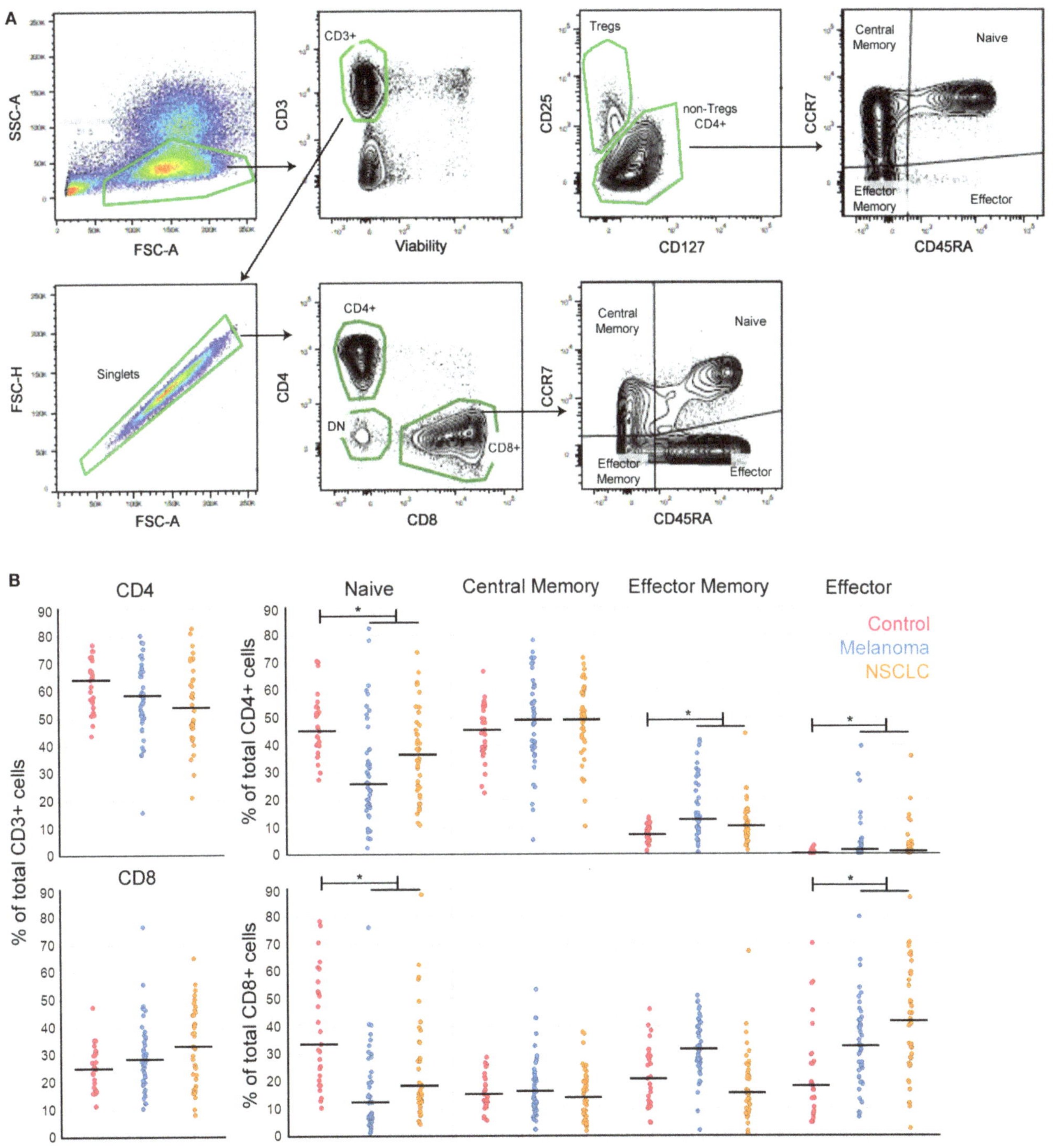

FIGURE 1 | Continued

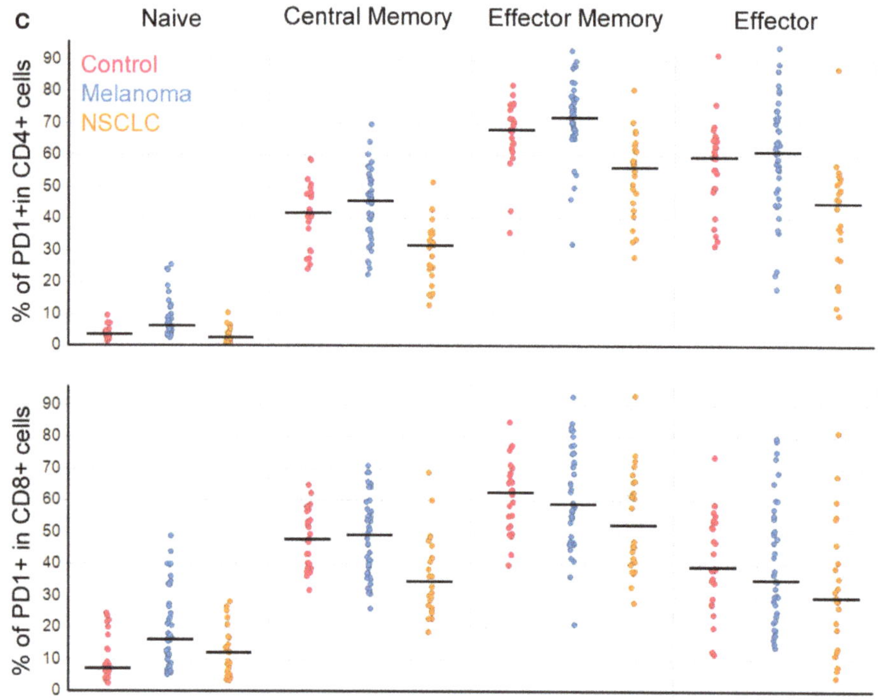

FIGURE 1 | Peripheral T cell subpopulations show evidence of an ongoing immune response in cancer patients. **(A)** Gating strategy to define T cell subpopulations in PBMC. **(B)** CD4+ and CD8+ T cell subpopulations in PBMC from melanoma and NSCLC patients. **(C)** Percentage of PD1+ cells per T cell subpopulation (controls *n* = 27, melanoma *n* = 43, NSCLC *n* = 40; Bonferroni-corrected *p*-values: *<0.001). Line marks the median.

Fischer's exact test was used for the analysis of 2 × 2 contingency tables for CM/Eff T cell ratios by inflammation state and PDL1 tumor proportion score (TPS) (separately).

For PFS analysis of patients undergoing treatment with nivolumab, all patients had at least 90 days of follow-up after first dose. PFS was calculated from the first day of nivolumab infusion until physician-confirmed disease progression (clinical or CT confirmed) by a scientist blind to the patient's biomarkers characteristics. Right-censored data were used to obtain Kaplan–Meier survival estimates and Wilcoxon *p*-values.

All statistical analysis were performed in JMP 13 (SAS, NC).

RESULTS

Circulating T Cells in Melanoma and Nonsquamous NSCLC Patients Show Evidence of Ongoing Immune Responses

Patients with cancer have circulating T cells specific for tumor antigens (13). Consequently, we hypothesized that the circulating T cell pool would reflect the immune responses to melanoma and NSCLC. To evaluate this premise in the absence of checkpoint inhibitors, we performed a cross-sectional, retrospective study of T cell subpopulations in archived PBMC from 43 melanoma and 40 NSCLC patients (all of them nonsquamous NSCLC). All of the patients had available matched tumor tissue, and none of them had prior treatment with checkpoint agents (**Table 1**; **Figure 1**).

Analysis of T cell subpopulations revealed that as a group, PBMC from cancer patients presented a decrease in the percentages of both $CD4^+$ and $CD8^+$ naïve T cells, accompanied by an increase in the percentages of EM and Eff $CD4^+$ and Eff $CD8^+$ T cells compared to control samples (**Figure 1B**). These findings are consistent with the presence of an ongoing immune response in these patients similar to that observed in patients with autoimmunity (14).

Association of Circulating T Cell Profiles With the Local Immune Response in Melanoma and Nonsquamous NSCLC

To assess the T cell differentiation patterns present in these patients, we implemented SPADE on the flow cytometry data (see Materials and Methods). Clustering of either $CD4^+$ or $CD8^+$ T cells using the differentiation markers CD45RA, CCR7, and CD28 showed that in cancer patients, the circulating antigen-experienced T cells present either CM-early Effector Memory or Eff phenotypes (**Figure 2A**), also reflected by the inverse relationships between CM and Eff subpopulations.

Next, we evaluated how the circulating T cell subpopulations reflect the local immune state observed in the tumors. We used matched frozen tumor tissues to evaluate gene expression profiles of immune-associated genes. We defined the tumors as inflamed, intermediate, and non-inflamed based on quantiles of inflammation gene signature scores. Through further analysis of

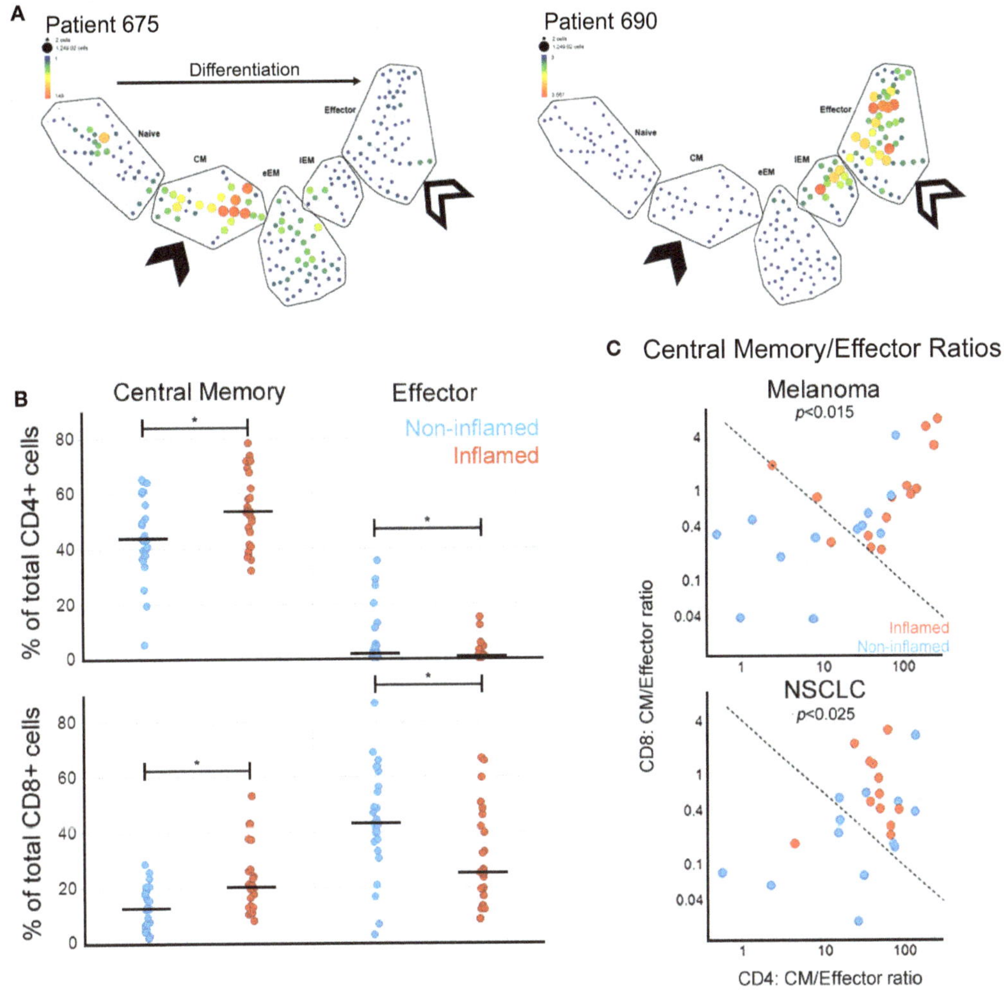

FIGURE 2 | Local immune responses in melanoma and NSCLC correlate with circulating central memory (CM)/effector (Eff) T cell ratios. **(A)** SPADE-generated maturation profiles of CD8⁺ T cells for two melanoma samples showing the divergent patterns of T cell subpopulations. Both have a reduction in naïve CD8⁺ T cells but show an expansion in either CM (solid arrow) or the Eff (open arrow) compartments. eEM, early Effector Memory; EM, Effector Memory. **(B)** Correlation between circulating CM and Eff CD4⁺ and CD8⁺ T cells and tumor inflammation state (*$p < 0.05$). **(C)** Correlation between CM/Eff T cell ratios by inflammation state in melanoma and NSCLC. Fisher's exact test p-value for a 0.05 significance level. Dividing line generated based on the 90th percentile of controls.

the inflamed vs. non-inflamed tumors we observed a correlation between tumor inflammation and the percentages of circulating central memory and effector T cells, which while similar in magnitude, showed a different direction. Surprisingly, the peripheral blood populations which showed a positive correlation with inflamed tumors were not the effector T cell subpopulations, but CM, for both CD4⁺ and CD8⁺ T cells (**Figure 2B**).

Given the inverse relationship between CM and Eff T cells, we calculated CM/Eff ratios for both CD4⁺ and CD8⁺ T cells (**Figure 2C**). Patients with inflamed tumors by gene expression had a tendency toward high CM/Eff ratios (upper right corner). Interestingly, CM/Eff ratios in patients with high inflammation scores are similar to those of the healthy control samples used in this study. Consequently, we used the 90th percentile of control samples to distinguish between low and high CM/Eff ratios (dotted line), observing that the inflamed melanoma and NSCLC tumors have high CM/Eff ratios compared to those with non-inflamed tumors.

Circulating CM/Eff T Cell Ratios in NSCLC Are Associated With Longer PFS in Response to Checkpoint Inhibitors

To evaluate CM/Eff T cell ratios as a tool to evaluate the status of the T cell arm of the immune system, we collected blood from a second cohort of NSCLC patients ($n = 57$). We were able to observe that the reduction of the naïve compartment and the expansion of Eff T cell subpopulations, both in CD4⁺ and CD8⁺ T cells is a reproducible finding (**Figure 3A**).

We then hypothesized that the interferon gamma produced during anti-tumor immune responses would lead to the upregulation of PDL1, as this is an interferon gamma-induced gene

(15). In the 23 patients where PDL1 expression was measured, we observed a bimodal distribution in the percentage of PDL1 tumor proportion score (%TPS) (**Figure 3B**). This pattern made us divide the patients at the antimode (25% TPS) as PDL1$^{neg/low}$ and PDL1^{high}. High CM/Eff T cell ratios, which we had previously found associated with higher inflammatory signature (**Figure 2C**), correlate with high PDL1 expression in the tumor (**Figure 3C**, Fisher's exact $p < 0.025$).

A subset of these NSCLC patients went on to receive nivolumab as part of their clinical care ($n = 22$). Those patients with high CM/Eff T cell ratios at baseline had an extended PFS compared to those patients with low CM/Eff T cell ratios (**Figure 3D**, Wilcoxon test $p < 0.05$, median survival time "*low*" ratio: 91 days, "*high*" ratio 215 days). A second blood sample, obtained around 3 months after the initiation of nivolumab treatment did not show major changes in CM/Eff T cell ratios in patients categorized as

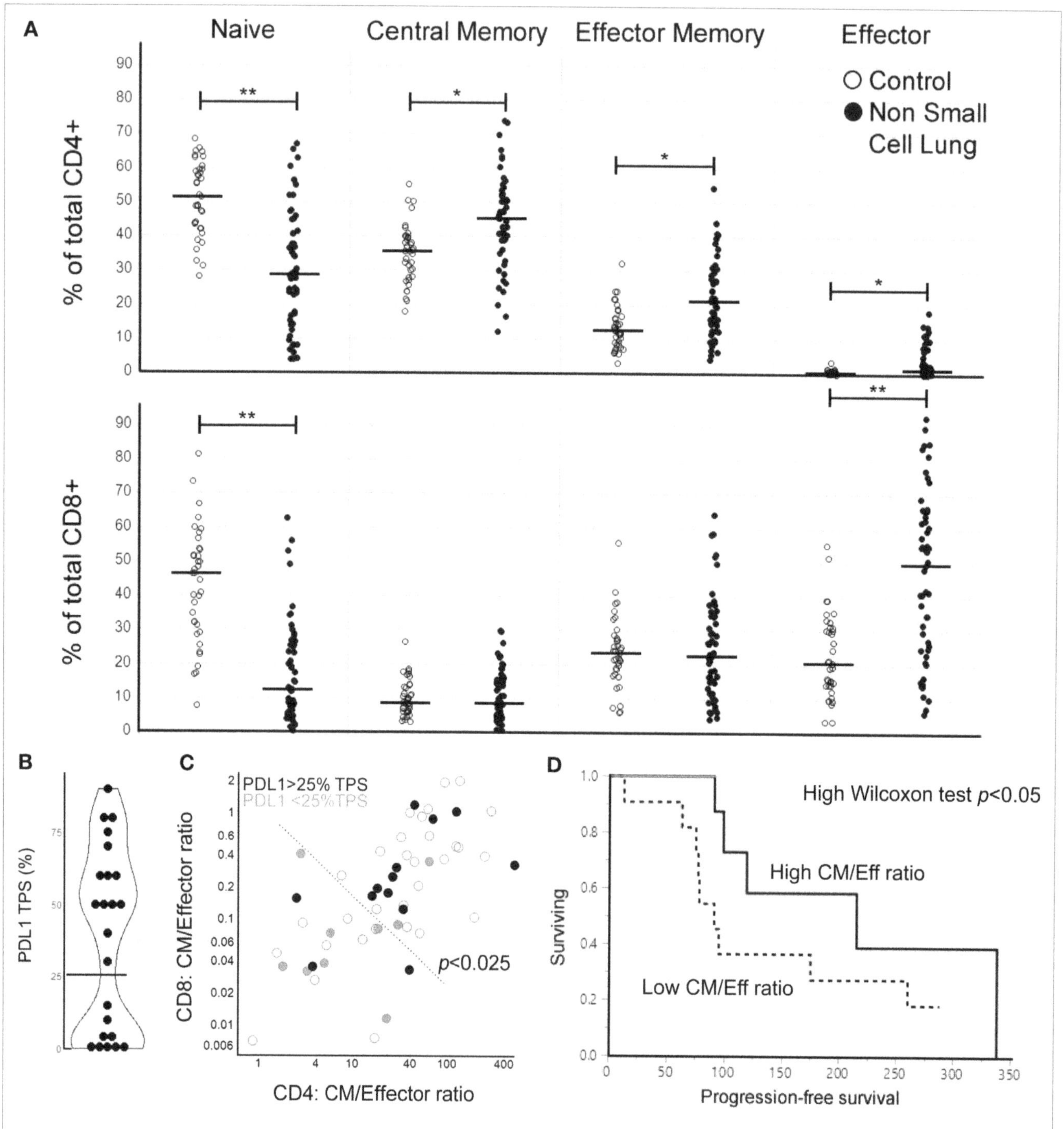

FIGURE 3 | Continued

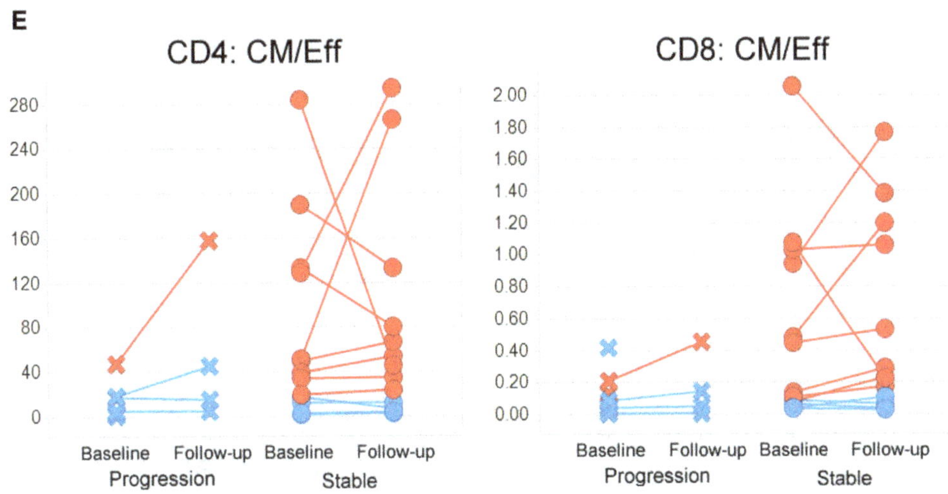

FIGURE 3 | High central memory (CM)/effector (Eff) T cell ratios at baseline are associated with longer progression-free survival (PFS) in response to nivolumab treatment for NSCLC. **(A)** Peripheral T cell profiles in a second cohort of NSCLC and control samples (Bonferroni-corrected *p*-values: *<0.001, **<0.0001, line marks the median for subpopulation). **(B)** Distribution of PDL1 tumor proportion score (TPS) ($n = 23$, the horizontal line marks the cutoff at the antimode: 25% TPS). **(C)** CM/Eff T cell ratios in the NSCLC cohort coded by PDL1 TPS (open circles: PDL1 expression not evaluated). CM/Eff T cell ratios high vs. low division line is drawn using the 90th percentile of the control samples. Fischer's p-value <0.025. **(D)** PFS after nivolumab treatment ($n = 22$) (p-value < 0.05, median survival by CM/Eff ratio: low, 91 days; high 215 days). **(E)** Change in CM/Eff T cell ratios three months after nivolumab-treatment initiation. Patients are classified by physician-reported response to treatment at three months.

"*low*," in contrast to those patients classified as "*high*" (**Figure 3E**). It is important to mention that because of disease progression, only 7 of the 11 "*low*" patients were still in nivolumab treatment, in contrast to 10 of the 11 "high" patients.

DISCUSSION

Here, we report that high circulating CM/Eff T cell ratios associate with tumor inflammation in melanoma and NSCLC, as well as with increased PDL1 expression at the tumor and longer PFS in response to nivolumab treatment in NSCLC. To the best of our knowledge, this is the first time that circulating T cell subpopulations are proposed as predictive biomarkers of response to checkpoint inhibitors in NSCLC.

The association between higher frequency of CM T cells (CD4 and CD8) and an increased tumor inflammatory profile is congruent with reports that CM T cells are the primary repository of the immunogenic experiences of a lifetime (16, 17). The inverse relationship between the frequency of Eff T cells in circulation and the inflammation signature in the tumor was nevertheless surprising and could reflect the presence of terminally differentiated T cells that are unable to reach the tumor. Rather than reflecting the immune response against the tumor, we hypothesize that CM/Eff ratios are a way to evaluate the status of the immune system. In this model, immune state evaluated by CM/Eff ratios would be associated with the capacity of a subject to mount an immune response against the tumor that checkpoint inhibitors can potentiate. This model is consistent with the high sensitivity of this analysis to detect cancer patients who have inflamed tumors (>90%, **Figure 2C**). Nevertheless, its low specificity highlights the multifactorial nature of the anti-tumor response, as other factors, such as TMB, also play a role in the anti-tumor response (18).

These findings provide a window into how the status of the immune system affects the anti-tumor response. Extended clinical responses to checkpoint inhibitors depend on the presence of tumor-specific T cells, and the ability of the immune system to co-evolve with the tumor. Thus, the predominant T cell response shifts as the dominant antigen disappears or mutates (9, 19). Under this model, increased immunological pressure toward the tumor (increased inflammation signature) may drive the upregulation of PDL1 as an immunosuppressive tumor-survival mechanism (20), as observed in the patients with high CM/Eff T cell ratios.

These results align with previous reports that the percentages of CD4 and $CD8^+$ T cell memory correlate with clinical response in melanoma patients treated with ipilimumab (21, 22). Moreover, a recent analysis of four melanoma patients (two with stable disease, one progressive disease, and one partial response) show an increase of central memory $CD4^+$ T cells in the two patients with longer survival times (23). These data are in line with a recent report of peripheral immune cells and its correlation with response to checkpoint inhibitors in melanoma which also found an association between increased $CD8^+$ CM T cells and clinical response (24). However, the highly overlapping ranges of the populations limit their use to identify patients with higher probabilities of responding to checkpoint inhibitors. Our data show how $CD4^+$ and $CD8^+$ CM and effector T cells are a bellwether of responses to checkpoint inhibitors, presumably because all of them contribute to the anti-tumor responses (25, 26). The integration of all these correlates of T cell status into a simple and novel parameter (CM/Eff T cell rations), allows a better separation between responders and non-responders and identification of those NSCLC patients most likely to experience clinical benefit from checkpoint inhibitor therapy.

There is a clear need to elucidate the mechanisms underlying primary resistance and short-lived clinical responses to checkpoint inhibitors. Our data suggest that the state of the T cell arm of the immune system, measured by the relative frequency of CM/Eff T cell ratios can be a contributing mechanism. Even more, improving the number of patients who can benefit from immune therapy requires a comprehensive analysis of the relative contributions of T cell subpopulations to anti-tumor responses. This challenge includes understanding whether a reduced naïve T cell repertoire contributes to functional T cell depletion, and the capacity of CM T cells to replenish the T cell repertoire (26). At a functional level, high levels of the pro-apoptotic molecule Bim in $PD1^{+}CD11a^{+}CD8^{+}$ T cells of melanoma patients associate with shorter survival after anti-PD1 treatment, presumably because Bim may induce apoptosis of anti-tumor-specific T cells (27). Early pharmacodynamics effects of anti-PD1 associated with clinical benefit are the extent of expression of the proliferation marker ki67 in $PD1^{+}$ T cells (28, 29) or of particular memory subtypes (30). An integrated analysis of these T cell subpopulations and their relationship to each other would provide a better understanding of the mechanisms behind primary resistance to anti-PD1 therapy. Along this line, a comprehensive analysis of the TCR repertoire together with gene expression in patients during checkpoint therapy would shed light on this particular question. Although there are still unanswered questions, this method to evaluate the immune system provides an easily accessible circulating biomarker to add to a comprehensive evaluation that already includes TMB and PDL1. Altogether, these assays may enable a better prediction of which patients will respond to checkpoint inhibitors, as well as those who may obtain more benefit from other agents.

ETHICS STATEMENT

This study was carried out in accordance with the recommendations of The Moffitt Cancer Center's Institutional Review Board and the Bristol-Myers Squibb Institutional Biosafety Committee. The protocol was approved by the Moffitt Cancer Center's Institutional Review Board and the Bristol-Myers Squibb Institutional Biosafety Committee. All subjects gave written informed consent in accordance with the Declaration of Helsinki.

AUTHOR CONTRIBUTIONS

NM-O, LM, SK, PF, BK, CJ, JC, PK, PK, SB, SS, and SN planned and designed experiments; SK, PF, BK, CJ, VP, and MY performed experiments; NM-O, LM, SK, PF, BK, SS, MC, DG, RG, SB, and SN analyzed data; DG, PK, SL, and HD performed gene expression analysis; SS and SN provided intellectual input and helped preparing this manuscript; all authors approved the final version.

ACKNOWLEDGMENTS

The authors are thankful to all the research volunteers and the coordination efforts of Henry Kao, Melissa Mitchell, Joanne P. Olivieri, Cheryl Rizzo, and Dawn Stetsko.

REFERENCES

1. Hodi FS, Chesney J, Pavlick AC, Robert C, Grossmann KF, McDermott DF, et al. Combined nivolumab and ipilimumab versus ipilimumab alone in patients with advanced melanoma: 2-year overall survival outcomes in a multicentre, randomised, controlled, phase 2 trial. *Lancet Oncol* (2016) 17(11):1558–68. doi:10.1016/S1470-2045(16)30366-7
2. Hui R, Garon EB, Goldman JW, Leighl NB, Hellmann MD, Patnaik A, et al. Pembrolizumab as first-line therapy for patients with PD-L1-positive advanced non-small cell lung cancer: a phase 1 trial. *Ann Oncol* (2017) 28(4): 874–81. doi:10.1093/annonc/mdx008
3. Boutros C, Tarhini A, Routier E, Lambotte O, Ladurie FL, Carbonnel F, et al. Safety profiles of anti-CTLA-4 and anti-PD-1 antibodies alone and in combination. *Nat Rev Clin Oncol* (2016) 13(8):473–86. doi:10.1038/nrclinonc.2016.58
4. Herbst RS, Soria J-C, Kowanetz M, Fine GD, Hamid O, Gordon MS, et al. Predictive correlates of response to the anti-PD-L1 antibody MPDL3280A in cancer patients. *Nature* (2014) 515(7528):563–7. doi:10.1038/nature14011
5. Snyder A, Makarov V, Merghoub T, Yuan J, Zaretsky JM, Desrichard A, et al. Genetic basis for clinical response to CTLA-4 blockade in melanoma. *N Engl J Med* (2014) 371(23):2189–99. doi:10.1056/NEJMoa1406498
6. Spranger S, Bao R, Gajewski TF. Melanoma-intrinsic beta-catenin signalling prevents anti-tumour immunity. *Nature* (2015) 523(7559):231–5. doi:10.1038/nature14404
7. Callea M, Albiges L, Gupta M, Cheng S-C, Genega EM, Fay AP, et al. Differential expression of PD-L1 between primary and metastatic sites in clear-cell renal cell carcinoma. *Cancer Immunol Res* (2015) 3(10):1158–64. doi:10.1158/2326-6066.CIR-15-0043
8. Chen Daniel S, Mellman I. Oncology meets immunology: the cancer-immunity cycle. *Immunity* (2013) 39(1):1–10. doi:10.1016/j.immuni.2013.07.012
9. Gatenby R, Brown J. The evolution and ecology of resistance in cancer therapy. *Cold Spring Harbor Perspect Med* (2018) 8(3). doi:10.1101/cshperspect.a033415
10. Qiu P, Simonds EF, Bendall SC, Gibbs KD Jr, Bruggner RV, Linderman MD, et al. Extracting a cellular hierarchy from high-dimensional cytometry data with SPADE. *Nat Biotechnol* (2011) 29(10):886–91. doi:10.1038/nbt.1991
11. Riley J. *Star Cluster*. Cambridge, MA: Massachusetts Institute of Technology (2018). Available from: http://star.mit.edu/cluster/ (Accessed: September, 2017).
12. Li B, Dewey CN. RSEM: accurate transcript quantification from RNA-Seq data with or without a reference genome. *BMC Bioinformatics* (2011) 12(1):323. doi:10.1186/1471-2105-12-323
13. Gros A, Parkhurst MR, Tran E, Pasetto A, Robbins PF, Ilyas S, et al. Prospective identification of neoantigen-specific lymphocytes in the peripheral blood of melanoma patients. *Nat Med* (2016) 22(4):433–8. doi:10.1038/nm.4051
14. Manjarrez-Orduño N, Menard LC, Carman JA, Suchard SJ, Casano F, Lee D, et al. A systemic lupus erythematosus endophenotype characterized by increased CD8 cytotoxic signature associates with renal involvement. *ImmunoHorizons* (2017) 1(7):124–32. doi:10.4049/immunohorizons.1700028
15. Garcia-Diaz A, Shin DS, Moreno BH, Saco J, Escuin-Ordinas H, Rodriguez GA, et al. Interferon receptor signaling pathways regulating PD-L1 and PD-L2 expression. *Cell Rep* (2017) 19(6):1189–201. doi:10.1016/j.celrep.2017.04.031
16. Berger C, Jensen MC, Lansdorp PM, Gough M, Elliott C, Riddell SR. Adoptive transfer of effector CD8+ T cells derived from central memory cells establishes persistent T cell memory in primates. *J Clin Invest* (2008) 118(1):294–305. doi:10.1172/JCI32103
17. Wherry EJ, Teichgraber V, Becker TC, Masopust D, Kaech SM, Antia R, et al. Lineage relationship and protective immunity of memory CD8 T cell subsets. *Nat Immunol* (2003) 4(3):225–34. doi:10.1038/ni889

18. Goodman AM, Kato S, Bazhenova L, Patel SP, Frampton GM, Miller V, et al. Tumor mutational burden as an independent predictor of response to immunotherapy in diverse cancers. *Mol Cancer Ther* (2017) 16(11):2598–608. doi:10.1158/1535-7163.MCT-17-0386
19. Purroy N, Wu CJ. Coevolution of leukemia and host immune cells in chronic lymphocytic leukemia. *Cold Spring Harbor Perspect Med* (2017) 7(4). doi:10.1101/cshperspect.a026740
20. Taube JM, Anders RA, Young GD, Xu H, Sharma R, McMiller TL, et al. Colocalization of inflammatory response with B7-h1 expression in human melanocytic lesions supports an adaptive resistance mechanism of immune escape. *Sci Transl Med* (2012) 4(127):127ra37. doi:10.1126/scitranslmed.3003689
21. Tietze JK, Angelova D, Heppt MV, Reinholz M, Murphy WJ, Spannagl M, et al. The proportion of circulating CD45RO(+)CD8(+) memory T cells is correlated with clinical response in melanoma patients treated with ipilimumab. *Eur J Cancer* (2017) 75:268–79. doi:10.1016/j.ejca.2016.12.031
22. Subrahmanyam PB, Dong Z, Gusenleitner D, Giobbie-Hurder A, Severgnini M, Zhou J, et al. Distinct predictive biomarker candidates for response to anti-CTLA-4 and anti-PD-1 immunotherapy in melanoma patients. *J Immunother Cancer* (2018) 6(1):18. doi:10.1186/s40425-018-0328-8
23. Takeuchi Y, Tanemura A, Tada Y, Katayama I, Kumanogoh A, Nishikawa H. Clinical response to PD-1 blockade correlates with a sub-fraction of peripheral central memory CD4+ T cells in patients with malignant melanoma. *Int Immunol* (2018) 30(1):13–22. doi:10.1093/intimm/dxx073
24. Krieg C, Nowicka M, Guglietta S, Schindler S, Hartmann FJ, Weber LM, et al. High-dimensional single-cell analysis predicts response to anti-PD-1 immunotherapy. *Nat Med* (2018) 24(2):144–53. doi:10.1038/nm.4466
25. Ahrends T, Spanjaard A, Pilzecker B, Babała N, Bovens A, Xiao Y, et al. CD4+ T cell help confers a cytotoxic T cell effector program including coinhibitory receptor downregulation and increased tissue invasiveness. *Immunity* (2017) 47(5):848–61.e5. doi:10.1016/j.immuni.2017.10.009
26. Klebanoff CA, Gattinoni L, Torabi-Parizi P, Kerstann K, Cardones AR, Finkelstein SE, et al. Central memory self/tumor-reactive CD8+ T cells confer superior antitumor immunity compared with effector memory T cells. *Proc Natl Acad Sci U S A* (2005) 102(27):9571–6. doi:10.1073/pnas.0503726102
27. Dronca RS, Liu X, Harrington SM, Chen L, Cao S, Kottschade LA, et al. T cell Bim levels reflect responses to anti–PD-1 cancer therapy. *JCI Insight* (2016) 1(6). doi:10.1172/jci.insight.86014
28. Huang AC, Postow MA, Orlowski RJ, Mick R, Bengsch B, Manne S, et al. T-cell invigoration to tumour burden ratio associated with anti-PD-1 response. *Nature* (2017) 545:60. doi:10.1038/nature22079
29. Kamphorst AO, Pillai RN, Yang S, Nasti TH, Akondy RS, Wieland A, et al. Proliferation of PD-1+ CD8 T cells in peripheral blood after PD-1–targeted therapy in lung cancer patients. *Proc Natl Acad Sci U S A* (2017) 114(19): 4993–8. doi:10.1073/pnas.1705327114
30. Yan Y, Cao S, Liu X, Harrington SM, Bindeman WE, Adjei AA, et al. CX3CR1 identifies PD-1 therapy–responsive CD8+ T cells that withstand chemotherapy during cancer chemoimmunotherapy. *JCI Insight* (2018) 3(8):e97828. doi:10.1172/jci.insight.97828

15

Engineered T Cell Therapy for Cancer in the Clinic

*Lijun Zhao and Yu J. Cao**

State Key Laboratory of Chemical Oncogenomics, Key Laboratory of Chemical Genomics, Peking University Shenzhen Graduate School, Shenzhen, China

Edited by:
Weidong Han,
PLA General Hospital, China

Reviewed by:
Pin Wang,
University of Southern California, United States
Zong Sheng Guo,
University of Pittsburgh School of Medicine, United States

***Correspondence:**
Yu J. Cao
joshuacao@pku.edu.cn

T cells play a key role in cell-mediated immunity, and strategies to genetically modify T cells, including chimeric antigen receptor (CAR) T cell therapy and T cell receptor (TCR) T cell therapy, have achieved substantial advances in the treatment of malignant tumors. In clinical trials, CAR-T cell and TCR-T cell therapies have produced encouraging clinical outcomes, thereby demonstrating their therapeutic potential in mitigating tumor development. This article summarizes the current applications of CAR-T cell and TCR-T cell therapies in clinical trials worldwide. It is predicted that genetically engineered T cell immunotherapies will become safe, well-tolerated, and effective therapeutics and bring hope to cancer patients.

Keywords: engineered T cells, CAR-T cell, TCR-T cell, clinic, immunotherapy

INTRODUCTION

The microenvironment of solid tumors contains an abundant fibrous matrix and immunosuppressive cells, which can protect the tumor tissue and resist immune cell attack (1). For example, in the pancreatic cancer microenvironment, the content of hyaluronan (HA) increases significantly, which impedes the infiltration of the immune cells (2). Immune checkpoint receptors on tumor cells or immunosuppressive cells can inhibit T cells, by binding to negative regulatory ligands on T cells (3). In this low-oxygen, acidic tumor microenvironment (TME) that lack essential amino acids, infiltrating T cells experience anergy, exhaustion, senescence, and stemness, making it challenging to achieve the desired tumor killing effect (4). There is still no cure for these diseases, and treatments only control their malignant development in various ways. Traditional methods of cancer treatment include surgical resection, radiotherapy and chemotherapy, small molecule targeted drugs, monoclonal antibodies, and hematopoietic stem cell transplantation. Surgical resection is effective for early-stage patients but not for metastatic cancer cells; radiotherapy and chemotherapy are more common but have poor selectivity and produce substantial damage to normal tissues, and targeted drugs (including small molecules and monoclonal antibodies) have better comprehensive efficacy and fewer toxic side effects but can also encourage gene mutation of tumor cells, drug tolerance, and so on (5). Hematopoietic stem cell transplantation is effective; however, choosing a donor is often difficult, and the graft is prone to rejection after the operation. Cellular immunotherapy is at the forefront of cancer therapy (6).

In recent years, great progress has been made in cancer treatment. Researchers not only have a better understanding of various solid and blood cancers but also have expanded the scope and impact of various immunotherapy strategies (7). Immunotherapy is the fastest and most remarkable developing field. Immunotherapy has generated new therapeutic options for a series of solid tumor and blood cancer patients; as such, the 2018 Nobel Prize in Physiology or Medicine was awarded to James P. Allison and Tasuku Honjo, who discovered how to harness the body's immune system to fight cancer, highlighting the importance of research progress in the field of immunotherapy (8).

Among immunotherapies, the programmed cell death protein 1 (PD-1) and programmed cell death ligand 1 (PD-L1) checkpoint inhibitors have been shown to be the primary treatment for advanced lung cancer (9–11). Immunotherapy combined with antibody therapy targeting PD-1 or PD-L1 (ClinicalTrials.gov number: NCT02366143 and NCT02578680) significantly increased median progression-free survival and 1-year overall survival (9–11). On September 30, 2018, the U.S. Food and Drug Administration (FDA) approved a new anti-PD-1 checkpoint inhibitor (Cemiplimab; Libtayo) for skin squamous cell carcinoma (**Table 1**).

A phase III clinical trial (ClinicalTrials.gov number: NCT02231749) has demonstrated that combined immunotherapy can improve the survival rate of renal cell carcinoma. Compared with the use of the tyrosine kinase inhibitor sunitinib, a monoclonal antibody drug, the combination of nivolumab and ipilimumab in the treatment of melanoma, increased the overall survival rate to 18 months in patients with high-risk renal cell carcinoma (12, 13). A second-stage study (ClinicalTrials.gov number: NCT02320058) showed that the complete response rate and partial response rate were 26 and 30%, respectively, after treatment with nivolumab and ipilimumab and that 82.8% of patients were alive 9 months later (14).

In the past 2 years, the most popular chimeric antigen receptor (CAR) T cell immunotherapy has mainly focused on targeting CD19 in lymphoma. FDA-approved CAR-T cell therapies such as tisagenlecleucel (Kymriah, CTL019) and axicabtagene ciloleucel (Yescarta, KET-C10) (ClinicalTrials.gov number: NCT03123939) have shown long-term benefits (15, 16). Anti-CD19 CAR-T cell therapy is a promising option for patients with relapsed and refractory B cell acute lymphoblastic leukemia (15).

Unlike systemic chemotherapy, targeted drug therapies make use of specific gene mutations in cancer cells, unlike systemic chemotherapy. For example, osimertinib, a new epidermal growth factor receptor inhibitor (ClinicalTrials.gov number: NCT01802632), can delay the progression of lung cancer in response to drug resistance mutations (17). Osimertinib has become the preferred initial treatment for some non-small-cell lung cancer patients with epidermal growth factor receptor mutations (18). A targeted therapy for human epidermal growth factor receptor-2 (HER2)/neu mutation, trastuzumab, was developed to treat breast cancer (19). Abemaciclib (Verzenio) is a novel drug (ClinicalTrials.gov number: NCT02102490, NCT02107703, and NCT02246621) that inhibits the activity of the CDK4/6 (cyclin-dependent kinases 4/6) protein, which

TABLE 1 | The FDA has approved a variety of new immunotherapies.

Trade name	Generic name	Target	Disease	Approved by FDA
Provenge	Sipuleucel-T	PAP	Asymptomatic or minimally symptomatic metastatic castrate resistant (hormone refractory) prostate cancer	2010.4
Yervoy	Ipilimumab	CTLA-4	Adult patients with inoperable or metastatic melanoma	2011.3
			Pediatric patients aged 12 years and older with unresectable or metastatic melanoma	2017.7
Keytruda	Pembrolizumab	PD-1	Advanced or unresectable melanoma	2014.9
			Classic Hodgkin's lymphoma	2017.3
			Recurrent or metastatic cervical cancer	2018.6
Blincyto	Blinatumomab	CD19, CD3	B-cell precursor ALL	2014.1
			MRD positive B cell precursor ALL	2018.3
Opdivo	Nivolumab	PD-1	Advance melanoma	2014.1
			NSCLC	2015.3
			Colorectal cancer	2017.8
Tecentriq	Atezolizumab	PD-L1	NSCLC	2018.1
			First-line treatment for extensive stage small cell lung cancer	2019.3
Bavencio	Avelumab	PD-L1	Metastatic MCC	2017.3
			Locally advanced or metastatic urothelial carcinoma	2017.5
Imfinzi	Durvalumab	PD-L1	Locally advanced or metastatic bladder carcinoma	2017.5
			Stage 3 non-small cell lung cancer that is stable after surgery, chemotherapy, or radiation	2018.2
Kymriah	Tisagenlecleucel	CD19	B-cell precursor ALL	2017.8
Yescarta	Axicabtagene Ciloleucel	CD19	Adults with relapsed or refractory large B-cell lymphoma	2017.1
Opdivo & Yervoy	Nivolumab & Ipilimumab	PD-1, CTLA-4	Intermediate and poor-risk advanced renal cell carcinoma	2018.4
Keytruda & Inlyta	Pembrolizumab & Axitinib	PD-1, VEGFR	Advanced RCC	2019.4

PAP, prostate acid phosphatase; CTLA-4, cytotoxic T-lymphocyte-associated protein 4; VEGFR, vascular endothelial growth factor receptor; ALL, acute lymphoblastic leukemia; MRD, minimal residual lesions; NSCLC, non-small cell lung cancer; MCC, Merkel cell carcinoma; RCC, renal cell carcinoma.

regulates the cell division rate, rather than targeting specific gene mutations (20–22).

ENGINEERED T CELL THERAPY

Early adoptive immunotherapy mainly transfuses autologous or allogeneic tumor-responsive T cells back into the patient's body to attack the patient's tumors. This method has been successful (6, 23, 24). However, this therapy has not been widely used, mainly because of the small number of invasive lymphocytes and the fact that it cannot improve the anti-tumor ability of the body's autoimmune system (6). T cell genetic engineering therapies can overcome the challenges of low survival and migration of T cells and immune escape to a certain extent (25, 26). T cells are extracted from the patient's blood and genetically modified to encode receptors that recognize cancer-specific antigens (**Figure 1**). Additional genes, such as those encoding cytokines, can also be modified to prolong survival and promote T cell penetration into cancer tissue (26). CAR-T cell therapy and T cell receptor (TCR)-T cell therapy, as the latest and most effective immunotherapy technologies, have been widely studied in recent years. Clinical research regarding therapies using genetically engineered T cells has shown remarkable success.

CAR-T CELL THERAPY

CAR-T cell therapy is a novel tumor immunotherapy technique for cancer treatment (17, 27–29). The efficacy of CAR-T cells for the treatment of acute B lymphocytic leukemia has been widely recognized, and several clinical trials using CAR-T cell therapy in the treatment of various types of tumors have been reported (17, 27–29). This approach is also more specific and more customizable because the antigen-binding domain can be changed to target various tumor targets (17, 27–29). Moreover, CAR-T cells can also establish memory in patients with advanced leukemia (30).

A CAR is the core component of CAR-T cells, making T cells MHC unrestricted. This phenomenon enables the modified T cells to recognize more extensive targets than the natural TCR on T cell surface and is not restricted by major histocompatibility complex (MHC) molecules. A CAR is a recombinant receptor with both tumor-antigen-binding and T cell-activating functions (**Figure 2**) (31, 32). The extracellular domain is a single-chain variable antibody domain (scFv), which can recognize specific antigens of tumors (25). The heavy-chain variable region (VH) and light-chain variable region (VL) of antibodies are linked by a small segment of polypeptide. Via the scFv, CAR-T cells can directly recognize and bind to tumor-specific antigens (25, 33). The hinge domain is composed of immunoglobulin superfamily members, such as CD8, CD28, or IgG, which play a role in signal transduction (25). The intracellular signal transduction region is mainly composed of the CD3ζ chain of the TCR (25). In addition to intracellular signaling domains, costimulatory molecules such as CD28 or 4-1BB (CD137) can improve cell proliferation and survival time *in vivo* and enhance the anti-tumor activity of CAR-T cells (25, 34). CAR-T cells directly recognize tumor surface antigens, and are not restricted by MHC class. When CAR-T cells bind to tumor surface antigen, they proliferate and kill tumor cells.

The activation of T cells mediated by first-generation CARs is accomplished through the tyrosine activation motif on the CD3ζ chain (**Figure 2**) or FcRγ (25, 35, 36). The CD3ζ chain can provide signals for T cell activation and target cell lysis, regulation of IL-2 secretion, and anti-tumor activity *in vivo* (36). However, the anti-tumor activity of first-generation CAR-modified T cells is limited *in vivo*, and this decreased T cell proliferation ultimately leads to T cell apoptosis (35, 36). Second-generation CARs incorporate an additional costimulatory signal. Experiments show that this signal amplifies the original "signal 1" derived from the TCR/CD3 complex and increases T cell proliferation and cytokine secretion, promoting the secretion of anti-apoptotic proteins (37). A commonly used costimulatory molecule is CD28 or CD137(4-1BB). To further improve the design of CARs, many research groups have focused on the development of third-generation CARs, which include not only CD3ζ and one costimulatory domain but also an additional costimulatory signal (34). Based on these second or third-generation CARs, fourth-generations CAR-T cells coexpress some key cytokines or costimulatory ligands, such as IL-12, IL-15, and IL-7, or suicide genes, which significantly enhance the expansion activity of T cells. For fifth generation CAR-T cells, it has been proposed to knock out the human leukocyte antigen (HLA) and TCR genes of T cells obtained from healthy donors to avoid host immune rejection or graft-vs.-host disease against transplanted CAR-T cells (3, 18, 38). Because it does not need to be modified according to the patient, this strategy can be used for the treatment of multiple patients (18).

Different researchers have used different targets and costimulatory signals to compare the results of second-generation and third-generation CARs. Some studies have reported that recombinant T cells expressing third-generation CARs have significantly increased anti-tumor activity, survival, and cytokine release abilities (34). It is worth noting that the above differences are conclusions obtained from only ex vivo mice experiments, and there are no *in vivo* comparisons of second-generation and third-generation CARs. The difference between the two generations of CARs may originate not only from the signal transduction domain but also from the extracellular antigen-binding domain (scFv), the transfection method used for the recombinant T cells (Lentivirus vs. Retrovirus), and the transfusion mode of recombinant T cells (intravenous transfusion vs. peritoneal infusion vs. intratumor infusion).

CAR-T Cell Therapy Process

CAR-T cell therapy is a revolutionary targeted immunotherapy (17, 27–29). It necessitates modification of patient T cells outside the body and retransfusion of these cells back into the human body to fight the target cancer cells. The typical CAR-T cell production process is divided into five steps (**Figure 1**) (25). The first step is to isolate T cells from cancer patients. The second step is to modify the T cells with CARs so that the T cells can simultaneously recognize tumor cells and activate

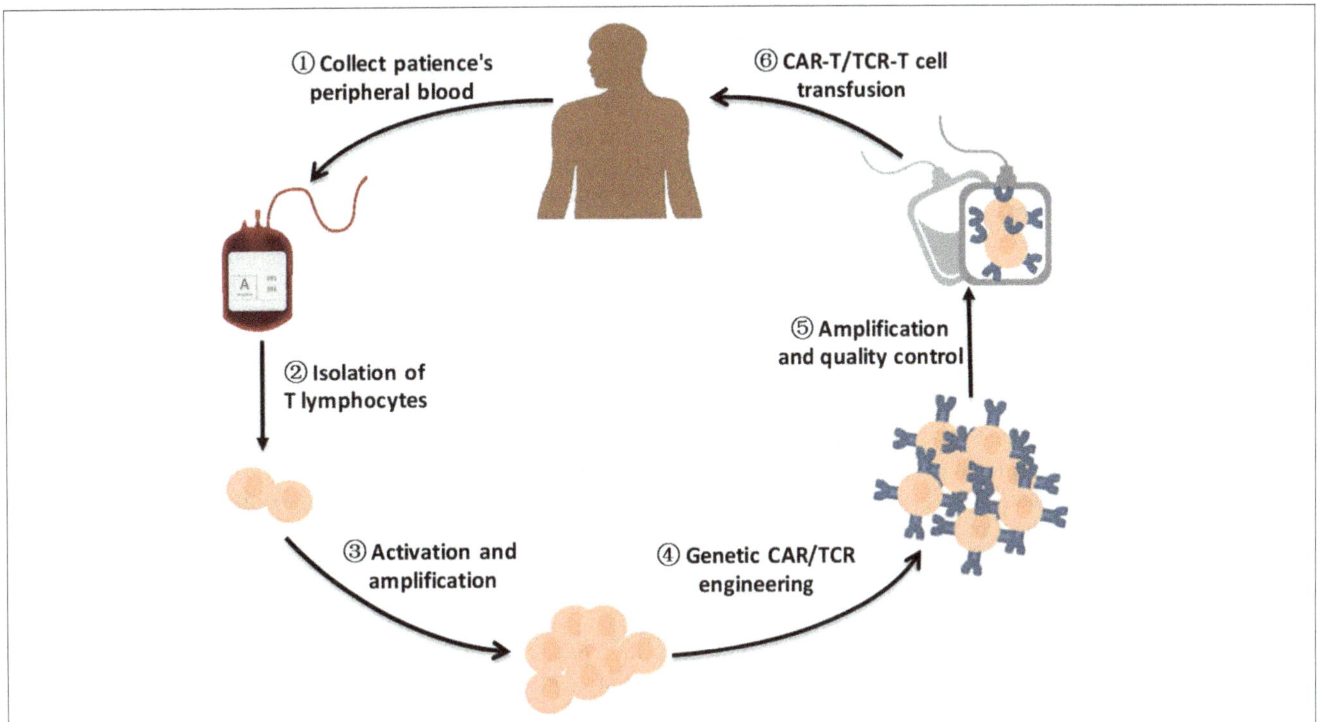

FIGURE 1 | A brief flow chart of engineered-T cell therapy. A sufficient amount of blood is drawn from patients to obtain enough peripheral blood mononeuclear cells (PBMCs) for engineered T cell manufacturing. The T cells are purified from patients PBMCs. After activation and amplification *in vitro*, T cells are modified by viral vector transfection, such as lentivirus transfection or retrovirus transfection, to express specific CARs/TCRs on the T cell surface. Following amplification and quality control, CAR-T cells/TCR-T cells are infused into the patient body to improvo antitumor ability.

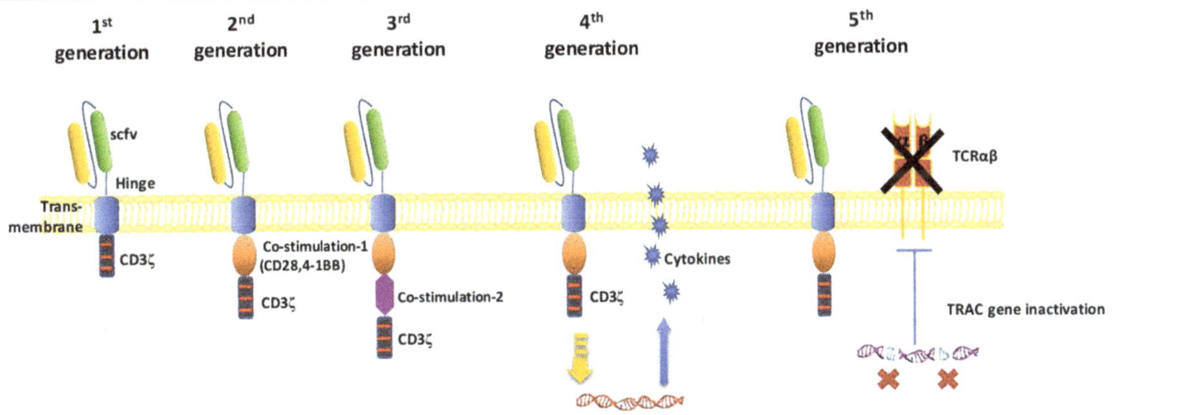

FIGURE 2 | Schematic diagram of the CAR-T cell structure. In the first generation of CARs, there was only one intracellular signal component CD3ζ. The second generation of CAR added one costimulatory molecule on the basis of the first generation. Based on the second generation of CARs, the third generation of CAR added another costimulatory molecule. Fourth-generation of CAR T cells can activate the downstream transcription factor to induce cytokine production after the CAR recognizes the target antigens. The fifth-generation of CARs, based on the second generation, uses gene editing to inactivate the TRAC gene, leading to the removal of the TCR alpha and beta chains.

T cells, creating CAR-T cells (6, 25). In the third step, CAR-T cells are cultured ex vivo and stimulated by cytokines to produce a large number of CAR-T cells (25). The fourth step is to transfuse the expanded CAR-T cells back into the patient at an appropriate dose (25). Finally, patients need to be closely monitored, especially to monitor and control severe physical reactions in the following few days (6). The whole process lasts approximately 3 weeks, and the preparation of CAR-T cells requires approximately 2 weeks, making the cell preparation step the most time-consuming step (25).

CAR-T cells are expanded ex vivo and frozen for future administration. Patients are given preconditioning chemotherapy (6). Following tumor burden reassessment, CAR-T cells are infused. When the antigen-binding domain recognizes malignant antigen, it stimulates the downstream activation signal and produces specific killing effects. The use of such CAR-T cell therapies in B cell lymphoma/leukemia in the clinic has achieved complete remission in a number of relapsed and refractory advanced patients (15).

Recruited Patients

To lay a foundation for the application of CAR-T cell therapy, clinical trials recruit suitable patients, and they must satisfy certain conditions. Patients aged older than 75 years or younger than 1 year will be detrimental to clinical trials, and the survival time should be at least 3 or 6 months. The recruited patients are usually relapsed or refractory, or they have experienced chemotherapy failure, bone marrow transplantation failure, or autologous, allogeneic hemopoietic stem cell transplantation failure, or have been unable to find an effective treatment. Although patients are widely recruited, some patients are excluded, such as those who have clinically significant cardiovascular disease or those who are pregnant or lactating. Patients who have participated in any other clinical trials in the past 30 days are excluded. Additionally, patients with any type of primary immunodeficiency are excluded from the clinical studies. Other symptoms are not applicable for CAR-T cell therapy because they may increase patient risk or interfere with clinical test results. The main goal of trials is to evaluate the safety, effectiveness, and feasibility of CAR-T cell immunotherapy.

Pretreatment of the Patient

In addition to killing cancer cells directly, the use of some chemotherapeutic drugs, such as fludarabine (FA) and cyclophosphamide (CTX), as pretreatment regimens before immunotherapy, may produce synergistic immunobiological effects, thereby enhancing the effects of anti-tumor immunotherapy (39). Pretreatment chemotherapy can remove existing lymphocytes in lymphoid tissue or bone marrow tissue, establish implantation space for newly implanted antitumor immune cells, and induce the production of bone marrow cytokines, thus promoting the recovery and proliferation of immune cells (28, 40). CTX is the most commonly used drug for pretreatment in cancer immunotherapy. In addition, other commonly used pretreatment chemotherapy drugs include FA, gemcitabine (GEM), lenalidomide, and docetaxel (DTX). For example, when FRα (Folate receptor α) CAR-T cells were used to treat patients with end-stage ovarian cancer, the pretreatment regimen was CTX 300 mg/m^2/day for three consecutive days and FA 30 mg/m^2/day for three consecutive days (41). For melanoma patients, Deniger et al. of the National Cancer Institute (NCI) formulated a routine regimen of 60 mg/kg/day CTX for 2 days and 25 mg/m^2/day FA for 5 days (42). However, the dosage, mode, and sequence of pretreatment still need further optimization and verification by more clinical trials.

Injection Dose

In clinical treatment, CAR-T cells are injected at a wide range of doses, sometimes with dose-increasing regimens. Some reports suggest that there is a correlation between the dose of CAR-T cells injected and the incidence and severity of the cytokine release storms (CRS) (43). The total number of CAR-T cells ranges from 1×10^5/kg to 1×10^{10}/kg CAR-T cells or more. Sometimes, to investigate the patient's tolerance, the total number of cells is injected over three courses, 10% on the first day, 30% on the second day, and 60% on the third day (44). One patient with chronic lymphoblastic leukemia who was treated with CAR-T cell therapy has been cancer free for 5 years (45). More importantly, that study found that the minimum cell number required for CAR-T cell therapy to exert its anticancer effects was only one cell (45).

Success and Advantages of CAR-T Cell Therapy

Emily Whitehead was the first pediatric ALL patient to receive CAR-T cell treatment. The University of Pennsylvania CAR-T cell clinical trial completely cured Emily's leukemia, and Emily has become a spokesperson for CAR-T cells. Here, we present three recent successful cases to illustrate the potential of CAR-T cell immunotherapy in cancer treatment. In a clinical trial for children and young adults with cancer, none of whom had responses to standard therapy, a CAR-T cell therapy called tisagenlecleucel (Kymriah) was successful in 52 of 63 patients. In the study, three out of every four patients did not relapse after 6 months (46). According to the results of this study, FDA approved tisagenlecleucel in August 2017 for the treatment of relapsed or refractory B cell precursor ALL in patients ≤25 years old.

Another study used CAR-T cell therapy to treat refractory large B-cell lymphoma. The CAR-T cell therapy used in this study is called axicabtagene ciloleucel (Yescarta) (28). Immunotherapy slowed or stopped the growth of cancer in 82% of patients, and more than half (54%) of the cancers disappeared completely (28). Nearly 15.4 months later, approximately 40% of patients still showed no signs of cancer. In October 2017, the FDA approved axicabtagene ciloleucel for the treatment of adults with relapsed or refractory large B-cell lymphoma, including diffuse large B-cell lymphoma (DLBCL), after two or more lines of systemic therapy.

Multiple myeloma is an incurable disease, and only approximately half of patients are still alive 5 years after diagnosis. Early clinical trials presented at the 2017 American Society of Clinical Oncology (ASCO) annual meeting showed that CAR-T cell therapy using B cell maturation antigen (BCMA) as a biomarker could prevent the development of multiple myeloma. The study included 35 patients with multiple myeloma who relapsed after treatment or were resistant to treatment. Of these 35 patients, 74% experienced a complete response of multiple myeloma after receiving BCMA CAR-T cells (47).

CAR-T cells are not restricted by MHC molecules. They specifically recognize antigens and kill tumor cells more effectively. Tumor infiltrating lymphocytes (TILs) and TCRs can recognize only the antigens presented by specific MHC molecules and tumors may escape immune surveillance due to downregulation or mutation of MHC molecules in tumor cells, resulting in clinical limitations (47).

Failures and Challenges of CAR-T Cell Therapy

The first third-generation CAR-T cell clinical studies included HER2-targeted CAR-T cell therapy and indications for metastatic melanoma. The NCI chose to make use of an scFv targeting HER2 in a CAR-T cell for therapy for HER2+ melanoma (48). The first patient received a high concentration of CAR-T cells, with a total dose of 1×10^{11} cells. After treatment, the patient experienced extreme pain within a few minutes and soon fell into a coma. Doctors administered a high-dose hormone intervention, and the patient died 5 days later. Subsequently, CAR-T cells were found throughout the patient's body, and the lungs were the most seriously infiltrated organ. Further analysis may find that HER2 expression in pulmonary epithelial cells was the main cause of this fatal lung T cell infiltration (48).

Some types of immunotherapy can attack cancer or slow its spread to other parts of the body. Others make it easier for the immune system to destroy cancer cells, but immunotherapy sometimes leads to the immune system attacking healthy cells, resulting in side effects. Different types of immunotherapy can cause different side effects. The occurrence of many side effects depends on the type of treatment, the type and location of the cancer, and the patient's overall health. Skin redness, blistering, and dryness are common reactions associated with immunotherapy. Fatigue, fever, chills, weakness, nausea, vomiting, dizziness, body pain, and hypertension or hypotension are also side effects of immunotherapy. This new approach to cancer treatment is powerful, and serious risks need to be considered before starting treatment. In particular, there are always possible side effects of treatment, including CRS and neurological problems.

CRS

CRS is caused by the production of a large number of inflammatory molecules by CAR-T cells. CRS can cause long-term fever, hypotension, dyspnea, and organ problems. Severe CRS can be a life-threatening problem, requiring intensive medical care, including the use of ventilators, drugs to increase blood pressure, and antiepilepsy drugs. The FDA approved intravenous injection of tocilizumab (Actemra), an IL-6 receptor inhibitor, for the treatment of CAR-T cell-induced severe or life-threatening CRS in patients 2 years of age and older. CRS is the most frequently mentioned adverse reaction in CAR-T cell treatment. After infusion of CAR-T cells, a systemic inflammatory reaction caused by a rapid rise in cytokines such as IL-1 and IL-6 was observed in a mouse model (49, 50). CRS usually occurs within 2 days after CAR-T cell infusion, and the worst part of the reaction occurs within 1–2 weeks after CAR-T cell infusion (51). It is worth noting that in the pathophysiological process of CRS, not only activated CAR-T cells but also monocytes, macrophages, and dendritic cells participate in the synthesis and release of cytokines, which leads to the corresponding clinical symptoms (50). Studies have shown that patients with massive lesions, patients with a high tumor burden, patients with complications, and patients with CRS after 3 days of CAR-T cell infusion are prone to severe CRS (50). Therefore, treatment evaluation before CAR-T cell infusion is of great significance for CRS control and prognostication. For tocilizumab, a dosage of 4 to 8 mg/kg should be infused intravenously (51). It should be noted that tocilizumab cannot effectively improve the neurotoxicity of CRS due to the blood–brain barrier (50). Methylprednisolone has been used in patients with severe CRS who did not receive tocilizumab.

Neurotoxicity

The overall incidence of neurotoxicity is 40% (52). The most common symptoms include decreased consciousness, confusion, seizures, and brain edema. Neurotoxicity can occur alone or simultaneously with CRS (31). Mild clinical signs can spontaneously regress within a few days. Severe symptoms may require treatment with single agents or combination with dexamethasone (10 mg intravenously or orally) (51, 53). Strategies to reduce CRS and neurotoxicity fall into two categories: preventive strategies aimed at reducing the occurrence of severe toxicity and remedial strategies aimed at minimizing toxicity once lethal toxicity occurs. Preventive strategies include reducing the burden of cancer by chemotherapy and reducing the dose of CAR-T cells in patients with high cancer burden before receiving CAR-T cell infusion (52). Without affecting the treatment of CAR-T cells, early intervention with tocilizumab and dexamethasone seems to reduce the incidence of severe CRS (51).

On-Target–Off-Tumor Toxicity

The ideal target antigen is tumor-specific and expressed only on the surface of cancer cells. Unfortunately, most of the antigens expressed in tumors are not specific to tumors; For example, most CARs target tumor-associated antigens, but this often leads to the possibility of mistargeting. Additionally, attention should be paid to the selection of secretory antigens to avoid the possibility of mistargeting by CAR-T cells. As long as the target is not 100% tumor-specific, there will be an off-target effect, which is the main source of CAR-T cell side effects. This means that these targets are expressed not only in cancer tissues but also in normal tissue (52). Specific antigens expressed only on the surface of cancer cells can be selected, or multiple antigen complex CAR structures can be designed to identify antigens. The best example of remedial strategies is the addition of suicide or elimination genes to CAR-T cells, which can be activated to selectively deplete CAR-T cells in the event of severe toxicity (54). Thus, "on-target–off-tumor" toxicity can be efficiently avoided.

Exhaustion of CAR-T Cells

Because of T cell exhaustion, T cells entering solid tumors may stop working. Coexpression of some cytokines, such as IL-15, promotes T cell proliferation and persistence in a mouse model (55). The Nr4a (nuclear receptor transcription factors) family of transcription factors plays a prominent role in regulating genes related to T cell exhaustion (56). Scientists have used melanoma mouse models to demonstrate that treatment with

CAR-T cells lacking these Nr4a transcription factors can reduce tumor sizes and improve survival in mice (57). These results suggest that the nuclear factor of activated T cells (NFAT) and Nr4a proteins are helpful in resisting T cell exhaustion in cancer and are "exhaustion markers" of T cells in a mouse model (57). However, the results of this experiment cannot be used in clinical practice because the consequences of editing multiple genes in human cells are unknown. Understanding the roles of Nr4a transcription factors provides cancer researchers with new targets for designing better therapies. The molecular design of CARs also has a significant effect on the proliferation and persistence of CAR-T cells. A CAR carrying the inducible costimulatory molecule (ICOS) costimulatory domain (ICOS-CAR) shows an improved ability to maintain the persistence of CD4+ T cells in a mouse model costimulatory (58). By injecting a mixture of CD4+ and CD8+ T cells expressing different CARs into mice at a ratio of 1:1, researchers found that CD4+ T cells expressing an ICOS-CAR not only increased their own persistence but also increased the persistence of the CD8+ T cells (58). The anticancer effect of this cell combination was also strongest in mice with non-small-cell lung cancer. When ICOS and 4-1BB costimulatory domains were added to the intracellular costimulatory domain of a third-generation CAR-T cell (ICOSBBz-CAR-T cell), and both CD4+ and CD8+ T cells expressed this ICOSBBz-CAR, the resulting T cells not only had better persistence but also had a better anticancer effect than a combination of CD4+ T cells expressing ICOS-CAR and CD8+ T cells expressing BBz-CAR (58). The expression level of ICOSBBz-CAR on the T cell surface was lower than that of ICOS-CAR or BBz-CAR. A possible reason for this finding is that the expression of the CAR was too high, which can cause T cells to be continuously activated, leading to their early depletion.

Tumor Escape

Although the patient response rate to CAR-T cells is very high, many patients treated with CAR-T cells will have disease recurrence. There are many reasons for this recurrence, such as antigen downregulation on tumor cells or low antigen levels. The mechanism of cancer evasion is closely related to the TME. The TME can influence the heterogeneity of tumors and play a key role in the subsequent development and metastasis of tumors (59). Mechanisms of immune escape include alterated of the expression of G1 regulatory proteins; production of inhibitors such as IL-10, transforming growth factor-beta (TGF-β), and indoleamine 2,3-dioxygenase (IDO); overexpression of immunosuppressive receptors such as PD-L1; and recruitment of Tregs (60). Therefore, combination therapies with immunological checkpoint inhibitors (such as a PD-1/PD-L1 antibody) should be adopted.

Treatment for Solid Tumors

The unprecedented success of CAR-T cell therapy in the treatment of hematological tumors has inspired people to extend this technology to solid tumors. Increasing numbers of clinical trials using CAR-T cell therapy for solid tumors have been carried out. However, the results of clinical trials are often unsatisfactory. The therapeutic effect of CAR-T cell therapy for solid tumors is greatly inferior to that of CAR-T therapy for hematological tumors and is often accompanied by toxicities (61). Hematological tumor cells are dispersed, and solid tumors usually form solid masses in certain organs early in the cancer process, which not only causes many obstacles for the recruitment of immune cells to the affected area but also results in the accumulation of many kinds of immunosuppressive cells and molecules (60). The antigens of hematological tumors are often specific and not expressed in other normal tissues, while the antigens of solid tumors are generally expressed in small amounts in other locations, such as the heart, lung, and liver, leading to mistargeted effects after treatment.

Encephaledema

In May 2016, one patient treated with JCAR015 died of cerebral edema, and two died of the same symptoms in July, so the experiment was suspended (61). Juno's researchers explained that the pretreatment scheme used CTX and FA and reported that FA would be eliminated from the pretreatment regimen in the subsequent attempt. Two more patients died of brain edema after the trial was restarted, and the trial was suspended again (61). In fact, the problem was not FA. It may have occurred because the costimulatory signal of CD28 is too strong, resulting in immune side effects and leading to brain edema. While 4-1BB is not as strong as CD28 as a costimulatory molecule, it provides late-acting signals to regulate T cell poliferation and survival (62). In the late stage of the immune response, T cells express inhibitory receptors such as CTLA-4, while CD28 expression is downregulated, leading to T cell loss of the second activation signal of the CD28-B7 pathway. However, 4-1BB is still expressed in the late stage of the T cell response, indicating that it persists longer.

The Cost of CAR-T Cell Therapy

The two available CAR-T cell therapies are currently very expensive. Novartis's CAR-T cell therapy, Kymriah, costs an average of ~$510,963, and Yescarta costs an average of approximately $402,647 (63, 64). If the patient does not experience an effect after CAR-T treatment for 1 month, the medical expenses can be waived. It takes approximately half a month to 1 month to make a specific CAR-T cell product for use in patients. Many enterprises are now studying more efficient and stable production strategies for CAR-T cells. For example, ThermoGenesis, a U.S. automation equipment company, has developed a platform called CAR-TXpress™ that specializes in producing CAR-T cells. The production cost of CAR-T cells can be greatly reduced. CAR-T cells are produced faster, and the quality of the cells is better. Thus, companies not only can use higher-quality cells for clinical research, allowing faster development of CAR-T cell therapies for more diseases, but also can achieve faster commercialization, making CAR-T cell therapies more readily available on the market (65). Because the cost of CAR-T cell immunotherapy is very high, many patients with leukemia who cannot afford such therapies are excluded from treatment, but with the development of this production strategy and the implementation of a series of national medical

TABLE 2 | Current clinical targets of CAR-T therapy for hematological malignancies (ClinicalTrials.gov).

Target	Disease	Stage	Phase	NCT number	Country
CD19	Refractory CD19+ lymphoma and leukemia	Completed	I	NCT01626495	United States
	B-cell leukemia or lymphoma		I	NCT01029366	United States
	Refractory B cell malignancy		I/II	NCT02132624	Sweden
	B cell leukemia or lymphoma		I	NCT01593696	United States
	ALL		I	NCT01551043	United States
	Resistant or refractory CD19+ ALL		I	NCT02975687	China
	Resistant or refractory CD19+ ALL		II	NCT02030847	United States
CD19 + CD22	Relapsed or refractory lymphoma and leukemia	Recruiting	I/II	NCT03398967	China
	CD19 positive diffuse large B-cell lymphoma or B ALL		I	NCT03233854	United States
	CD19 +CD22+ leukemia		I	NCT03330691	United States
	Refractory and/or Recurrent B cell malignancies		I/II	NCT03098355	China
	Children or young adults with CD19 positive B ALL		I	NCT03241940	United States
	B-cell ALL		I/II	NCT03614858	China
	B-cell ALL		I/II	NCT03289455	United Kingdom
	B-cell hematologic malignancy		I/II	NCT02903810	China
	CD19/CD22-expressing B cell malignancies		I	NCT03448393	United States
CD19 + CD20	Relapsed or refractory lymphoma and leukemia	Recruiting	I/II	NCT03398967	China
CD22	CD22+ leukemia and lymphoma	Active	I	NCT03244306	United States
	Chemotherapy resistant or refractory ALL	Terminated	I	NCT02588456	United States
	B cell malignancies	Recruiting	I/II	NCT02935153	China
	B cell malignancies	Recruiting	I/II	NCT03262298	China
	ALL	Recruiting	I	NCT03620058	United States
	ALL	Recruiting	I	NCT02650414	United States
CD20	Refractory or relapsed B lymphocyte lymphoma	Recruiting	I	NCT03576807	China
	B cell malignancies	Recruiting	I/II	NCT02710149	China
	Relapsed or refractory B cell non-Hodgkin lymphomas	Recruiting	I/II	NCT03277729	United States
ROR1R	ROR1+ malignancies	Recruiting	I	NCT02706392	United States
	CLL	Withdrawn	I	NCT02194374	United States
CD4	CD4+ lymphoma and leukemia	Recruiting	I	NCT03829540	United States
CD7	High risk T cell malignancies	NR	I	NCT03690011	United States
CD38	Relapsed B-cell ALL after anti-CD19 CAR-T therapy	Recruiting	I/II	NCT03754764	China
CD30	Lymphocyte malignancies	Recruiting	I/II	NCT02958410	China
	Hodgkin lymphoma, adult	NA	–	NCT03914885	United States
BCMA	High-risk multiple myeloma	Recruiting	I/II	NCT03455972	China
	B-cell lymphoma and leukemia	Recruiting	I/II	NCT02954445	China

CLL, chronic lymphocytic leukemia; ROR1R, receptor tyrosine kinase-like orphan receptor; NA, not available; NR, not yet recruiting.

policies, it is believed that an increasing number of patients will benefit from this therapy.

Current Clinical Target of CAR-T Cell Therapy in Hematological Malignancies

The expression of CD molecules as surface markers can be used for the identification of cell types. Several clinical studies using CD19 as the target of CAR-T cells have been registered. In addition to CD19, which is the most widely reported target, there are many tumor-related targets that have entered phase I and phase II clinical trails. In currently registered clinical trials and published research results, B cell maturation antigen (BCMA) has been presented as a particularly important target. At present, there are many targets involved in clinical CAR-T cell projects. Current clinical trials of CAR-T cell therapies mainly focus on CD19, CD20, CD22, GPC3 (Glypican-3), BCMA, and other promising targets (**Table 2** and **Figure 3**).

As of May 2018, 19 clinical applications for CAR-T cell projects from 13 enterprises had been accepted by the CDE (Drug evaluation center of state drug administration) in China; most of these applications targeted CD19. The clinical application of the LCAR-B38M CAR-T cell preparation submitted by Nanjing Legend was formally accepted by the CDE, and it became the first CAR-T cell product to be clinically accepted in China. This product is a BCMA-targeted CAR-T cell product that is mainly used for relapsed or refractory multiple myeloma. A total of 57 patients with multiple myeloma from the Second Affiliated Hospital of Xi'an Jiaotong University

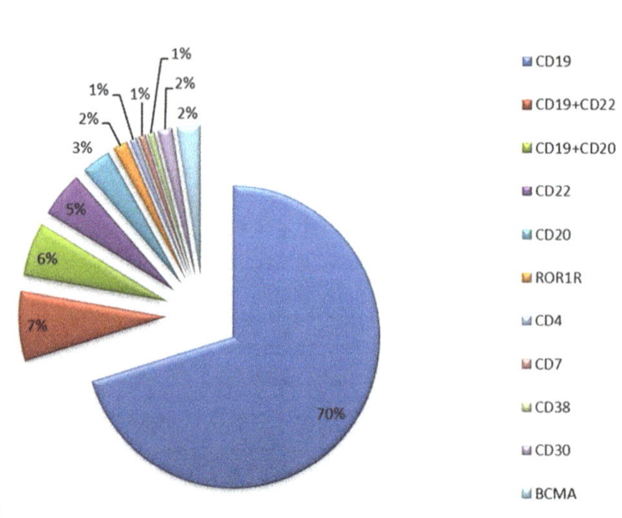

FIGURE 3 | Current clinical targets for CAR-T treatment of hematologic malignancies. The pie chart is based on the statistical result of CAR-T clinical trials for hematologic malignancies registered on ClinicalTrials.gov.

participated in the LCAR-B38M clinical trial (66). The overall response rate was 88%, and 68% of patients achieved a complete response.

The Department of Hematology, Jiangsu Institute of Hematology, China, conducted the first clinical study to treat relapsed/refractory acute lymphoblastic leukemia by sequential transfusion of two types of CAR-T cells: CD19-CAR-T cells and CD22-CAR-T cells (67). Infusion of mixed second-generation CAR-T cells is feasible and safe for patients with refractory/recurrent ALL. Combination therapy against multiple target antigens should be an effective way to overcome recurrence after antigen escape.

Current Clinical Targets of CAR-T Cell Therapy in Solid Tumors

Because of their relatively isolated physiological locations and special immunosuppressive microenvironments, immunotherapy is less effective for solid tumors than for hematological tumors (**Table 3** and **Figure 4**) (68). Regulating the level of chemical flooding factors on the surface of T cells can encourage these cells to enter solid tumors. The immunosuppressive microenvironment of solid tumors is mainly caused by cytokines such as IL-6 and TGF-beta and immunosuppressive cells such as Tregs and myeloid-derived suppressor cells (MDSCs). The use of neutraling (blocking) antibodies against these cytokines and immunosuppressive cells can reverse the immunosuppressive microenvironment to some extent (69). Moreover, the use of nonspecific PD-1 and CTLA-4 antibodies to reverse T cell inhibition can also resolve the poor efficacy of T cell immunotherapy for solid tumors to a certain extent (68, 69).

Published Clinical Targets of CAR-T Cell Therapy in Hematological Malignancies

CAR-T cell immunotherapy has been proven to be a breakthrough in the treatment of hematological tumors, showing good targeting, lethality, and persistence (**Table 4**). The two CAR-T cell products (17, 29) approved by Novartis and Kite Pharma are suitable for acute lymphoblastic leukemia and B cell lymphoma, respectively, and their application is being investigated in blood cancers (17, 29). The application of CAR-T cell therapy in solid tumors has been relatively slow. Statistics show that approximately 75% of CAR-T cell clinical trials in the world are used for leukemia, lymphoma, and other blood cancers, and only a small number of CAR-T cell projects target solid tumors such as liver cancer and lung cancer.

The FDA announced approval of Kite Pharma's CAR-T cell therapy Yescarta for adult patients with specific types of large B cell lymphoma in October 2017. These patients had received at least two other treatments, but no remissions occurred. It is worth mentioning that this is the first non-Hodgkin lymphoma-specific CAR-T cell therapy approved by the FDA (17, 29) and the second approved CAR-T cell therapy. In a multicenter clinical trial, more than 100 adult patients were treated with Yescarta and showed surprising results: complete remissions (CRs) with Yescarta was observed in 51% of patients.

Researchers from the University of Texas M.D. Anderson Cancer Center in Houston conducted a CAR-T cell study involving 111 patients who had a specific type of B cell lymphoma and relapsed after other treatments. In this study, the researchers collected T cells from patients, genetically modified them under laboratory conditions to target lymphoma cells, and eventually transfused them back into the patients after amplification. After a median follow-up of 15.4 months, 42% of patients continued to have a response and 40% of patients had a complete response (28). As expected, 13% had grade 3 or higher CRS, which led to fever, and 28% had neurological disorders, among other adverse reactions (ClinicalTrials.gov number: NCT02348216).

A new CAR-T cell therapy targeting the surface molecule CD22 has been designed. A phase I trial of this CAR-T cell platform recruited 21 children and young adults (aged 7–30) with B-ALL who had relapsed or had not responded to previous treatments (79). Fifteen of these patients also received CAR-T cell therapy targeting CD19, but no significant improvements were achieved. These patients were given different doses of the CD22-targeting CAR-T cell therapy. A total of 73% patients achieved complete remission after receiving $\geq 1 \times 10^6$ CD22 CAR-T cells (79).

Published Clinical Targets of CAR-T Cell Therapy in Solid Tumors

There are many reasons for the remarkable progress of CAR-T cell therapy in hematological tumors and the slow progress in solid tumors (82). On the one hand, there are major differences between solid tumors and hematological tumors. The high heterogeneity makes treatment of solid tumors with CAR-T cell therapy much more difficult. Additionally, tumor antigens associated with solid tumors are expressed not only in tumor

TABLE 3 | Current clinical targets of CAR-T therapy for solid tumors (ClinicalTrials.gov).

Target	Disease	Stage	Phase	NCT number	Country
Mesothelin	Recurrent or metastatic malignant tumors	Recruiting	I	NCT02930993	China
	Malignant pleural mesothelioma	Completed	I	NCT01355965	United States
	Metastatic pancreatic (ductal) adenocarcinoma	Completed	I	NCT02159716	United States
	Epithelial ovarian cancer	Completed	I	NCT01897415	United States
EGFR	EGFR+ advanced solid tumor	Recruiting	I/II	NCT03182816	China
	EGFR+ colorectal cancer	Recruiting	I/II	NCT03152435	China
	Metastatic colorectal cancer	NR	I	NCT03542799	China
	Recurrent or refractory pediatric CNS tumors	Recruiting	I	NCT03638167	United States
	Recurrent glioblastoma multiforme'	Recruiting	I	NCT02844062	China
GPC3	Advanced HCC	Completed	I/II	NCT03130712	China
	HCC	Recruiting	I	NCT02905188	United States
MUC1	Intrahepatic cholangiocarcinoma	Recruiting	I/II	NCT03633773	China
	NSCLC	Recruiting	I/II	NCT03525782	China
	Esophageal cancer	Recruiting	I/II	NCT03706326	China
HER2	Brain or leptomeningeal metastases	Recruiting	I	NCT03696030	United States
	HER2+ cancer	Recruiting	I/II	NCT02713984	China
	Breast cancer	Completed	I/II	NCT02547961	China
	HER2+ CNS tumors	Recruiting	I	NCT02442297	United States
	Recurrent/refractory pediatric CNS tumors	Recruiting	I	NCT03500991	United States
	Advanced solid tumors	Unknown	I/II	NCT01935843	China
GD2	High risk and/or relapsed/refractory neuroblastoma	Recruiting	I/II	NCT03373097	Italy
	Glioma	Recruiting	I	NCT02761915	United Kingdom
	Glioma	Completed	I/II	NCT03252171	China
CEA	Metastatic pancreatic carcinoma	Recruiting	I	NCT03818165	United States
	Liver metastases	Completed	I	NCT02416466	United States
EpCAM	Nasopharyngeal carcinoma	Recruiting	I	NCT02915445	China
	Advanced gastric cancer with peritoneal metastasis	Recruiting	I	NCT03563326	China
LeY	Advanced cancer	Recruiting	I	NCT03851146	Australia
	Myeloid malignancies	Recruiting	I/II	NCT02958384	China
PSCA	Metastatic castration resistant prostate cancer	Recruiting	I	NCT03873805	United States

CNS, central nervous system; EGFR, epidermal growth factor receptor; GD2, ganglioside; CEA, carcino-embryonic antigen; EpCAM, epithelial cell adhesion molecule; Ley, Lewis Y antigen; PSCA, prostate stem cell antigen; HCC, hepatocellular carcinoma; NR, not yet recruiting.

tissues but also in normal tissues. This poses another challenge in the treatment of solid tumors with CAR-T cells (61). In addition, the homing and activation of CAR-T cells in solid tumors are also challenging. How to make CAR-T cells accurately home from the peripheral blood to function at the tumor site needs to be solved urgently, but a single CAR-T cell therapy will not solve this problem. Moreover, CAR-T cells can coexpress some cytokines to enhance their killing activity and homing function, such as IL-2, IL-7, and chemokine (C-C motif) ligand 19 (CCL19) (**Table 5**).

Researchers from the Department of Neurosurgery, Perelman School of Medicine at the University of Pennsylvania used CAR-T cells to target the tumor-specific antigen EGFRvIII to treat patients (43). In this study, the authors found two major challenges with this technique: one problem is that the expression of EGFRvIII in the tumor tissues of patients is quite variable; the other is that the TME has a strong immunosuppressive effect, which will gradually become more concerning over the course of treatment. Therefore, the authors believe that it is necessary to search for new tumor antigens and drugs to overcome these immunosuppressive effects simultaneously to achieve the killing of tumor tissue. This also explains why CAR-T cell therapy is ineffective in treating gliomas: the immunosuppressive effects of the TME and the complexity of gene mutations (43).

T cells are picky about their environment and die within a few days without proper nutrients. In addition, tumor tissue releases self-defensive chemicals that block the normal functioning of T cells. Researchers at the Fred Hutchinson Cancer Research Center used a synthetic receptor "skeleton" to coat cancer-specific T cells and nutrients to kill tumor cells in mouse model (99). The results showed that the cytoskeleton coated T cells could effectively reduce tumor size in mice with pancreatic cancer and melanoma, and the therapeutic effect was stronger than that of injecting T cells alone. Of course, this approach is still a long way from clinical application (99).

Future Improvements

Scientists have developed a variety of ways to improve the anticancer efficacy of CAR-T cell therapy. CAR-T cells were

Current clinical target of CAR-T therapy in solid tumor

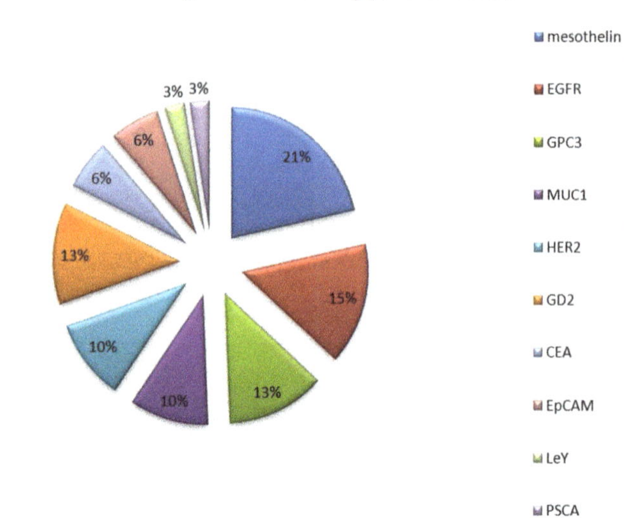

FIGURE 4 | Current clinical targets for CAR-T therapy in solid tumors. The pie chart is based on the statistical result of CAR-T clinical trials for solid tumors registered on ClinicalTrials.gov.

further modified to secrete proinflammatory cytokines, thus protecting CAR-T cells in the inhibitory TME. Modified CAR-T cells secreting IL-12 have achieved encouraging results in a mouse model (100). To improve the persistence of CAR-T cells, scientists constructed a dual-receptor CAR, which enables engineered T cells to express two artificial receptors, one for TAA recognition and the other for cytokine-mediated growth stimulation of T cells. CAR-T cells are subject to suppressive immune checkpoint signals in the TME, such as PD-L1 or CTLA-4. These inhibitory receptor–ligand interactions can be blocked by monoclonal antibodies, thus eliminating the inhibition of T cells. CAR-T cells targeting tumor vessels are being studied for the treatment of melanoma and renal cancer. The presence of angiogenic growth factors (such as VEGF) in the TME and the overexpression of their receptors in tumor cells are associated with poor prognosis and metastasis (101). One potential reason for the failure of CAR-T cell therapy relates to the persistence of CAR-T cells; strategies such as the replacement of the costimulatory domain of 4-1BB and increased production of cytokines that stimulate T cell proliferation and activation have potential.

New CAR-T targets are necessary for the treatment of patients with hematological malignancies that do not express CD19. In addition, some patients treated with CD19-CAR-T cell therapy will relapse due to mutations that allow tumor escape. Currently, the most promising targets for the treatment of hematological malignancies include CD22, CD20, ROR1, immunoglobulin kappa chain, BCMA, and CD138 (for plasma malignancies) as well as CD33, CD123, and LeY (for myeloid malignancy).

There are many gene-editing tools, including zinc finger nucleases (ZFNs), meganucleases, transcription activator-like (TAL) effector nucleases (TALENs), and the Clustered regularly interspaced short palindromic repeats-associated protein 9

TABLE 4 | Published clinical targets of CAR-T therapy for hematological malignancies.

Target	Disease	Costimulatory domain	Vector	Pretreatment	Dose	No. of patients	Phage	Response	Country	References
CD19	B-ALL	CD28	Lentivirus	FLU, CY	5×10^4–1×10^6/kg	3	I	Grade 2 or 3 CRS;	China	(70)
CD19	B-ALL	4-1BB	Lentivirus	FLU, CY	Total dose of 1.19×10^6/kg	2	–	Acute GVHD	China	(71)
CD19	B-ALL	CD28 + 4-1BB	Lentivirus	CE, FLU	2×10^5–2×10^7/kg	30	I/II	93% remission	United States	(72)
CD19	HL	4-1BB	Lentivirus	FLU, CY	Median dose of 1.56×10^7/kg	18	I/II	2/18 grade ≥3 toxicities; 13/18 remission	China	(73)
CD19	CLL; DLBCL	CD28	Retrovirus	FLU, CY	1×10^6/kg	15	–	80% remission; 1 died	United States	(74)
CD19	B-ALL	4-1BB	Lentivirus		7.6×10^5–2.06×10^7/kg	30	I/II	90% remission; 27% seriously CRS	United States	(53)
CD19	B-ALL	4-1BB	Lentivirus	FLU, CY	1.4×10^7–1.1×10^9/person	14	I	57% remission; 4/14 complete remission	United States	(75)
CD19	B-ALL	CD28	Retrovirus	CY	Total dose of 3×10^6/kg	16	I	88% regression;	United States	(76)
CD19	NHL	CD28 + 4-1BB	Lentivirus	CY, VP	2×10^6–2×10^7/kg	32	I	13/32 grade ≥3 CRS; 72% remission	United States	(77)
CD20	DLBCL	4-1BB	Lentivirus	CY, VCR	1×10^7/person	7	I	5 tumor regression	China	(78)
CD22	B-ALL	4-1BB	Lentivirus	CY, FLU	3×10^5–3×10^6/kg	21	I	73% complete remission; 8 relapsed	United States	(79)
CD30	HL	CD28	Retrovirus	–	2×10^7–2×10^8/m^2	9	I	1/9 complete remission	United States	(80)
LeY	AML	CD28	Retrovirus	FLU	5×10^8–1.3×10^9 /person	5	I	1 relapse; 1 long-term remission	Australia	(81)

B-ALL, B-cell precursor acute lymphoblastic leukemia; FLU, fludarabine; CY, cyclophosphamide; CNS, cytokine release syndrome; GVHD, graft-vs.-host disease; CE, cyclophosphamide and etoposide; HL, Hodgkin's lymphoma; DLBCL, diffuse large B cell lymphoma; VP, etoposide; VCR, vincristine; AML, acute myelocytic leukemia.

TABLE 5 | Published clinical targets of CAR-T therapy for solid tumors.

Target	Disease	Costimulatory domain	Vector	Pretreatment	Dose	No. of patients	Phage	Response	Country	References
EGFRvIII	Glioblastoma	4-1BB	Lentivirus	Temozolomide radiation	1–5 × 10^8/person	10	I	5 remission	United States	(43)
EGFR	NSCLC	4-1BB	Lentivirus	CY, CDDP	4.5 × 10^6–1.09 × 10^7/kg	11	I/II	7/11 remission;	China	(83)
GD2	NB	NA	Retrovirus	–	2 × 10^7–1 × 10^8/m^2	19	I	11/19 remission	United States	(84)
GD2	Metastatic melanoma	CD28 + OX40	Retrovirus	FLU, CY	1–2 × 10^7/m^2	4	I	4 partial response	South Australia	(85)
IL13Rα2	GBM	NA	DNA electroporation	–	10.6 × 10^8/person	13	I	3 relapse	United States	(86)
IL13Rα2	GBM	4-1BB	Lentivirus	–	Total dose of 5.2–9.2 × 10^7/person	1	I	1 relapse	United States	(87)
HER2	PNET; DSRCT	CD28	Retrovirus	Chemotherapy	1 × 10^4–1 × 10^8/m^2	19	I/II	1 necrosis; 4/19 remission;	United States	(88)
CAIX	RCC	NA	Retrovirus	–	3 × 10^8–2.1 × 10^9/person	11	–	–	Netherlands	(89)
CAIX	RCC	NA	Retrovirus	–	6 × 10^8–4 × 10^9/person	12	–	–	Netherlands	(90)
Mesothelin	PAC; MPM	4-1BB	mRNA electroporation	–	Total dose of 1.2 × 10^9/person	4	–	1 allergic reactions and cardiac arrest	United States	(91)
Mesothelin	MPM; PDA	4-1BB	mRNA electroporation	Chemotherapy	4.4 × 10^9 of one patient; 3.1 × 10^9/m^2 of another	2	I	1 partial response	United States	(92)
MUC1	Seminal vesicle cancer	CD28 + 4-1BB	Lentivirus	–	Intratumoral injection of 5 × 10^5 cells at two sites, respectively	1	I	no side effects	China	(93)
CEA	mCRC	CD28	Lentivirus	CY, FLU	2.5 × 10^7-1.52 × 10^{10}/person	10	I	70% remission	China	(44)
CEA	Liver metastases	CD28	Retrovirus	–	1 × 10^8–3 × 10^{10}/person	6	I	5 patients died of progressive disease;	United States	(94)
CEA	Adenocarcinoma; PMP	NA	–	FLU, CY	1 × 10^9–5 × 10^{10}/person	14	I	Transient acute respiratory toxicity	United Kingdom	(40)
BCMA	MM	CD28	Retrovirus	CY, FLU	3 × 10^5–9 × 10^6/kg	12	I	1 relapse after 17 weeks; 1 complete remission	United States	(95)
c-Met	Breast cancer	4-1BB	mRNA electroporation	–	3 × 10^7–3 × 10^8/person	6	–	Tumor necrosis at the injection site	United States	(96)
PSMA	PCa	NA	Retrovirus	Chemotherapy	1 × 10^9–1 × 10^{10}/person	5	I	2/5 partial remission	United States	(97)
TAG72	CRC	NA	Retrovirus	–	3–3.11 × 10^{10}/person	16	I	Low-grade CRS	United States	(98)

CDDP, cis-diamminedichoro platinum; NB, neuroblastoma; GBM, glomerular basement membrane; PNET, primitive neuroectodermal tumors; DSRCT, desmoplastic small round cell tumor; PAC, perennial allergic colitis; MPM, malignant pleural mesothelioma; PDA, patent ductus arteriosus; mCRC, metastatic colorectal cancer; PMP, pseudomyxoma peritonei; MM, multiple myeloma; PCa, prostate cancer; CRC, colorectal cancer; CAIX, carbonic anhydrase IX, c-Met, c-mesenchymal–epithelial transition; PSMA, prostate-specific membrane antigen; TAG72, tumor-associated glycoproteins-72; NA, not applicable. The first generation of CAR contains a CD3 signaling domain.

(CRISPR-Cas9 nuclease) (38). These techniques have been successfully applied in the study of engineered T cells. Due to the rapid development of this field, universal CAR-T cells may eventually be widely used. The manufacturing process for universal CAR-T cell therapy is simpler, and it is expected to achieve faster and more inexpensive off-the-shelf cell therapy products.

Challenges in this process include the selection of target antigens, the management of toxicity, and the regulation of the immunosuppressive TME. Many researchers are actively developing CAR-T cell therapies to achieve the same success in other hematological malignancies and solid tumors.

TCR-T CELL THERAPY

Both TCR and CAR-therapies modify the patient's own T lymphocytes *ex vivo* and then inject them back into the patient's body to kill cancer, but their mechanisms for recognizing antigens are quite different. TCRs use heterodimers consisting of alpha and beta peptide chains to recognize polypeptide fragments presented by MHC molecules (**Figure 5**) (102). CAR-T cells, on the other hand, use antibody fragments that bind to specific antigens on the surface of cancer cells. The target antigens identified by CAR-T cell therapy are all cell surface proteins, while TCR-T cell therapy can recognize intracellular antigen fragments presented by MHC molecules (102), so TCR-T cell therapy has a wider range of targets. However, TCR-T cell therapy is MHC restricted and depends on presentation by MHC molecules to recognize targets and activate T cell function, so these traits are also a disadvantage of TCR-T cell therapy.

Dr. Michael Steinmetz first transferred TCR genes from one T cell to another, giving the second T cell the same antigen specificity (103). This process is the origin of current TCR gene therapy. The TCR is a specific receptor and a characteristic marker on the surface of T cells. TCR-T cells are genetically engineered TCR products that can recognize specific antigens. The core goal behind TCR-T cell technology is to directly modify TCR binding to tumor antigens. The affinity of human TCRs to these antigens is relatively low, which makes it impossible to recognize and kill tumors effectively. The artificially designed high-affinity TCR is encoded in T cells by genetic engineering technology (54), which enhances both specificity recognition and affinity during the recognition of tumor cells by T cells.

The construction of high-affinity TCR-T cells requires the identification of specific targets. First, the polypeptides presented by cancer cells are identified, and then the polypeptides presented in normal tissues are screened out. After the target is confirmed, a TCR phage display library is established to screen TCRs with high affinity and specificity. A preclinical safety test is then performed to ensure minimal off-target effects and cross-reactivity.

In one report, after modifying several key amino acids, the resulting TCR had a greatly increased affinity for a common cancer antigen [tumor-associated antigen (TAA)], New York esophageal squamous cell carcinoma (NY-ESO-1), and this TCR can be used to attack NY-ESO-1-overexpressing cancers, such as multiple myeloma (104). In this clinical trial, 80% of patients with multiple myeloma had a good clinical response, and 70% of them had a complete or near-complete response (104).

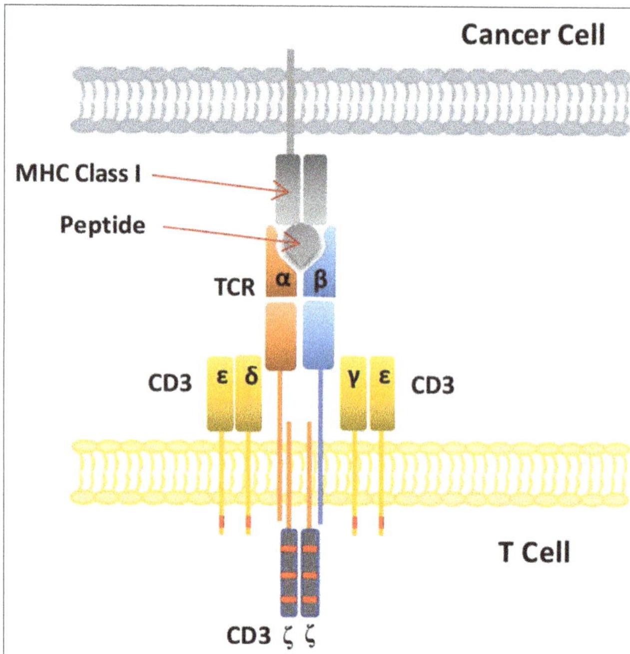

FIGURE 5 | Schematic diagram of the CAR-T cell structure. The TCR complex is a heterodimer consisting of two different peptide chains, TCRα and TCRβ, and is surrounded by four CD3 chains. The MHC class I molecules present intracellular antigenic peptides of cancer cells for recognition bt the T cell receptor.

Advantages and Challenges of TCR-T Cell Therapy

Any antigen that can be presented by MHC molecules can be recognized by TCR-T cells, whether it is an intracellular or cell surface antigen or a neo-antigen produced by tumor cells after mutation. TCRs can recognize the internal molecules of cancer cells, and TCR-T cells can have greatly improved affinity for cancer cells through genetic engineering. Because they retain all the auxiliary molecules of the TCR signal transduction pathway, TCR-T cells can be fully activated when a small amount of antigen is present, resulting in a killing effect (26, 82).

Difficulties in the development of TCR-T cell technology include the selection of good targets, the search for specific TCRs, screening for optimal TCR affinity, safety evaluation, time, and cost. Target selection is one of the most important aspects (82). These problems have become barriers to TCR-T cell therapy, and finding a solution to these problems has become the key to determining the success of TCR-T cells.

Most TCR-T cell therapy targets are limited by MHC class. In addition, there is a risk of hybridization (mismatch) between exogenous and endogenous chains, which may induce harmful recognition of autoantigens, leading to graft-vs.-host disease. Increased TCR affinity poses a risk of false targeting, so TCR-T cell therapy should be applied carefully. TCR-T cell therapy has shown some therapeutic potential, but there are still many limitations, such as the matching of histocompatibility antigens and the need for antigens to be presented on the cell surface.

TABLE 6 | Current clinical targets of TCR-T therapy for hematological malignancies (ClinicalTrials.gov).

Target	Disease	Stage	Phase	NCT number	Country
HA-1	Relapsed or refractory acute leukemia after donor stem cell	Recruiting	I	NCT03326921	United States
WT1	Myelodysplastic syndromes and acute myeloid leukemia patients	Completed	I/II	NCT02550535	Germany
WT1	Acute myeloid leukemia	Active	I/II	NCT02770820	United States
CMV	Hematological malignancies and CMV infection	Suspended	I	NCT02988258	United Kingdom

CMV, cytomegalovirus; HA-1, a protein that present on the surface of blood cells; WT1, Wilms tumor 1.

TABLE 7 | Current clinical targets of TCR-T therapy for solid tumors (ClinicalTrials.gov).

Target	Disease	Stage	Phase	NCT number	Country
MAGE	Solid and hematological malignancies;	Enrolling	–	NCT03391791	Canada
	Metastatic renal cancer and melanoma;	Terminated	I/II	NCT01273181	United States
Gp100	Metastatic melanoma;	Completed	II	NCT00923195	United States
	Malignant melanoma;	Terminated	II	NCT02889861	United Kingdom
MART-1	Skin metastatic melanoma	Completed	I	NCT00091104	United States
HPV-16 E6	HPV+ NHSCC or cervical cancer;	Recruiting	I	NCT03578406	China
	HPV-associated cancer;	Completed	I/II	NCT02280811	United States
NY-ESO-1	Ovarian, fallopian tube, or primary peritoneal cancer;	Recruiting	I	NCT03691376	United States
	Advanced NSCLC;	Recruiting	I	NCT03029273	China
	Sarcoma;	Recruiting	I	NCT03462316	China
HBV	Hepatocellular	Recruiting	I	NCT02719782	China
P53	Metastatic cancer that overexpresses p53	Completed	II	NCT00393029	United States
CEA	Metastatic cancer;	Terminated	I	NCT00923806	United States
HPV E7	Human papillomavirus-associated cancers	Recruiting	I/II	NCT02858310	United States
SL9	HIV	Completed	I	NCT00991224	United States
TGFβII	Metastatic colorectal cancer	Terminated	I/II	NCT03431311	Norway
MCPyV	Metastatic or unresectable Merkel cell cancer	Recruiting	I/II	NCT03747484	United States
TRAIL	Metastatic renal cancer	Terminated	I	NCT00923390	United States
PRAME	AML/MDS or metastatic uveal melanoma	Active	I/II	NCT02743611	United States
EBV	Recurrent or metastatic NPC	NR	II	NCT03648697	China
CMV	Hematological malignancies and CMV infection	Suspended	I	NCT02988258	United Kingdom
KRAS	KRAS G12V + tumor;	Recruiting	I/II	NCT03190941	United States
	KRAS G12D + tumor;	Recruiting	I/II	NCT03745326	United States

NHSCC, head and neck squamous cell carcinoma; MDS, myelodysplastic syndromes; NPC, nasopharyngeal carcinoma; MAGE, melanoma antigen; Gp100, melanoma associated antigen; MART1, melanoma antigen recognized by T cells 1; HPV-16-E6, human papillomavirus-16 E6 protein; NR, not yet recruiting.

Current Clinical Targets of TCR-T Cell Therapy in Hematological Malignancies

Specific targeted immunotherapy of leukemic stem cells is an ideal method for the treatment of malignant myeloid tumors (**Table 6**), but the appropriate epitopes are still unclear. The comparative proteomic characteristics of hematopoietic stem cells and progenitor cells from healthy stem cell donors and patients with acute myeloid leukemia may reveal differentially expressed proteins that can be used as surface markers or as substitutes for affected molecular pathways.

Current Clinical Targets of TCR-T Cell Therapy in Solid Tumors

T cells activated by TCRs can target most tumor-specific antigens, especially those antigens that are intracellular. Therefore, many TCR-T cell techniques have been applied in clinical trials of solid tumors (**Table 7** and **Figure 6**). Because of their relatively isolated physiological locations and unique immunosuppressive microenvironments, immunotherapy is less effective for solid tumors than for hematological tumors. To overcome the isolated physiological locations of solid tumors, local injection of T cells into tumors was used in a mouse model (105). The effect from local injection is better than that achieved by systemic drug administration, such as injecting T cells into the cerebrospinal fluid in brain tumors.

Published Clinical TCR-T Cell Therapies in Hematological Malignancies

The clinical application of gene-modified T cell therapy has led to unprecedented response rates in leukemia and lymphoma patients treated with anti-CD19 CAR-T cells. Although CAR-T cell therapy has shown significant efficacy in CD19+

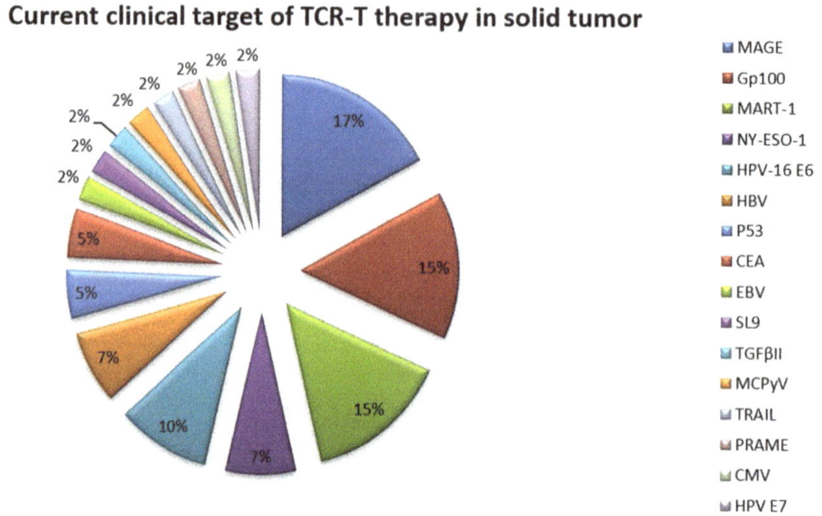

FIGURE 6 | Current clinical targets for TCR-T therapy in solid tumors (ClinicalTrials.gov). The pie chart is based on the statistical result of TCR-T clinical trials for solid tumors registered on ClinicalTrials.gov.

TABLE 8 | Published clinical TCR-T therapy for hematological malignancies.

Target	Disease	Vector	Pretreatment	Dose	No. of patients	Phage	Response	Country	Reference
WT1	Acute myeloid leukemia; MDS	Retrovirus	Cytosine arabinoside and aclarubicin	2×10^8–5×10^9/person	8	I	50% remission	Japan	(106)

hematological cancers such as lymphoma and leukemia, life-threatening side effects such as CRS and neurotoxicity limit the clinical application of CAR-T cell therapy. Eureka Therapeutics has published preclinical data on its proprietary antibody-TCR (AbTCR) platform, proving that AbTCR-T cells have the same anticancer effects as existing anti-CD19 CAR-T cells in a mouse model (102); however, the production of inflammatory cytokines is significantly reduced in AbTCR-T cells, reducing the risk of CRS. Safer T cell therapy can provide patients with a larger therapeutic window while reducing the direct and indirect costs for patients and the entire health care system (**Table 8**).

Published Clinical TCR-T Cell Therapies in Solid Tumors

Researchers isolated endogenous TCRs, engineered them, and introduced these modified T cells into the human body. In this way, the number of T cells with the ability to target cancer cells will increase, and this is expected to help identify and target multiple solid tumors and hematological tumors (**Table 9**).

Differences Between CAR-T Cell and TCR-T Cell Therapies

CARs can recognize not only peptide antigens but also carbohydrate and glycolipid antigens, which enlarges the pool of targetable cancer antigens. CAR-T cell therapy is not restricted by MHC class. CAR-T cells can target nonprotein glycolipid antigens of cancer cells to recognize antigens in multiple dimensions. The problem with the treatment of solid and hematological tumors by CAR-T cells is that the target antigens are all cell surface proteins. Even if CAR-T cells have a potent killing effect on tumor cells, without appropriate, specific cell surface target proteins, CAR-T cell therapy cannot have a real impact. Because MHC molecules can present peptide chains obtained from the cell surface or intracellular proteins, TCRs can target more antigens than CARs. These antigens, including CEA, HER-2, CD19, gp100, MART-1, MAGA-A3, and NY-ESO-1, are suitable for TCR-T cell therapy. TCRs target intracellular proteins with tumor specificity. These antigens include neo-antigens generated by random mutations in tumor DNA and so-called cancer testis antigens (82). These antigens are usually expressed in only some tumors and genital tissues, while MHC molecules are not expressed in genital tissues. TILs and TCRs can recognize only the antigens presented by specific MHC molecules and may escape immune surveillance due to the downregulation or mutation of MHC molecules in tumor cells, resulting in clinical limitations (25). TCR-based therapies may be superior to CAR-based therapies because TCR-T cells use natural T cell signaling mechanisms (112).

The dosage of CAR-T cell therapy is two to three orders of magnitude lower than that needed with TILs and TCR-T cells. Because CAR-T cell therapies have a clear target and a high specificity for recognizing tumor surface antigen and are able to overcome MHC restriction, the number of single transfusion cells needed for CAR-T cell therapy is far smaller than that needed for TCR-T cell therapy or TIL therapy to generate the same therapeutic effect.

TABLE 9 | Published clinical TCR-T therapy for solid tumors.

Target	Disease	Vector	Pretreatment	Dose	No. of patients	Phage	Response	Country	References
MART-1	Metastatic melanoma	Retrovirus	Chemotherapy	1.5×10^9–1.07×10^{11} /person	20	II	30% objective antitumor response	United States	(107)
Gp100	Metastatic melanoma	Retrovirus	Chemotherapy	1.8×10^9–1.1×10^{11} /person	16	II	19% objective antitumor response	United States	(107)
CEA	Metastatic colorectal	Retrovirus	Chemotherapy	2–4 $\times 10^8$/person	3	–	Grade 2/3 diarrhea	United States	(108)
NY-ESO-1	Metastatic melanoma/synovial cell sarcoma	Retrovirus	Chemotherapy	1.6×10^{10}–1.3×10^{11}/person	17	I	2 complete remission; 1 partial remission	United States	(109)
NY-ESO-1	Multiple myeloma	Lentivirus	Chemotherapy	Average dose of 2.4 $\times 10^9$/person	20	I/II	80% remission;	United States	(104)
MAGE-A3	Metastatic melanoma/multiple myeloma	Lentivirus	CY	2.4–5.3 $\times 10^9$/person	2	III/IV	2 died for cardiac toxicity	United States	(110)
MAGE-A4	Esophageal cancer	Retrovirus	Surgery; radiotherapy; chemotherapy	2×10^8–5×10^9/person	10	I	7/10 tumor progression	Japan	(111)

DISCUSSION

Immunotherapy, unlike traditional therapies, directly acts on cancer cells by recruiting the autoimmune system and using it to attack tumors. The anti-tumor immune response can continuously recognize and memorize tumor antigens and increasingly expand with time; this cycle can be repeated to strengthen the anti-tumor immune response. With expansion of the immune response, some cytotoxic T cells differentiate into mature memory T cells, which can provide long-term immune memory even when primary antigen stimulation does not exist. Therefore, immunotherapy can bring lasting benefits and long-term survival to patients.

The development of a new drug or therapy is not easy, and it often costs billions of dollars. Juno Therapeutics is committed to the research of tumor cell immunity and is one of the pioneers in this field. At present, research on CAR-T cell products targeting CD19 is relatively extensive, and the two approved products target CD19 for the treatment of hematological tumors. Globally, the R&D pipeline of CAR-T cells has expanded rapidly, including the exploration of new targets, such as BCMA, CD123, and CD33, as well as the expansion to new indications, such as the progression of hematological tumors to solid tumors. A number of companies around the world have been pushing their projects to the clinical stage, and it is expected that there will be CAR-T cell products for different tumors in the future. With the promotion of new structures in clinical trials and improvements in production technology, the third and fourth generations of CAR-T cell products are expected to have better efficacy. TCR-T therapies targeting solid tumor targets such as WT-1, L1CAM, ROR-1, MUC-16, LewisY, HPV-16, etc. are also undergoing clinical trials. For solid tumors, TCR-T therapies may be more advantageous. Many companies around the world such as Kite Pharma, JunoTherapeutics, Adaptimmune Therapeutics, etc. are all committed to the development of TCR-T immunotherapy, hoping to bring feasible treatment plans.

The preparation of engineered T cells still depends on traditional manual operation, such that cell quality and stability are difficult to guarantee. Moreover, the curative effect is greatly reduced. With the continuous improvement of engineered T cell technologies, it is foreseeable that automatic production of engineered T cells will be a major trend in the future. We also look forward to engineered T cell therapy becoming more technically mature, safer, and efficient. Tumor immunotherapy will bring hope to many cancer patients soon. Some of the greatest challenges in developing cell therapies include the lack of preclinical models to assess the safety and efficacy of these complex therapies and the responses to safety issues identified in early clinical studies. In addition, there are still many obstacles in the treatment of solid tumors.

It is expected that, due to technological advances in engineering T cells, gene editing, and cell manufacturing, the foundations of T cell-based therapies will be extended to other cell types in the future, such as induced pluripotent stem cells, hematopoietic stem cells, and NK cells. The indications will also transcend cancer and are expected to include infectious diseases, organ transplantation, and autoimmune diseases.

AUTHOR CONTRIBUTIONS

LZ drafted the manuscript, during which she received carefully guidance and support from YC. All authors read and approved the final manuscript.

FUNDING

This work was supported by the National Natural Science Foundation of China (Grants 31741042 and 81872783), the Guangdong Natural Science Foundation (Grant 2018A030313916), and the Shenzhen Science and Technology Innovation Program (Grants JCYJ20170818090043031 and JCYJ20180504165501371).

REFERENCES

1. Scarfò I, Maus MV. Current approaches to increase CAR T cell potency in solid tumors: targeting the tumor microenvironment. *J Immunother Cancer.* (2017) 5:28. doi: 10.1186/s40425-017-0230-9
2. Hendifar AE, Hingorani SR, Harris WP, Seery TE, Sigal D, Wu W, et al. LBA-02 high response rate and PFS with PEGPH20 added to Nab-Paclitaxel/Gemcitabine in stage IV previously untreated pancreatic cancer patients with high-HA tumors: interim results of a randomized phase 2 study. *Ann Oncol.* (2015) 26(Suppl. 4):iv117. doi: 10.1093/annonc/mdv262.02
3. Ren J, Liu X, Fang C, Jiang S, June CH, Zhao Y. Multiplex genome editing to generate universal CAR T cells resistant to PD1 inhibition. *Clin Cancer Res.* (2017) 23:2255–66. doi: 10.1158/1078-0432.CCR-16-1300
4. Crespo J, Sun H, Welling TH, Tian Z, Zou W. T cell anergy, exhaustion, senescence, and stemness in the tumor microenvironment. *Curr Opin Immunol.* (2013) 25:214–21. doi: 10.1016/j.coi.2012.12.003
5. Andrikou K, Peterle C, Pipitone S, Salati M, Cascinu S. Emerging antibodies for the treatment of pancreatic cancer. *Exp Opin Emerg Drugs.* (2017) 22:39–51. doi: 10.1080/14728214.2017.1293649
6. Perica K, Varela JC, Oelke M, Schneck J. Adoptive T cell immunotherapy for cancer. *Rambam Maimonides Med J.* (2015) 6:e0004. doi: 10.5041/RMMJ.10179
7. Renfro LA, An MW, Mandrekar SJ. Precision oncology: a new era of cancer clinical trials. *Cancer Lett.* (2016) 387:121–6. doi: 10.1016/j.canlet.2016.03.015
8. Bernadic M Jr, Duchon R, Aziri R, Mladosievicova B. New principles of cancer therapy give new hope for oncological patients. *Bratisl Lek Listy.* (2019) 120:15–8. doi: 10.4149/BLL_2019_002
9. Reck M, Mok TSK, Nishio M, Jotte RM, Cappuzzo F, Orlandi F, et al. Atezolizumab plus bevacizumab and chemotherapy in non-small-cell lung cancer (IMpower150): key subgroup analyses of patients with EGFR mutations or baseline liver metastases in a randomised, open-label phase 3 trial. *Lancet Respir Med.* (2019) 7:387–401 doi: 10.1016/S2213-2600(19)30084-0
10. Frederickson AM, Arndorfer S, Zhang I, Lorenzi M, Insinga R, Arunachalam A, et al. Pembrolizumab plus chemotherapy in metastatic non-small-cell lung cancer. *N Engl J Med.* (2018) 378:2078–92. doi: 10.1056/NEJMoa1801005
11. Socinski MA, Jotte RM, Cappuzzo F, Orlandi F, Stroyakovskiy D, Nogami N, et al. Atezolizumab for first-line treatment of metastatic nonsquamous NSCLC. *N Engl J Med.* (2018) 378:2288–301. doi: 10.1056/NEJMoa1716948
12. Cella D, Grünwald V, Escudier B, Hammers HJ, George S, Nathan P, et al. Patient-reported outcomes of patients with advanced renal cell carcinoma treated with nivolumab plus ipilimumab versus sunitinib (CheckMate 214): a randomised, phase 3 trial. *Lancet Oncol.* (2019) 20:297–310. doi: 10.1016/S1470-2045(18)30778-2
13. Motzer RJ, Tannir NM, McDermott DF, Arén Frontera O, Melichar B, Choueiri TK, et al. Nivolumab plus Ipilimumab versus sunitinib in advanced renal-cell carcinoma. *N Engl J Med.* (2018) 378:1277–90. doi: 10.1056/NEJMoa1712126
14. Tawbi HA, Forsyth PA, Algazi A, Hamid O, Hodi FS, Moschos SJ, et al. Combined nivolumab and ipilimumab in melanoma metastatic to the brain. *New Engl J Med.* (2018) 379:722–30. doi: 10.1056/NEJMoa1805453
15. Heyman B, Yang Y. New developments in immunotherapy for lymphoma. *Cancer Biol Med.* (2018) 15:189–209. doi: 10.20892/j.issn.2095-3941.2018.0037
16. Vairy S, Garcia JL, Teira P, Bittencourt H. CTL019 (tisagenlecleucel): CAR-T therapy for relapsed and refractory B-cell acute lymphoblastic leukemia. *Drug Des Devel Ther.* (2018) 12:3885–98. doi: 10.2147/DDDT.S138765
17. Ramalingam SS, Yang JC, Lee CK, Kurata T, Kim DW, John T, et al. Osimertinib as first-line treatment of EGFR mutation–positive advanced non–small-cell lung cancer. *J Clin Oncol.* (2018) 36:841–9. doi: 10.1200/JCO.2017.74.7576
18. Soria JC, Ohe Y, Vansteenkiste J, Reungwetwattana T, Chewaskulyong B, Lee KH, et al. Osimertinib in untreated EGFR-mutated advanced non-small-cell lung cancer. *N Engl J Med.* (2018) 378:113–25. doi: 10.1056/NEJMoa1713137
19. Mohan N, Shen Y, Endo Y, ElZarrad MK, Wu WJ. Trastuzumab, but not pertuzumab, dysregulates HER2 signaling to mediate inhibition of autophagy and increase in reactive oxygen species production in human cardiomyocytes. *Mol Cancer Ther.* (2016) 15:1321–31. doi: 10.1158/1535-7163.MCT-15-0741
20. Sammons SL, Topping DL, Blackwell KL. HR+, HER2- advanced breast cancer and CDK4/6 inhibitors: Mode of action, clinical activity, and safety profiles. *Curr Cancer Drug Targets.* (2017) 17:637–49. doi: 10.2174/1568009617666170330120452
21. McCain J. First-in-class CDK4/6 inhibitor palbociclib could usher in a new wave of combination therapies for HR+, HER2- breast cancer. *P&T.* (2015) 40:511–20.
22. Sledge GW, Toi M, Neven P, Sohn J, Inoue K, Pivot X, et al. MONARCH 2: abemaciclib in combination with fulvestrant in women with HR+/HER2- advanced breast cancer who had progressed while receiving endocrine therapy. *J Clin Oncol.* (2017) 35:2875–84. doi: 10.1200/JCO.2017.73.7585
23. Maus MV, Fraietta JA, Levine BL, Kalos M, Zhao Y, June CH. Adoptive immunotherapy for cancer or viruses. *Ann Rev Immunol.* (2014) 32:189–225. doi: 10.1146/annurev-immunol-032713-120136
24. Gattinoni L, Powell DJ, Rosenberg SA, Restifo NP. Adoptive immunotherapy for cancer: building on success. *Nat Rev Immunol.* (2006) 6:383–93. doi: 10.1038/nri1842
25. Sadelain M, Riviere I, and Riddell S. Therapeutic T cell engineering. *Nature.* (2017) 545:423–31. doi: 10.1038/nature22395
26. Kershaw MH, Westwood JA, and Darcy PK. Gene-engineered T cells for cancer therapy. *Nat Rev Cancer.* (2013) 13:525–41. doi: 10.1038/nrc3565
27. Maude SL, Laetsch TW, Buechner J, Rives S, Boyer M, Bittencourt H, et al. Tisagenlecleucel in children and young adults with B-cell lymphoblastic leukemia. *New Engl J Med.* (2018) 378:439–45. doi: 10.1056/NEJMoa1709866
28. Neelapu SS, Locke FL, Bartlett NL, Lekakis LJ, Miklos DB, Jacobson CA, et al. Axicabtagene ciloleucel CAR T-cell therapy in refractory large B-cell lymphoma. *N Engl J Med.* (2017) 377:2531–44. doi: 10.1056/NEJMoa1707447
29. Mullard A. FDA approves first CAR T therapy. *Nat Rev Drug Discov.* (2017) 16:669. doi: 10.1038/nrd.2017.196
30. Kalos M, Levine BL, Porter DL, Katz S, Grupp SA, Bagg A, et al. T cells with chimeric antigen receptors have potent antitumor effects and can establish memory in patients with advanced leukemia. *Sci Transl Med.* (2011) 3:95ra73. doi: 10.1126/scitranslmed.3002842
31. Wang Z, Guo Y, Han W. Current status and perspectives of chimeric antigen receptor modified T cells for cancer treatment. *Protein Cell.* (2017) 8:896–925. doi: 10.1007/s13238-017-0400-z
32. Maus MV, June CH. Making better chimeric antigen receptors for adoptive T-cell therapy. *Clin Cancer Res.* (2016) 22:1875–84. doi: 10.1158/1078-0432.CCR-15-1433
33. Kenderian SS, Porter DL, Gill S. Chimeric antigen receptor T cells and hematopoietic cell transplantation: how not to put the CART before the horse. *Biol Blood Marrow Transplant.* (2017) 23:235–46. doi: 10.1016/j.bbmt.2016.09.002
34. Tang XY, Sun Y, Zhang A, Hu GL, Cao W, Wang DH, et al. Third-generation CD28/4-1BB chimeric antigen receptor T cells for chemotherapy relapsed or refractory acute lymphoblastic leukaemia: A non-randomised, open-label phase I trial protocol. *BMJ Open.* (2016) 6:e013904. doi: 10.1136/bmjopen-2016-013904
35. Zhang C, Liu J, Zhong, JF, Zhang X. Engineering CAR-T cells. *Biomark Res.* (2017) 5:22. doi: 10.1186/s40364-017-0102-y
36. Sadelain M, Brentjens R, Rivière I. The basic principles of chimeric antigen receptor design. *Cancer Discov.* (2013) 3:388–98. doi: 10.1158/2159-8290.CD-12-0548
37. Lee DW, Kochenderfer JN, Stetler-Stevenson M, Cui YK, Delbrook C, Feldman SA, et al. T cells expressing CD19 chimeric antigen receptors for acute lymphoblastic leukaemia in children and young adults: A phase 1 dose-escalation trial. *Lancet.* (2015) 385:517–28. doi: 10.1016/S0140-6736(14)61403-3
38. Zhao J, Lin Q, Song Y, Liu D. Universal CARs, universal T cells, and universal CAR T cells. *J Hematol Oncol.* (2018) 11:132. doi: 10.1186/s13045-018-0677-2

39. Gardner RA, Finney O, Annesley C, Brakke H, Summers C, Leger K, et al. Intent-to-treat leukemia remission by CD19 CAR T cells of defined formulation and dose in children and young adults. *Blood.* (2017) 129:3322–31. doi: 10.1182/blood-2017-02-769208
40. Thistlethwaite FC, Gilham DE, Guest RD, Rothwell DG, Pillai M, Burt DJ, et al. The clinical efficacy of first-generation carcinoembryonic antigen (CEACAM5)-specific CAR T cells is limited by poor persistence and transient pre-conditioning-dependent respiratory toxicity. *Cancer Immunol Immunother.* (2017) 66:1425–36. doi: 10.1007/s00262-017-2034-7
41. Kandalaft LE, Powell DJ, Coukos G. A phase I clinical trial of adoptive transfer of folate receptor-alpha redirected autologous T cells for recurrent ovarian cancer. *J Transl Med.* (2012) 10:157. doi: 10.1186/1479-5876-10-157
42. Deniger DC, Kwong ML, Pasetto A, Dudley ME, Wunderlich JR, Langhan MM, et al. A pilot trial of the combination of vemurafenib with adoptive cell therapy in patients with metastatic melanoma. *Clin Cancer Res.* (2017) 23:351–362. doi: 10.1158/1078-0432.CCR-16-0906
43. O'Rourke DM, Nasrallah MP, Desai A, Melenhorst JJ, Mansfield K, Morrissette JJD, et al. A single dose of peripherally infused EGFRvIII-directed CAR T cells mediates antigen loss and induces adaptive resistance in patients with recurrent glioblastoma. *Sci Transl Med.* (2017) 9:eaaa0984. doi: 10.1126/scitranslmed.aaa0984
44. Zhang C, Wang Z, Yang Z, Wang M, Li S, Li Y, et al. Phase I escalating-dose trial of CAR-T therapy targeting CEA(+) metastatic colorectal cancers. *Mol Ther.* (2017) 25:1248–58. doi: 10.1016/j.ymthe.2017.03.010
45. Fraietta JA, Nobles CL, Sammons MA, Lundh S, Carty SA, Reich TJ, et al. Disruption of TET2 promotes the therapeutic efficacy of CD19-targeted T cells. *Nature.* (2018) 558:307–12. doi: 10.1038/s41586-018-0178-z
46. Ruella M, Kenderian SS. Next-generation chimeric antigen receptor T-cell therapy: going off the shelf. *Bio Drugs.* (2017) 31:473–81. doi: 10.1007/s40259-017-0247-0
47. Cohen AD. CAR T cells and other cellular therapies for multiple myeloma: 2018 update. *Am Soc Clin Oncol Educ Book.* 2018:e6–15. doi: 10.1200/EDBK_200889
48. Johnson LA, June CH. Driving gene-engineered T cell immunotherapy of cancer. *Cell Res.* (2016) 27:38–58. doi: 10.1038/cr.2016.154
49. Norelli M, Camisa B, Barbiera G, Falcone L, Purevdorj A, Genua M, et al. Monocyte-derived IL-1 and IL-6 are differentially required for cytokine-release syndrome and neurotoxicity due to CAR T cells. *Nat Med.* (2018) 24:739–48. doi: 10.1038/s41591-018-0036-4
50. Giavridis T, van der Stegen SJC, Eyquem J, Hamieh M, Piersigilli A, Sadelain M. CAR T cell-induced cytokine release syndrome is mediated by macrophages and abated by IL-1 blockade. *Nat Med.* (2018) 24:731–8. doi: 10.1038/s41591-018-0041-7
51. Hay KA, Hanafi LA, Li D, Gust J, Liles WC, Wurfel MM, et al. Kinetics and biomarkers of severe cytokine release syndrome after CD19 chimeric antigen receptor-modified T-cell therapy. *Blood.* (2017) 130:2295–306. doi: 10.1182/blood-2017-06-793141
52. Wang Z, Han W. Biomarkers of cytokine release syndrome and neurotoxicity related to CAR-T cell therapy. *Biomarker Res.* (2018) 6:4. doi: 10.1186/s40364-018-0116-0
53. Maude SL, Frey N, Shaw PA, Aplenc R, Barrett DM, Bunin NJ, et al. Chimeric antigen receptor T cells for sustained remissions in leukemia. *N Engl J Med.* (2014) 371:1507–17. doi: 10.1056/NEJMoa1407222
54. Barrett DM, Grupp SA, June CH. Chimeric antigen receptor- and TCR-modified T cells enter main street and wall street. *J Immunol.* (2015) 195:755–61. doi: 10.4049/jimmunol.1500751
55. Krenciute G, Prinzing BL, Yi Z, Wu MF, Liu H, Dotti G, et al. Transgenic expression of IL15 improves antiglioma activity of IL13Ralpha2-CAR T cells but results in antigen-loss variants. *Cancer Immunol Res.* (2017) 19(Suppl. 4):iv31. doi: 10.1093/neuonc/nox083.127
56. Seo H, Chen J, González-Avalos E, Samaniego-Castruita D, Das A, Wang YH, et al. TOX and TOX2 transcription factors cooperate with NR4A transcription factors to impose $CD8^+$ T cell exhaustion. *Proc Natl Acad Sci.* (2019) 116:12410–5. doi: 10.1073/pnas.1905675116
57. Chen J, López-Moyado IF, Seo H, Lio CJ, Hempleman LJ, Sekiya T, et al. NR4A transcription factors limit CAR T cell function in solid tumours. *Nature.* (2019) 567:530–4. doi: 10.1038/s41586-019-0985-x
58. Guedan S, Posey AD, Shaw C, Wing A, Da T, Patel PR, et al. Enhancing CAR T cell persistence through ICOS and 4-1BB costimulation. *JCI Insight.* (2018) 3:96976. doi: 10.1172/jci.insight.96976
59. Brodt P. Role of the microenvironment in liver metastasis: From pre- to prometastatic niches. *Clin Cancer Res.* (2016) 22:5971–82. doi: 10.1158/1078-0432.CCR-16-0460
60. Kasakovski D, Xu L, Li Y. T cell senescence and CAR-T cell exhaustion in hematological malignancies. *J Hematol Oncol.* (2018) 11:91. doi: 10.1186/s13045-018-0629-x
61. Newick K, Moon E, Albelda SM. Chimeric antigen receptor T-cell therapy for solid tumors. *Mol Ther Oncol.* (2016) 3:E191. doi: 10.1038/mto.2016.6
62. Zhong XS, Matsushita M, Plotkin J, Riviere I, Sadelain M. Chimeric antigen receptors combining 4-1BB and CD28 signaling domains augment PI 3 kinase/AKT/Bcl-X L activation and CD8 + T cell–mediated tumor eradication. *Mol Ther.* (2010) 18:413–20. doi: 10.1038/mt.2009.210
63. Hernandez I, Prasad V, Gellad WF. Total costs of chimeric antigen receptor T-cell immunotherapy. *JAMA Oncol.* (2018) 4:E1–3. doi: 10.1001/jamaoncol.2018.0977
64. Whittington MD, Ollendorf DA, Campbell JD. Accounting for all costs in the total cost of chimeric antigen receptor T-cell immunotherapy accounting for all costs in the total cost of chimeric antigen receptor T-cell immunotherapy letters. *JAMA Oncol.* (2018) 4:1784–5. doi: 10.1001/jamaoncol.2018.4625
65. Calmels B, Mfarrej B, Chabannon C. From clinical proof-of-concept to commercialization of CAR T cells. *Drug Discov Today.* (2018) 23:758–62. doi: 10.1016/j.drudis.2018.01.024
66. Zhao WH, Liu J, Wang BY, Chen YX, Cao XM, Yang Y, et al. A phase 1, open-label study of LCAR-B38M, a chimeric antigen receptor T cell therapy directed against B cell maturation antigen, in patients with relapsed or refractory multiple myeloma. *J Hematol Oncol.* (2018) 11:141. doi: 10.1186/s13045-018-0681-6
67. Yang F, Zhang J, Zhang X, Tian M, Wang J, Kang L, et al. Delayed remission following sequential infusion of humanized CD19- and CD22-modified CAR-T cells in a patient with relapsed/refractory acute lymphoblastic leukemia and prior exposure to murine-derived CD19-directed CAR-T cells. *Onco Targets Ther.* (2019) 12:2187–91. doi: 10.2147/OTT.S189103
68. Kosti P, Maher J, Arnold JN. Perspectives on chimeric antigen receptor T-cell immunotherapy for solid tumors. *Front Immunol.* (2018) 9:1104. doi: 10.3389/fimmu.2018.01104
69. Scott EM, Duffy MR, Freedman JD, Fisher KD, Seymour LW. Solid tumor immunotherapy with T cell engager-armed oncolytic viruses. *Macromol Biosci.* (2017) 18:1700187. doi: 10.1002/mabi.201700187
70. Weng J, Lai P, Qin L, Lai Y, Jiang Z, Luo C, et al. A novel generation 1928zT2 CAR T cells induce remission in extramedullary relapse of acute lymphoblastic leukemia. *J Hematol Oncol.* (2018) 11:25. doi: 10.1186/s13045-018-0572-x
71. Zhu YM, Wu Z, Tan YP, Du YY, Liu Z, Ou RM, et al. Anti-CD19 chimeric antigen receptor T-cell therapy for adult Philadelphia chromosome-positive acute lymphoblastic leukemia: two case reports. *Medicine.* (2016) 95:e5676. doi: 10.1097/MD.0000000000005676
72. Turtle CJ, Hanafi LA, Berger C, Gooley TA, Cherian S, Hudecek M, et al. CD19 CAR-T cells of defined CD4+:CD8+ composition in adult B cell ALL patients. *J Clin Invest.* (2016) 126:2123–38. doi: 10.1172/JCI85309
73. Wang CM, Wu ZQ, Wang Y, Guo YL, Dai HR, Wang XH, et al. Autologous T cells expressing CD30 chimeric antigen receptors for relapsed or refractory Hodgkin lymphoma: an open-label phase I trial. *Clin Cancer Res.* (2017) 23:1156–66. doi: 10.1158/1078-0432.CCR-16-1365
74. Kochenderfer JN, Dudley ME, Kassim SH, Somerville RP, Carpenter RO, Stetler-Stevenson M, et al. Chemotherapy-refractory diffuse large B-cell lymphoma and indolent B-cell malignancies can be effectively treated with autologous T cells expressing an anti-CD19 chimeric antigen receptor. *J Clin Oncol.* (2015) 33:540–9. doi: 10.1200/JCO.2014.56.2025
75. Porter DL, Hwang WT, Frey NV, Lacey SF, Shaw PA, Loren AW, et al. Chimeric antigen receptor T cells persist and induce sustained remissions

in relapsed refractory chronic lymphocytic leukemia. *Sci Transl Med.* (2015) 7:303ra139. doi: 10.1126/scitranslmed.aac5415
76. Davila ML, Riviere I, Wang X, Bartido S, Park J, Curran K, et al. Efficacy and toxicity management of 19-28z CAR T cell therapy in B cell acute lymphoblastic leukemia. *Sci Transl Med.* (2014) 6:224ra225. doi: 10.1126/scitranslmed.3008226
77. Turtle CJ, Hanafi LA, Berger C, Hudecek M, Pender B, Robinson E, et al. Immunotherapy of non-Hodgkin's lymphoma with a defined ratio of $CD8^+$ and $CD4^+$ CD19-specific chimeric antigen receptor–modified T cells. *Sci Translat Med.* (2016) 8:355ra116. doi: 10.1126/scitranslmed.aaf8621
78. Wang Y, Zhang WY, Han QW, Liu Y, Dai HR, Guo YL, et al. Effective response and delayed toxicities of refractory advanced diffuse large B-cell lymphoma treated by CD20-directed chimeric antigen receptor-modified T cells. *Clin Immunol.* (2014) 155:160–75. doi: 10.1016/j.clim.2014.10.002
79. Fry TJ, Shah NN, Orentas RJ, Stetler-Stevenson M, Yuan CM, Ramakrishna S, et al. CD22-targeted CAR T cells induce remission in B-ALL that is naive or resistant to CD19-targeted CAR immunotherapy. *Nat Med.* (2017) 24:20–8. doi: 10.1038/nm.4441
80. Ramos CA, Ballard B, Zhang H, Dakhova O, Gee AP, Mei Z, et al. Clinical and immunological responses after CD30-specific chimeric antigen receptor-redirected lymphocytes. *J Clin Investig.* (2017) 127:3462–71. doi: 10.1172/JCI94306
81. Ritchie DS, Neeson PJ, Khot A, Peinert S, Tai T, Tainton K, et al. Persistence and efficacy of second generation CAR T cell against the LeY antigen in acute myeloid leukemia. *Mol Ther.* (2013) 21:2122–9. doi: 10.1038/mt.2013.154
82. Garber K. Driving T-cell immunotherapy to solid tumors. *Nat Biotechnol.* (2018) 36:215–9. doi: 10.1038/nbt.4090
83. Feng K, Guo Y, Dai H, Wang Y, Li X, Jia H, et al. Chimeric antigen receptor-modified T cells for the immunotherapy of patients with EGFR-expressing advanced relapsed/refractory non-small cell lung cancer. *Sci China Life Sci.* (2016) 59:468–79. doi: 10.1007/s11427-016-5023-8
84. Louis CU, Savoldo B, Dotti G, Pule M, Yvon E, Myers GD, et al. Antitumor activity and long-term fate of chimeric antigen receptor-positive T cells in patients with neuroblastoma. *Blood.* (2011) 118:6050–6. doi: 10.1182/blood-2011-05-354449
85. Gargett T, Yu W, Dotti G, Yvon ES, Christo SN, Hayball JD, et al. GD2-specific CAR T cells undergo potent activation and deletion following antigen encounter but can be protected from activation-induced cell death by PD-1 blockade. *Mol Ther.* (2016) 24:1135–49. doi: 10.1038/mt.2016.63
86. Brown CE, Badie B, Barish ME, Weng L, Ostberg JR, Chang WC, et al. Bioactivity and safety of IL13Ralpha2-redirected chimeric antigen receptor CD8+ T cells in patients with recurrent glioblastoma. *Clin Cancer Res.* (2015) 21:4062–72. doi: 10.1158/1078-0432.CCR-15-0428
87. Brown CE, Alizadeh D, Starr R, Weng L, Wagner JR, Naranjo A, et al. Regression of glioblastoma after chimeric antigen receptor T-cell therapy. *N Engl J Med.* (2016) 375:2561–9. doi: 10.1056/NEJMoa1610497
88. Ahmed N, Brawley VS, Hegde M, Robertson C, Ghazi A, Gerken C, et al. Human epidermal growth factor receptor 2 (HER2)-specific chimeric antigen receptor-modified T cells for the immunotherapy of HER2-positive sarcoma. *J Clin Oncol.* (2015) 33:1688–96. doi: 10.1200/JCO.2014.58.0225
89. Lamers CH, Willemsen R, van Elzakker P, van Steenbergen-Langeveld S, Broertjes M, Oosterwijk-Wakka J, et al. Immune responses to transgene and retroviral vector in patients treated with *ex vivo*-engineered T cells. *Blood.* (2011) 117:72–82. doi: 10.1182/blood-2010-07-294520
90. Lamers CH, Sleijfer S, van Steenbergen S, van Elzakker P, van Krimpen B, Groot C, et al. Treatment of metastatic renal cell carcinoma with CAIX CAR-engineered T cells: Clinical evaluation and management of on-target toxicity. *Mol Ther.* (2013) 21:904–12. doi: 10.1038/mt.2013.17
91. Maus MV, Haas AR, Beatty GL, Albelda SM, Levine BL, Liu X, et al. T cells expressing chimeric antigen receptors can cause anaphylaxis in humans. *Cancer Immunol Res.* (2013) 1:26–31. doi: 10.1158/2326-6066.CIR-13-0006
92. Beatty GL, Haas AR, Maus MV, Torigian DA, Soulen MC, Plesa G, et al. Mesothelin-specific chimeric antigen receptor mRNA-engineered T cells induce anti-tumor activity in solid malignancies. *Cancer Immunol Res.* (2014) 2:112–20. doi: 10.1158/2326-6066.CIR-13-0170
93. You F, Jiang L, Zhang B, Lu Q, Zhou Q, Liao X, et al. Phase 1 clinical trial demonstrated that MUC1 positive metastatic seminal vesicle cancer can be effectively eradicated by modified anti-MUC1 chimeric antigen receptor transduced T cells. *Sci China Life Sci.* (2016) 59:386–97. doi: 10.1007/s11427-016-5024-7
94. Katz SC, Burga RA, McCormack E, Wang LJ, Mooring W, Point GR, et al. Phase I hepatic immunotherapy for metastases study of intra-arterial chimeric antigen receptor-modified T-cell therapy for CEA+ liver metastases. *Clin Cancer Res.* (2015) 21:3149–59. doi: 10.1158/1078-0432.CCR-14-1421
95. Ali SA, Shi V, Maric I, Wang M, Stroncek DF, Rose JJ, et al. T cells expressing an anti-B-cell maturation antigen chimeric antigen receptor cause remissions of multiple myeloma. *Blood.* (2016) 128:1688–700. doi: 10.1182/blood-2016-04-711903
96. Tchou J, Zhao Y, Levine BL, Zhang PJ, Davis MM, Melenhorst JJ, et al. Safety and efficacy of intratumoral injections of chimeric antigen receptor (CAR) T cells in metastatic breast cancer. *Cancer Immunol Res.* (2017) 5:1152–61. doi: 10.1158/2326-6066.CIR-17-0189
97. Junghans RP, Ma Q, Rathore R, Gomes EM, Bais AJ, Lo AS, et al. Phase I trial of anti-PSMA designer CAR-T cells in prostate cancer: Possible role for interacting interleukin 2-T cell pharmacodynamics as a determinant of clinical response. *Prostate.* (2016) 76:1257–70. doi: 10.1002/pros.23214
98. Hege KM, Bergsland EK, Fisher GA, Nemunaitis JJ, Warren RS, McArthur JG, et al. Safety, tumor trafficking and immunogenicity of chimeric antigen receptor (CAR)-T cells specific for TAG-72 in colorectal cancer. *J Immunother Cancer.* (2017) 5:22. doi: 10.1186/s40425-017-0222-9
99. Smith TT, Moffett HF, Stephan SB, Opel CF, Dumigan AG, Jiang X, et al. Biopolymers codelivering engineered T cells and STING agonists can eliminate heterogeneous tumors. *J Clin Investig.* (2017) 127:2176–91. doi: 10.1172/JCI87624
100. Kueberuwa G, Kalaitsidou M, Cheadle E, Hawkins RE, Gilham DE. CD19 CAR T-cells expressing IL-12 eradicate lymphoma in fully lymphoreplete mice through induction of host immunity. *Mol Ther Oncol.* (2018) 8:41–51. doi: 10.1016/j.omto.2017.12.003
101. Zhang N, Chen J, Ferraro GB, Wu L, Datta M, Jain RK, et al. Anti-VEGF treatment improves neurological function in tumors of the nervous system. *Exp Neurol.* (2017) 299(Pt B):326–33. doi: 10.1016/j.expneurol.2017.09.008
102. Xu Y, Yang Z, Horan LH, Zhang P, Liu L, Zimdahl B, et al. A novel antibody-TCR (AbTCR) platform combines Fab-based antigen recognition with gamma/delta-TCR signaling to facilitate T-cell cytotoxicity with low cytokine release. *Cell Discov.* (2018) 4:62. doi: 10.1038/s41421-018-0066-6
103. Blüthmann H, Kisielow P, Uematsu Y, Malissen M, Krimpenfort P, Berns A, et al. T-cell-specific deletion of T-cell receptor transgenes allows functional rearrangement of endogenous α- and β-genes. *Nature.* (1988) 334:156–9. doi: 10.1038/334156a0
104. Rapoport AP, Stadtmauer EA, Binder-Scholl GK, Goloubeva O, Vogl DT, Lacey SF, et al. NY-ESO-1-specific TCR-engineered T cells mediate sustained antigen-specific antitumor effects in myeloma. *Nat Med.* (2015) 21:914–21. doi: 10.1038/nm.3910
105. Kavunja HW, Lang S, Sungsuwan S, Yin Z, Huang X. Delivery of foreign cytotoxic T lymphocyte epitopes to tumor tissues for effective antitumor immunotherapy against pre-established solid tumors in mice. *Cancer Immunol Immunother.* (2017) 66:451–60. doi: 10.1007/s00262-016-1948-9
106. Tawara I, Kageyama S, Miyahara Y, Fujiwara H, Nishida T, Akatsuka Y, et al. Safety and persistence of WT1-specific T-cell receptor gene-transduced lymphocytes in patients with AML and MDS. *Blood.* (2017) 130:1985–94. doi: 10.1182/blood-2017-06-791202
107. Johnson LA, Morgan RA, Dudley ME, Cassard L, Yang JC, Hughes MS, et al. Gene therapy with human and mouse T-cell receptors mediates cancer regression and targets normal tissues expressing cognate antigen. *Blood.* (2009) 114:535–46. doi: 10.1182/blood-2009-03-211714
108. Parkhurst MR, Yang JC, Langan RC, Dudley ME, Nathan DA, Feldman SA, et al. T cells targeting carcinoembryonic antigen can mediate regression of metastatic colorectal cancer but induce severe transient colitis. *Mol Ther.* (2011) 19:620–6. doi: 10.1038/mt.2010.272
109. Robbins PF, Morgan RA, Feldman SA, Yang JC, Sherry RM, Dudley ME, et al. Tumor regression in patients with metastatic synovial cell sarcoma and melanoma using genetically engineered lymphocytes reactive with NY-ESO-1. *J Clin Oncol.* (2011) 29:917–24. doi: 10.1200/JCO.2010.32.2537
110. Linette GP, Stadtmauer EA, Maus MV, Rapoport AP, Levine BL, Emery L, et al. Cardiovascular toxicity and titin cross-reactivity of

affinity-enhanced T cells in myeloma and melanoma. *Blood.* (2013) 122:863–71. doi: 10.1182/blood-2013-03-490565

111. Kageyama S, Ikeda H, Miyahara Y, Imai N, Ishihara M, Saito K, et al. Adoptive transfer of MAGE-A4 T-cell receptor gene-transduced lymphocytes in patients with recurrent esophageal cancer. *Clin Cancer Res.* (2015) 21:2268–77. doi: 10.1158/1078-0432.CCR-14-1559

112. Peng PD, Cohen CJ, Yang S, Hsu C, Jones S, Zhao Y, et al. Efficient nonviral Sleeping Beauty transposon-based TCR gene transfer to peripheral blood lymphocytes confers antigen-specific antitumor reactivity. *Gene Ther.* (2009) 16:1042–9. doi: 10.1038/gt.2009.54

16

Expression of the Circadian Clock Gene *BMAL1* Positively Correlates with Antitumor Immunity and Patient Survival in Metastatic Melanoma

Leonardo Vinícius Monteiro de Assis[1*†], *Gabriela Sarti Kinker*[2*†], *Maria Nathália Moraes*[1], *Regina P. Markus*[2], *Pedro Augusto Fernandes*[2] *and Ana Maria de Lauro Castrucci*[1,3]

[1] Laboratory of Comparative Physiology of Pigmentation, Department of Physiology, Institute of Biosciences, University of São Paulo, São Paulo, Brazil, [2] Laboratory of Neuroimmunemodulation, Department of Physiology, Institute of Biosciences, University of São Paulo, São Paulo, Brazil, [3] Department of Biology, University of Virginia, Charlottesville, VA, United States

Edited by:
Svetlana Karakhanova,
Universität Heidelberg, Germany

Reviewed by:
Derre Laurent,
Centre Hospitalier Universitaire Vaudois (CHUV), Switzerland
Zsuzsanna Lengyel,
University of Pécs, Hungary

***Correspondence:**
Leonardo Vinícius Monteiro de Assis
deassis.leonardo@usp.br;
Gabriela Sarti Kinker
gabriela.kinker@usp.br

†These authors have contributed equally to this work.

Introduction: Melanoma is the most lethal type of skin cancer, with increasing incidence and mortality rates worldwide. Multiple studies have demonstrated a link between cancer development/progression and circadian disruption; however, the complex role of tumor-autonomous molecular clocks remains poorly understood. With that in mind, we investigated the pathophysiological relevance of clock genes expression in metastatic melanoma.

Methods: We analyzed gene expression, somatic mutation, and clinical data from 340 metastatic melanomas from The Cancer Genome Atlas, as well as gene expression data from 234 normal skin samples from genotype-tissue expression. Findings were confirmed in independent datasets.

Results: In melanomas, the expression of most clock genes was remarkably reduced and displayed a disrupted pattern of co-expression compared to the normal skins, indicating a dysfunctional circadian clock. Importantly, we demonstrate that the expression of the clock gene aryl hydrocarbon receptor nuclear translocator-like protein 1 (*BMAL1*) positively correlates with patient overall survival and with the expression of T-cell activity and exhaustion markers in the tumor bulk. Accordingly, high *BMAL1* expression in pretreatment samples was significantly associated with clinical benefit from immune checkpoint inhibitors. The robust intratumoral T-cell infiltration/activation observed in patients with high *BMAL1* expression was associated with a decreased expression of key DNA-repair enzymes, and with an increased mutational/neoantigen load.

Conclusion: Overall, our data corroborate previous reports regarding the impact of *BMAL1* expression on the cellular DNA-repair capacity and indicate that alterations in the tumor-autonomous molecular clock could influence the cellular composition of the surrounding microenvironment. Moreover, we revealed the potential of *BMAL1* as a clinically relevant prognostic factor and biomarker for T-cell-based immunotherapies.

Keywords: skin cancer, melanoma, circadian rhythms, clock genes, ARNTL/BMAL1 immunotherapy

SIGNIFICANCE

Here, we provide a first glimpse regarding the impact of a disrupted tumor-autonomous molecular clock on the cellular composition of the tumor microenvironment through the modulation of DNA-repair capacity. Within this line, our data revealed the potential of *BMAL1* as a clinically relevant biomarker for immunotherapy response and overall survival of patients with metastatic melanoma.

INTRODUCTION

Melanoma is the most lethal type of skin cancer, with increasing incidence and mortality rates worldwide (1, 2). It represents only 4% of skin cancer but accounts for approximately 80% of skin cancer-related death (3). Although complete surgical resection is often curative for melanomas detected at initial stages, patients with metastatic disease have an overall survival of approximately 5 months (4). Therapeutic options for patients with metastatic melanoma have dramatically changed in the past years, with the introduction of more effective agents such as proto-oncogene, serine/theronine kinase (BRAF), mitogen activated protein kinase kinase (MAPK), and immunotherapeutic antibodies directed to cytotoxic T-lymphocyte-associated antigen 4 (CTLA-4), programmed cell-death protein 1 (PD-1) and its ligand (PD-L1) (5–8). Melanoma etiology is multifactorial and includes risk factors such as ultraviolet radiation exposure, genetic susceptibility, high nevus density, reduced skin pigmentation, and immunosuppression (9, 10).

Proper temporal control of physiological functions is crucial for maintaining the homeostasis of multi-cellular organisms (11–13). In mammals, the molecular machinery of timekeeping and circadian rhythm generation is based on interconnected positive and negative transcriptional–translational feedback loops. The central hypothalamic clock (suprachiasmatic nuclei, SCN) and clocks located in peripheral tissues share the same molecular architecture, engaging core genes such as aryl hydrocarbon receptor nuclear translocator-like protein 1 (*BMAL1* also known as *ARNTL*), cryptochrome 1 and 2 (*CRY1/2*), circadian locomotor output cycles kaput (*CLOCK*), period 1, 2, and 3 (*PER1/2/3*), receptor subfamily 1, group D, member 1/2 (*NRD1/2* also known as *REV-ERBα/β*), and RAR-related orphan receptor A and B (*RORA/B* also known as NR1F1/2). In healthy conditions, CLOCK–BMAL1 heterodimers translocate to the nucleus and induce the gene expression of their own inhibitors, PER and CRY proteins. This core oscillatory pathway is augmented and stabilized by a secondary loop involving *NRD1/2* and *RORA/B*, nuclear receptors that modulate *BMAL1* expression. Importantly, CLOCK–BMAL1 heterodimers also regulate the expression of several clock-controlled genes, which are tissue- and cell type-specific (11–13).

Many epidemiologic studies have demonstrated that the disturbance of biological rhythms through shift work, increased light exposure at night, and irregular feeding regimens (14–16) is associated with increased risk of developing several types of cancers (17–19). In fact, alterations in the cellular circadian machinery have been shown to affect cancer-related processes such as cell proliferation (20, 21), DNA damage response (22, 23), and metabolism (24–27) in a tumor-specific manner. Accordingly, the aberrant expression of clock core genes such as *CRY1*, *PER1*, and *PER2* has been shown to impact tumor progression in colorectal, prostate, and breast cancers, respectively (28–30).

In melanoma, mRNA levels and nuclear immunopositivity for CLOCK, CRY1, and PER1 are reduced compared to adjacent non-tumorous skin and present a significant association with clinicopathological features such as Breslow thickness (31). Moreover, the expression of RORA is lower in melanomas than in nevi, and positively correlates with overall survival and disease-free survival (32). Interestingly, enhancing the circadian clock function of melanoma cells impairs cell cycle progression and inhibits tumor growth *in vivo* (21). In this sense, we have previously demonstrated that the expression of clock core genes in murine melanoma cells can be activated by different stimulus, such as white light exposure (33), UVA radiation (34), estradiol (35), and thermal energy (36). Recently, we have demonstrated that a non-metastatic model of melanoma leads to a systemic chronodisruption in tumor-adjacent skin, lungs, liver, and SCN, as in these tissues the rhythmic expression of *Bmal1* was lost in tumor-bearing mice (37). These data reinforce that the modulation of tumor-autonomous clock might represent a novel and promising therapeutic strategy.

To further characterize the pathophysiological relevance of the molecular clock in skin cancer, we investigated the clinical value of clock core genes expression in metastatic melanoma, using public high-throughput molecular data. Overall, we revealed the robust prognostic power of *BMAL1* expression and provided evidence into its underlying biological processes.

MATERIALS AND METHODS

Datasets of Melanoma and Normal Skin Samples

Gene expression, somatic mutation, and clinical data from 340 metastatic melanomas from The Cancer Genome Atlas (TCGA) and gene expression data from 234 Genotype-Tissue Expression (GTEx) normal skin (not sun exposed) samples were downloaded from the UCSC XENA Browser (http://xena.ucsc.edu) in January of 2017. TCGA and GTEx gene expression data were originally generated by TCGA (38) and GTEx consortia (39), respectively, using the Illumina HiSeq 2000 RNA sequencing platform, quantified using RSEM, upper quartile normalized and $\log_2(x + 1)$ transformed. TCGA somatic mutation data were generated using the Illumina GAIIx DNA sequencing platform and somatic variants (SNPs and small indels) were identified using MuTect2. Neoantigen load information for TCGA metastatic melanoma samples was obtained from Rooney et al. (40). Briefly, for each metastatic melanoma patient, all novel amino acid 9–10mers resulting from missense mutations in expressed genes (median > 10 TPM) were identified. Mutant peptides with a HLA-binding affinity <500 nM, predicted by NetMHCpan (v2.4), were considered antigenic (41). Clinical information and gene expression data of pretreatment biopsies from 49 patients who received anti-PD1 immunotherapy (nivolumab) were obtained from Riaz et al. (42). Expression data were generated using the Illumina HiSeq 2000 RNA sequencing platform, counted using Rsamtools v3.2, upper quartile normalized and $\log_2(x + 1)$ transformed. Treatment response for patients was defined by RECIST v1.1.

Co-Expression Network Analysis

Undirected weighted co-expression networks were constructed based on the pairwise Spearman's correlation coefficients between the expression of clock core genes *BMAL1*, *CRY1*, *CRY2*, *NRD1*, *PER1*, *PER2*, *PER3*, and *RORA*. Using the CoGA R package (43), we compared the structural properties of co-expression networks from normal skin and metastatic melanomas by testing the equality in their spectral distributions (44, 45). The spectrum of a graph, defined as the set of eigenvalues of its adjacency matrix, describes several structural features and represents a comprehensive characterization of networks (44, 46). *P*-values were calculated based on 1,000 phenotype permutations and networks were visualized using the gplots R package.

Gene Set Enrichment Analysis (GSEA)

Genes in the TCGA expression dataset were ranked according to the Spearman's correlation coefficient between their expression and the expression of *BMAL1*. GSEA was performed using GSEA v3.0 and Reactome pathways (47, 48). Enrichment scores (ES) were calculated based on a weighted Kolmogorov–Smirnov-like statistic and normalized (NES) to account for the size of each gene set. *P*-values corresponding to each NES were calculated based on 1,000 phenotype permutations and corrected for multiple comparisons using the false discovery rate (FDR) procedure. Adjusted *P*-values < 0.05 were considered statistically significant.

Single Sample Gene Set Enrichment Analysis (ssGSEA)

Single sample gene set enrichment analysis, an extension of GSEA, was used to estimate the degree of enrichment of gene sets in individual samples within the TCGA gene expression dataset (49). For each sample, gene expression values were rank-normalized, and ESs were calculated based on the difference between weighted Empirical Cumulative Distribution Functions of genes inside and outside the gene sets. We performed ssGSEA using the GSVA R package (50) and DNA repair-related KEGG pathways (51), namely: base excision repair (hsa03410), nucleotide excision repair (hsa03420), mismatch repair (hsa03430), homologous recombination (hsa03440), and non-homologous end joining (hsa0345).

Statistical Analysis

We used the two-sided Wilcoxon–Mann–Whitney test to perform two-group comparisons, the Spearman's correlation test to assess ordinal associations, and the Chi-square test to analyze the relationship between two categorical variables. The impact of clock core genes expression on patient overall survival was evaluated using univariate Cox regressions. The prognostic power of *BMAL1* expression was further investigated using Kaplan–Meier curves, combined to the log-rank test, and multivariate Cox regressions. Hazard Ratios, including 95% confidence intervals, were calculated. Statistical analyses were performed with GraphPad Prism 6 and R (www.r-project.org). *P*-values < 0.05 were considered statistically significant. Where indicated, *P*-values were adjusted for multiple comparisons using the FDR procedure.

RESULTS

Clinical Relevance of Clock Core Genes Expression in Metastatic Melanomas

We first analyzed the expression of clock core genes in normal skin and in metastatic melanomas. Compared to normal skin, metastatic melanomas demonstrated a remarkably decreased expression of *BMAL1*, *CRY1*, *CRY2*, *NRD1*, *PER1*, *PER2*, *PER3*, and *RORA* and an increased expression of *CLOCK* (**Figure 1A**). In normal skin, we have found a classic pattern of clock gene expression: *PER*s and CRYs are concomitantly expressed (in phase) and are in antiphase with *BMAL1* and *CLOCK* expression, as expected; on the other hand, in metastatic melanomas such correlations are severely attenuated (**Figure 1B**), which further corroborates a dysfunctional circadian clock within the tumor. In metastatic melanomas, male presented increased percentage of tumor showing high expression of *NRD1*, *PER2*, and *PER3* ($P = 0.015$, $P = 0.028$, and $P < 0.001$, respectively; **Table 1**; Table S1 in Supplementary Material). Patients with high *PER3* expression were also significantly older and more frequently diagnosed with stage I–II tumors ($P = 0.002$ and $P = 0.037$, respectively; **Table 1**; Table S1 in Supplementary Material).

Next, using univariate Cox regressions we evaluated the clinical relevance of clock core genes in metastatic melanoma. Among all nine genes analyzed, only *BMAL1* showed a significant prognostic value: high *BMAL1* expression was associated with longer overall survival (HR = 0.678, $P = 0.002$; **Figures 1C,D**). Importantly, multivariate Cox regression adjusting for age, gender, tumor pathologic stage, ulceration status, mitotic count, and Breslow thickness revealed *BMAL1* expression as an independent prognostic factor (**Table 2**). Additionally, the prognostic value of *BMAL1* expression in metastatic melanomas was confirmed in two other independent datasets (GSE6590 and GSE54467; Figures S1A,B and Table S2 in Supplementary Material).

BMAL1 Expression and the Overall Biological Profile of Metastatic Melanoma

To investigate the biological mechanisms that likely underlie the impact of *BMAL1* expression on patient survival, we performed GSEA using genes ranked according to their Spearman's correlation with *BMAL1* expression. Significantly enriched pathways presented positive NES and were mainly involved in the activation of the immune system (**Figure 2A**). In fact, in metastatic

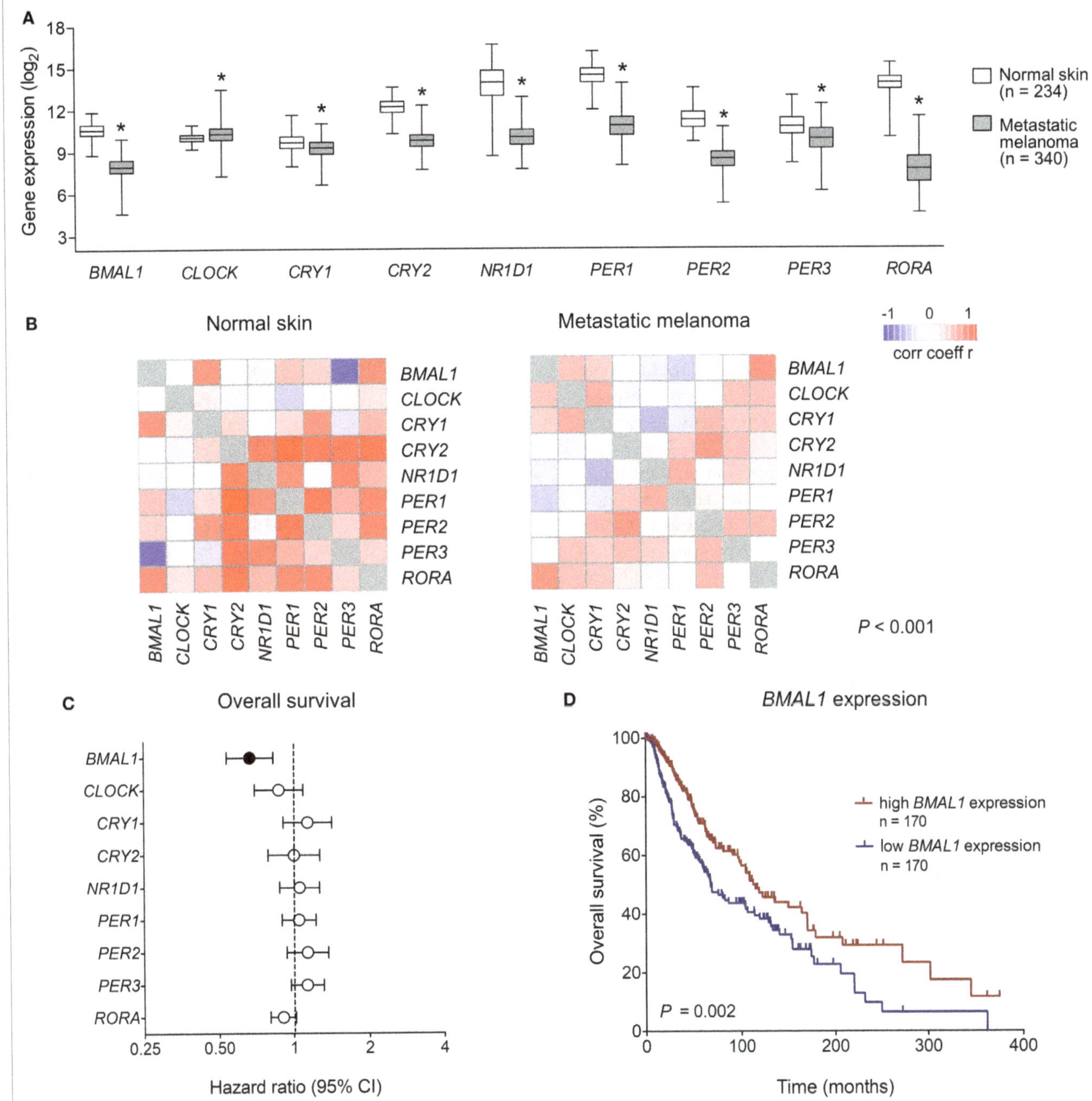

FIGURE 1 | Clinical relevance of clock genes expression in metastatic melanomas. **(A)** RNAseq analysis of clock genes expression in genotype-tissue expression (GTEx) normal skins (n = 234) and The Cancer Genome Atlas (TCGA) metastatic melanoma (n = 340). Expression values were estimated using RSEM and $\log_2(x + 1)$ transformed. The boxes extend from the 25th to the 75th percentile, the central bold line shows the median, and whiskers are drawn from minimum to maximum values. Comparisons were performed using the two-sided Wilcoxon–Mann–Whitney test. *Significantly different from normal skin ($P < 0.05$). **(B)** Co-expression matrix showing pairwise Spearman's correlation coefficients of clock core genes in GTEx normal skins (n = 234) and TCGA metastatic melanomas (n = 340). Networks were compared using the CoGA software. **(C)** Univariate Cox analysis of overall survival according to the expression of clock core genes in TCGA metastatic melanomas. Hazard Ratios including 95% confidence intervals are shown. Genes with a significant prognostic value ($P < 0.05$) are marked in black. **(D)** Kaplan–Meier survival curve according to the expression of aryl hydrocarbon receptor nuclear translocator-like protein 1 (*BMAL1*) in TCGA metastatic melanomas. The median expression of *BMAL1* was used as the cutoff to dichotomize the population. Comparisons were performed using the log-rank test.

melanomas, *BMAL1* expression exhibited a strong positive correlation with the expression of dendritic cell markers, T-cell markers *CD4* and *CD8A*, and T-cell activation/differentiation markers (**Figure 2B**). This robust intratumoral activation of leukocytes was accompanied by the expression of T-cells exhaustion markers (**Figure 2B**), such as *CTLA4*, *PD1*, and *PDL1*,

TABLE 1 | Clinicopathological features according to the expression of clock genes in The Cancer Genome Atlas metastatic melanomas.

	P-values*								
Variables	***BMAL1***	***CRY1***	***CRY2***	***CLOCK***	***NR1D1***	***PER1***	***PER2***	***PER3***	***RORA***
Age	0.59	0.592	0.998	0.151	0.057	0.19	0.754	**0.002**	0.286
Gender	0.659	0.271	0.269	0.269	**0.015**	0.06	**0.028**	**<0.001**	0.269
Pathologic stage	0.817	0.643	0.644	0.083	0.247	0.418	0.132	**0.037**	0.417
Ulceration status	1	0.404	0.094	0.889	1	0.78	0.267	0.889	1
Mitotic count	0.769	0.175	0.07	0.801	0.465	0.256	0.276	0.613	0.963
Breslow thickness	0.731	0.545	0.65	0.847	0.179	0.816	0.823	0.961	0.838

P-values in bold are statistically significant.
**Two-sided Wilcoxon–Mann–Whitney (continuous variables) or Chi-square exact test (categorical variable) comparing tumors with high vs. low expression.*

corroborating the fact that T-cell were chronically exposed to antigens (52, 53). Accordingly, patients with high *BMAL1* expression in pretreatment biopsies demonstrated improved response to anti-PD1 immunotherapy in comparison to patients expressing low *BMAL1* levels (**Figure 2C**).

The correlation between *BMAL1* expression and antitumor immune response was also confirmed in two additional independent datasets (GSE6590 and GSE54467; Figures S1C,D in Supplementary Material). Importantly, the expression of *BMAL1* was a prognostic factor independent of the percentage of leukocyte, monocyte, and neutrophil infiltration in TCGA melanomas (**Table 3**).

TABLE 2 | Multivariate Cox regression analysis of survival in The Cancer Genome Atlas metastatic melanomas.

	Overall survival	
Variables	**HR (95%CI)**	***P*-value**
Age	1.024 (1.007–1.041)	**0.006**
Gender		
Male vs. female	1.158 (0.655–2.051)	0.612
Pathologic stage		
III-IV vs. I-II	2.405 (1.427–4.053)	**<0.001**
Ulceration status		
Present vs. absent	0.994 (0.556–1.769)	0.985
Mitotic count	1.015 (0.986–1.045)	0.301
Breslow thickness	1.080 (1.004–1.161)	**0.038**
BMAL1 expression	0.525 (0.369–0.746)	**<0.001**

P-values in bold are statistically significant.
HR, hazard ratio; CI, confidence interval.

BMAL1 Expression and the Mutational Load in Metastatic Melanomas

Tumor somatic mutations can generate major histocompatibility complex Class I-associated neoantigens expression that plays a central role in inducing T-cell meditated antitumor cytolytic activity (54, 55). Interestingly, in metastatic melanomas, *BMAL1* expression positively correlated with the number of total somatic mutations and predicted neoantigens (**Figure 3A**). With that in mind, we investigated whether the expression of *BMAL1* was associated with the activation of different DNA-repair pathways. Using ssGSEA, we demonstrated that base excision repair is likely impaired in tumors expressing high *BMAL1* (**Figure 3B**). No significant differences were observed regarding the nucleotide excision repair, mismatch repair, homologous recombination, and non-homologous end joining DNA-repairing mechanisms. Importantly, the expression of base excision repair-related genes, such as *NTHL1*, *XRCC1*, and *SMUG1*, and the expression of general DNA repair-related genes, such as *POLD1*, *POLD2*, and *LIG1*, were downregulated in tumors expressing high *BMAL1* in all three datasets analyzed (**Figure 3C**; Figure S2 in Supplementary Material). High *BMAL1* expression was also associated with impaired DNA-repair capacity in human melanoma cell lines from the Cancer Cell Line Encyclopedia (Figure S3 in Supplementary Material).

DISCUSSION

Cancer onset, development, and progression have been linked to circadian disruption (17–19); however, the complex role of the tumor-autonomous molecular clock within these processes is yet poorly understood. Here, confirming previous reports in humans and in mice (32, 33, 35, 37), we showed that the expression of core components of the molecular clock machinery is severely repressed in melanomas. Moreover, we demonstrated that, for such tumors, high mRNA levels of *BMAL1* are associated with decreased gene expression of base excision repair enzymes and increased mutation load and predicted neoantigen presentation. The high incidence of antigenic peptides observed in metastatic melanomas with high *BMAL1* expression was accompanied by increased expression of cytotoxic T-cell activity markers in the tumor bulk and better prognosis. Even though our data do not provide a detailed mechanistic perspective, the present findings strongly support a role for *BMAL1* as a clinically relevant biomarker of DNA damage repair deficiency and intratumoral T-cell response. Thus, confirming such findings using common molecular techniques would be of great relevance for prognosis prediction and proposition of personalized therapeutic strategies.

Accumulating evidence implicates cell autonomous-circadian clocks in cancer development, as the disruption of peripheral systems of timekeeping seems to be a common event in malignant tissues (17, 18). As demonstrated here for metastatic melanomas, the expression of most clock core genes is downregulated in several types of cancers when compared to normal tissue (28, 32,

A

Reactome pathway	NES	Adjusted *P*-value
CYTOKINE SIGNALING IN IMMUNE SYSTEM	2.355	0.027
SIGNALING BY ILS	2.314	0.021
NUCLEOTIDE BINDING DOMAIN LEUCINE RICH REPEAT CONTAINING RECEPTOR NLR SIGNALING PATHWAYS	2.275	0.023
INNATE IMMUNE SYSTEM	2.256	0.024
NOD1 2 SIGNALING PATHWAY	2.212	0.035
IL1 SIGNALING	2.211	0.030
ADAPTIVE IMMUNE SYSTEM	2.210	0.025
TOLL RECEPTOR CASCADES	2.201	0.026
ACTIVATED TLR4 SIGNALLING	2.200	0.023
INTERFERON SIGNALING	2.194	0.023
MYD88 MAL CASCADE INITIATED ON PLASMA MEMBRANE	2.170	0.027
TCR SIGNALING	2.156	0.030
G ALPHA1213 SIGNALLING EVENTS	2.135	0.037
DOWNSTREAM TCR SIGNALING	2.135	0.034
REGULATION OF SIGNALING BY CBL	2.116	0.042
G ALPHA I SIGNALLING EVENTS	2.112	0.041
GASTRIN CREB SIGNALLING PATHWAY VIA PKC AND MAPK	2.105	0.041
TRAF6 MEDIATED INDUCTION OF NFKB AND MAP KINASES UPON TLR7 8 OR 9 ACTIVATION	2.093	0.045
INTERFERON GAMMA SIGNALING	2.080	0.049
IL 3 5 AND GM CSF SIGNALING	2.078	0.048
RIG I MDA5 MEDIATED INDUCTION OF IFN ALPHA BETA PATHWAYS	2.077	0.046
TRIF MEDIATED TLR3 SIGNALING	2.075	0.045

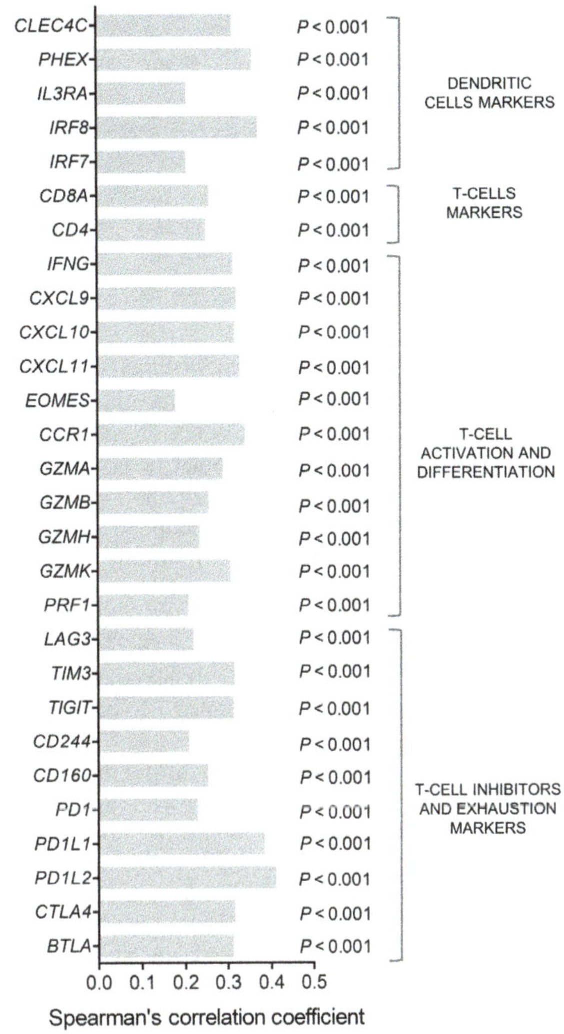

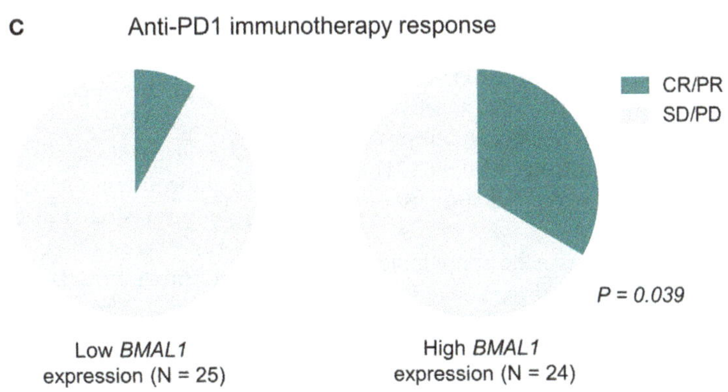

FIGURE 2 | Aryl hydrocarbon receptor nuclear translocator-like protein 1 (*BMAL1*) expression positively correlates with antitumor immunity in metastatic melanomas. **(A)** Gene Set Enrichment Analysis (GSEA) using genes ranked according to the Spearman's correlation coefficient between their expression and the expression of *BMAL1* in The Cancer Genome Atlas (TCGA) metastatic melanomas ($n = 340$). Normalized enrichment scores (NES) and *P*-values corrected by false discovery rate (FDR) were calculated using GSEA v3.0 and Reactome pathways. Only significantly enriched pathways (adjusted $P < 0.05$) are shown. **(B)** Spearman's correlation coefficient between the expression of *BMAL1* and immune cells markers in TCGA metastatic melanomas. *P*-values were corrected by FDR. **(C)** Association between *BMAL1* expression (pretreatment biopsies) and clinical benefit of melanoma patients from anti-PD1 immunotherapy (nivolumab). RNAseq data and treatment response information were obtained from Ref. (42). Comparisons were performed using the Chi-square test. CR, complete response; PR, partial response; SD, stable disease; PD, progressive disease.

TABLE 3 | Multivariate Cox regression analysis of overall survival in metastatic melanomas adjusted for the percentage of immune cell infiltration in The Cancer Genome Atlas metastatic melanomas.

Variables	Overall survival	
	HR (95% CI)	***P*-value**
% Lymphocyte infiltration	0.975 (0.932–1.019)	0.261
% Monocyte infiltration	1.001 (0.902–1.111)	0.974
% Neutrophil infiltration	0.956 (0.673–1.357)	0.901
BMAL1 expression	0.685 (0.550–0.854)	**<0.001**

P-values in bold are statistically significant.
HR, hazard ratio; CI, confidence interval.

56–61). Moreover, the overexpression of *PER1* and *PER2* has been shown to impair tumor proliferation and induce apoptosis in lung, prostate, and pancreatic cancer (29, 62, 63), reinforcing the idea that the molecular clock machinery may be considered as a new therapeutic target.

The protein encoded by *BMAL1* belongs to the family of the bHLH-PAS structural domain transcription factors and it is estimated to control the expression of more than 150 target genes, including the clock genes *CRY1*, *CRY2*, *NR1D1*, *PER1*, *PER2*, and *PER3* (64). *BMAL1* has also been revealed as a candidate gene for susceptibility to hypertension, diabetes, and obesity, and mutations in *BMAL1* have been linked to infertility and metabolic dysfunctions (65–70). Here, we demonstrated that, in metastatic melanomas, the expression of *BMAL1* is a robust positive prognostic factor of overall survival and has a negative association with the expression of key DNA-repair enzymes, such as *POLD1*, *POLD2*, and *LIG1*. Accordingly, in colorectal cancer, downregulation of *BMAL1* gene expression accelerates cell proliferation *in vitro*, promotes tumor growth in mice, and decreases DNA damage induced by cisplatin (71). Moreover, high *BMAL1* expression is associated with increased sensitivity of colorectal cancer cells to oxaliplatin *in vitro* and *in vivo*, and predicts favorable outcome for patients treated with oxaliplatin-based chemotherapy (72). *BMAL1* expression also positively correlates with patient survival in pancreatic ductal adenocarcinomas (61), causes growth inhibition in lymphoma/leukemia cells (58), negatively impacts DNA-repair capacity of mice fibroblast (73), but promotes proliferation in malignant pleura mesothelioma (74), suggesting that its role in tumorigenesis is complex and tissue-specific.

Although it has been shown that alterations in the tumor molecular clock impact some parameters of tumor progression (28–30, 62, 63), the influence of endogenous oscillatory systems on the cellular composition of the tumor microenvironment is largely unknown. In this sense, our data indicate that the prolonged survival of metastatic melanoma patients with high *BMAL1* bulk expression is associated with a robust intratumoral T-cell infiltration/activation, which can be partially explained by the increased neoantigen load that likely reflects the impaired DNA-repair capacity. Previous reports have also linked DNA-repair deficiency to increased mutational load and antitumor immune response in melanomas, lung, colorectal, and endometrial cancers (75–78). It is now clear that DNA repair and genomic instability have a pivotal role in the modulation of antitumor immune responses (79); thus, understanding their interplay with tumor-autonomous clocks may provide clinically relevant insights.

Immunotherapies that boost the ability of T lymphocytes to combat tumor cells have demonstrated therapeutic efficiency in a variety of solid tumors. Monoclonal antibodies against T-cell checkpoint proteins, such as CTLA-4, PD-1, and PD-L1, have now been approved for melanoma treatment and are associated with robust durable responses, but only in a subset of tumors (80–82). Thus, there is a need to identify biomarkers that will allow the selection of treatment-responsive patients, avoid unnecessary toxicity, and help personalize therapy regimens (83). Metastatic melanomas presenting high *BMAL1* expression have impaired DNA-repair capacity combined with increased mutation/neoantigen load, T-cell intratumoral infiltration, and T-cell expression of exhaustion markers, all of which have been shown to predict good clinical response to the treatment with immune checkpoint inhibitors (78, 84–87). In fact, we showed that high *BMAL1* expression in pretreatment melanoma samples is associated with clinical benefit from anti-PD1 immunotherapy. Considering that whole-genome and -transcriptome sequencing is expensive and time-consuming, profiling a smaller fraction of genes could serve as a useful tool to help translate those findings into routine clinical practices (88). Therefore, the present data indicate that *BMAL1* expression in melanoma patients must be considered as a relevant marker for immunotherapy efficacy. Nevertheless, larger clinical studies are necessary to validate the potential of *BMAL1* alone, or along with other biomarkers, in discriminating responders from non-responders in immunotherapy regiments.

CONCLUSION

The molecular characterization of melanomas using high-throughput approaches has the potential to generate insights into their biological heterogeneity, having important implications for prognosis and therapy. In this sense, our data highlight the relevance of further studies focusing on the biological and clinical relevance of the tumor-autonomous molecular clock machinery. Overall, we demonstrated that, in metastatic melanoma, a high bulk *BMAL1* expression seems to be associated with a "too tumorigenic" program and could be a marker for immunotherapy response.

ETHICS STATEMENT

All data presented in this manuscript are public and freely available. We did not perform any human or animal related experiments. All analyses and conclusions were drawn from the following public datasets: The Cancer Genome Atlas (TCGA), Genotype-Tissue Expression (GTEx), Gene Expression Omnibus, and datasets from Ref. (40, 42). In all mentioned

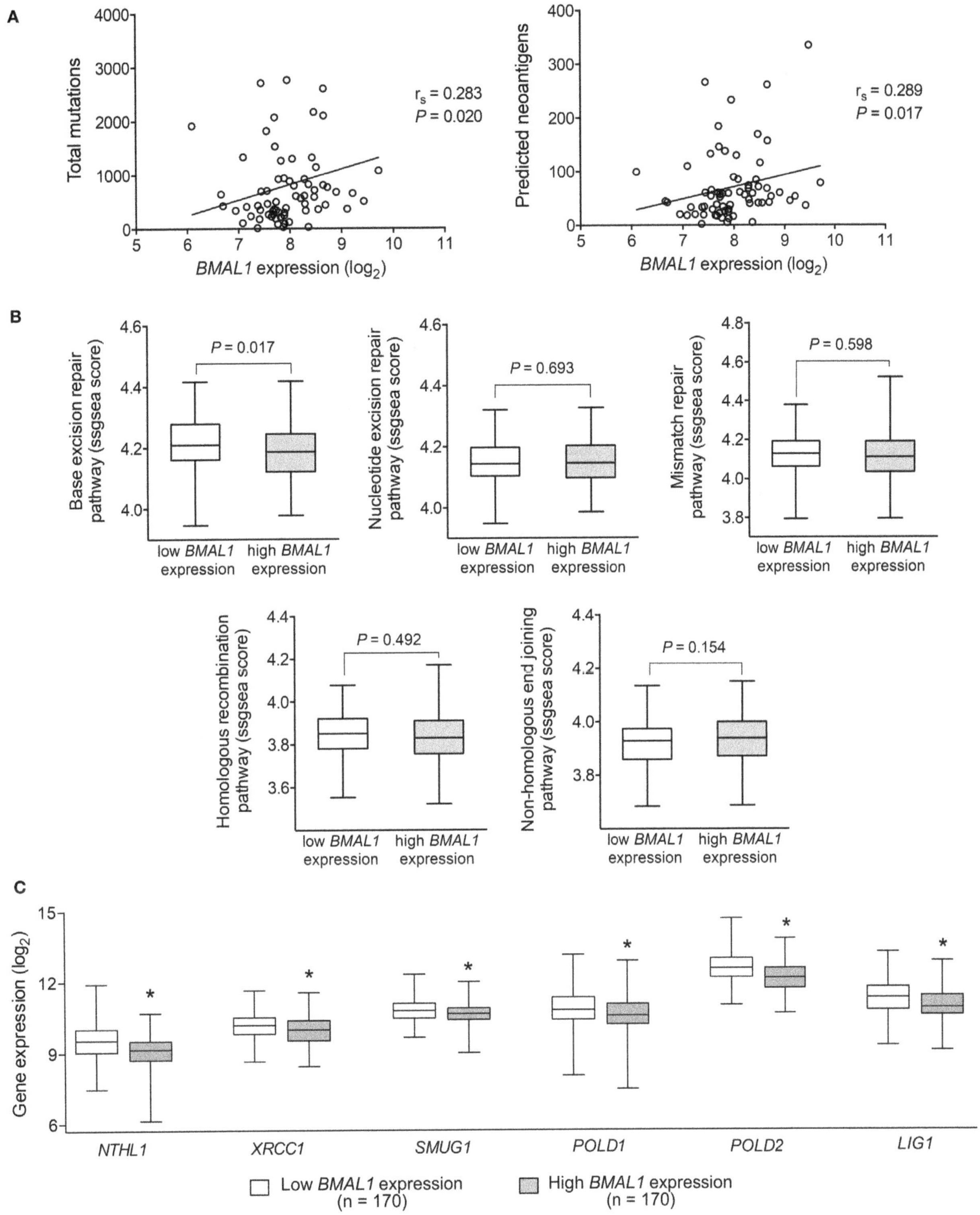

FIGURE 3 | Aryl hydrocarbon receptor nuclear translocator like protein 1 (*BMAL1*) expression positively correlates with the mutational and neoantigen load in metastatic melanomas. **(A)** Spearman's correlation between the expression of *BMAL1* and the number of total mutations and predicted neoantigens in The Cancer Genome Atlas (TCGA) metastatic melanomas (n = 68). NetMHCpan-predicted neoantigens were obtained from Ref. (40). Gene expression of **(B)** DNA-repair programs and **(C)** selected base excision repair enzymes according to the expression of *BMAL1* in TCGA metastatic melanomas (n = 340). Pathway scores were calculated using single sample Gene Set Enrichment Analysis available in the GSVA R package. The median expression of *BMAL1* was used as the cutoff to dichotomize the population. The boxes extend from the 25th to the 75th percentile, the central bold line shows the median, and whiskers are drawn from minimum to maximum values. Comparisons were performed using the two-sided Wilcoxon–Mann–Whitney test. *Significantly different from the low *BMAL1* group.

papers, the authors stated that all procedures were carried out according ethical rules.

AUTHOR CONTRIBUTIONS

LA and GK designed the study, analyzed the data, and drafted the manuscript. All authors provided insightful discussion during data acquisition and aided in the writing process of the manuscript. All authors critically revised the manuscript. All authors have approved the definitive version of the manuscript and agreed to be accountable for all aspects of the study in ensuring that questions related to the accuracy or integrity of any part of the study are appropriately investigated and resolved. All persons designated as authors qualify for authorship, and all those who qualify for authorship are listed.

REFERENCES

1. Garbe C, Leiter U. Melanoma epidemiology and trends. *Clin Dermatol* (2009) 27:3–9. doi:10.1016/j.clindermatol.2008.09.001
2. Erdei E, Torres SM. A new understanding in the epidemiology of melanoma. *Expert Rev Anticancer Ther* (2010) 10:1811–23. doi:10.1586/era.10.170
3. Jemal A, Siegel R, Ward E, Hao Y, Xu J, Murray T, et al. Cancer statistics, 2008. *CA Cancer J Clin* (2008) 58:71–96. doi:10.3322/CA.2007.0010
4. Song X, Zhao Z, Barber B, Farr AM, Ivanov B, Novich M. Overall survival in patients with metastatic melanoma. *Curr Med Res Opin* (2015) 31:987–91. doi:10.1185/03007995.2015.1021904
5. Chapman PB, Hauschild A, Robert C, Haanen JB, Ascierto P, Larkin J, et al. Improved survival with vemurafenib in melanoma with BRAF V600E mutation. *N Engl J Med* (2011) 364:2507–16. doi:10.1056/NEJMoa1103782
6. Grimaldi AM, Simeone E, Ascierto PA. The role of MEK inhibitors in the treatment of metastatic melanoma. *Curr Opin Oncol* (2014) 26:196–203. doi:10.1097/CCO.0000000000000050
7. Long GV, Stroyakovskiy D, Gogas H, Levchenko E, De Braud F, Larkin J, et al. Combined BRAF and MEK inhibition versus BRAF inhibition alone in melanoma. *N Engl J Med* (2014) 371:1877–88. doi:10.1056/NEJMoa1406037
8. Redman JM, Gibney GT, Atkins MB. Advances in immunotherapy for melanoma. *BMC Med* (2016) 14:20. doi:10.1186/s12916-016-0571-0
9. Markovic SN, Erickson LA, Rao RD, Weenig RH, Pockaj BA, Bardia A, et al. Malignant melanoma in the 21st century, part 1: epidemiology, risk factors, screening, prevention, and diagnosis. *Mayo Clin Proc* (2007) 82:364–80. doi:10.1016/S0025-6196(11)61033-1
10. Vuong K, Armstrong BK, Weiderpass E, Lund E, Adami HO, Veierod MB, et al. Development and external validation of a melanoma risk prediction model based on self-assessed risk factors. *JAMA Dermatol* (2016) 152:889–96. doi:10.1001/jamadermatol.2016.0939
11. Brown SA, Azzi A. Peripheral circadian oscillators in mammals. *Handb Exp Pharmacol* (2013) 217:45–66. doi:10.1007/978-3-642-25950-0_3
12. Buhr ED, Takahashi JS. Molecular components of the mammalian circadian clock. *Handb Exp Pharmacol* (2013) 217:3–27. doi:10.1007/978-3-642-25950-0_1
13. Takahashi JS. Transcriptional architecture of the mammalian circadian clock. *Nat Rev Genet* (2017) 18:164–79. doi:10.1038/nrg.2016.150
14. Baron KG, Reid KJ. Circadian misalignment and health. *Int Rev Psychiatry* (2014) 26:139–54. doi:10.3109/09540261.2014.911149
15. West AC, Bechtold DA. The cost of circadian desynchrony: evidence, insights and open questions. *Bioessays* (2015) 37:777–88. doi:10.1002/bies.201400173
16. Potter GD, Skene DJ, Arendt J, Cade JE, Grant PJ, Hardie LJ. Circadian rhythm and sleep disruption: causes, metabolic consequences, and countermeasures. *Endocr Rev* (2016) 37:584–608. doi:10.1210/er.2016-1083
17. Savvidis C, Koutsilieris M. Circadian rhythm disruption in cancer biology. *Mol Med* (2012) 18:1249–60. doi:10.2119/molmed.2012.00077
18. Kelleher FC, Rao A, Maguire A. Circadian molecular clocks and cancer. *Cancer Lett* (2014) 342:9–18. doi:10.1016/j.canlet.2013.09.040
19. Masri S, Kinouchi K, Sassone-Corsi P. Circadian clocks, epigenetics, and cancer. *Curr Opin Oncol* (2015) 27:50–6. doi:10.1097/CCO.0000000000000153
20. Yang X, Wood PA, Ansell CM, Quiton DF, Oh EY, Du-Quiton J, et al. The circadian clock gene Per1 suppresses cancer cell proliferation and tumor growth at specific times of day. *Chronobiol Int* (2009) 26:1323–39. doi:10.3109/07420520903431301
21. Kiessling S, Beaulieu-Laroche L, Blum ID, Landgraf D, Welsh DK, Storch KF, et al. Enhancing circadian clock function in cancer cells inhibits tumor growth. *BMC Biol* (2017) 15:13. doi:10.1186/s12915-017-0349-7
22. Gaddameedhi S, Selby CP, Kaufmann WK, Smart RC, Sancar A. Control of skin cancer by the circadian rhythm. *Proc Natl Acad Sci U S A* (2011) 108:18790–5. doi:10.1073/pnas.1115249108
23. Gaddameedhi S, Selby CP, Kemp MG, Ye R, Sancar A. The circadian clock controls sunburn apoptosis and erythema in mouse skin. *J Invest Dermatol* (2015) 135:1119–27. doi:10.1038/jid.2014.508
24. Albrecht U. The circadian clock, metabolism and obesity. *Obes Rev* (2017) 18(Suppl 1):25–33. doi:10.1111/obr.12502
25. Krishnaiah SY, Wu G, Altman BJ, Growe J, Rhoades SD, Coldren F, et al. Clock regulation of metabolites reveals coupling between transcription and metabolism. *Cell Metab* (2017) 25(5):1206. doi:10.1016/j.cmet.2017.04.023
26. Moraes MN, De Assis LVM, Henriques FDS, Batista ML Jr., Guler AD, Castrucci AML. Cold-sensing TRPM8 channel participates in circadian control of the brown adipose tissue. *Biochim Biophys Acta* (2017) 1864:2415–27. doi:10.1016/j.bbamcr.2017.09.011
27. Moraes MN, Mezzalira N, De Assis LV, Menaker M, Guler A, Castrucci AM. TRPV1 participates in the activation of clock molecular machinery in the brown adipose tissue in response to light-dark cycle. *Biochim Biophys Acta* (2017) 1864:324–35. doi:10.1016/j.bbamcr.2016.11.010
28. Chen ST, Choo KB, Hou MF, Yeh KT, Kuo SJ, Chang JG. Deregulated expression of the PER1, PER2 and PER3 genes in breast cancers. *Carcinogenesis* (2005) 26:1241–6. doi:10.1093/carcin/bgi075
29. Cao Q, Gery S, Dashti A, Yin D, Zhou Y, Gu J, et al. A role for the clock gene per1 in prostate cancer. *Cancer Res* (2009) 69:7619–25. doi:10.1158/0008-5472.CAN-08-4199
30. Yu H, Meng X, Wu J, Pan C, Ying X, Zhou Y, et al. Cryptochrome 1 overexpression correlates with tumor progression and poor prognosis in patients with colorectal cancer. *PLoS One* (2013) 8:e61679. doi:10.1371/journal.pone.0061679
31. Lengyel Z, Lovig C, Kommedal S, Keszthelyi R, Szekeres G, Battyani Z, et al. Altered expression patterns of clock gene mRNAs and clock proteins in human skin tumors. *Tumour Biol* (2013) 34:811–9. doi:10.1007/s13277-012-0611-0
32. Brozyna AA, Jozwicki W, Skobowiat C, Jetten A, Slominski AT. RORalpha and RORgamma expression inversely correlates with human melanoma progression. *Oncotarget* (2016) 7(39):63261–82. doi:10.18632/oncotarget.11211
33. de Assis LV, Moraes MN, da Silveira Cruz-Machado S, Castrucci AM. The effect of white light on normal and malignant murine melanocytes: a link between opsins, clock genes, and melanogenesis. *Biochim Biophys Acta* (2016) 1863:1119–33. doi:10.1016/j.bbamcr.2016.03.001
34. de Assis LV, Moraes MN, Castrucci AM. Heat shock antagonizes UVA-induced responses in murine melanocytes and melanoma cells: an unexpected interaction. *Photochem Photobiol Sci* (2017) 16(5):633–48. doi:10.1039/c6pp00330c
35. Poletini MO, De Assis LV, Moraes MN, Castrucci AM. Estradiol differently affects melanin synthesis of malignant and normal melanocytes: a relationship with clock and clock-controlled genes. *Mol Cell Biochem* (2016) 421:29–39. doi:10.1007/s11010-016-2781-3
36. Moraes MN, De Assis LVM, Magalhaes-Marques KK, Poletini MO, De Lima L, Castrucci AML. Melanopsin, a canonical light receptor, mediates thermal activation of clock genes. *Sci Rep* (2017) 7:13977. doi:10.1038/s41598-017-13939-3
37. de Assis LVM, Moraes MN, Magalhães-Marques KK, Kinker GS, da Silveira Cruz-Machado S, Castrucci AM. Non-metastatic cutaneous melanoma induces chronodisruption in central and peripheral circadian clocks. *Int J Mol Sci* (2018) 19(4):E1065. doi:10.3390/ijms19041065
38. Cancer Genome Atlas Network. Genomic classification of cutaneous melanoma. *Cell* (2015) 161:1681–96. doi:10.1016/j.cell.2015.05.044
39. Consortium GT. Human genomics. The Genotype-Tissue Expression (GTEx) pilot analysis: multitissue gene regulation in humans. *Science* (2015) 348:648–60. doi:10.1126/science.1262110

40. Rooney MS, Shukla SA, Wu CJ, Getz G, Hacohen N. Molecular and genetic properties of tumors associated with local immune cytolytic activity. *Cell* (2015) 160:48–61. doi:10.1016/j.cell.2014.12.033
41. Nielsen M, Lundegaard C, Blicher T, Lamberth K, Harndahl M, Justesen S, et al. NetMHCpan, a method for quantitative predictions of peptide binding to any HLA-A and -B locus protein of known sequence. *PLoS One* (2007) 2:e796. doi:10.1371/journal.pone.0000796
42. Riaz N, Havel JJ, Makarov V, Desrichard A, Urba WJ, Sims JS, et al. Tumor and microenvironment evolution during immunotherapy with nivolumab. *Cell* (2017) 171:934–49. doi:10.1016/j.cell.2017.09.028
43. Santos SDS, Galatro TFDA, Watanabe RA, Oba-Shinjo SM, Nagahashi Marie SK, Fujita A. CoGA: an R package to identify differentially co-expressed gene sets by analyzing the graph spectra. *PLoS One* (2015) 10:e0135831. doi:10.1371/journal.pone.0135831
44. Takahashi DY, Sato JR, Ferreira CE, Fujita A. Discriminating different classes of biological networks by analyzing the graphs spectra distribution. *PLoS One* (2012) 7:e49949. doi:10.1371/journal.pone.0049949
45. Kinker GS, Thomas AM, Carvalho VJ, Lima FP, Fujita A. Deletion and low expression of NFKBIA are associated with poor prognosis in lower-grade glioma patients. *Sci Rep* (2016) 6:24160. doi:10.1038/srep24160
46. Van Mieghem P. *Graph Spectra for Complex Networks*. Cambridge: Cambridge University Press (2010).
47. Subramanian A, Tamayo P, Mootha VK, Mukherjee S, Ebert BL, Gillette MA, et al. Gene set enrichment analysis: a knowledge-based approach for interpreting genome-wide expression profiles. *Proc Natl Acad Sci U S A* (2005) 102:15545–50. doi:10.1073/pnas.0506580102
48. Croft D, O'kelly G, Wu G, Haw R, Gillespie M, Matthews L, et al. Reactome: a database of reactions, pathways and biological processes. *Nucleic Acids Res* (2011) 39:D691–7. doi:10.1093/nar/gkq1018
49. Barbie DA, Tamayo P, Boehm JS, Kim SY, Moody SE, Dunn IF, et al. Systematic RNA interference reveals that oncogenic KRAS-driven cancers require TBK1. *Nature* (2009) 462:108–12. doi:10.1038/nature08460
50. Hänzelmann S, Castelo R, Guinney J. GSVA: gene set variation analysis for microarray and RNA-Seq data. *BMC Bioinformatics* (2013) 14:7. doi:10.1186/1471-2105-14-7
51. Kanehisa M, Goto S. KEGG: kyoto encyclopedia of genes and genomes. *Nucleic Acids Res* (2000) 28:27–30. doi:10.1093/nar/28.1.27
52. Wherry EJ, Kurachi M. Molecular and cellular insights into T cell exhaustion. *Nat Rev Immunol* (2015) 15:486–99. doi:10.1038/nri3862
53. Catakovic K, Klieser E, Neureiter D, Geisberger R. T cell exhaustion: from pathophysiological basics to tumor immunotherapy. *Cell Commun Signal* (2017) 15:1. doi:10.1186/s12964-016-0160-z
54. Gajewski TF, Schreiber H, Fu YX. Innate and adaptive immune cells in the tumor microenvironment. *Nat Immunol* (2013) 14:1014–22. doi:10.1038/ni.2703
55. Coulie PG, Van Den Eynde BJ, Van Der Bruggen P, Boon T. Tumour antigens recognized by T lymphocytes: at the core of cancer immunotherapy. *Nat Rev Cancer* (2014) 14:135–46. doi:10.1038/nrc3670
56. Yeh KT, Yang MY, Liu TC, Chen JC, Chan WL, Lin SF, et al. Abnormal expression of period 1 (PER1) in endometrial carcinoma. *J Pathol* (2005) 206:111–20. doi:10.1002/path.1756
57. Kuo SJ, Chen ST, Yeh KT, Hou MF, Chang YS, Hsu NC, et al. Disturbance of circadian gene expression in breast cancer. *Virchows Arch* (2009) 454:467–74. doi:10.1007/s00428-009-0761-7
58. Taniguchi H, Fernandez AF, Setien F, Ropero S, Ballestar E, Villanueva A, et al. Epigenetic inactivation of the circadian clock gene BMAL1 in hematologic malignancies. *Cancer Res* (2009) 69:8447–54. doi:10.1158/0008-5472.CAN-09-0551
59. Huisman SA, Ahmadi AR, Jn IJ, Verhoef C, Van Der Horst GT, De Bruin RW. Disruption of clock gene expression in human colorectal liver metastases. *Tumour Biol* (2016) 37(10):13973–81. doi:10.1007/s13277-016-5231-7
60. Jiang W, Zhao S, Jiang X, Zhang E, Hu G, Hu B, et al. The circadian clock gene Bmal1 acts as a potential anti-oncogene in pancreatic cancer by activating the p53 tumor suppressor pathway. *Cancer Lett* (2016) 371:314–25. doi:10.1016/j.canlet.2015.12.002
61. Li W, Liu L, Liu D, Jin S, Yang Y, Tang W, et al. Decreased circadian component Bmal1 predicts tumor progression and poor prognosis in human pancreatic ductal adenocarcinoma. *Biochem Biophys Res Commun* (2016) 472:156–62. doi:10.1016/j.bbrc.2016.02.087
62. Hua H, Wang Y, Wan C, Liu Y, Zhu B, Wang X, et al. Inhibition of tumorigenesis by intratumoral delivery of the circadian gene mPer2 in C57BL/6 mice. *Cancer Gene Ther* (2007) 14:815–8. doi:10.1038/sj.cgt.7701061
63. Oda A, Katayose Y, Yabuuchi S, Yamamoto K, Mizuma M, Shirasou S, et al. Clock gene mouse period2 overexpression inhibits growth of human pancreatic cancer cells and has synergistic effect with cisplatin. *Anticancer Res* (2009) 29:1201–9.
64. Hatanaka F, Matsubara C, Myung J, Yoritaka T, Kamimura N, Tsutsumi S, et al. Genome-wide profiling of the core clock protein BMAL1 targets reveals a strict relationship with metabolism. *Mol Cell Biol* (2010) 30:5636–48. doi:10.1128/MCB.00781-10
65. Rudic RD, Mcnamara P, Curtis AM, Boston RC, Panda S, Hogenesch JB, et al. BMAL1 and CLOCK, two essential components of the circadian clock, are involved in glucose homeostasis. *PLoS Biol* (2004) 2:e377. doi:10.1371/journal.pbio.0020377
66. Woon PY, Kaisaki PJ, Braganca J, Bihoreau MT, Levy JC, Farrall M, et al. Aryl hydrocarbon receptor nuclear translocator-like (BMAL1) is associated with susceptibility to hypertension and type 2 diabetes. *Proc Natl Acad Sci U S A* (2007) 104:14412–7. doi:10.1073/pnas.0703247104
67. Marcheva B, Ramsey KM, Buhr ED, Kobayashi Y, Su H, Ko CH, et al. Disruption of the clock components CLOCK and BMAL1 leads to hypoinsulinaemia and diabetes. *Nature* (2010) 466:627–31. doi:10.1038/nature09253
68. Milagro FI, Gomez-Abellan P, Campion J, Martinez JA, Ordovas JM, Garaulet M. CLOCK, PER2 and BMAL1 DNA methylation: association with obesity and metabolic syndrome characteristics and monounsaturated fat intake. *Chronobiol Int* (2012) 29:1180–94. doi:10.3109/07420528.2012.719967
69. Hodzic A, Ristanovic M, Zorn B, Tulic C, Maver A, Novakovic I, et al. Genetic variation in circadian rhythm genes CLOCK and ARNTL as risk factor for male infertility. *PLoS One* (2013) 8:e59220. doi:10.1371/journal.pone.0059220
70. Kettner NM, Katchy CA, Fu L. Circadian gene variants in cancer. *Ann Med* (2014) 46:208–20. doi:10.3109/07853890.2014.914808
71. Zeng ZL, Wu MW, Sun J, Sun YL, Cai YC, Huang YJ, et al. Effects of the biological clock gene Bmal1 on tumour growth and anti-cancer drug activity. *J Biochem* (2010) 148:319–26. doi:10.1093/jb/mvq069
72. Zeng ZL, Luo HY, Yang J, Wu WJ, Chen DL, Huang P, et al. Overexpression of the circadian clock gene Bmal1 increases sensitivity to oxaliplatin in colorectal cancer. *Clin Cancer Res* (2014) 20:1042–52. doi:10.1158/1078-0432.CCR-13-0171
73. Khapre RV, Kondratova AA, Susova O, Kondratov RV. Circadian clock protein BMAL1 regulates cellular senescence in vivo. *Cell Cycle* (2011) 10:4162–9. doi:10.4161/cc.10.23.18381
74. Elshazley M, Sato M, Hase T, Yamashita R, Yoshida K, Toyokuni S, et al. The circadian clock gene BMAL1 is a novel therapeutic target for malignant pleural mesothelioma. *Int J Cancer* (2012) 131:2820–31. doi:10.1002/ijc.27598
75. Le DT, Uram JN, Wang H, Bartlett BR, Kemberling H, Eyring AD, et al. PD-1 blockade in tumors with mismatch-repair deficiency. *N Engl J Med* (2015) 372:2509–20. doi:10.1056/NEJMoa1500596
76. Rizvi NA, Hellmann MD, Snyder A, Kvistborg P, Makarov V, Havel JJ, et al. Cancer immunology. Mutational landscape determines sensitivity to PD-1 blockade in non-small cell lung cancer. *Science* (2015) 348:124–8. doi:10.1126/science.aaa1348
77. van Gool IC, Eggink FA, Freeman-Mills L, Stelloo E, Marchi E, De Bruyn M, et al. POLE proofreading mutations elicit an antitumor immune response in endometrial cancer. *Clin Cancer Res* (2015) 21:3347–55. doi:10.1158/1078-0432.CCR-15-0057
78. Hugo W, Zaretsky JM, Sun L, Song C, Moreno BH, Hu-Lieskovan S, et al. Genomic and transcriptomic features of response to anti-PD-1 therapy in metastatic melanoma. *Cell* (2016) 165:35–44. doi:10.1016/j.cell.2016.02.065
79. Mouw KW, Goldberg MS, Konstantinopoulos PA, D'andrea AD. DNA damage and repair biomarkers of immunotherapy response. *Cancer Discov* (2017) 7:675–93. doi:10.1158/2159-8290.CD-17-0226
80. Hodi FS, O'day SJ, Mcdermott DF, Weber RW, Sosman JA, Haanen JB, et al. Improved survival with ipilimumab in patients with metastatic melanoma. *N Engl J Med* (2010) 363:711–23. doi:10.1056/NEJMoa1003466
81. Topalian SL, Sznol M, Mcdermott DF, Kluger HM, Carvajal RD, Sharfman WH, et al. Survival, durable tumor remission, and long-term safety in patients with

advanced melanoma receiving nivolumab. *J Clin Oncol* (2014) 32:1020–30. doi:10.1200/JCO.2013.53.0105

82. Schadendorf D, Hodi FS, Robert C, Weber JS, Margolin K, Hamid O, et al. Pooled analysis of long-term survival data from phase II and phase III trials of ipilimumab in unresectable or metastatic melanoma. *J Clin Oncol* (2015) 33:1889–94. doi:10.1200/JCO.2014.56.2736
83. Spencer KR, Wang J, Silk AW, Ganesan S, Kaufman HL, Mehnert JM. Biomarkers for immunotherapy: current developments and challenges. *Am Soc Clin Oncol Educ Book* (2016) 35:e493–503. doi:10.14694/EDBK_160766
84. Ji RR, Chasalow SD, Wang L, Hamid O, Schmidt H, Cogswell J, et al. An immune-active tumor microenvironment favors clinical response to ipilimumab. *Cancer Immunol Immunother* (2012) 61:1019–31. doi:10.1007/s00262-011-1172-6
85. Snyder A, Makarov V, Merghoub T, Yuan J, Zaretsky JM, Desrichard A, et al. Genetic basis for clinical response to CTLA-4 blockade in melanoma. *N Engl J Med* (2014) 371:2189–99. doi:10.1056/NEJMoa1406498
86. Taube JM, Klein A, Brahmer JR, Xu H, Pan X, Kim JH, et al. Association of PD-1, PD-1 ligands, and other features of the tumor immune microenvironment with response to anti-PD-1 therapy. *Clin Cancer Res* (2014) 20:5064–74. doi:10.1158/1078-0432.CCR-13-3271
87. Van Allen EM, Miao D, Schilling B, Shukla SA, Blank C, Zimmer L, et al. Genomic correlates of response to CTLA-4 blockade in metastatic melanoma. *Science* (2015) 350:207–11. doi:10.1126/science.aad0095
88. Johnson DB, Frampton GM, Rioth MJ, Yusko E, Xu Y, Guo X, et al. Targeted next generation sequencing identifies markers of response to PD-1 blockade. *Cancer Immunol Res* (2016) 4:959–67. doi:10.1158/2326-6066.CIR-16-0143

17

An IL-4/21 Inverted Cytokine Receptor Improving CAR-T Cell Potency in Immunosuppressive Solid-Tumor Microenvironment

Yi Wang[1], *Hua Jiang*[2], *Hong Luo*[1], *Yansha Sun*[2], *Bizhi Shi*[2], *Ruixin Sun*[2] *and Zonghai Li*[1,2*]

[1] *State Key Laboratory of Oncogenes and Related Genes, School of Biomedical Engineering, Renji Hosptial, Shanghai Jiao Tong University, Shanghai, China,* [2] *State Key Laboratory of Oncogenes and Related Genes, Renji Hospital, Shanghai Cancer Institute, Shanghai Jiao Tong University School of Medicine, Shanghai, China*

Edited by:
Weidong Han,
PLA General Hospital, China

Reviewed by:
Limin Zheng,
Sun Yat-sen University, China
Jan Joseph Melenhorst,
University of Pennsylvania, United States

***Correspondence:**
Zonghai Li
zonghaili@shsmu.edu.cn

Incorporation of inverted cytokine receptor (ICR) such as interleukin (IL)-4 vs. IL-7 (4/7) ICR is one strategy to improve the antitumor activities of chimeric antigen receptor (CAR) modified T (CAR-T) cells facing immunosuppressive cytokines. Here we report a novel interleukin (IL)-4 vs. IL-21 ICR (4/21 ICR) that enhanced CAR-T cell potency in IL-4^+ tumor milieu via a different working-mechanism from 4/7 ICR. Upon IL-4 stimulation, 4/21 ICR activated the STAT3 pathway and promoted Th17-like polarization and tumor-targeted cytotoxicity in CAR-T cells *in vitro*. Furthermore, 4/21 ICR-CAR T cells persisted and eradicated established IL-4^+ tumors *in vivo*. Thus, 4/21 ICR is a promising clinical CAR-T cell therapeutics for solid tumors rich in IL-4.

Keywords: CAR-T cells, inverted cytokine receptors, interleukin-4, interleukin-21, immunosuppressive tumor microenvironment

INTRODUCTION

Although the adoptive transfer of T cells genetically engineered with a chimeric antigen receptor (CAR) has shown great promise as a therapeutic for hematological malignancies (1, 2), limited success has been made in the application of CAR-T cells for the treatment of solid tumors. Existing theories believe that the immunosuppressive microenvironment of solid tumors, which features limited nutrients and oxygen, accumulation of inhibitory cells and cytokines, vascular disturbances, and endothelial dysfunction, poses a major obstacle for cancer immunotherapy including CAR-T cell therapy (3, 4).

To increase T cell potency in the suppressive microenvironment, CAR-T cells could be modified to become intrinsically resistant to anti-inflammatory cytokines. Notably, an inverted cytokine receptor (ICR), in which the ectodomain of the interleukin (IL)-4 receptor is fused to the endodomain of the IL-7 receptor (4/7 ICR), has been designed to protect CAR-T cells from IL-4 suppression (5, 6). 4/7 ICR could accept immunosuppressive IL-4 but convert the downstream signal to that of the immunostimulatory IL-7 receptor. Upon IL-4 engagement, CAR-T cells armored with 4/7 ICR retained the Th1 phenotype and cell viability *in vitro*, and persisted with powerful antitumor activity *in vivo* (5).

In addition to IL-7, IL-21 has also been reported to promote T cell-mediated tumor rejection. Tumor-directed T cells expanded in IL-21 conditional media showed enhanced antitumor efficacy in a B16-melanoma mouse model (7). Human CAR-T cells engineered to express IL-21, efficiently eliminated tumor cells with long-term persistence in immunodeficient mice (8). Thus, as a γ-chain cytokine like IL-7, IL-21 could be a hopeful candidate to constitute a novel IL-4-related ICR. IL-21 is a pleiotropic cytokine that plays critical roles in modulating the effector functions of $CD8^+$ T cells and polarization of naïve $CD4^+$ T helper (Th) cells (9). Hence, it is interesting to investigate the different efficacy and working-mechanisms in CAR-T cells between 4/7 ICR and 4/21 ICR.

In the current study, 4/21 ICR-CAR T cells achieved rapid tumor eradication in the presence of IL-4, with a comparable efficiency to that of 4/7 ICR-CAR T cells. Evidences indicated that 4/21 ICR-CAR T cells polarized to the Th17-like phenotype rather than the Th1 phenotype of 4/7 ICR-CAR T cells (5), suggesting a distinct mechanism on promoting antitumor activities between 4/7 ICR and 4/21 ICR.

MATERIALS AND METHODS

Mice

Female 6-week-old NOD.Cg-*Prkdc*^{scid}Il2*rg*^{tm1Sug}/JicCrl (NOG) mice were introduced by Vital River Co. (Beijing, China) from Central Institute for Experimental Animals (CIEA) of Japan and housed under specific pathogen-free conditions.

Cell Lines

Huh-7, PLC/PRF/5, and HEK-293T were obtained from the ATCC. SMMC-7721 cells were obtained from the Cell Bank of the Shanghai Institute of Cell Biology, Chinese Academy of Sciences. The HCC cells were engineered to produce IL-4 by transduction with the GFP-F2A-IL-4 lentivirus. For the transduction, 2×10^5 /ml cells were placed in a 24-well plate with lentiviral supernatant. The transgene expression was analyzed by GFP fluorescence using flow cytometry. The IL-4 secretion was further confirmed by ELISA (**Supplementary Figure S1**). All these cells were cultured in DMEM supplemented with 10% FBS.

Generation of Lentiviral Vector Encoding CAR and ICR

The nucleotide sequence encoding for the signal peptide and extracellular domain of the IL-4 receptor α was fused to the transmembrane and intracellular domain of IL-7 or IL-21, respectively, to generation 4/7 or 4/21 ICR coding sequences. Then the ICR sequences were linked with the sequence encoding anti-GPC-3-28zCAR by a self-cleaving 2A (F2A) sequence with the restriction sites MluI and SalI. Finally, the CAR-F2A-ICR DNA fragments were integrated into pRRLSIN vector after enzymatic digestion with MluI and SalI.

Lentivirus Production

The lentiviral supernatants were produced by HEK-293T cells, which were transfected with 5.4 μg of vectors that encoded CAR and ICR, 6.2 μg of Prre, and pREV vector and 2.4 μg of pVSVG vector for envelope expression, by 60 μg of polyethylenimine (PEI, Polysciences, Inc.). The supernatants were collected 48 h after transfection and further concentrated 80-fold by polyethylene glycol 8000 (PEG 8000, Sigma-Aldrich) precipitation at 4°C overnight.

Transduction and Expansion of Human T Cells

The activation, transduction, and expansion of human T cells have been described in the previous study (10). Briefly, T cells in peripheral blood mononuclear cells (PBMCs) were activated by Dynabeads (ThermoFisher Scientific) for 48 h. Then 1×10^6/ml cells were transduced with lentivirus in a RetroNectin-precoated 24-well plate by centrifugation under 1,800 rpm for 40 min. Human T cells were cultured in AIM-V (Gibco) supplemented with 2% ABS added IL-2 (500 U/ml, Huaxin Biotech., Shanghai, China).

Flow Cytometry

CAR-T cells treated with IL-4 were harvested and washed with ice-cold phosphate buffered saline (PBS) followed by incubation with antibodies for 30 min on ice. After being washed twice, cells were subjected to analysis by flow cytometry. For plasma samples, Lysing Solution (BD) was added to lyse red blood cells after antibody incubation.

Western Blot Analysis

CAR-T cells were rested in serum-free AIM-V without cytokines overnight, and subsequently stimulated with IL-4 (20 ng/ml, Peprotech) for 30 min. The cell lysates were denatured for SDS-PAGE and immunoblotted with monoclonal antibodies listed in **Supplementary Table S1**.

Quantitative Real-Time Polymerase Chain Reaction (qPCR)

CAR-T cells were treated with IL-4 (20 ng/ml) for 72 h and collected for RNA extraction by TriZol (Life Tech.). The total RNA was further reverse transcribed to cDNA using GoScript Reverse Transcrition System (Promega). The mRNA expression was analyzed by qPCR using SYBR Premix Ex Taq II (TaKaRa) with primers listed in **Supplementary Table S2**. The relative quantification of targeted genes was calculated with the ΔΔCt method.

Cytotoxicity Assays *in vitro*

The cytotoxicity assay has been described in the previous study (11). In brief, CAR-T cells pre-treated with IL-4 (20 ng/ml) were co-cultured with target tumor cells for 18 h and the lactate dehydrogenase activity in supernatant was detected by the CytoTox 96 Non-Radioactive Cytotoxicity Assay (Promega).

Tumor Re-challenging Assays

CAR-T cells were co-cultured with IL-4-producing Huh-7 cells at the effector: target ratio of 1:1 for the first round of stimulation. Tumor clearance was confirmed as no adherent cell appeared in the microscopic field after 48 h. CAR-T cells were then analyzed for the expression of inhibitory receptors or further cultured with IL-4-producing Huh-7 cells at the effector: target ratio of 1:20 for another 48 h. CAR-T cells were collected to re-analyze the expression of inhibitory receptors. Wells were gently rinsed by PBS twice to remove non-adhesive T cells and the tumor cells in wells were stained by crystal violet.

Tumor Xenograft Models

NOG mice were subcutaneously inoculated with 3×10^6 tumor cells on the right flank. When tumor burden reached the scheduled level (~100 mm^3 for SMMC-7721 and 200 mm^3 for PLC/PFR/5), mice were randomly subdivided into four treatment groups and intravenously injected with 3×10^6 CAR-T or untransduced T cells. Tumor dimensions were measured with calipers every 3–4 days. The tumor volumes were calculated by the formula: V= (length × width^2)/2. The peripheral blood samples were collected for the analysis of T-cell survival on day 14 after T-cell infusion.

Statistical Analysis

Statistical analysis was performed using GraphPad Prism 5.0 and SPSS 17.0. The Unpaired Student's *t*-test was used to compare the two groups. The One-way ANOVA with Tukey *post-test* was used to determine the statistical significance for three-group comparisons. All experimental data are presented graphically or by mean ± standard deviation (SD).

RESULTS

IL-4 Induced a Transformed STAT3 Phosphorylation in 4/21 ICR-CAR T Cells

Similar to the design of 4/7 ICR (5), 4/21 ICR was constructed by fusing the extracellular domain of the IL-4 receptor to the transmembrane and intracellular domain of the IL-21 receptor (**Figure 1A**). The transduction efficiency of 4/7 ICR CAR and 4/21 ICR CAR is around 50% and relatively lower than that of CAR alone (**Figure 1B**). Tumor-associated IL-4 can induce Th2 differentiation via STAT6 phosphorylation to directly inhibit T-cell cancer immunity. In our assumption, IL-4 recognition by 4/21 ICR should result in STAT3 phosphorylation, a hallmark of IL-21 signaling, and increase the T cell activities (**Figure 1C**). As shown in **Figure 1D**, in the presence of IL-4, STAT3 was strongly phosphorylated in 4/21 ICR-CAR T cells, accompanied with a weak phosphorylation of STAT5, which was reported to transiently occur in IL-21 signaling (12), and as previously reported, increased STAT5 phosphorylation was observed in 4/7 ICR-CAR T cells exposed to IL-4 (5).

4/21 ICR-CAR T Cells Demonstrated Th17-Like Phenotypes in the Presence of IL-4

We next measured the mRNA expression of IL-21 target genes in T cells after IL-4 exposure. The expression of Bcl-6, a transcriptional regulator that maintains memory cell properties (13), was significantly increased in 4/21 ICR-CAR T cells, while the expression of Blimp-1, a transcriptional repressor associated with effector functions and memory responses (14), was reserved. In addition, the elevated expression level of Granzyme B was also observed (**Figure 2A**). These results indicate that 4/21 ICR-CAR T cells might sustain memory T cell homeostasis with enhanced effector functions, which is not surprising in light of the multifaceted roles of IL-21 in T cell differentiation (9).

Unlike the IL-7-STAT5 axis that facilitates Th1 polarization, IL-21 regulates the differentiation of almost every major subset of CD4$^+$ T cells (9). Upon IL-4 engagement, the expression of the Th1 cell master regulator, T-bet, was down-regulated in control CAR-T cells but not in both ICR-expressing T cells. Th2-specific GATA3 expression was up-regulated in control cells while little affected in ICR-expressing T cells. Intriguingly, RORγt expression was dramatically elevated in 4/21 ICR-CAR T cells (**Figure 2B**). RORγt is the critical transcriptional factor that orchestrates the differentiation of the Th17 cell lineage, whose expression is induced in an IL-21/STAT3-dependent manner (15). To further confirm the Th17 phenotypes of 4/21 ICR-CAR T cells, the expression of CD26, one of the distinguished markers of Th17 cells (16), was assessed and found to be highly expressed in most 4/21 ICR-CAR T cells exposed to IL-4 (**Figure 2C**). Consistently, CXCR3, the chemokine receptor generally expressed on Th1/Th17 cells (17), was highly expressed on the 4/21 ICR-CAR T cells in the presence of IL-4 (**Figure 2D**). As expected, 4/21 ICR-CAR T cells secreted higher levels of IL-17A after antigen stimulation, compared with control cells (**Supplementary Figure S2**). These data support that 4/21 ICR can activate the analogous downstream signaling of native IL-21R and thereby promote Th17-like differentiation in CAR-T cells upon IL-4 engagement.

4/21 ICR-CAR T Cells Efficiently Killed Tumor Cells With Attenuated Exhaustion *in vitro*

The previous study declared that 4/7 ICR-CAR T cells maintained a CD25$^+$ activated phenotype in IL-4-rich condition (6). A similar activated phenotype was also observed in 4/21 ICR-CAR T cells (**Figure 3A**). However, unlike the control and 4/7 ICR-CAR T cells whose cytotoxicity's were significantly compromised by IL-4, 4/21 ICR-CAR T cells retained cytotoxicity in the presence of IL-4 (**Figure 3B**). Consistent with the data of mRNA quantification, the Granzyme B expression in 4/21 ICR-CAR T cells was higher than in the control and 4/7 ICR-CAR T cells, especially in the CD4$^+$ subset, after tumor cell stimulation (**Figure 3C**). Furthermore, 4/21 ICR-CAR T cells exhibited a larger subset of CD45RA$^-$ CD62L$^+$ cells (**Figure 3D**), which is considered to retain the central memory (Tcm) phenotype (18).

To determine the long-term anti-tumor effects of 4/21 ICR-CAR T cells, we constructed tumor cells producing human IL-4. After being repeatedly challenged with IL4-Huh7 cells, 4/21 ICR-CAR T cells displayed an improved tumor-cell elimination than the control CAR and 4/7 ICR-CAR T cells (**Figures 4A,B**). Analyses of inhibitory molecule expression revealed that PD-1 and TIM3 expression were minimally induced after two antigen stimulations in 4/21 ICR-CAR T cells, while being greatly upregulated in both the control and 4/7 ICR-CAR T cells (**Figure 4C**). Thus, our data suggests that in the IL-4$^+$ tumor milieu, 4/21 ICR-CAR T cells can maintain an activated but less exhausted status and persistently eliminate tumor cells.

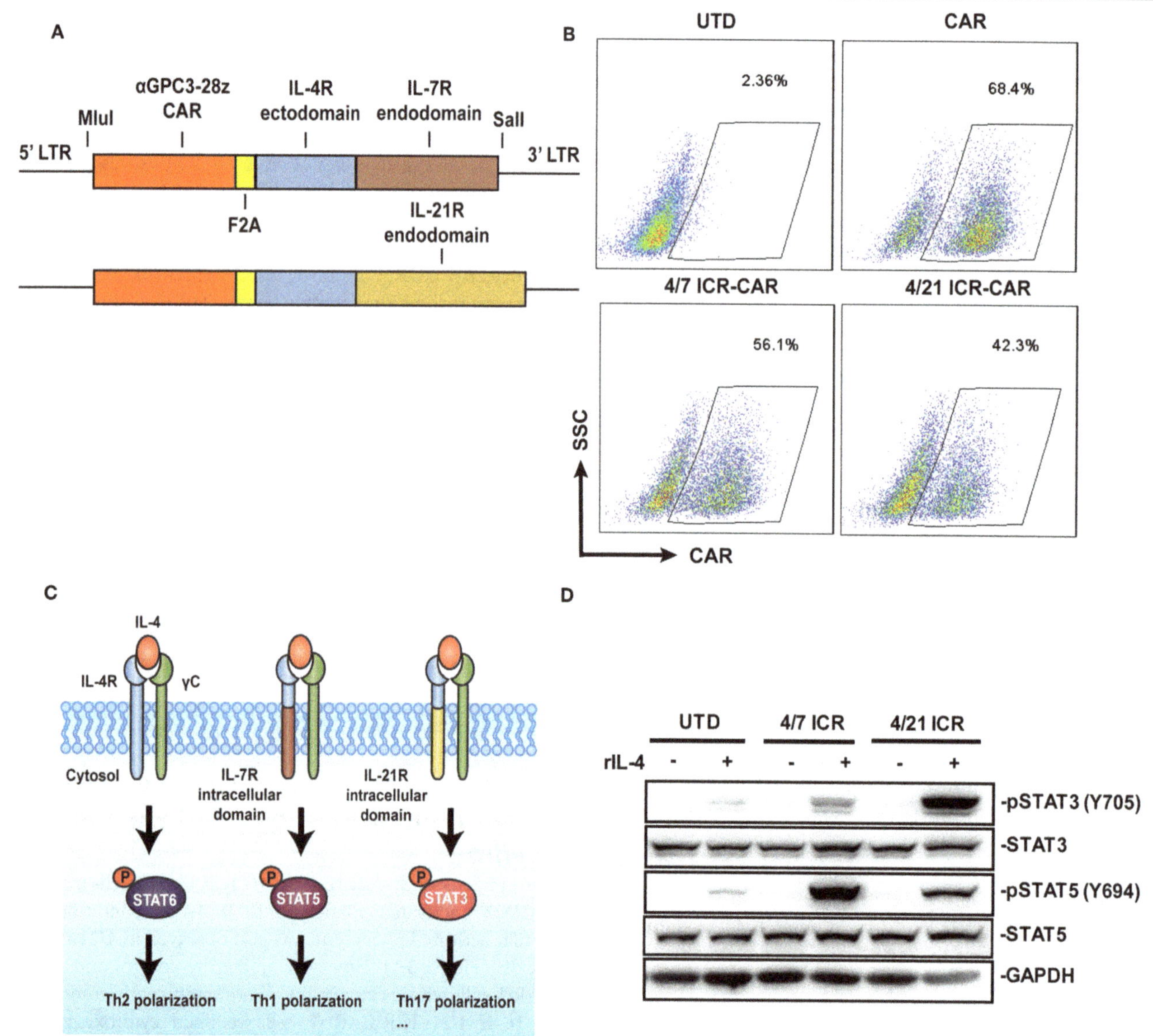

FIGURE 1 | Generation of 4/21 ICR-CAR T cells. **(A)** Schematic representation of 4/7 and 4/21 ICR CARs. **(B)** Flow cytometric analysis of the transgenic efficiency of 4/7 and 4/21 ICR CARs. **(C)** Simplified model for IL-4 signaling pathway through native IL-4 receptors or 4/7 and 4/21 ICR. **(D)** Altered downstream signaling of 4/7 and 4/21 ICR as determined by STAT3/5 phosphorylation using Western blot. Representative results from one of three or more independent experiments are shown.

4/21 ICR-CAR T Cells Survived and Eradicated Established IL-4$^+$ Tumors *in vivo*

To investigate the therapeutic effects of 4/21 ICR-CAR T cells *in vivo*, we resorted to a tumor xenograft mouse model. Since Huh-7 tumors had been efficiently cleared by CAR-T cells in our previous animal experiment (11), we adopted two tumor cell lines that were less sensitive to CAR-T cells. In one xenograft model, IL-4-producing SMMC-7721 tumor cells were subcutaneously transplanted into immunodeficient mice. After the tumors had grown to ~100 mm^3, the mice were administrated CAR-T or untransduced (UTD) control T cells intravenously. In this tumor model, both 4/7 and 4/21 ICR-CAR T cells showed superior anti-tumor effects compared with control CAR-T cells (**Figure 5A**). A number of CD3$^+$ T cells were still detectable in both ICR-CAR T cell-treated mice 2 weeks after infusion, indicating the enhanced persistence of the ICR-CAR T cells *in vivo* (**Figure 5B**). Interestingly, the proportion of the CD4$^+$ subset in the survived T cells was significantly higher in the 4/21 ICR group, which could be explained by the long-lived subset of Th17 cells (19, 20).

In the IL-4-PLC/PRF/5 tumor model, CAR-T cells were challenged with a larger tumor burden (~200 mm^3). We observed that tumors treated with 4/21 ICR-CAR T cells were rapidly eradicated compared with those in the control group,

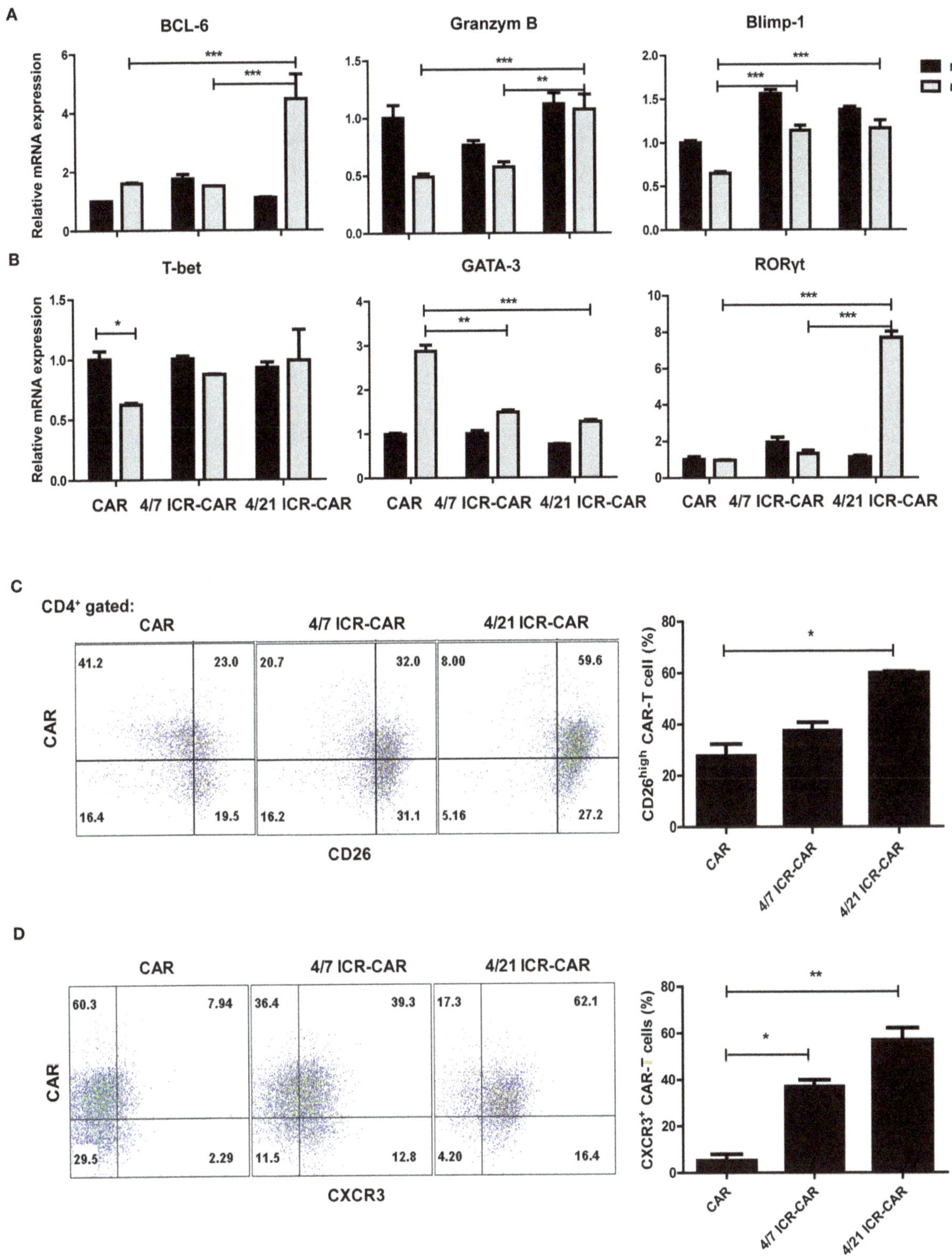

FIGURE 2 | Th17-like polarization of 4/21 ICR-CAR T cells. **(A,B)** Relative mRNA expression of IL-21 target genes and specific transcriptional factors for T helper subsets (T-bet for Th1, GATA3 for Th2, and RORγt for Th17) after IL-4 exposure (20 ng/ml for 48 h) were measured by qPCR. **(C,D)** Flow cytometric analysis of CD26 and CXCR3 expression of 4/7 and 4/21 ICR CARs after IL-4 exposure (20 ng/mL for 48 h). Representative results from one of three independent experiments are shown. $n = 3$ samples for each group; Graphic results are presented as mean ± SD; *$p < 0.05$; **$p < 0.01$; ***$p < 0.001$, one-way ANOVA with Tukey *post-test* for multiple comparison.

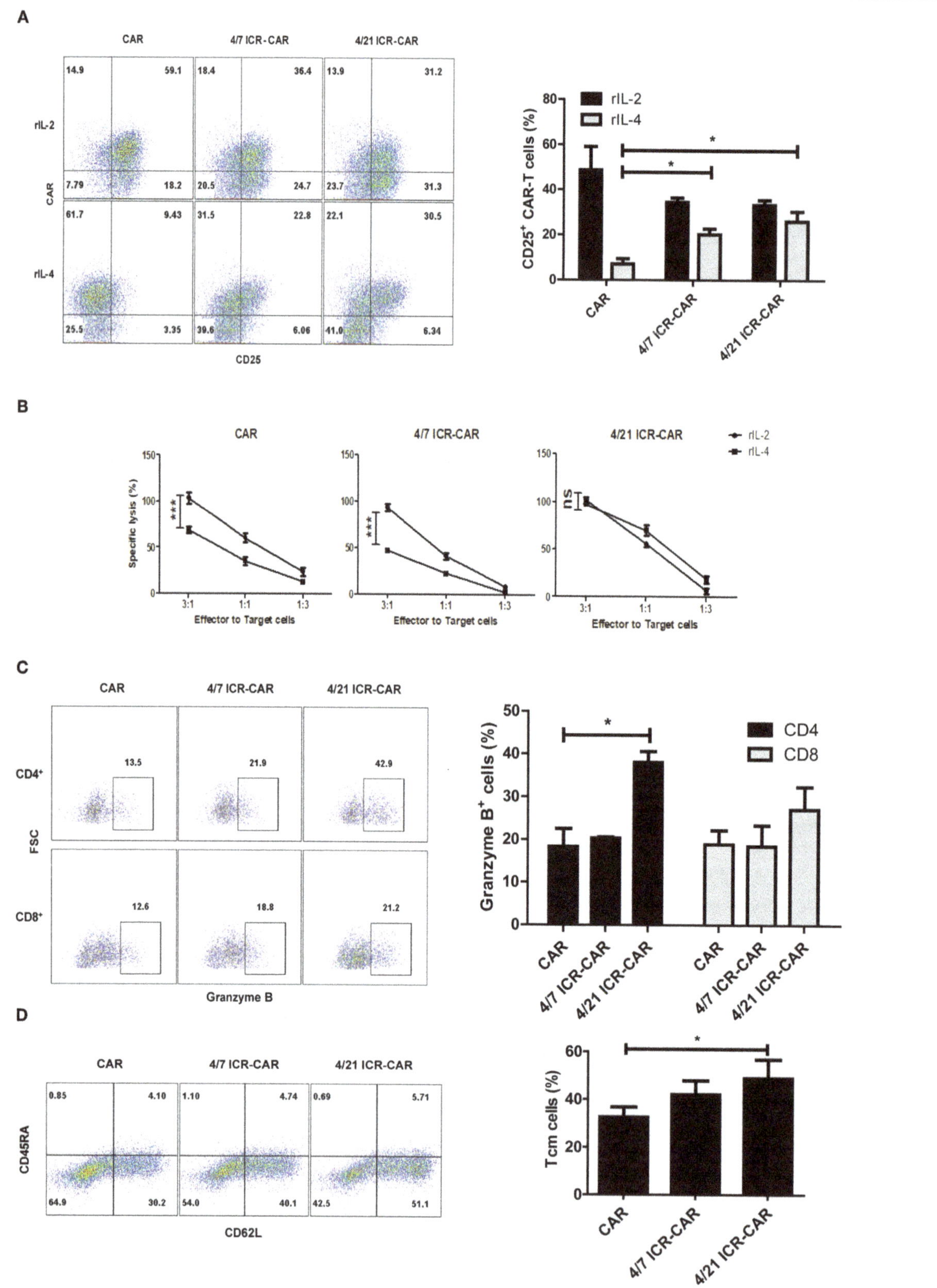

FIGURE 3 | Anti-tumor activities of 4/21 ICR-CAR T cells *in vitro*. **(A)** T cell activation marker, CD25 expression upon IL-4 treatment (20 ng/ml for 48 h) was determined by flow cytometry. **(B)** Following IL-4 exposure, control, 4/7 ICR or 4/21 ICR-CAR T cells were co-incubated with Huh-7 cells at different E:T ratios for 18 h.

(Continued)

FIGURE 3 | Cytotoxicity was measured using a standard non-radioactive cytotoxicity assay. **(C)** Granzyme B expression of CAR-T cells was measured by flow cytometry after Huh-7 cell stimulation for 24 h. **(D)** The CD45RA$^-$ CD62L$^+$ subset of CAR-T cells was detected 3 days after Huh-7 cell stimulation. Representative results from one of three independent experiments are shown. $n = 3$ samples for each group; Graphic results are presented as mean ± SD; ns: not significant; $^*p < 0.05$; $^{***}p < 0.001$, one-way ANOVA with Tukey *post-test* for multiple comparison.

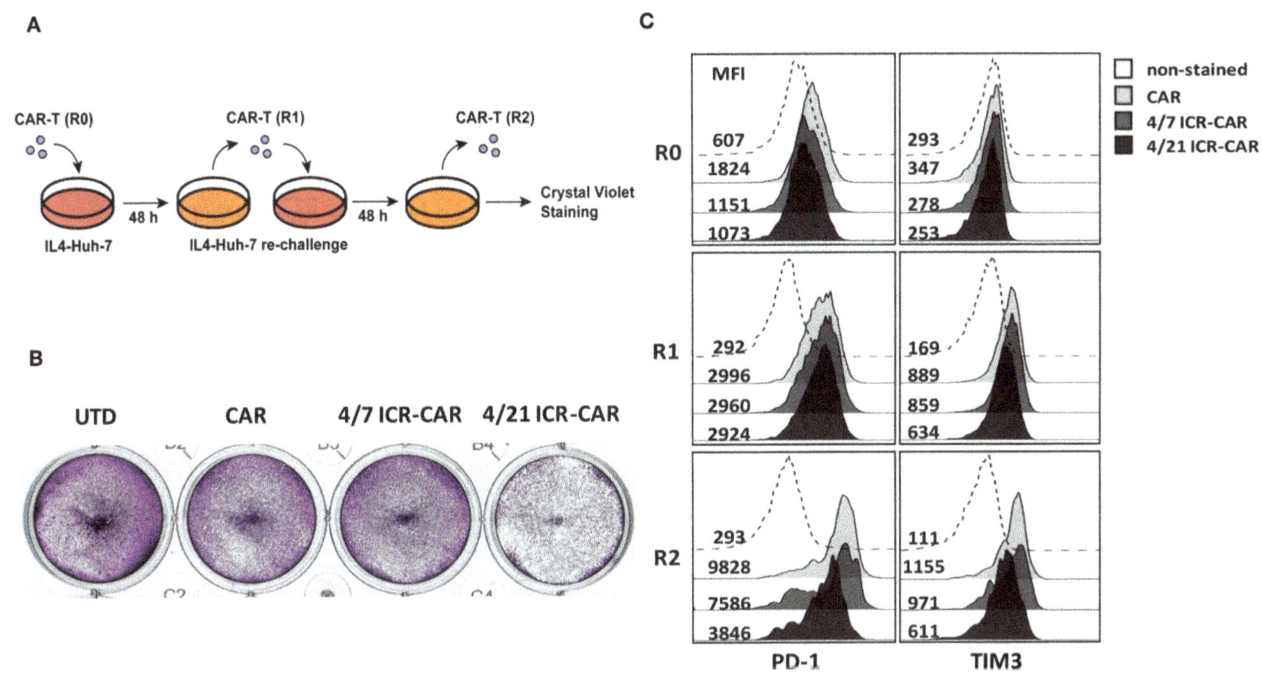

FIGURE 4 | (A,B) After 48 h antigen stimulation by IL-4-Huh7 cells (E:T ratio=1:1), control, 4/7 ICR or 4/21 ICR-CAR T cells were re-challenged with IL-4-Huh7 cells at an E:T ratio of 1:20 for another 48 h. **(C)** T cells were collected for PD-1 and TIM3 expression analysis at indicated time points and tumor cells were stained by crystal violet at the end point. Representative results from one of three independent experiments are shown.

whereas the tumor clearance was not that efficient by 4/7 ICR-CAR T cells (**Figures 5C,D**).

DISCUSSION

4/7 ICR has been invented to reinforce CAR-T cells to withstand the immunosuppressive tumor microenvironment, but whether other combinations of the cytokine receptors could be equally or more effective remains to be explored. Inspired by this, we constructed the novel 4/21 ICR which combines the ectodomain of the IL-4 receptor and endodomain of the IL-21 receptor. 4/21 ICR expressing CAR-T cells achieved enhanced resistance to IL-4, exhibiting the comparable, if not improved, anti-tumor activities to the 4/7 ICR-CAR T cells *in vivo*.

Our findings indicate that 4/7 and 4/21 ICR fundamentally differed in the phospho-STAT signaling cascade. 4/7 ICR activation leads to STAT5 phosphorylation, while 4/21 ICR prefers to activate STAT3 phosphorylation. Importantly, activation of STAT3 is supposed to be one of the critical determinants of CAR-T cell potency. A transcriptomic study has revealed that the genes of STAT3 signatures were enriched in CAR-T cells from complete-responding patients (21). Furthermore, a newly designed CAR with superior anti-tumor capacity has involved the STAT3 signal by integrating the YXXQ motif from IL-21 receptors, which is essential for its optimal functions (22). Therefore, 4/21 ICR would be a new trigger to activate the STAT3 pathway in response to immunosuppressive IL-4, to produce potent antitumor functions in CAR-T cells.

4/21 ICR-CAR T cells presented superior functional activities in our *in vitro* assays. Although IL-4 impaired the cytotoxicity of the control and 4/7 ICR-CAR T cells, 4/21 ICR-CAR T cells retained the cytotoxicity in the presence of IL-4 (**Figure 3B**). This could be attributed to the increased expression of Granzyme B (**Figures 2A, 3C**), an important effector molecule that has been reported as a target gene of IL-21 signaling (23). In addition, 4/21 ICR-CAR T cells displayed sustained cytotoxicity with an attenuated exhaustion phenotype in the tumor re-challenge assay. These results could be explained by the Th17-like polarization of 4/21 ICR-CAR T cells, since Th17 cells has been demonstrated to retain a stem cell-like molecular signature with lower expression of exhaustion markers than Th1 cells (20).

Th17 cells have been discovered as a new CD4$^+$ effector subset independent of other helper cells. Although CD8$^+$ T cells have been recognized as the major effector cells for T-cell cancer immunity, it has become controversial to adopt CD4$^+$

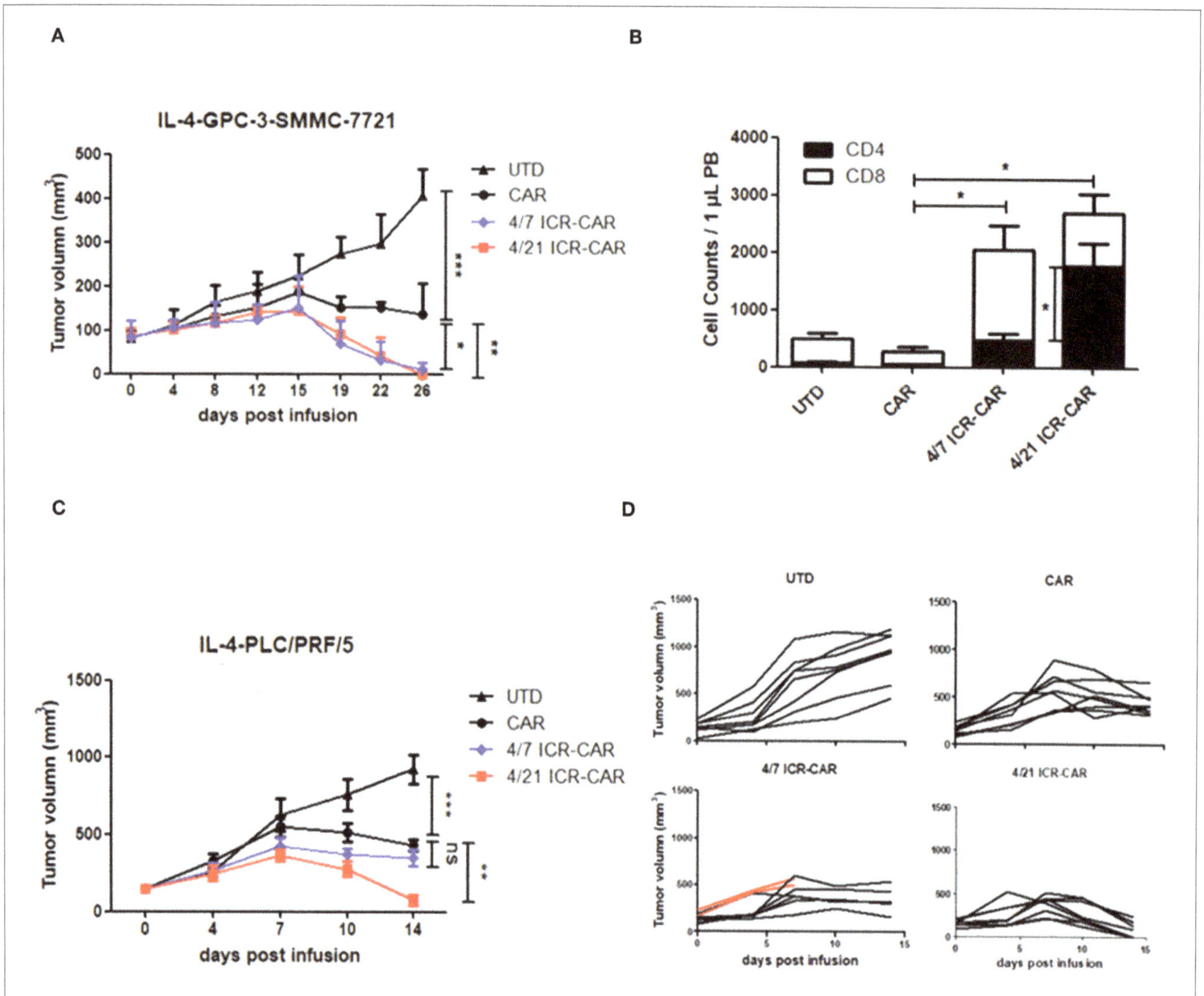

FIGURE 5 | Anti-tumor activities of 4/21 ICR-CAR T cells in established cancer xenografts *in vivo.* **(A)** Mice were subcutaneously inoculated with 3×10^6 IL-4-SMMC-7721 tumor cells on the right flank. 3×10^6 UTD T cells, control, 4/7 ICR or 4/21 ICR-CAR T cells were intravenously injected when tumors had grown to ~100 mm^3. $n = 4$ mice for each group; **(B)** Peripheral blood samples were collected on 14 days after T cell infusion to determine the T cell survival. T cells were analyzed by anti-CD3/CD4/CD8 antibodies and enumerated. **(C,D)** Mice were subcutaneously inoculated with 3×10^6 IL-4-PLC/PRF/5 tumor cells on the right flank. 3×10^6 UTD T cells, control, 4/7 ICR or 4/21 ICR-CAR T cells were intravenously injected when tumor burden had reached ~200 mm^3. Red lines in **(D)** indicate the tumor volume of two mice died after T cell infusion. $n = 8$ mice for each group; Data are presented as mean ± SD; ns: not significant; $^*p < 0.05$; $^{**}p < 0.01$; $^{***}p < 0.001$, one-way ANOVA with Tukey *post-test* for multiple comparison.

or CD8$^+$ T cells to generate CAR-T cells. A recent study on glioblastoma-targeted CAR-T cells claimed that CD4$^+$ CAR-T cells performed a long-term antitumor response superior to CD8$^+$ CAR-T cells (24). In line with this, CD8$^+$ CAR-T cells have been demonstrated to be prone to exhaustion and apoptosis upon TCR engagement (25). C. June and his colleagues first explored the efficacy of CD4$^+$ ICOS-CAR-T cells generated in the Th17-redirected condition (26). They further raised that the CD26^{high}-ICOS-CAR-T cells with Th1/Th17 phenotypes elicited potent tumor elimination and durable persistence, and even outperformed CD8 CAR-T cells in the mesothelioma animal model (27). In the present study, 4/21 ICR-CAR T cells highly expressed RORγt and displayed Th17-like phenotypes *in vitro* and performed potent anti-tumor activities with persistence of CD4$^+$ T cells *in vivo.* These results suggest that 4/21 ICR enhances CAR-T cell functions upon IL-4 exposure in a Th17-promoting manner, which is distinct from 4/7 ICR.

As a cytokine driving homeostatic expansion, IL-7 can stimulate T cell proliferation in an antigen-independent manner. A constitutively active form of the IL-7 receptor (C7R) has been engineered for CAR-T cells to improve proliferation, survival and anti-tumor activity (28). Although the investigators did not observe autonomous T cell expansion *in vitro*, the potential safety risk could not be completely obviated. Considering this, the

IL-7R mutant has been associated with T-cell acute lymphoblastic leukemia (29). Similarly, given that IL-7 signaling could be over-activated in 4/7 ICR-CAR T cells, if IL-4 is available in abundance outside tumors, it might induce unwarranted expansion. By contrast, IL-21 synergistically induces T cell proliferation with TCR signaling, but has little effect alone (30). Our data also indicates that IL-4 alone did not enhance the expansion of 4/21 ICR-CAR T cells but did in the presence of antigen (**Supplementary Figure S3**). In our animal experiments, we observed the lethal toxicity of 4/7 ICR-CAR T cells in mice with heavier tumor burdens (**Figure 5D**, **Supplementary Figure S4**) early after T cell infusion, while all mice that received 4/21 ICR-CAR T cells survived at the end point of the experiment. The mechanism for 4/7 ICR induced toxicity is currently unclear. Nonetheless, IL-4 levels in patients must be carefully monitored when ICR constructs are clinically translated.

Admittedly, the present research is limited by the immunodeficient mouse model, which lacks the crosstalk between CAR-T cells and the native immune cells. Especially, considering that IL-21 has pleiotropic effects synergizing with various cytokines in T cells, it must be closely scrutinized whether 4/21 ICR could achieve an expected outcome in immune-competent models and clinical trials.

Altogether, in the presence of the inhibitory IL-4 signal, CAR-T cells expressing 4/21 ICR polarized into Th17-like phenotypes and showed potent anti-tumor effects and long-term persistence *in vivo*. Thus, 4/21 ICR is promising to be an alternative design for next-generation CAR-T therapy in IL-4-rich cancers.

ETHICS STATEMENT

This study was carried out in accordance with the recommendations of' the Animal Research: Reporting *in vivo* Experiments (ARRIVE) criteria. The protocol was approved by Shanghai Cancer Institute Experimental Animal Care Commission.

AUTHOR CONTRIBUTIONS

ZL, YW, and HJ contributed to the conception and design of the study. YW, HL, YS, and RS contributed to data acquisition and statistical analysis. YW wrote the first draft of the manuscript. ZL, HJ, and BS contributed to the manuscript review and editing. All authors approved the submitted version.

FUNDING

This study is supported by funding from the National Natural Science Foundation of China (No. 81872483), the 13th Five-Year Plan National Science and Technology Major Project of China (No. 2017ZX10203206006), the Program of Shanghai Subject Chief Scientist (No.16XD1402600), the Grant from the State Key Laboratory of Oncogenes and Related Genes (No. 91-17-23) and the Grant-in-Aid for Young Scientists Foundation of Shanghai Cancer Institute (No. SB18-05).

REFERENCES

1. Schuster SJ, Svoboda J, Chong EA, Nasta SD, Mato AR, Anak O, et al. Chimeric antigen receptor T cells in refractory B-cell lymphomas. *N Engl J Med.* (2017) 377:2545–54. doi: 10.1056/NEJMoa1708566
2. Maude SL, Laetsch TW, Buechner J, Rives S, Boyer M, Bittencourt H, et al. Tisagenlecleucel in children and young adults with B-cell lymphoblastic leukemia. *N Engl J Med.* (2018) 378:439–48. doi: 10.1056/NEJMoa1709866
3. Beatty GL, Moon EK. Chimeric antigen receptor T cells are vulnerable to immunosuppressive mechanisms present within the tumor microenvironment. *Oncoimmunology.* (2014) 3:e970027. doi: 10.4161/21624011.2014.970027
4. Anderson KG, Stromnes IM, Greenberg PD. Obstacles posed by the tumor microenvironment to T cell activity: a case for synergistic therapies. *Cancer Cell.* (2017) 31:311–25. doi: 10.1016/j.ccell.2017.02.008
5. Leen AM, Sukumaran S, Watanabe N, Mohammed S, Keirnan J, Yanagisawa R, et al. Reversal of tumor immune inhibition using a chimeric cytokine receptor. *Mol Ther.* (2014) 22:1211–20. doi: 10.1038/mt.2014.47
6. Mohammed S, Sukumaran S, Bajgain P, Watanabe N, Heslop HE, Rooney CM, et al. Improving chimeric antigen receptor-modified T cell function by reversing the immunosuppressive tumor microenvironment of pancreatic cancer. *Mol Ther.* (2017) 25:249–58. doi: 10.1016/j.ymthe.2016.10.016
7. Hinrichs CS, Spolski R, Paulos CM, Gattinoni L, Kerstann KW, Palmer DC, et al. IL-2 and IL-21 confer opposing differentiation programs to CD8+ T cells for adoptive immunotherapy. *Blood.* (2008) 111:5326–33. doi: 10.1182/blood-2007-09-113050
8. Markley JC, Sadelain M. IL-7 and IL-21 are superior to IL-2 and IL-15 in promoting human T cell-mediated rejection of systemic lymphoma in immunodeficient mice. *Blood.* (2010) 115:3508–19. doi: 10.1182/blood-2009-09-241398
9. Tian Y, Zajac AJ. IL-21 and T cell differentiation: consider the context. *Trends Immunol.* (2016) 37:557–68. doi: 10.1016/j.it.2016.06.001
10. Wu X, Shi B, Zhang J, Shi Z, Di S, Fan M, et al. A fusion receptor as a safety switch, detection, and purification biomarker for adoptive transferred T cells. *Mol Ther.* (2017) 25:2270–9. doi: 10.1016/j.ymthe.2017.06.026
11. Gao H, Li K, Tu H, Pan X, Jiang H, Shi B, et al. Development of T cells redirected to glypican-3 for the treatment of hepatocellular carcinoma. *Clin Cancer Res.* (2014) 20:6418–28. doi: 10.1158/1078-0432.CCR-14-1170
12. Zeng R, Spolski R, Casas E, Zhu W, Levy DE, Leonard WJ. The molecular basis of IL-21-mediated proliferation. *Blood.* (2007) 109:4135–42. doi: 10.1182/blood-2006-10-054973
13. Crotty S, Johnston RJ, Schoenberger SP. Effectors and memories: Bcl-6 and Blimp-1 in T and B lymphocyte differentiation. *Nat Immunol.* (2010) 11:114–20. doi: 10.1038/ni.1837
14. Kallies A, Xin A, Belz GT, Nutt SL. Blimp-1 transcription factor is required for the differentiation of effector CD8(+) T cells and memory responses. *Immunity.* (2009) 31:283–95. doi: 10.1016/j.immuni.2009.06.021
15. Korn T, Bettelli E, Gao W, Awasthi A, Jager A, Strom TB, et al. IL-21 initiates an alternative pathway to induce proinflammatory T(H)17 cells. *Nature.* (2007) 448:484–7. doi: 10.1038/nature05970
16. Bengsch B, Seigel B, Flecken T, Wolanski J, Blum HE, Thimme R. Human Th17 cells express high levels of enzymatically active dipeptidylpeptidase IV (CD26). *J Immunol.* (2012) 188:5438–47. doi: 10.4049/jimmunol.1103801
17. Lim HW, Lee J, Hillsamer P, Kim CH. Human Th17 cells share major trafficking receptors with both polarized effector T cells and FOXP3+ regulatory T cells. *J Immunol.* (2008) 180:122–9. doi: 10.4049/jimmunol.180.1.122
18. Gattinoni L, Speiser DE, Lichterfeld M, Bonini C. T memory stem cells in health and disease. *Nat Med.* (2017) 23:18–27. doi: 10.1038/nm.4241

19. Kryczek I, Zhao E, Liu Y, Wang Y, Vatan L, Szeliga W, et al. Human TH17 cells are long-lived effector memory cells. *Sci Transl Med.* (2011) 3:104ra100. doi: 10.1126/scitranslmed.3002949
20. Muranski P, Borman ZA, Kerkar SP, Klebanoff CA, Ji Y, Sanchez-Perez L, et al. Th17 cells are long lived and retain a stem cell-like molecular signature. *Immunity.* (2011) 35:972–85. doi: 10.1016/j.immuni.2011.09.019
21. Fraietta JA, Lacey SF, Orlando EJ, Pruteanu-Malinici I, Gohil M, Lundh S, et al. Determinants of response and resistance to CD19 chimeric antigen receptor (CAR) T cell therapy of chronic lymphocytic leukemia. *Nat Med.* (2018) 24:563–71. doi: 10.1038/s41591-018-0010-1
22. Kagoya Y, Tanaka S, Guo T, Anczurowski M, Wang CH, Saso K, et al. A novel chimeric antigen receptor containing a JAK-STAT signaling domain mediates superior antitumor effects. *Nat Med.* (2018) 24:352–9. doi: 10.1038/nm.4478
23. Zeng R, Spolski R, Finkelstein SE, Oh S, Kovanen PE, Hinrichs CS, et al. Synergy of IL-21 and IL-15 in regulating CD8+ T cell expansion and function. *J Exp Med.* (2005) 201:139–48. doi: 10.1084/jem.20041057
24. Wang D, Aguilar B, Starr R, Alizadeh D, Brito A, Sarkissian A, et al. Glioblastoma-targeted CD4+ CAR T cells mediate superior antitumor activity. *JCI Insight.* (2018) 3:e99048. doi: 10.1172/jci.insight.99048
25. Yang Y, Kohler ME, Chien CD, Sauter CT, Jacoby E, Yan C, et al. TCR engagement negatively affects CD8 but not CD4 CAR T cell expansion and leukemic clearance. *Sci Transl Med.* (2017) 9:eaag1209. doi: 10.1126/scitranslmed.aag1209
26. Guedan S, Chen X, Madar A, Carpenito C, McGettigan SE, Frigault MJ, et al. ICOS-based chimeric antigen receptors program bipolar TH17/TH1 cells. *Blood.* (2014) 124:1070–80. doi: 10.1182/blood-2013-10-535245
27. Bailey SR, Nelson MH, Majchrzak K, Bowers JS, Wyatt MM, Smith AS, et al. Human CD26(high) T cells elicit tumor immunity against multiple malignancies via enhanced migration and persistence. *Nat Commun.* (2017) 8:1961. doi: 10.1038/s41467-017-01867-9
28. Shum T, Omer B, Tashiro H, Kruse RL, Wagner DL, Parikh K, et al. Constitutive signaling from an engineered IL7 receptor promotes durable tumor elimination by tumor-redirected T cells. *Cancer Discov.* (2017) 7:1238–47. doi: 10.1158/2159-8290.CD-17-0538
29. Zenatti PP, Ribeiro D, Li W, Zuurbier L, Silva MC, Paganin M, et al. Oncogenic IL7R gain-of-function mutations in childhood T-cell acute lymphoblastic leukemia. *Nat Genet.* (2011) 43:932–9. doi: 10.1038/ng.924
30. Parrish-Novak J, Dillon SR, Nelson A, Hammond A, Sprecher C, Gross JA, et al. Interleukin 21 and its receptor are involved in NK cell expansion and regulation of lymphocyte function. *Nature.* (2000) 408:57–63. doi: 10.1038/35040504

18

Mitochondria-Targeting Immunogenic Cell Death Inducer Improves the Adoptive T-Cell Therapy Against Solid Tumor

Qingzhi Jiang[1,2†], Chi Zhang[2†], Huilan Wang[1,2], Tao Peng[3], Li Zhang[3], Yang Wang[3], Weidong Han[4*] and Chunmeng Shi[1,2*]*

[1] Department of Oncology, The Affiliated Hospital of Southwest Medical University, Luzhou, China, [2] State Key Laboratory of Trauma, Burns and Combined Injury, Institute of Rocket Force Medicine, Third Military Medical University, Chongqing, China, [3] Department of Blood Transfusion, The General Hospital of Western Theater Command, Chengdu, China, [4] Department of Molecular Biology, School of Life Sciences, Institute of Basic Medicine, Chinese PLA General Hospital, Beijing, China

Edited by:
Brian J. Czerniecki,
Moffitt Cancer Center, United States

Reviewed by:
Guilan Shi,
Old Dominion University, United States
Thorbald Van Hall,
Leiden University, Netherlands

***Correspondence:**
Yang Wang
200616wy@163.com
Weidong Han
hanwdrsw69@yahoo.com
Chunmeng Shi
shicm@sina.com

† These authors have contributed equally to this work

Cancer immunotherapy including adoptive T cell therapy (ACT) is widely used in the clinic and is highly beneficial for patients with hematological malignancies; however, it remains a challenge to develop effective immunotherapy strategies for the treatment of solid cancers, due to the inefficiency of the immune response and the immunosuppressive tumor microenvironment (TME). Immunogenic cell death (ICD) converts dying cancer cells into a therapeutic vaccine and stimulate a systemic antigen-specific antitumor immune response, which can effectively subvert the immunosuppressive TME and enhance the efficiency of immune responses, relative to conventional immunotherapeutic regimens. However, the application of traditional inducers of ICD in anti-cancer immunotherapy has been limited because of low levels of ICD induction and a lack of tumor-targeting accumulation. Mitochondria are important for tumor-targeting strategies and have emerged as organelles with key roles in the immune system. We hypothesized that the alteration of mitochondria in cancer cells could be an important target for the development of an efficient ICD inducer for use in cancer immunotherapy. Here, we report the evaluation of a mitochondria-targeted small molecule, IR-780, that acts as an ICD inducer and exhibits exceptional antineoplastic activity. IR-780 specifically accumulated in tumor cells to elicit ICD *in vitro* and *in vivo*, effectively suppressed tumor growth and lung metastasis, and enhanced adoptive T-cell therapy effects against solid tumors in mouse models. These anticancer effects were linked to dendritic cell maturation and synergistic effector T cell priming and infiltration into tumors. The underlying mechanism involves the direct targeting of the mitochondria by IR-780, to destroy cancer cells, including drug-resistant cancer cells, leading to the full exposure of tumor-associated antigens (TAAs), thereby enhancing antigen-specific antitumor immune responses. These features of IR-780 suggest that it has the advantage of leading to complete TAA exposure and the stimulation of efficient antitumor immune responses in the TME. IR-780 has potential for use as a preparative ICD inducer, in combination with conventional immunostimulatory regimens for cancer immunotherapy, particularly in the context of solid tumor treatment.

Keywords: tumor targeting, mitochondria, immunogenic cell death, adoptive T-cell therapy, immunotherapy

INTRODUCTION

In the last decade, immunotherapy has emerged as the most promising cancer treatment strategy, alongside chemotherapy, radiation therapy, and surgery (1). Immunotherapy enhances the specificity and power of the immune response, to eradicate cancer cells in a variety of human malignancies, resulting in durable antitumor responses, which reduce tumor metastasis and recurrence more effectively than traditional treatments (2, 3). One cancer immunotherapy strategy, using adoptive T cell therapy (ACT), with either allogeneic or autologous immune cells, has shown unequivocal therapeutic benefits in a substantial fraction of cancer patients (4, 5). More recently, ACT has been developed to use genetically engineered T cells, with the introduction of an additional chimeric antigen receptor (CAR) or T cell receptor (TCR) to crosslink target and effector cells. CAR T therapy in particular has been widely used in the clinic and is highly beneficial for patients with B cell malignancies (6); however, it remains a challenge to develop effective ACT strategies for the treatment of solid cancers, due to the inefficiency of effector T cell activation and the immunosuppressive tumor microenvironment (TME), resulting from chronic, but suboptimal exposure to tumor-associated antigens (TAAs) (7). Hence, there has been considerable interest in the development of complementary approaches, including therapeutic chemotherapy, which can fully expose TAAs and stimulate an antitumor microenvironment (8), to induce increased and prolonged adoptive T cell responses at tumor sites, exerting strong antitumor immunity against solidtumors (9).

Notably, recent studies have shown that a special form of cancer cell death, known as immunogenic cell death (ICD) (10), caused by specific types of chemotherapeutic drugs, radiotherapy, or photodynamic therapy, may contribute to antitumor T cell responses. Tumor cells undergoing ICD up-regulate the expression of calreticulin (CRT) on their surfaces, where CRT provides "eat me" and "danger" signals, which induce dendritic cells (DCs) to devour tumor cells and present TAAs. The subsequent release of ATP and high-mobility group box 1 (HMGB1) by tumor cells undergoing ICD promotes DC activation and triggers antigen-specific T cell responses (11, 12). Thus, the use of ICD-inducing agents may offer a convenient strategy for killing cancer cells, while simultaneously eliciting broad antitumor T cell responses (13); however, the immunogenic consequences largely depend on cancer cell targeting therapeutic effects, exposure of TAAs, and the level of the antitumor immune response. The application of traditional ICD inducers in anti-cancer immunotherapy is limited because of their lack of tumor-targeting and accumulation, as well as their weak induction of ICD (14).

Recent reports have emphasized the emergence of mitochondrial alterations as a hallmark of cancer cell biology (15, 16). In addition to their involvement in bioenergetic and biosynthetic processes, mitochondria are integral to stress sensing, which allows cellular adaptation to the microenvironment, and confer vital roles in the regulation of tumorigenesis and tumor progression (17). Many studies have indicated that some types of tumor, or cancer cell subpopulations, rely more heavily on mitochondrial functions. Thus, targeting mitochondria in cancer cells provides an opportunity for development of tumor-targeting treatment strategies, particularly for cancer stem cells or drug-resistant cancer cell subpopulations, which may be more dependent on mitochondria (18, 19). Mitochondria are the only organelles that retain a small DNA genome, which encodes proteins essential for respiration. Cancer cells harbor alterations in mitochondria, including mutations of mtDNA and proteins, which contribute to the cellular adaptation of the complex TME (20). Important roles for mitochondria in regulation of the human immune system have also emerged, including the control of signaling pathways involved in the stimulation of innate and adaptive immunity, as well as the metabolic regulation of immune function and the establishment of immune cell phenotypes (21). These characteristics provide a rationale for targeting aberrant mitochondria and tumor-associated mitochondrial antigens, which meet all the criteria of ideal targets for the effective induction of ICD (22). Therefore, we hypothesize that agents targeting mitochondria could be important candidates for development as efficient tumor-targeted ICD inducers for application in solid tumor immunotherapy. In previous work, we have identified a class of heptamethine cyanine dyes characterized with a tumor-targeted ability and which prefer to accumulate at the mitochondria in a manner that is dependent on the proton gradient of the inner mitochondrial membrane (23, 24). These dyes also induce apoptosis in drug-resistant cancer cells (25, 26) and mediate multimodal tumor therapeutic activities by targeting mitochondria (27, 28). In the present study, we describe the assessment of a mitochondria-targeting small molecule, IR-780, for use as an ICD inducer that can effectively suppress tumor growth and lung metastasis of colorectal cancer (CRC) in a mouse model. IR-780 directly targets mitochondria to destroy cancer cells, including drug-resistant cells, leading to the improved exposure of TAAs and thereby enhancing the effects of ACT, when combined with OT-1 T cell transfer in the B16F10-OVA mouse tumor model. These findings suggest that the mitochondria-targeting small molecule, IR-780, has immense advantages as an ICD inducer, which can mediate tumor-targeted accumulation, full exposure of TAAs, and stimulate strong antitumor immune responses.

MATERIALS AND METHODS

Cell Lines and Animals

Mouse colon cancer cells (CT26) and melanoma cancer cells (B16F10 OVA) were cultured in 1640 medium and DMEM medium with 10% FBS at 37°C with 5% CO_2. BALB/c and C57BL/6 mice (6 to 8 weeks old) were purchased from the laboratory animal center of the Third Military Medical University. Mice transgenic for a T cell receptor specific for ovalbumine (OT-1) were obtained from the Jackson laboratory and were bred in our SPF laboratory animal room.

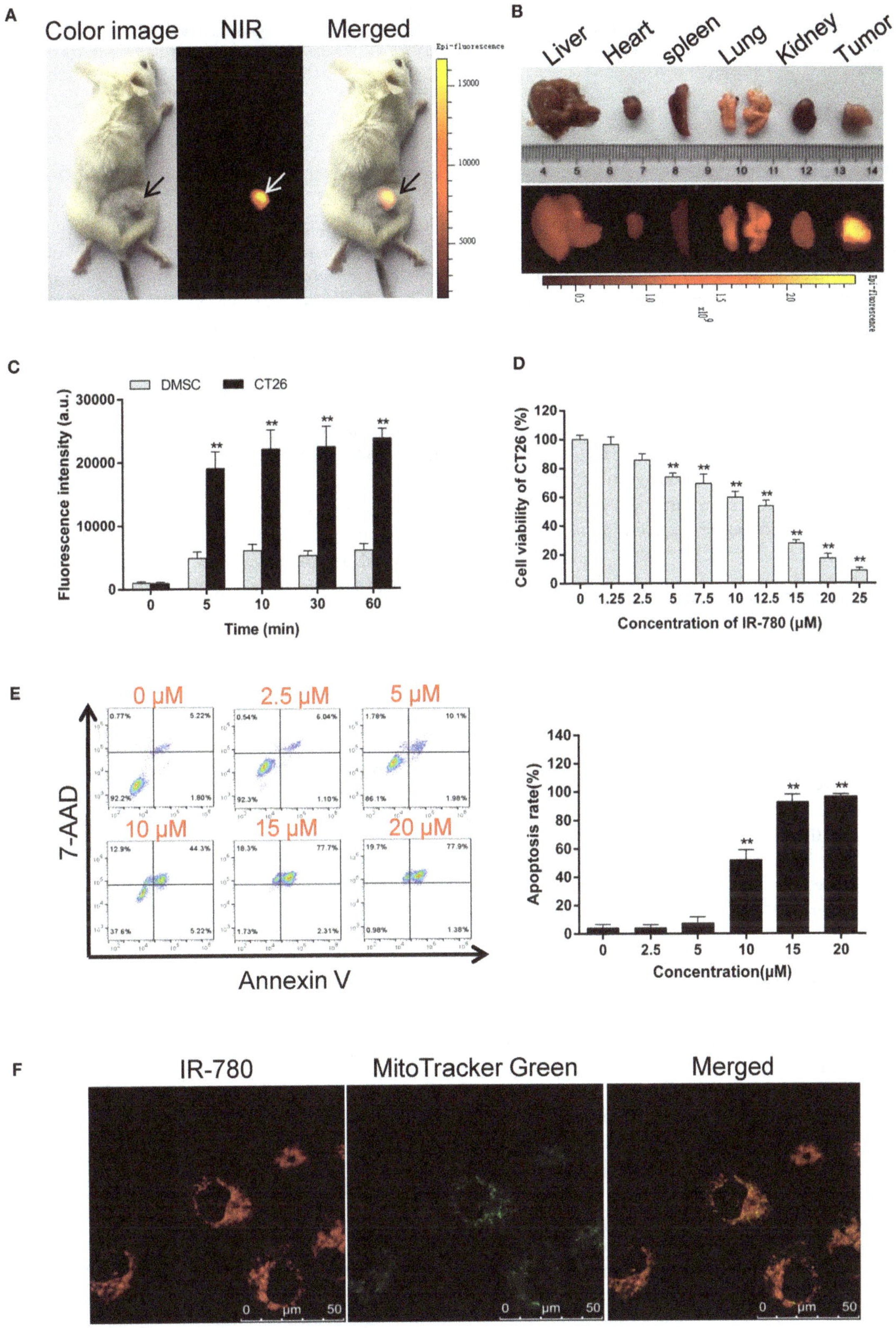

FIGURE 1 | IR-780 selectively accumulates in mitochondria of cancer cells and induces apoptosis. **(A)** Preferential accumulation of IR-780 in the tumor pre-established with CT26 cells. **(B)** The fluorescent imaging of dissected organs. The animal and dissected organs were subjected to imaging with the Kodak *in vivo* *(Continued)*

FIGURE 1 | FX Pro imaging system. **(C)** NIR fluorescent intensity in mouse dermal mesenchymal stromal cells (DMSCs) and CT26 cells were compared after incubated with 2.0 μM IR-780 for various minutes ($n = 3$). **(D)** CT26 cells viability was tested after treated with different concentration of IR-780 for 24 h ($n = 5$). **(E)** CT26 cells were treated with IR-780 for 24 h and stained with Annexin V/7-AAD to detect cell apoptosis by flow cytometry. **(F)** Co-localization of IR-780 with a mitochondria-specific tracker (Mito Tracker Green) in CT26 cells, imaged using a confocal microscope (scale bars = 50 μm). All the data are presented as mean ± SD. $^{**}p < 0.01$.

Detection of ICD Markers

CT26 colorectal cancer cells were treated with 10 μM IR-780 for 24 h, then CRT and HSP90 expression levels were determined using an immunofluorescence assay. After washing with PBS, cells were fixed in 4% of paraformaldehyde for 5 min and incubated with anti-calreticulin antibody (Cat# ab2907, Abcam) or anti-Hsp90 antibody (Cat# ab13492, Abcam) at 4°C overnight. After washing with PBS three times, cells were stained with secondary antibody (Cat# ab150077, Abcam) at 37°C for 40 min. Nuclei were stained with DAPI, then observed using fluorescence microscopy. CRT-positive cells were also analyzed by flow cytometry following staining. ATP and HMGB1 released in culture supernatants were detected using an enhanced ATP assay kit (Cat# S0027, Beyotime Biotechnology) and an HMGB1 ELISA kit (Cat# 6010, Chondrex), respectively, according to the manufacturer's instructions.

Evaluation of DC Maturation *in vitro*

To evaluate DC maturation *in vitro*, bone marrow cells were obtained from BALB/c mice and cultured in complete 1640 medium, supplemented with mouse recombinant macrophage colony stimulating factor (GMCSF, 20 ng/ml, Cat# 576304, Biolegend) and IL-4 (10 ng/ml, Cat# 574304, Biolegend) for 6 days to generate bone marrow-derived DCs. Then, IR-780 treated CT26 cancer cells were co-cultured with the DCs for 24 h. Next, the cells were collected and stained with APC anti-mouse CD11c Antibody (Cat# 117310, Biolegend), Brilliant Violet 421™ FITC anti-mouse CD80 Antibody (Cat# 104706, Biolegend), PE anti-mouse CD86 Antibody (Cat# 105008, Biolegend), or anti-mouse I-A/I-E Antibody (Cat# 107632, Biolegend), and analyzed by flow cytometry.

Mouse Tumor Models and Treatments

Vaccination Assays

The same number of CT26 cells were treated with 10 μM IR-780, 1 μM mitoxantrone (MTX), or 20 μM cisplatin (CIS), respectively for 24 h. After being washed with PBS, 1×10^6 treated cells were injected into the left flanks of each BALB/c mouse (s.c. vaccination site). PBS was injected as the control. One week later, mice were challenged with a subcutaneous injection of 1×10^6 living CT26 cells into the right flanks of mice (re-challenge site). Tumor incidence and growth in each group of mice were routinely monitored for 30 days after the re-challenge. Tumor volumes were calculated as: volume = length × width ^{2} × 0.5.

Effects of IR-780 in Tumor Metastasis Inhibition

1×10^6 CT26 cells were treated with 10 μM IR-780 for 24 h and subcutaneously injected into the right flanks of BALB/c mice (IR-780 group). PBS was injected as the control group. After 1 week, each group of mice were injected with 2×10^6 CT26 cells through the tail veins, and then sacrificed at day 20. The tumor sites in the lungs of each group of mice were examined and compared. To investigate immune memory effects, the spleen cells of each group of mice were separated and stained using a Zombie Green™ Fixable Viability Kit (Cat# 423102), CD8a (Cat# 100722), CD44 (Cat# 103040), or CD62L (Cat# 104432) antibodies, and analyzed by flow cytometry. All these antibodies were purchased from Biolegend.

Combination Treatment of B16F10-OVA Mouse Tumor Models

B16F10-OVA cells (5×10^5) were suspended in PBS (100 μl) and inoculated subcutaneously into the right flanks of C57BL/6 mice. Four days later, mice were treated with IR-780 (intra-peritoneal, 3 mg/kg) five times, every 2 days. On day 7 after tumor inoculation, mice were injected with OT-1 cells (intra-venous, 2×10^6), which were obtained from OT-1 mice. Cells isolated from tumors and tumor-draining lymph nodes were stained using a Zombie Green™ Fixable Viability Kit and the following fluorochrome-conjugated antibodies: CD45, CD8a, CD69, or KLRG1. For staining of intracellular cytokines (IFN-γ, TNF-α, and Granzyme B), cell suspensions were stimulated with a cell activation cocktail (including Brefeldin A) (Cat# 423303, Biolegend) for 6 h, then fixed and stained with intracellular antigen antibodies (IFN-γ, Granzyme B, and TNF-α), according to the manufacturer's instructions. All antibodies were purchased from Biolegend.

Statistical Analyses

All the data were presented as mean ± standard deviation. One-way analysis of variance was used to determine significance among groups. Statistical significance was set at $^{*}p < 0.05$ and $^{**}p < 0.01$. All the statistical analyses were conducted using the SPSS 13.0 statistical software.

RESULTS

Identification of a Tumor-Targeted Small Molecule as a Potential Inducer of ICD

Tumor-targeted ICD inducers stimulate a high level of immune responses in accumulating tumor tissues, which is more necessary and needed for immunotherapy. In our previous study, we found that the near-infrared fluorescent small-molecule, IR-780, could directly target mitochondria in the cancer cells (24), and induce apoptosis in drug-resistant cancer cells (25). Here, we confirmed that IR-780 specifically targeted tumor tissues *in vivo* (**Figures 1A,B**) and preferentially accumulated in CT26 mouse colorectal cancer cells, relative to normal mouse dermal mesenchymal stromal cells (DMSCs, **Figure 1C**). IR-780 could efficiently and dose-dependently decrease the viability of CT26 cells (**Figure 1D**) and induce cell apoptosis (**Figure 1E**). Moreover, IR-780 exclusively accumulated in the mitochondria of cancer cells and co-localized with the mitochondria-specific fluorescent probe, Mito Tracker Green (**Figure 1F**), which may help to release mitochondrial antigens and stimulate an efficient antitumor response. All these results indicate that IR-780 may act

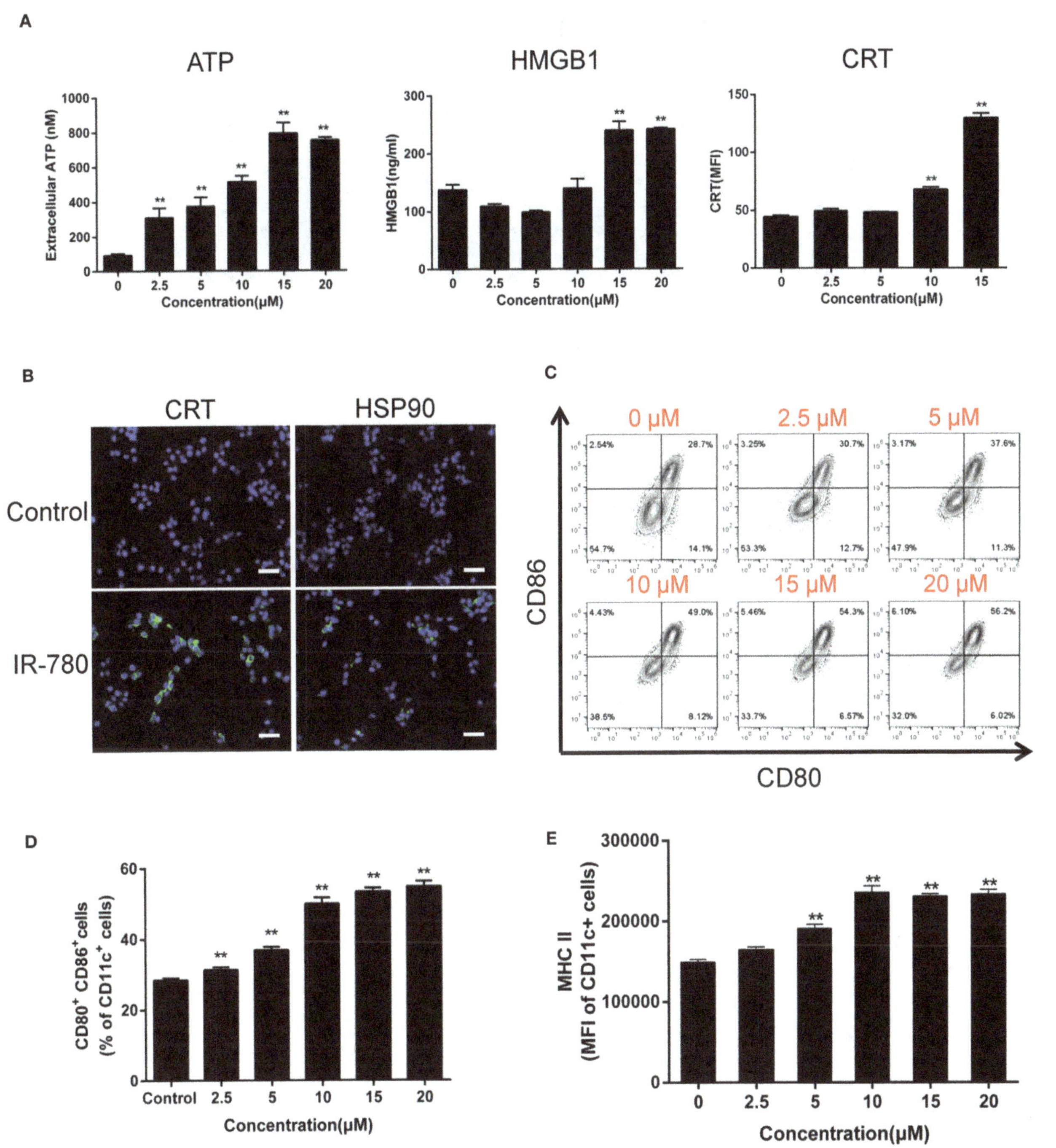

FIGURE 2 | IR-780 induces immunogenic cell death (ICD) *in vitro*. **(A)** Graphical data show the released of ATP, HMGB1, and surface expression of CRT on viable CT26 cells after treated with the indicated concentration of IR-780 ($n = 3$). **(B)** Immunofluorescence detection of CRT and HSP90 expression on the surface of CT26 cells after treated with 10 mM IR-780 for 24 h; scale bars = 20 μm. **(C, D)** Flow cytometry analysis of DC maturation by the markers ($CD80^+CD86^+$ of $CD11c^+$ cells) after the immature DCs were cultured with IR-780-treated CT26 cells ($n = 3$). **(E)** Flow cytometry analysis the expression of MHCII in the $CD11c^+$ cell population after the immature DCs were cultured with IR-780-treated CT26 cells ($n = 3$). All the data are presented as mean ± SD. $^{**}p < 0.01$.

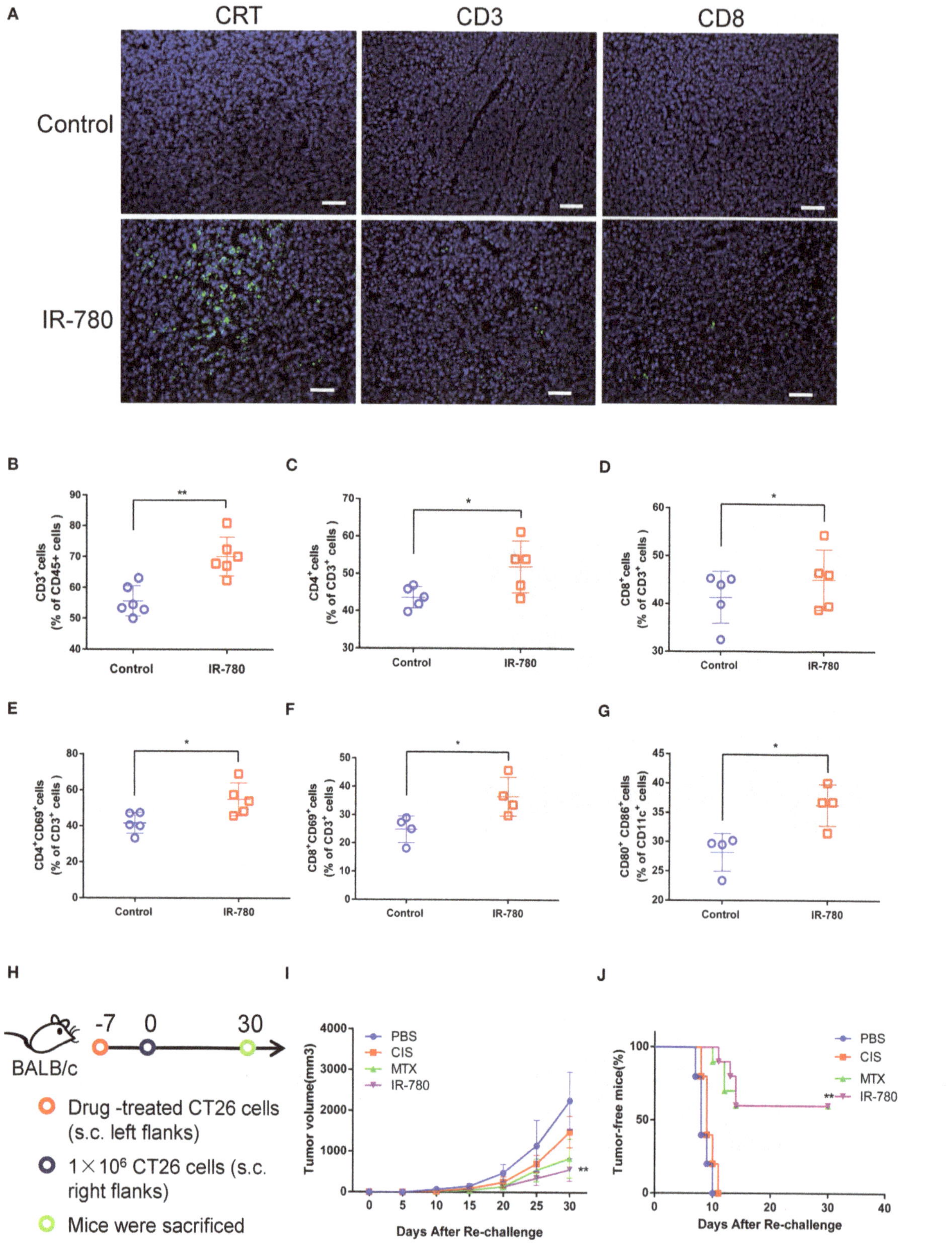

FIGURE 3 | IR-780 induces immunogenic cell death (ICD) *in vivo*. **(A)** Immunofluorescence detection of CRT, CD3, and CD8 expression in tumor sections; scale bar = 20 μm. The percentages of tumor-infiltrating **(B)** $CD3^+$, **(C)** $CD4^+$, and **(D)** $CD8^+$ T cells were analyzed by flow cytometry. And the activation of T cell populations *(Continued)*

FIGURE 3 | was measured by detecting the percentage of **(E)** $CD4^+CD69^+$ and **(F)** $CD8^+$ $CD69^+$ T cells populations. **(G)** The activation of $CD80^+CD86^+$ DCs was analyzed by flow cytometry. **(H)** Schedule representation of different treatment-mediated antitumor vaccination effects in CT26 tumor models. **(I)** After subcutaneous injection of different treated CT26 cells (10 μM IR-780, 1 μM MTX, and 20 μM CIS, respectively) in the left flank of mice, the tumor volumes in the right flank of each group mice were detected and compared (tumor volume = length × width ^{2} × 0.5). **(J)** The frequency of tumor-free mice in each group after vaccinated with different pretreated CT26 cells ($n = 10$). All the data are presented as mean ± SD. $^*p < 0.05$; $^{**}p < 0.01$ as comparing with control group.

as a potential inducer of ICD, with tumor-targeting properties and the release of mitochondrial antigens, and could assist in stimulating an antitumor response to kill drug-resistant cancer cells.

IR-780 Induces ICD and Enhances DC Function *in vitro*

ICD induces the activation of antitumor immune responses, accompanied by a sequence of changes in the cell surface composition and release of soluble mediators. Here, we tested the hallmarks of ICD in IR-780 treated cancer cells and observed dose-dependent increases in ATP and HMGB1 secretion, as well as the expression of the ER/cytosolic chaperone, CRT, on the surface of cancer cells (**Figure 2A**). Immunofluorescent assays also indicate cell surface exposure of CRT and the mitochondrial protein, HSP90 (**Figure 2B**). As DCs have key roles in the recognition of damage associated molecular patterns associated with ICD, and the subsequent uptake and presentation of TAAs, we tested the activation of mouse bone marrow-derived DCs (**Supplementary Figure 1**) after co-culture with IR-780 treated CT26 cancer cells. IR-780 treatment efficiently increased DC activation and maturation, with up-regulated surface expression of CD80, CD86, and MHCII on DCs (**Figures 2C–E**). To test whether cancer cell antigen presentation was also enhanced, the peptide antigen transporter gene expression was evaluated, and the results indicated that *Tap1*, *Tap2*, *Tapbp*, *B2m*, *H2D1*, and *H2K1* mRNA expression levels in cancer cells were increased after IR-780 treatment (**Supplementary Figure 2**). Altogether, these data clearly demonstrate that IR-780 treatment can induce ICD in cancer cells and increase DC activation and maturation, to enhance the processing and presentation of TAAs.

IR-780 Induces an ICD Response *in vivo*

To discriminate between ICD and non-ICD inducers, a systematic analysis of the results of vaccination of immunocompetent and antitumor adaptive immune responses in syngeneic mice treated with dying cancer cells is the gold standard for determining ICD induction (29). In this study, IR-780 was intraperitoneally injected into BALB/c mice bearing CT26 tumors, to evaluate the adaptive immune response *in vivo*. IR-780 effectively inhibited tumor growth, increased the expression of CRT on cancer cells, and increased T cell infiltration into tumor tissue (**Figure 3A**). On day 10, after treatment with IR-780, tumors were harvested and analyzed by flow cytometry. Compared to the control group, we found that IR-780 treatment clearly increased the infiltration of both $CD4^+$ and $CD8^+$ T cells into tumor tissues (**Figures 3B–D**). Additionally, a high proportion of tumor-infiltrating T cells in the treatment groups expressed CD69, a marker of T cell activation (**Figures 3E,F**). Moreover, IR-780 treatment also increased the number of activated $CD11c^+$ DCs infiltrating tumor tissues, which are important for the stimulation of tumor cell-specific immune responses (**Figure 3G**). Further, we studied the immunogenic potential of IR-780 treatment in the context of a mouse vaccination model. We treated CT26 cancer cells with PBS, CIS (proven not to induce an ICD response), MTX (proven to induce ICD) (30), and IR-780 *in vitro* and then injected them into the left flank of immunocompetent BALB/c mice. Mice were re-challenged with live CT26 cancer cells by subcutaneous (s.c.) injection into the right flank at day 7 (**Figure 3H**). Tumor growth and tumor-free survival were measured and compared among mice (**Figures 3I,J**). All these results clearly establish that IR-780 acts as an ICD inducer *in vivo*.

IR-780 Effectively Suppresses Tumor Metastasis in a CRC Mouse Model

We next assessed the immunotherapeutic effects of IR-780 on tumor metastasis in a mouse model. CT26 cancer cells were treated with IR-780 *in vitro* and then injected (s.c.) into the right flank of immunocompetent BALB/c mice. Then, 2 × 10^6 live CT26 cancer cells were injected into the mouse tail veins at day 7. Twenty days after injection, mice were sacrificed, and their lungs collected, and metastatic foci analyzed (**Figure 4A**). Mice vaccinated with IR-780 treated CT26 cells had significantly less tumor metastases in the lungs, relative to the control group (**Figures 4B,C**). Hematoxylin and eosin staining of lung tissues also indicated that vaccination with IR-780 treated CT26 cells led to decreased tumor metastasis, with fewer and smaller metastatic lesions in the lungs, relative to the control group (**Figures 4D–F**). To verify that IR-780 treatment can induce a systemic immune response to inhibit distant tumor metastasis and generate immune-memory effects, spleen effector memory T cells ($CD8^+$ $CD44^+$ $CD62L^-$) were analyzed by flow cytometry. Vaccination with IR-780 treated CT26 cells led to a significantly increased frequency of effector memory T cells (**Figure 4G**), suggesting that a memory immune response was established in mice treated with IR-780.

IR-780 Enhances the Effects of ACT in the B16F10-OVA Mouse Tumor Model

Given the great advantages of IR-780 in tumor targeting and eliciting antitumor immune responses, it was combined with ACT to evaluate its effects in this context. First, CT26 tumor mouse models were treated using a combination of IR-780 and T cells [mouse spleen T cells stimulated using plate-bound anti-CD3 and IL-2, and soluble anti-CD28, for 4 days (31)]. The results indicated that IR-780

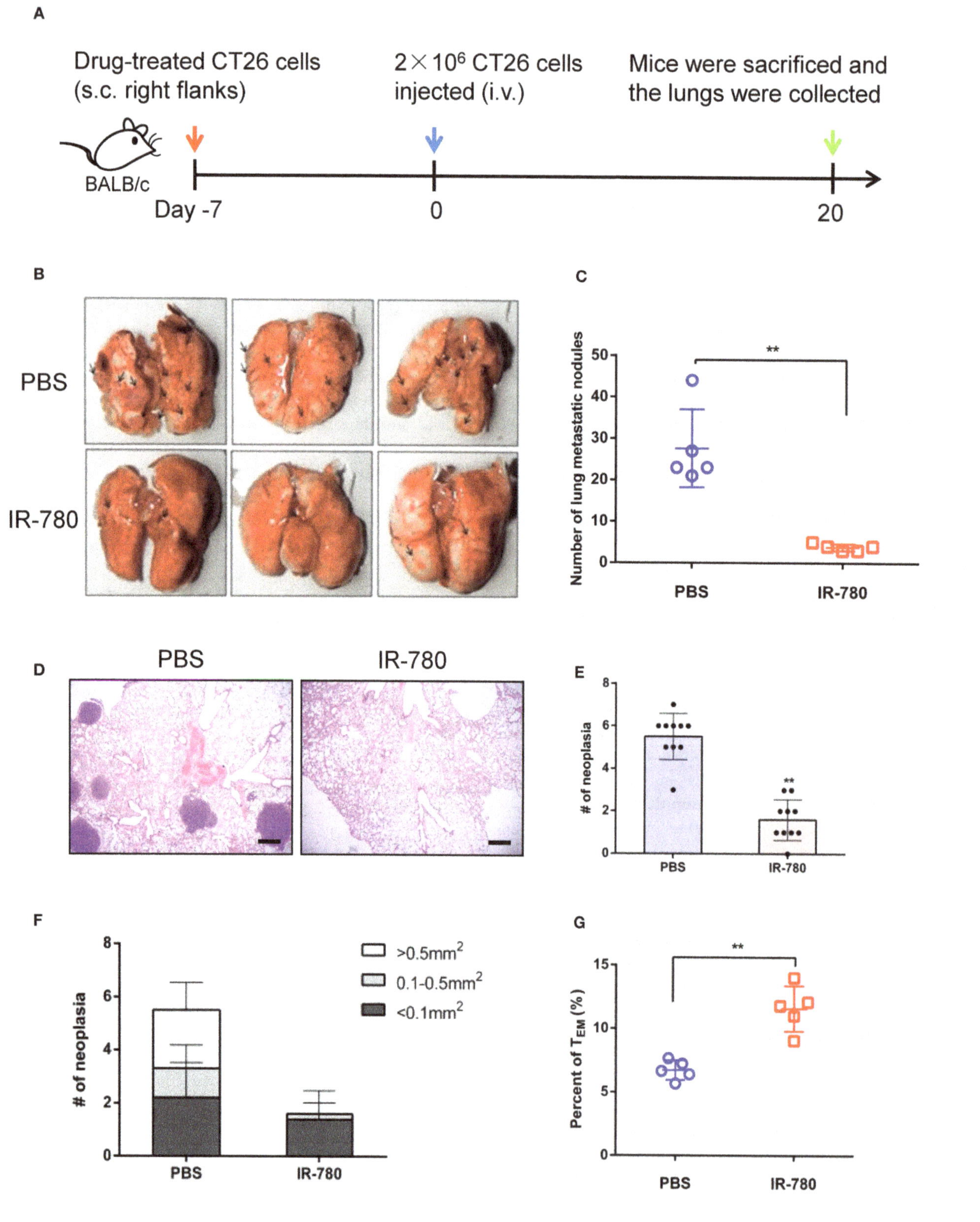

FIGURE 4 | Tumor metastasis prevention effects via IR-780 induced long-term immune memory. **(A)** Therapeutic schedule for IR-780 mediated inhibition of tumor metastasis in mouse model. **(B)** Representative photographs of lung tissue in different group mice. **(C)** Quantification of pulmonary metastasis nodules

(Continued)

FIGURE 4 | on control mice or mice pre-vaccinated with IR-780 treated CT26 cancer cells. **(D)** H&E staining of the lung tissue collected at day 20; Scale bars = 200 μm. **(E, F)** Quantification of pulmonary metastasis neoplasia and tumor sizes on pulmonary sections. **(G)** The proportions of effector memory T cells ($CD8^+CD44^+CD62L^-$) in the spleen of different group mice detected by flow cytometry. All the data are presented as mean ± SD. $^{**}p < 0.01$.

significantly enhanced the antitumor effects of T cells in the CT26 tumor model (**Supplementary Figure 3**). Next, a B16F10-OVA mouse tumor model was established by s.c. injection of the B16F10-OVA melanoma cell line (5×10^5 cells), which stably expresses chicken ovalbumin, in the right flanks of mice. Cognate peptide-activated OT-1 T cells, designed to recognize B16F10-OVA cells, were used alone, or combined with IR-780, to treat B16F10-OVA tumor model mice (**Figure 5A**). OT-1 T cell treatment (2×10^6 $CD8^+$ $V\alpha2^+$ cells, **Supplementary Figure 4**) exhibited a minor therapeutic impact in this model, indicating the substantial negative effect of immunosuppression in the TME. In contrast, combination treatment with 3.0 mg/kg IR-780 and OT-1 T cells significantly reduced tumor growth (**Figures 5B,C**) without induced obvious toxicity in mice (**Supplementary Figure 5**). Further, on day 10 of combination treatment, the number of activated ($CD8^+$ $CD69^+$) T cells in the tumor were increased (**Figure 5D**) and T-cell functions were enhanced, with an up-regulated expression of the effector T-cell markers, IFN-γ, Granzyme B, and KLRG1 (**Figures 5E–G**). We also stained for intracellular expression of CD69, IFN-γ, and TNF-α in inguinal lymph node $CD8^+$ T cells. Combined treatment induced higher levels of activated $CD8^+$ T cells in the lymph nodes, leading to an improved therapeutic outcome (**Figures 5H–J**). Further evidence that IR-780 induced a more pronounced effector phenotype was attained by the assessment of multiple CTL effector markers through real-time qPCR of the whole tumor mRNA, demonstrating increased expression of *IFN-γ*, *TNF-α*, *Granzyme B*, *EOMES*, *Perforin*, *BLIMP-1*, *FOXO3*, and *CXCL10* (**Supplementary Figure 6**). All these data indicate that a combined treatment strategy, including the tumor-targeted ICD inducer, IR-780, increased tumor infiltration of T cells and their function, and significantly enhanced the effects of ACT in solid tumors.

DISCUSSION

ACT involves the infusion of autologous or non-autologous lymphocytes into patients after expansion *ex vivo*. Given its remarkable early results, the Food and Drug Administration has approved ACT for certain types of tumors. ACT has recently been adapted to use gene-modified T cells, with both TCR- and CAR-based therapy achieving tremendous success against B cell malignancies (32); however, this approach has been less successful against solid cancer, partly due to the immunosuppressive TME (4, 33). The TME comprises a stromal compartment, which helps to establish the appropriate network required to support tumor development, including immunosuppressive cells, such as regulatory T cells, myeloid-derived suppressor cells, tumor-associated macrophages, neutrophils, and stromal fibroblasts, which secrete immunosuppressive factors and up-regulate inhibitory ligands, including PD-L1, which can suppress the effectiveness of ACT (34–36). TMEs are also characterized by T cell exhaustion, resulting from chronic, but suboptimal, exposure to TAAs, without sufficient co-stimulation (37). Excitingly, with the growth of knowledge of immune cells and their interaction with the TME, newly developed combinatorial strategies have allowed us to identify key requirements for overcoming the challenges imposed by the immunosuppressive TME. Combination strategies that promote ACT antitumor responses, persistence, and trafficking, will greatly improve therapeutic effects in solid tumors. The main combinatorial strategies used in ACT include targeting immune checkpoints, using immune agonists to boost immune responses in ACT, regulating the cytokine and/or chemokine milieu to enhance ACT, and enhancing T cell activity against solid tumors by vaccine boosting. These approaches have demonstrated tremendous potential in various preclinical models and are in the process of being translated to the clinic (38).

ICD can convert dying cancer cells into a therapeutic vaccination and induce the release of key immunostimulatory factors or signals to drive efficient antitumor immune responses (39, 40). Therefore, ICD inducers are widely-studied in clinical practice and are often used in combinatorial approaches aimed at subverting the highly immunosuppressive TME of solid tumors, since the induction of ICD can facilitate an initial T cell-driven anticancer immunity by resetting the TME to favor T cell infiltration. Combination approaches, using an ICD inducer alongside checkpoint blockade immunotherapies, are widely demonstrated in preclinical models as having superior benefits against various malignant tumors. In addition, ICD inducers can be used as neoadjuvants to increase tumor-infiltrating lymphocytes in tumor tissues, which can serve as a source of T cells for subsequent ACT (41, 42). Moreover, ICD inducers can be administered following ACT, to re-stimulate the effective antitumor activity of ACT cells, by fully exposing TAAs. While applications of ICD inducers combined with immunotherapy are widely reported to exhibit superior performance, how optimal therapeutic outcomes can be achieved using ICD inducers remains to be determined, particularly given the limited intra-tumoral accumulation and inadequate circulation half-life time of conventional ICD inducers, as well as their induction of off-tumor inflammatory responses (14, 43). To address these challenges, strategies to develop tumor-targeted ICD inducers have the potential to provide safe and effective approaches for use in combination immunotherapy (44). Given the important roles of mitochondria in tumorigenesis and tumor progression, and the recognition of mitochondrial damage as a hallmark of cancer, in this study we assessed the ICD inducer, IR-780, which targets cancer cell mitochondria. IR-780 specifically

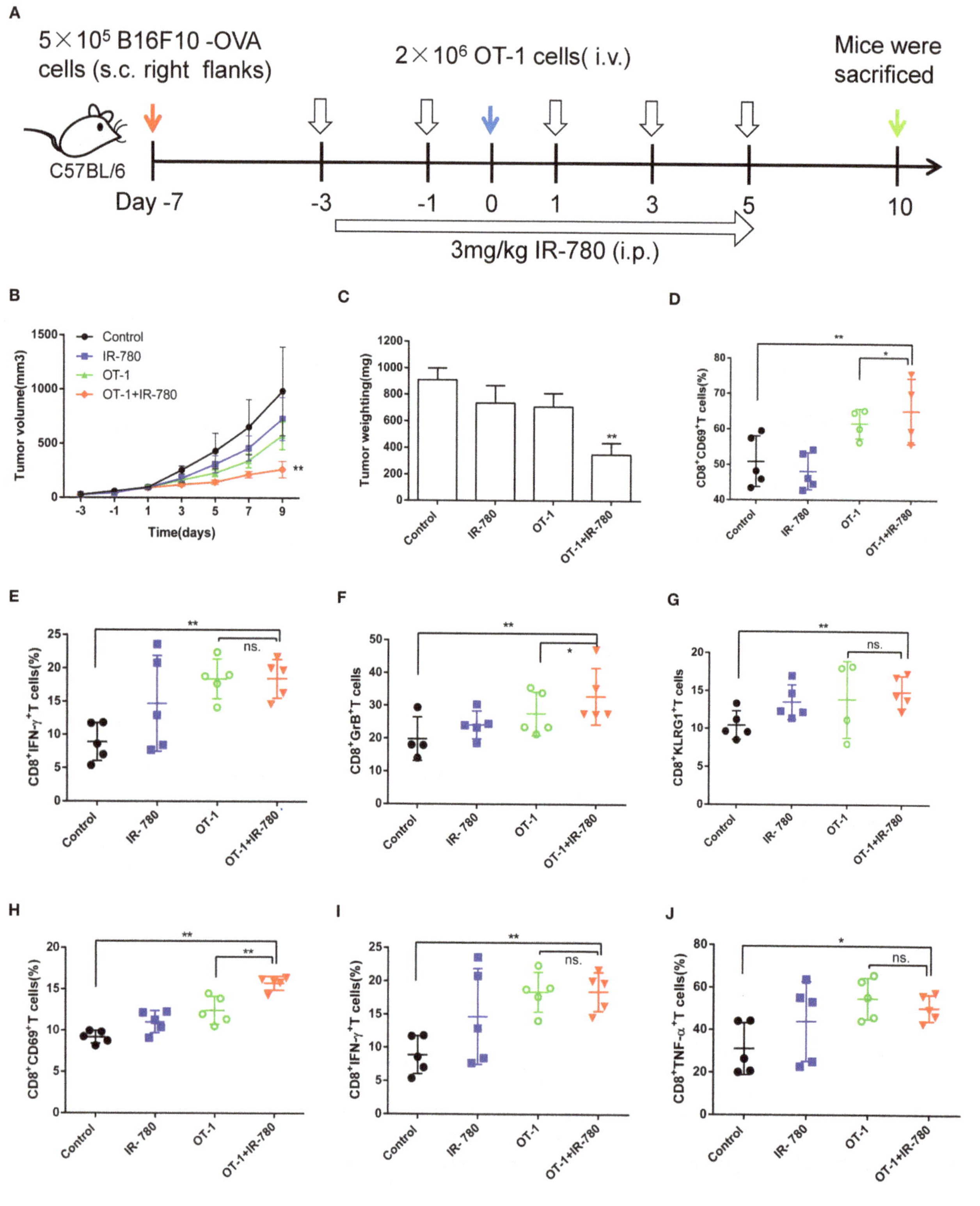

FIGURE 5 | Combinatorial treatment of IR-780 with OT-1 cells therapy in B16F10-OVA tumor mouse models. **(A)** Therapeutic schedule for combination therapy in mouse models. **(B)** The tumor volumes were detected every 2 days in different groups (volume = length × width^2 × 0.5; $n = 8$). **(C)** The tumor weight in different groups at day 10. The percentage of activation of CD8$^+$ T cells in tumors **(D)** and tumor-draining lymph nodes **(H)**. Flow cytometry analysis of the functional CD8$^+$ T cells **(E)** IFN-γ $^+$, **(F)** GzB$^+$, and **(G)** KLRG1$^+$ cells in tumor tissue, and **(I)** IFN-γ$^+$, **(J)** TNF-α$^+$ cells in tumor-draining lymph nodes. All the data are presented as mean ±SD. $^*p < 0.05$; $^{**}p < 0.01$.

accumulates in tumor cells to elicit ICD *in vitro* and *in vivo* and effectively suppresses the growth of tumors and lung metastases in a CRC mouse model. Specifically, IR-780 directly targets mitochondria to destroy cancer cells, including drug-resistant cancer cells, which can lead to complete exposure of TAAs, including tumor-specific mitochondrial antigens. IR-780 significantly enhanced the effects ACT in the B16F10-OVA mouse tumor model, when combined with OT-1 T cell transfer.

In conclusion, we present a new strategy for the development of tumor-targeted ICD inducers, by targeting tumor mitochondria and demonstrate its application in combination with ACT for the treatment of solid tumors. Our combination immunotherapy approach achieved potent antitumor efficacy, leading to the significant inhibition of solid tumors in animal models, representing a valuable reference in the field of tumor-targeted immunotherapy.

AUTHOR CONTRIBUTIONS

QJ, CZ, and HW performed the experiments. QJ and CZ interpreted data and drafted the manuscript. TP and LZ performed the data analysis. YW, WH, and CS conceived and designed the study and wrote the manuscript.

FUNDING

This work was supported by University Innovation Team Building Program of Chongqing (CXTDG201602020).

REFERENCES

1. Rosenberg SA. Decade in review-cancer immunotherapy: entering the mainstream of cancer treatment. *Nat Rev Clin Oncol.* (2014) 11:630–2. doi: 10.1038/nrclinonc.2014.174
2. Sharma P, Hu-Lieskovan S, Wargo JA, Ribas A. Primary, adaptive, and acquired resistance to cancer immunotherapy. *Cell.* (2017) 4:707–23. doi: 10.1016/j.cell.2017.01.017
3. Wang T, Wang D, Yu H, Feng B, Zhou F, Zhang H, et al. A cancer vaccine-mediated postoperative immunotherapy for recurrent and metastatic tumors. *Nat Commun.* (2018) 9:1532. doi: 10.1038/s41467-018-03915-4
4. Yeku O, Li X, Brentjens RJ. Adoptive T-cell therapy for solid tumors. *Am Soc Clin Oncol Educ Book.* (2017) 37:193–204. doi: 10.1200/EDBK_180328
5. Yang JC, Rosenberg SA. Adoptive T-cell therapy for cancer. *Adv Immunol.* (2016) 130:279–94. doi: 10.1016/bs.ai.2015.12.006
6. Brudno JN, Kochenderfer JN. Chimeric antigen receptor T-cell therapies for lymphoma. *Nat Rev Clin Oncol.* (2018) 15:31–46. doi: 10.1038/nrclinonc.2017.128
7. Gowrishankar K, Birtwistle L, Micklethwaite K. Manipulating the tumor microenvironment by adoptive cell transfer of CAR T-cells. *Mamm Genome.* (2018) 29:739–56. doi: 10.1007/s00335-018-9756-5
8. Aaes Tania L, Kaczmarek A, Delvaeye T, De Craene B, De Koker S, Heyndrickx L, et al. Vaccination with necroptotic cancer cells induces efficient anti-tumor immunity. *Cell Rep.* (2016) 15:274–87. doi: 10.1016/j.celrep.2016.03.037
9. Arina A, Corrales L, Bronte V. Enhancing T cell therapy by overcoming the immunosuppressive tumor microenvironment. *Semin Immunol.* (2016) 28:54–63. doi: 10.1016/j.smim.2016.01.002
10. Kroemer G, Galluzzi L, Kepp O, Zitvogel L. Immunogenic cell death in cancer therapy. *Annu Rev Immunol.* (2013) 31:51–72. doi: 10.1146/annurev-immunol-032712-100008
11. Galluzzi L, Buque A, Kepp O, Zitvogel L, Kroemer G. Immunogenic cell death in cancer and infectious disease. *Nat Rev Immunol.* (2017) 17:97–111. doi: 10.1038/nri.2016.107
12. Inoue H, Tani K. Multimodal immunogenic cancer cell death as a consequence of anticancer cytotoxic treatments. *Cell Death Differ.* (2014) 21:39–49. doi: 10.1038/cdd.2013.84
13. Garg AD, Vandenberk L, Koks C, Verschuere T, Boon L, Van Gool SW, et al. Dendritic cell vaccines based on immunogenic cell death elicit danger signals and T cell-driven rejection of high-grade glioma. *Sci Transl Med.* (2016) 8:328–27. doi: 10.1126/scitranslmed.aae0105
14. Lee EJ, Nam GH, Lee NK, Kih M, Koh E, Kim YK, et al. Nanocage-therapeutics prevailing phagocytosis and immunogenic cell death awakens immunity against cancer. *Adv Mater.* (2018) 30:1705581. doi: 10.1002/adma.201705581
15. Fulda S, Galluzzi L, Kroemer G. Targeting mitochondria for cancer therapy. *Nat Rev Drug Discov.* (2010) 9:447–64. doi: 10.1038/nrd3137
16. Wallace DC. Mitochondria and cancer. *Nat Rev Cancer.* (2012) 12:685–98. doi: 10.1038/nrc3365
17. Vyas S, Zaganjor E, Haigis MC. Mitochondria and cancer. *Cell.* (2016) 3:555–66. doi: 10.1016/j.cell.2016.07.002
18. Shi Y, Lim SK, Liang Q, Iyer SV, Wang HY, Wang Z, et al. Gboxin is an oxidative phosphorylation inhibitor that targets glioblastoma. *Nature.* (2019) 567:341–6. doi: 10.1038/s41586-019-0993-x
19. Molina JR, Sun Y, Protopopova M, Gera S, Bandi M, Bristow C, et al. An inhibitor of oxidative phosphorylation exploits cancer vulnerability. *Nat Med.* (2018) 24:1036–46. doi: 10.1038/s41591-018-0052-4
20. Buondonno I, Gazzano E, Jean SR, Audrito V, Kopecka J, Fanelli M, et al. Mitochondria-targeted doxorubicin: a new therapeutic strategy against doxorubicin-resistant osteosarcoma. *Mol Cancer Ther.* (2016) 15:2640–52. doi: 10.1158/1535-7163.MCT-16-0048
21. Pustylnikov S, Costabile F, Beghi S, Facciabene A. Targeting mitochondria in cancer: current concepts and immunotherapy approaches. *Transl Res.* (2018) 202:35–51. doi: 10.1016/j.trsl.2018.07.013
22. Pierini S, Fang C, Rafail S, Facciponte JG, Huang J, De Sanctis F, et al. A Tumor mitochondria vaccine protects against experimental renal cell carcinoma. *J Immunol.* (2015) 8:4020–7. doi: 10.4049/jimmunol.1500281
23. Zhang C, Liu T, Su Y, Luo S, Zhu Y, Tan X, et al. A near-infrared fluorescent heptamethine indocyanine dye with preferential tumor accumulation for *in vivo* imaging. *Biomaterials.* (2010) 31:6612–7. doi: 10.1016/j.biomaterials.2010.05.007
24. Zhang EL, Luo SL, Tan X, Shi CM. Mechanistic study of IR-780 dye as a potential tumor targeting and drug delivery agent. *Biomaterials.* (2014) 35:771–8. doi: 10.1016/j.biomaterials.2013.10.033
25. Wang Y, Liu T, Zhang E, Luo S, Tan X, Shi C. Preferential accumulation of the near infrared heptamethine dye IR-780 in the mitochondria of drug-resistant lung cancer cells. *Biomaterials.* (2014) 13:4116–24. doi: 10.1016/j.biomaterials.2014.01.061
26. Wang Y, Liao XY, Sun JG, Yi B, Luo SL, Liu T, et al. Characterization of HIF-1 alpha/glycolysis hyperactive cell population via small-molecule-based imaging of mitochondrial transporter activity. *Adv Sci.* (2018) 5:1700392. doi: 10.1002/advs.2017 00392
27. Luo SL, Tan X, Fang ST, Wang Y, Liu T, Wang X, et al. Mitochondria-targeted small-molecule fluorophores for dual modal cancer phototherapy. *Adv Funct Mater.* (2016) 26: 2826–35. doi: 10.1002/adfm.201600159
28. Tan X, Luo S, Long L, Wang Y, Wang D, Fang S, et al. Structure-guided design and synthesis of a mitochondria-targeting near-infrared fluorophore with multimodal therapeutic activities. *Adv Mater.* (2017) 29:1704196. doi: 10.1002/adma.2017 04196

29. Kepp O, Senovilla L, Vitale I, Vacchelli E, Adjemian S, Agostinis P, et al. Consensus guidelines for the detection of immunogenic cell death. *OncoImmunology.* (2014) 3:e955691. doi: 10.4161/21624011.2014.955691
30. Liu P, Zhao L, Pol J, Levesque S, Petrazzuolo A, Pfirschke C, et al. Crizotinib-induced immunogenic cell death in non-small cell lung cancer. *Nat Commun.* (2019) 10:1486. doi: 10.1038/s41467-019-09415-3
31. Sukumar M, Liu J, Ji Y, Subramanian M, Crompton JG, Yu Z, et al. Inhibiting glycolytic metabolism enhances CD8+ T cell memory and antitumor function. *J Clin Invest.* (2013) 10:4479–88. doi: 10.1172/JCI69589
32. Bonini C, Mondino A. Adoptive T-cell therapy for cancer: the era of engineered T cells. *Eur J Immunol.* (2015) 9:2457–69. doi: 10.1002/eji.201545552
33. Marina M, Edmund KM. CAR T cells for solid tumors: new strategies for finding, infiltrating, and surviving in the tumor microenvironment. *Front Immunol.* (2019) 10:128. doi: 10.3389/fimmu.2019.00128
34. Joyce JA, Fearon DT. T cell exclusion, immune privilege, and the tumor microenvironment. *Science.* (2015) 348:74–80. doi: 10.1126/science.aaa6204
35. Zhu J, Zhi Q, Zhou BP, Tao M, Liu J, Li W. The role of tumor associated macrophages in the tumor microenvironment: mechanism and functions. *Anticancer Agents Med Chem.* (2016) 16:1133–41. doi: 10.2174/1871520616666160520112622
36. Jiao S, Xia W, Yamaguchi H, Wei Y, Chen MK, Hsu JM, et al. PARP inhibitor upregulates PD-L1 expression and enhances cancer-associated immunosuppression. *Clin Cancer Res.* (2017) 23:3711–20. doi: 10.1158/1078-0432.CCR-16-3215
37. Rufo N, Garg AD, Agostinis P. The unfolded protein response in immunogenic cell death and cancer immunotherapy. *Trend Caner.* (2017) 3:643–58. doi: 10.1016/j.trecan.2017.07.002
38. Mahoney KM, Rennert PD, Freeman GJ. Combination cancer immunotherapy and new immunomodulatory targets. *Nat Rev Drug Discov.* (2015) 14:561–84. doi: 10.1038/nrd4591
39. Stevanović S, Pasetto A, Helman SR, Gartner JJ, Prickett TD, Howie B, et al. Landscape of immunogenic tumor antigens in successful immunotherapy of virally induced epithelial cancer. *Science.* (2017) 356:200–5. doi: 10.1126/science.aak9510
40. Lu J, Liu X, Liao YP, Salazar F, Sun B, Jiang W, et al. Nano-enabled pancreas cancer immunotherapy using immunogenic cell death and reversing immunosuppression. *Nat Commun.* (2017) 8:1811. doi: 10.1038/s41467-017-01651-9
41. Khalil DN, Smith EL, Brentjens RJ, Wolchok JD. The future of cancer treatment: immunomodulation, CARs and combination immunotherapy. *Nat Rev Clin Oncol.* (2016) 13:273–90. doi: 10.1038/nrclinonc.2016.25
42. Rui K, Wenmin Y, Sejin S, Jutaek N, Yao X, Yuchen F, et al. Elimination of established tumors with nanodisc-based combination chemoimmunotherapy. *Sci Adv.* (2018) 4:eaao1736. doi: 10.1126/sciadv.aao1736
43. Mardian S, Solomon BJ, Darcy PK, Beavis PA. Supercharging adoptive T cell therapy to overcome solid tumor–induced immunosuppression. *Sci Transl Med.* (2019) 11:eaaw2293. doi: 10.1126/scitranslmed.aaw2293
44. Allegrezza MJ, Conejo-Garcia JR. Targeted therapy and immunosuppression in the tumor microenvironment. *Trends Caner.* (2017) 3:19–27. doi: 10.1016/j.trecan.2016.11.009

Permissions

All chapters in this book were first published in ICMCI, by Frontiers; hereby published with permission under the Creative Commons Attribution License or equivalent. Every chapter published in this book has been scrutinized by our experts. Their significance has been extensively debated. The topics covered herein carry significant findings which will fuel the growth of the discipline. They may even be implemented as practical applications or may be referred to as a beginning point for another development.

The contributors of this book come from diverse backgrounds, making this book a truly international effort. This book will bring forth new frontiers with its revolutionizing research information and detailed analysis of the nascent developments around the world.

We would like to thank all the contributing authors for lending their expertise to make the book truly unique. They have played a crucial role in the development of this book. Without their invaluable contributions this book wouldn't have been possible. They have made vital efforts to compile up to date information on the varied aspects of this subject to make this book a valuable addition to the collection of many professionals and students.

This book was conceptualized with the vision of imparting up-to-date information and advanced data in this field. To ensure the same, a matchless editorial board was set up. Every individual on the board went through rigorous rounds of assessment to prove their worth. After which they invested a large part of their time researching and compiling the most relevant data for our readers.

The editorial board has been involved in producing this book since its inception. They have spent rigorous hours researching and exploring the diverse topics which have resulted in the successful publishing of this book. They have passed on their knowledge of decades through this book. To expedite this challenging task, the publisher supported the team at every step. A small team of assistant editors was also appointed to further simplify the editing procedure and attain best results for the readers.

Apart from the editorial board, the designing team has also invested a significant amount of their time in understanding the subject and creating the most relevant covers. They scrutinized every image to scout for the most suitable representation of the subject and create an appropriate cover for the book.

The publishing team has been an ardent support to the editorial, designing and production team. Their endless efforts to recruit the best for this project, has resulted in the accomplishment of this book. They are a veteran in the field of academics and their pool of knowledge is as vast as their experience in printing. Their expertise and guidance has proved useful at every step. Their uncompromising quality standards have made this book an exceptional effort. Their encouragement from time to time has been an inspiration for everyone.

The publisher and the editorial board hope that this book will prove to be a valuable piece of knowledge for researchers, students, practitioners and scholars across the globe.

List of Contributors

Yiming Wang, Rena Ma, Fang Liu, Seul A. Lee and Li Zhang
School of Biotechnology and Biomolecular Sciences, University of New South Wales, Sydney, NSW, Australia

Yiyi Yan and Svetomir N. Markovic
Division of Medical Oncology, Mayo Clinic, Rochester, MN, United States

Anagha Bangalore Kumar
Department of Immunology, Mayo Clinic, Rochester, MN, United States

Heidi Finnes
Department of Pharmacy, Mayo Clinic, Rochester, MN, United States

Sean Park
Department of Radiation Oncology, Mayo Clinic, Rochester, MN, United States

Roxana S. Dronca
Division of Hematology and Medical Oncology, Mayo Clinic, Jacksonville, FL, United States

Haidong Dong
Department of Immunology, Mayo Clinic, Rochester, MN, United States Department of Urology, Mayo Clinic, Rochester, MN, United States

Felicitas Rataj, Fabian B. T. Kraus, Michael Chaloupka, Simon Grassmann, Constanze Heise, Bruno L. Cadilha and Peter Duewell
Center of Integrated Protein Science Munich (CIPS-M) and Division of Clinical Pharmacology, Department of Medicine IV, Klinikum der Universität München, Member of the German Center for Lung Research (DZL), Munich, Germany

Stefan Endres and Sebastian Kobold
Center of Integrated Protein Science Munich (CIPS-M) and Division of Clinical Pharmacology, Department of Medicine IV, Klinikum der Universität München, Member of the German Center for Lung Research (DZL), Munich, Germany German Cancer Research Center (DKTK), Partner Site Munich, Heidelberg, Germany

Kristina Buder-Bakhaya and Jessica C. Hassel
Section of Dermatooncology, Department of Dermatology and National Center for Tumor Diseases (NCT), University Hospital Heidelberg, Heidelberg, Germany

Ivan Shevchenko
Institute for Immunology, Ludwig-Maximilians University, Munich, Germany

Alexandr V. Bazhin
Department of General, Visceral and Transplantation Surgery, Ludwig-Maximilians University, Munich, Germany German Cancer Consortium (DKTK), Partner Site Munich, Munich, Germany

Xiaoying Hu, Vasyl Nagibin, Christopher Groth, Peter Altevogt, Jochen Utikal and Viktor Umansky
Skin Cancer Unit, German Cancer Research Center (DKFZ), Heidelberg, Germany Department of Dermatology, Venereology and Allergology, University Medical Center Mannheim, Ruprecht-Karl University of Heidelberg, Mannheim, Germany

Rebekka Weber and Viktor Fleming
Skin Cancer Unit, German Cancer Research Center (DKFZ), Heidelberg, Germany Department of Dermatology, Venereology and Allergology, University Medical Center Mannheim, Ruprecht-Karl University of Heidelberg, Mannheim, Germany Faculty of Biosciences, Ruprecht-Karl University of Heidelberg, Heidelberg, Germany

Sajad A. Bhat, Disha Mohan Vedpathak and Shubhada V. Chiplunkar
Chiplunkar Laboratory, Advanced Centre for Treatment, Research and Education in Cancer (ACTREC), Tata Memorial Centre, Navi Mumbai, India HomiBhabha National Institute, Mumbai, India

Alexandr V. Bazhin and Jens Werner
Department of General, Visceral, and Transplant Surgery, Ludwig-Maximilians-University Munich, Munich, Germany German Cancer Consortium (DKTK), Partner Site Munich, Munich, Germany

Katharina von Ahn and Jasmin Fritz
Department of General, Visceral and Transplantation Surgery, University of Heidelberg, Heidelberg, Germany

Svetlana Karakhanova
Department of General, Visceral and Transplantation Surgery, University of Heidelberg, Heidelberg, Germany Section Surgical Research, University of

Heidelberg, Heidelberg, Germany

Angela Rita Elia, Sara Caputo and Matteo Bellone
Cellular Immunology Unit, Department of Immunology, Transplantation and Infectious Diseases, San Raffaele Scientific Institute, Milan, Italy

Wolfram Osen and Stefan B. Eichmüller
GMP & T Cell Therapy Unit, German Cancer Research Center (DKFZ), Heidelberg, Germany

Theresa Kordaß
GMP & T Cell Therapy Unit, German Cancer Research Center (DKFZ), Heidelberg, Germany Faculty of Biosciences, University Heidelberg, Heidelberg, Germany

Hui Zhang, Wen-Ting Gan, Wen-Ge Hao, Peng-Fei Wang and Zhuo-Yan Li
Department of Pediatric Hematology/Oncology, Guangzhou Women and Children's Medical Center, Guangzhou, China

Lung-Ji Chang
Shenzhen Geno-Immune Medical Institute, Shenzhen, China Department of Molecular Genetics and Microbiology, College of Medicine, University of Florida, Gainesville, FL, United States

Maryam Khelil, Debbie Ferns and Ekaterina S. Jordanova
Center Gynecological Oncology Amsterdam (CGOA), Department of Obstetrics and Gynecology, VU University Medical Center, Amsterdam, Netherlands

A. Marijne Heeren
Center Gynecological Oncology Amsterdam (CGOA), Department of Obstetrics and Gynecology, VU University Medical Center, Amsterdam, Netherlands Cancer Center Amsterdam, Departments of Medical Oncology & Radiation Oncology, VU University Medical Center, Amsterdam, Netherlands

Ilse van Dijk, Victor L. Thijssen and Tanja D. de Gruijl
Cancer Center Amsterdam, Departments of Medical Oncology & Radiation Oncology, VU University Medical Center, Amsterdam, Netherlands

Daniella R. A. I. Berry and Maaike C. G. Bleeker
Department of Pathology, VU University Medical Center, Amsterdam, Netherlands

Jeroen Kole and René J. P. Musters
Laboratory for Physiology, Institute for Cardiovascular Research, VU University Medical Center, Amsterdam, Netherlands

Constantijne H. Mom
Center Gynecological Oncology Amsterdam (CGOA), Department of Obstetrics and Gynecology, Academic Medical Center, Amsterdam, Netherlands

Gemma G. Kenter
Center Gynecological Oncology Amsterdam (CGOA), Department of Obstetrics and Gynecology, VU University Medical Center, Amsterdam, Netherlands Center Gynecological Oncology Amsterdam (CGOA), Department of Obstetrics and Gynecology, Academic Medical Center, Amsterdam, Netherlands Center Gynecological Oncology Amsterdam (CGOA), Department of Gynecology, Netherlands Cancer Institute - Antoni van Leeuwenhoek, Amsterdam, Netherlands

Derya Kabacaoglu, Katrin J. Ciecielski, Dietrich A. Ruess and Hana Algül
Internal Medicine II, Klinikum rechts der Isar, Technische Universität München, Munich, Germany

Nataly Manjarrez-Orduño, Laurence C. Menard, Selena Kansal, Paul Fischer, Bijal Kakrecha, Can Jiang, Mark Cunningham, Danielle Greenawalt, Vishal Patel, Minghui Yang, Ryan Golhar, Julie A. Carman, Paul S. Kayne, Suzanne J. Suchard, Steven H. Bernstein and Steven G. Nadler
Bristol-Myers Squibb, Princeton, NJ, United States

Sergey Lezhnin and Hongyue Dai
M2GEN, Tampa, FL, United States

Lijun Zhao and Yu J. Cao
State Key Laboratory of Chemical Oncogenomics, Key Laboratory of Chemical Genomics, Peking University Shenzhen Graduate School, Shenzhen, China

Leonardo Vinícius Monteiro de Assis and Maria Nathália Moraes
Laboratory of Comparative Physiology of Pigmentation, Department of Physiology, Institute of Biosciences, University of São Paulo, São Paulo, Brazil

Gabriela Sarti Kinker, Regina P. Markus and Pedro Augusto Fernandes
Laboratory of Neuroimmunemodulation, Department of Physiology, Institute of Biosciences, University of São Paulo, São Paulo, Brazil

Ana Maria de Lauro Castrucci
Laboratory of Comparative Physiology of Pigmentation, Department of Physiology, Institute of Biosciences, University of São Paulo, São Paulo, Brazil Department of Biology, University of Virginia, Charlottesville, VA, United States

Yi Wang and Hong Luo
State Key Laboratory of Oncogenes and Related1 State Key Laboratory of Oncogenes and Related Genes, School of Biomedical Engineering, Renji Hosptial, Shanghai Jiao Tong University, Shanghai, China

Hua Jiang, Yansha Sun, Bizhi Shi and Ruixin Sun
State Key Laboratory of Oncogenes and Related Genes, Renji Hospital, Shanghai Cancer Institute, Shanghai Jiao Tong University School of Medicine, Shanghai, China

Zonghai Li
State Key Laboratory of Oncogenes and Related Genes, School of Biomedical Engineering, Renji Hosptial, Shanghai Jiao Tong University, Shanghai, China State Key Laboratory of Oncogenes and Related Genes, Renji Hospital, Shanghai Cancer Institute, Shanghai Jiao Tong University School of Medicine, Shanghai, China

Qingzhi Jiang, Huilan Wang and Chunmeng Shi
Department of Oncology, The Affiliated Hospital of Southwest Medical University, Luzhou, China

Chi Zhang
State Key Laboratory of Trauma, Burns and Combined Injury, Institute of Rocket Force Medicine, Third Military Medical University, Chongqing, China

Tao Peng, Li Zhang and Yang Wang
Department of Blood Transfusion, The General Hospital of Western Theater Command, Chengdu, China

Weidong Han
Department of Molecular Biology, School of Life Sciences, Institute of Basic Medicine, Chinese PLA General Hospital, Beijing, China

Index

A

A2a Receptor, 111, 113

Adenosine, 111, 113-114, 116-117, 150, 163

Adoptive Cell Therapy, 108, 153, 156, 164

Adoptive T Cell Transfer, 28, 36-38

B

B Cells, 1, 37, 149-150, 152

Bladder Cancer, 43, 50, 52, 63, 67, 82, 86, 89, 100, 157

Blood Cancer, 118, 174

Blood Samples, 73, 122, 166, 212

Breast Cancer Cells, 25, 100, 113-114, 117

C

Cancer Genome Atlas, 125-126, 136-137, 139, 194-195, 197-202

Cancer Immunotherapy, 1-3, 14, 21, 23, 28, 37-38, 56, 60-63, 67, 87-88, 90, 100-101, 107-108, 110, 117, 143, 158-160, 162-164, 178, 203, 205, 215-216, 225-226

Car-t Cell Therapy, 122, 155, 176, 178-184, 186, 188, 191, 205

Cervical Cancer, 88, 125-126, 129-131, 133, 135-136, 138-140, 175, 187

Checkpoint Blockade, 10, 24, 28, 50-51, 53, 56, 60, 69-72, 88-89, 103, 105, 107, 151-153, 155, 158-160, 162-165, 223

Checkpoint Inhibition, 39, 43, 62-64, 69-70, 141-142, 144, 146-148, 150-151, 154, 156

Checkpoint Molecule, 111, 113

Chemotherapy, 4-6, 11-12, 14-18, 20-24, 42-43, 49-50, 53-54, 69, 86, 89, 91, 100-101, 104, 106-110, 119-120, 122, 126, 137-138, 142, 151-153, 155, 157, 166, 173-175, 178-179, 181, 185, 189-191, 200, 216

Chimeric Antigen Receptor, 37, 119, 123, 151, 155, 164, 174-175, 190-192, 205, 213-214, 216, 225

Chronic Infection, 9, 63, 135, 158

Circadian Rhythms, 194

Clock Genes, 194, 197-198, 200, 202

Combination Therapy, 14, 18-20, 22, 25, 45, 62, 64, 66, 101, 143, 152, 161, 182, 224

Costimulation, 10, 28, 57-58, 61, 122, 158, 191

D

Dendritic Cell, 10-11, 15, 25, 68-69, 90, 100-101, 158, 161, 197, 215, 225

E

Effector Functions, 23, 57, 61, 71-72, 75-76, 78, 80, 82-83, 85-86, 88-89, 104-105, 113, 206-207

Efficacy, 1, 3, 7-12, 15, 18, 21-25, 28, 32-33, 37-38, 43, 50-52, 54, 56, 58, 60, 63, 70, 80, 96, 119, 122, 142, 149-151, 154, 157, 160-161, 164-165, 174, 176, 182-183, 191-192, 200, 205-206, 212, 225

Engineered T Cells, 37, 174, 184, 186, 189-190, 192, 216, 226

Epacadostat, 135, 139, 152-153

G

Gene Expression, 8, 44, 46, 54, 71, 73, 80, 82, 98, 101, 105, 111, 125-126, 131, 154, 166-169, 172, 194-196, 198, 200-201, 203, 221

Glycolysis, 57-61, 106, 150, 162, 225

Granzyme B, 27, 30, 32-33, 71-76, 78, 82, 85-88, 207, 211, 218, 223

Gut Microbiota, 1, 3, 7-10, 12, 45, 51

H

Histone Deacetylases Inhibitors, 71-72, 83

Homeostasis, 56, 58, 61, 78, 158, 195, 203, 207

Hyaluronan, 147, 149, 161, 174

I

Immunocytochemistry, 92, 97

Immunogenicity, 23, 82, 107, 141-142, 144-146, 148-151, 154-155, 160, 192

Immunosuppression, 28, 37, 51, 62, 64, 67-68, 70, 90-91, 96, 100, 148, 160, 195, 223, 226

Immunotherapy, 1-3, 7, 9-10, 12, 14-16, 18-19, 21-28, 36-38, 40, 48-56, 60-63, 72, 78, 86-90, 96, 103, 107-108, 113, 126, 173-176, 182, 187, 194-196, 198-200, 202-205, 213, 218, 223, 225-226

Indoximod, 135, 139-140

Inflamed Tumors, 166, 169, 171

K

Kynurenine, 125-126, 129, 131-132, 135, 139-140, 150

L

Liquid Biopsy, 45, 52

Lung Cancer, 4, 6-8, 11-12, 14, 21, 23-26, 28, 37, 39-40, 47-48, 50, 52-54, 62, 64-67, 69, 86, 89, 101, 113, 115-118, 135, 139, 145-146, 157, 159-160, 163, 165, 172-173, 175, 180, 182, 190, 192, 203, 225-226

Lymphocytes, 10-11, 15, 24, 28, 36-39, 41, 43, 46-47, 51, 55, 58-60, 68, 87, 89, 94-95, 103, 105, 108-109, 113-114, 116, 121-122, 140, 142-146, 156, 158-164, 172, 176, 178, 186, 192-193, 200, 203, 223

M

Melanoma, 3-4, 6, 8, 10-14, 16, 18-26, 28, 36-55, 62-69, 72, 78, 86, 88-89, 91, 98, 100, 113, 115-118, 137, 142-143, 148, 160, 163-166, 168-169, 175, 178-179, 183-185, 187, 189-200, 202-205, 216, 223

Metabolic Checkpoints, 56-58

Microrna, 111, 118

Myelodysplastic Syndrome, 119

Myeloid-derived Suppressor Cells, 15, 23, 42-43, 62-64, 67-70, 87, 101, 126, 143-146, 160-162, 223

N

Neurotoxicity, 179, 188, 191

O

Oncolytic Viruses, 151-152, 154-155, 163, 191

Oxidative Phosphorylation, 150, 225

Oxygen Tension, 56-57

P

Patient Cohort, 126, 128-129

Peripheral Blood, 18, 28, 36, 39-40, iv

43-44, 49, 51, 62, 64, 67, 69, 71-72, 74, 87, 92, 120, 122, 166, 169, 172-173, 177, 183, 193, 206-207, 212

Peripheral T Cells, 41, 43, 166

Phosphoantigen, 71, 75-76, 82, 87

Polymerase, 19-20, 25, 206

Prognosis, 28, 40, 43-44, 52, 68, 89, 91, 100, 106, 109, 118-120, 122, 125, 135, 138-139, 141, 149, 156, 164, 184, 198, 200, 202-203

Programmed Death, 1-2, 4, 7-8, 10-12, 25, 27-28, 37, 50, 52, 54, 68-69, 71-72, 78, 84-85, 91, 96, 103-106, 157-158

Programmed Death Ligand-1, 1, 4, 7, 71, 84

Prostate Cancer, 63-64, 68-69, 103, 107-109, 113, 135, 137, 139, 163-164, 175, 183, 185, 192, 202

R

Radiotherapy, 14, 21-22, 25-26, 54, 106-107, 126, 142, 147, 151, 153, 163, 166, 174, 189

Rapamycin Pathway, 56

S

Serum, 13, 29, 39-40, 42-44, 51-52, 69, 73, 92, 100, 121-122, 125-126, 128-129, 131-132, 135, 137-140, 151, 206

Skin Cancer, 62, 194-195, 202

Stromal Remodeling, 148, 150

T

T-cell Therapy, 37-38, 87, 119-123, 155, 164, 190-192, 215, 225-226

Targeted Therapy, 14, 18-19, 22, 42, 45, 54, 65, 149, 152, 173, 175, 226

Transcription Factor, 59, 86, 88, 111, 115, 143, 158, 177, 213

Tryptophan, 58, 64, 68, 125-126, 129, 131-132, 135-140, 162-163

Tumor Antigens, 2, 28, 57, 82, 143, 156, 182-183, 186, 189, 226

Tumor Burden, 39-40, 42, 46, 147-148, 178-179, 207-208, 212

Tumor Cells, 2-4, 10, 19, 23, 32-37, 40, 49, 52, 58-59, 66, 78, 86-87, 98, 104, 106-108, 111, 126-130, 132-133, 135, 137, 142-146, 148, 152, 154-155, 164, 174, 176, 186, 188, 200, 211-212, 215-216, 225

Tumor Microenvironment, 1-2, 15, 19, 21, 23, 39, 42-43, 49, 53, 58, 63-65, 67-69, 103, 107, 113, 117, 128, 132, 135, 137-139, 141, 152, 158-162, 174, 190, 195, 200, 204-205, 211, 213, 216, 225-226

Tumorigenesis, 18-20, 65, 69, 71, 87, 108, 143, 162, 200, 216, 223

Z

Zoledronate, 74, 78, 83, 85-86, 89

www.ingramcontent.com/pod-product-compliance
Lightning Source LLC
LaVergne TN
LVHW060536210926
848485LV00005B/1213
* 9 7 8 1 6 3 9 8 7 0 1 6 5 *